D1381227

The Innate Immune Response to Infection

The Innate Immune Response to Infection

EDITED BY

Stefan H. E. Kaufmann
Max Planck Institute for Infection Biology
Berlin, Germany

Ruslan Medzhitov
Department of Immunobiology
Yale University School of Medicine
New Haven, Connecticut

Siamon Gordon
Sir William Dunn School of Pathology
University of Oxford
Oxford, United Kingdom

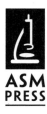

ASM PRESS WASHINGTON, D.C.

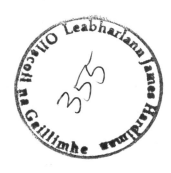

Cover image: mycobacteria in a macrophage phagosome.
Colorized transmission electron micrograph by Dr. Volker Brinkmann,
Max Planck Institute for Infection Biology, Berlin, Germany.

Copyright © 2004   ASM Press
                     American Society for Microbiology
                     1752 N Street, N.W.
                     Washington, DC 20036-2904

Library of Congress Cataloging-in-Publication Data

The innate immune response to infection / edited by Stefan H. E. Kaufmann, Ruslan
Medzhitov, Siamon Gordon.
     p. ; cm.
   Includes bibliographical references and index.
   ISBN 1-55581-291-0
   1. Natural immunity.
   [DNLM: 1. Bacterial Infections--immunology. 2. Immunity, Natural--physiology. 3.
Antibody Formation--physiology. 4. Immunity, Cellular--physiology. QW 541 I575 2004]
I. Kaufmann, S. H. E. (Stefan H. E.) II. Medzhitov, Ruslan. III. Gordon, Siamon.

   QR185.2.I486 2004
   616.07'9--dc22

                                         2004005850

All Rights Reserved
Printed in the United States of America

10 9 8 7 6 5 4 3 2 1

Address editorial correspondence to: ASM Press, 1752 N St., N.W., Washington, DC
20036-2904, U.S.A.

Send orders to: ASM Press, P.O. Box 605, Herndon, VA 20172, U.S.A.
Phone: 800-546-2416; 703-661-1593
Fax: 703-661-1501
Email: books@asmusa.org
Online: www.asmpress.org

CONTENTS

CONTRIBUTORS

Shizuo Akira   Department of Host Defense, Research Institute for Microbial Diseases, Osaka University, and SORST of Japan Science and Technology Corporation, 3-1 Yamada-oka, Suita, Osaka 565-0871, Japan

K. Frank Austen   Department of Medicine, Harvard Medical School, and Division of Rheumatology, Immunology and Allergy, Brigham and Women's Hospital, Boston, MA 02115

Winfried Barchet   Department of Pathology and Immunology, Washington University School of Medicine, Box 8118, 660 South Euclid Ave., St. Louis, MO 63110

Gregory M. Barton   Howard Hughes Medical Institute, Yale University School of Medicine, 300 Cedar St., TAC S660, New Haven, CT 06520

G. Bergsten   Department of Laboratory Medicine, Division of Microbiology, Immunology, and Glycobiology, Lund University, Sölvegatan 23, 223 62 Lund, Sweden

Christian Bogdan   Institute of Medical Microbiology and Hygiene, Department of Medical Microbiology and Hygiene, University of Freiburg, Hermann-Herder-Strasse 11, D-79104 Freiburg, Germany

Michael C. Carroll   Departments of Pathology and Pediatrics, Harvard Medical School, The CBR Institute for Biomedical Research, 800 Huntington Ave., Boston, MA 02115-5701

Devavani Chatterjea   Department of Pathology, Stanford University School of Medicine, 300 Pasteur Dr., L-235, Stanford, CA 94305-5324

Howard Clark   MRC Immunochemistry Unit, Department of Biochemistry, University of Oxford, Oxford O1 3QU, United Kingdom

Marco Colonna   Department of Pathology and Immunology, Washington University School of Medicine, Box 8118, 660 South Euclid Ave., St. Louis, MO 63110

Charles T. Esmon Cardiovascular Biology Research Program, Oklahoma Medical Research Foundation; Department of Pathology and Department of Biochemistry & Molecular Biology, University of Oklahoma Health Sciences Center; and Howard Hughes Medical Institute, Oklahoma City, OK 73104

Alan Ezekowitz Laboratory of Developmental Immunology, Harvard Department of Pediatrics, Massachusetts General Hospital, 15 Parkman St., Boston, MA 02114

S. Feau University of Milano-Bicocca, Department of Biotechnology and Bioscience, Piazza della Scienza 2, 20126 Milan, Italy

H. Fischer Department of Laboratory Medicine, Division of Microbiology, Immunology, and Glycobiology, Lund University, Sölvegatan 23, 223 62 Lund, Sweden

Stephen J. Galli Departments of Pathology and Microbiology and Immunology, Stanford University School of Medicine, 300 Pasteur Dr., L-235, Stanford, CA 94305-5324

Tomas Ganz CHS 37-055, Department of Medicine, David Geffen School of Medicine, University of California, Los Angeles, Los Angeles, CA 90095

Siamon Gordon Sir William Dunn School of Pathology, University of Oxford, South Parks Road, Oxford OX1 3RE, United Kingdom

F. Granucci University of Milano-Bicocca, Department of Biotechnology and Bioscience, Piazza della Scienza 2, 20126 Milan, Italy

Jules A. Hoffmann Réponse Immunitaire et Développement chez les Insectes, Institut de Biologie Moleculaire et Cellulaire UPR9022 CNRS, 15 rue René Descartes, 67084 Strasbourg, France

David A. Hume Institute for Molecular Bioscience, The University of Queensland, St. Lucia Q4072, Australia

Yoshihide Kanaoka Department of Medicine, Harvard Medical School, and Division of Rheumatology, Immunology and Allergy, Brigham and Women's Hospital, Boston, MA 02115

D. Karpman Department of Pediatrics, Lund University Hospital, Lund, Sweden

Stefan H. E. Kaufmann Max Planck Institute for Infection Biology, Schumannstr. 21/22, D-10117 Berlin, Germany

Satish Keshav Centre for Gastroenterology, Department of Medicine, Royal Free & University College Medical School, University College London, Upper 3rd Floor, Rowland Hill Street, London NW3 2PF, United Kingdom

Taco W. Kuijpers Emma Children's Hospital, Academic Medical Centre, University of Amsterdam, 1105 AZ Amsterdam, The Netherlands

Robert I. Lehrer   CHS 37-055, Department of Medicine, David Geffen School of Medicine, University of California, Los Angeles, Los Angeles, CA 90095

I. Leijonhufvud   Department of Laboratory Medicine, Division of Microbiology, Immunology, and Glycobiology, Lund University, Sölvegatan 23, 223 62 Lund, Sweden

Petros Ligoxygakis   Genetics Unit, Department of Biochemistry, University of Oxford, South Parks Road, Oxford OX1 3QU, United Kingdom

A. C. Lundstedt   Department of Laboratory Medicine, Division of Microbiology, Immunology, and Glycobiology, Lund University, Sölvegatan 23, 223 62 Lund, Sweden

John J. Marchalonis   Department of Microbiology and Immunology, University of Arizona, College of Medicine, P.O. Box 24-5049, Tucson, AZ 85724

Ruslan Medzhitov   Howard Hughes Medical Institute, Yale University School of Medicine, 300 Cedar St., TAC S660, New Haven, CT 06520

Bernhard Moser   Theodor-Kocher Institute, University of Bern, Freiestrasse 1, CH-3012 Bern, Switzerland

Chandrashekhar Pasare   Howard Hughes Medical Institute, Yale University School of Medicine, 300 Cedar St., TAC S660, New Haven, CT 06520

N. Pavelka   University of Milano-Bicocca, Department of Biotechnology and Bioscience, Piazza della Scienza 2, 20126 Milan, Italy

G. Raimondi   University of Milano-Bicocca, Department of Biotechnology and Bioscience, Piazza della Scienza 2, 20126 Milan, Italy

Kenneth Reid   MRC Immunochemistry Unit, Department of Biochemistry, University of Oxford, Oxford O1 3QU, United Kingdom

P. Ricciardi-Castagnoli   University of Milano-Bicocca, Department of Biotechnology and Bioscience, Piazza della Scienza 2, 20126 Milan, Italy

Dirk Roos   Sanquin Research at CLB, and Landsteiner Laboratory, Academic Medical Center, University of Amsterdam, 1105 AZ Amsterdam, The Netherlands

M. Samuelsson   Department of Laboratory Medicine, Division of Microbiology, Immunology, and Glycobiology, Lund University, Sölvegatan 23, 223 62 Lund, Sweden

P. Samuelsson   Department of Laboratory Medicine, Division of Microbiology, Immunology, and Glycobiology, Lund University, Sölvegatan 23, 223 62 Lund, Sweden

R. Tedjo Sasmono   Institute for Molecular Bioscience, The University of Queensland, St. Lucia Q4072, Australia

Samuel F. Schluter   Department of Biochemistry, University of Arizona, College of Medicine, P.O. Box 24-509, Tucson, AZ 85724

Peter Seiler   Max Planck Institute for Infection Biology, Schumannstr. 21/22, D-10117 Berlin, Germany

Thilo Stehle   Laboratory of Developmental Immunology, Harvard Department of Pediatrics, Massachusetts General Hospital, 15 Parkman St., Boston, MA 02114

Ulrich Steinhoff   Max Planck Institute for Infection Biology, Schumannstr. 21/22, D-10117 Berlin, Germany

C. Svanborg   Department of Laboratory Medicine, Division of Microbiology, Immunology, and Glycobiology, Lund University, Sölvegatan 23, 223 62 Lund, Sweden

M. L. Svensson   Department of Laboratory Medicine, Division of Microbiology, Immunology, and Glycobiology, Lund University, Sölvegatan 23, 223 62 Lund, Sweden

Kiyoshi Takeda   Department of Host Defense, Research Institute for Microbial Diseases, Osaka University, and SORST of Japan Science and Technology Corporation, 3-1 Yamada-oka, Suita, Osaka 565-0871, Japan

Mindy Tsai   Department of Pathology, Stanford University School of Medicine, 300 Pasteur Dr., L-235, Stanford, CA 94305-5324

Admar Verschoor   Departments of Pathology and Pediatrics, The CBR Institute for Biomedical Research, Harvard Medical School, 800 Huntington Ave., Boston, MA 02115-5701

C. Vizzardelli   University of Milano-Bicocca, Department of Biotechnology and Bioscience, Piazza della Scienza 2, 20126 Milan, Italy

G. Kerr Whitfield   Department of Biochemistry, University of Arizona, College of Medicine, Tucson, AZ 85724

B. Wullt   Department of Urology, Lund University Hospital, 223 62 Lund, Sweden

Wayne M. Yokoyama   Howard Hughes Medical Institute, Rheumatology Division, Box 8045, Washington University Medical Center, 660 South Euclid Ave., St. Louis, MO 63110

I. Zanoni   University of Milano-Bicocca, Department of Biotechnology and Bioscience, Piazza della Scienza 2, 20126 Milan, Italy

Michael Zasloff   Georgetown University Medical Center, 3900 Reservoir Rd., Washington, DC 20057

PREFACE

Concepts of dichotomy are frequently used in science. Even though such differences are sometimes artificial, they are often advantageous for creating comprehensible scientific working models. In immunology there are numerous examples such as the distinctions between B lymphocytes and T lymphocytes, between CD4 and CD8 T cells, between MHC class I and MHC class II, and so forth. The two earliest principles, however, are the divisions into innate versus acquired immunity and into humoral versus cellular immunity.

Since the birth of scientific immunology in the late 19th century, these two principles have coexisted. In fact, in the beginning the failure to separate the two general principles from each other led to confusion, since the "Berlin school" of immunologists, notably Paul Ehrlich and Emil von Behring—the proponents of the acquired immune response—emphasized humoral mechanisms, whereas the proponents of innate immune responses at the Pasteur Institute in Paris, headed by Elie Metchnikoff, concentrated on cellular mechanisms (see Fig. 1 and Color Plate P). This confusion, however, was soon resolved when Hans Buchner, and soon thereafter Paul Ehrlich, described alexins or complement, respectively, as the soluble components of the innate immune response, leading to a free combination of cellular and humoral immunity with specific (acquired) and nonspecific (innate) immunity.

A critical finding was that antibodies and complement could be distinguished by means of their temperature sensitivity, with complement being sensitive and antibodies being resistant to heating at 56°C. As a consequence, it was easily established, first by Paul Ehrlich and Julius Morgenroth in vitro and later by Richard Pfeiffer in vivo, that both elements, antibodies and complement, act together, with antibodies guaranteeing specificity and complement taking care of effector functions (typically, bacterial lysis) (see Fig. 2). Similarly, the capacity of complement to improve phagocytic activities was discovered by Elie Metchnikoff and Jules Bordet and propagated as a unifying view of specific (acquired) and

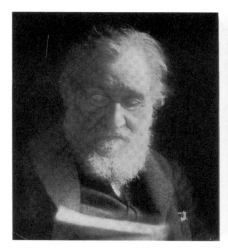 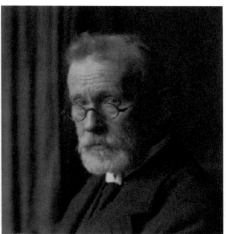

FIGURE 1   Elie Metchnikoff (Elias Metschnikow), 1914; Paul Ehrlich.

nonspecific (innate) immunity. In regard to the dichotomy between cellular and humoral responses, this was correct; in regard to innate and acquired immunity, it was false. This dilemma was solved by the Englishman Almroth Wright in 1903, who first described opsonization, showing that serum from naive animals contained weak opsonizing activity which was sensitive to 56°C, whereas that of immunized animals harbored potent opsonizing activity resistant to heating. Thus, the link between innate cellular and humoral acquired (specific) immune responses was made. The only missing link was the interaction between cells of the innate and cells of the acquired immune response.

It took another 50 years before cell-mediated acquired immune responses—which, as we all know now, are the function of T lymphocytes—were described. This late identification of T lymphocytes as mediators of the cell-mediated acquired immune response led to a conceptual shift which raised the interest of many immunologists in the second half of the 20th century. Innate immune responses of cellular or humoral type were increasingly treated like. stepchildren by mainstream immunologists, although several research areas pertinent to innate immunity, such as mechanisms of phagocytosis and antimicrobial effector molecules, were covered by cell biologists. As a corollary, the two research directions grew apart.

Above all, the acquired immune response was characterized by the unique hallmark of immunology, namely, the exquisite antigen specificity caused by rearrangement of the genes encoding T-cell receptors and immunoglobulins by RAG (recombinase activating genes). The discovery of the underlying mechanism as DNA transposition by RAG by the groups of D. G. Schatz and M. Gellert in 1998 allowed scientists to pinpoint the immunologic quantum leap in evolution: the jawless fish were primitive, i.e., without a specific immune system, whereas all higher vertebrates, starting with the jawed fish, were able to mount a specific immune response and therefore were considered more efficient in combating infectious diseases. It was somehow overlooked by mainstream immunology that the lower animals, way down to the protozoa, have to deal with microbes as well,

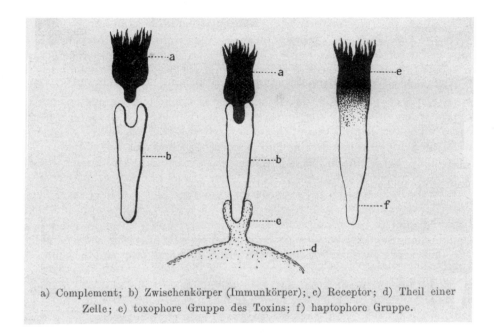

a) Complement; b) Zwischenkörper (Immunkörper); c) Receptor; d) Theil einer Zelle; e) toxophore Gruppe des Toxins; f) haptophore Gruppe.

and do so quite efficiently. This is because the innate immune system exists throughout evolution of the animal kingdom, starting with protozoa.

Only in the last decade of the 20th century did mainstream immunology turn its interest towards the innate immune responses as being equally important and interesting. The rediscovery that the innate immune response is highly conserved opened new avenues for comparative biology, best exemplified by the identification of the Toll-like receptors (TLR) as homologues of the molecules of the Toll-signaling cascade in insects. Again, it was the father of innate and cellular immunology, Elie Metchnikoff, who had foreseen this high conservation. He started his career as a zoologist and embryologist studying lower organisms, namely, coelenterata and echinodermata. Studying in Naples and later in Messina, he was interested in the intracellular digestion by cells in these organisms. These studies soon convinced him that the same mechanisms were also relevant to host defense, first shown by inflammatory responses against inert material in sea stars, and soon in the model of fungal infection in *Daphnia*. The word "phagocyte" was coined, and in 1884 Elie Metchnikoff extended his concepts to mammals, showing phagocytosis, killing, and degradation of *Bacillus anthracis* by macrophages from rabbits. At this stage he observed that phagocytosis was enhanced in immune animals, concluding that phagocytes become accustomed to phagocytosis—yet he did not realize fully the impact of the acquired on the innate immune response.

Studying Elie Metchnikoff's work of the 1880s readily reveals his genius. Although he himself was not the first to discover phagocytosis in protozoa, he was ready to extend his concept to all other animal species, and he was also ready to extend the concept from nutrition to host defense and even to immune surveillance. His colleague Kowalewsky had shown that macrophages also phagocytose host cells that become superfluous, e.g., during metamorphosis in insects or frogs. We now know about the important function of macrophages in removing apoptotic cell debris. Metchnikoff also achieved the first insight into the specifics of phagocytosis (see Color Plate P). Using neutral red dye, which was introduced into immunology by Paul Ehrlich, he found that the phagosomes containing bacteria such as streptococci or *Escherichia coli* soon became red as a sign of acidification. In contrast, using the intracellular bacterium *Mycobacterium tuberculosis*, Metchnikoff realized first that the bacteria survived within macrophages and second that the phagosomes became pink, suggesting to him that they did not acidify. We now know that *M. tuberculosis* survives in macrophages because it arrests phagosome maturation by preventing phagosome acidification.

Is there any need for a book on innate immunity 120 years after these phenomenal discoveries by Elie Metchnikoff, Paul Ehrlich, Almroth Wright, and others? Although for a long time innate immunity has been appreciated as a highly efficacious defense system, the most obvious is often taken for granted. We, the editors, are therefore convinced that a new look at innate immunity is timely.

After a long period of dormancy, innate immunity has reemerged into the center stage of immunology. This is for at least two main reasons. First, we now realize that the innate immune response also has to distinguish between self and nonself. Even though innate immunity does not achieve this by means of exquisite antigen specificity afforded by rearranged receptors, it succeeds by focusing on conserved structures typical for microbes using conventional receptors such as the TLR in the signaling pathway. The capacity to recognize and distinguish foreign physicochemical entities by a limited number of receptors is an ingenious mechanism which allows rapid defense responses against the foreign invader. Second, we increasingly appreciate that the innate immune system is not only an effector system which—by itself or under the guidance of the acquired immune response—defends us against invading microorganisms. The innate immune system also plays a central role in instructing the adaptive immune system as to which type of specific response should develop, in order to be optimally equipped to combat a particular infectious agent among the vast plethora of possible invaders.

In this book we have purposely made innate immunity central, even at the risk of some bias. It may appear ironic that in doing so we partly follow in the footsteps of Elie Metchnikoff. As he did, we emphasize evolutionary aspects as well as the host cells and humoral factors of innate immunity. Standing on the shoulders of recent achievements in molecular and cellular biology, we give equal room to the molecular receptors that equip the innate immune system and to the capacity to focus on foreign molecules while ignoring self-structures. Finally, the molecular mechanisms of phagocytosis as well as effector mechanisms afforded by the cells and molecules of innate immunity are being covered in equal depth.

We hope that this book fulfills its goal, namely, to represent a state-of-the-art review of innate immunity, looking at the oldest immune system through the eyes of the most timely concepts of cellular and molecular biology. In compiling the challenging aspects that are unique to innate immunity, as well as those underlying the cross-talk between innate immunity and foreign invaders on the one hand and the acquired immune system on the other hand, we hope to reestablish a closer relationship between the different disciplines. After all, the immune system has developed to combat infectious diseases, and in this endeavor it is the innate immune response that translates prokaryotic signatures into signals that are understood not only by its different members but also by the cells of the acquired immune system with their exquisite specificity.

We want to cordially express our thanks for the care given by the editorial staff of ASM Press, particularly Jeff Holtmeier (Director, ASM Press) and Ellie Tupper, as well as by our administrative assistants and secretaries, including Yvonne Bennett, Nancy Dometios, and Christine Holt, for their unique dedication. Last but not least, we would like to express our gratitude and appreciation to all our colleagues who generously shared their deep knowledge in innate immunity with us. In reviewing critically the current knowledge and describing their own concepts and ideas in their field of expertise, they allowed us to produce a book which we hope will be helpful to immunologists and biologists alike.

STEFAN H. E. KAUFMANN
RUSLAN MEDZHITOV
SIAMON GORDON

EVOLUTIONARY EMERGENCE AND INTERACTIONS AMONG ELEMENTS OF THE INNATE AND COMBINATORIAL RESPONSES

John J. Marchalonis, G. Kerr Whitfield, and Samuel F. Schluter

I

The foundations of the present concepts of innate and adaptive immunity were established during the latter decades of the 19th century when Metchnikoff (1905) observed phagocytosis in an echinoderm and in an arthropod and Ehrlich (1900) was carrying out pioneering studies on the properties of the specific serum molecules called antibodies. Macrophages lack antibodies or T-cell receptors (TCRs), which are the recognition units for antigen in the adaptive system, but can recognize various determinants by means of lectins and pattern-recognizing surface molecules. Furthermore, these cells of the innate immune system can cooperate with T and B lymphocytes via antigen presentation and immunomodulatory cytokine interactions. Here, we consider evolutionary factors regarding the emergence and phylogenetic distribution of the innate immune system and the combinatorial or adaptive immune system, as well as the interactions between the two.

Although analysis of relationships among individual molecules can be incisive, it is necessary to consider functionally interrelated systems rather than merely tracing the evolutionary history of single genes or related families of genes. To this end we consider two distinct, but interrelated, systems that can carry out specific recognition in defense against pathogens and mediate pathways of development and differentiation. Figure 1A presents a highly simplified schematic view of recognition, activation, and differentiation anchored through the nuclear receptor κB transcription factor (NF-κB). Similarly, Fig. 1B illustrates a recognition, defense, and effector situation involving complement as the central player. In the first case, products of the *Drosophila* Toll gene (Lemaitre et al., 1995; Rutschmann et al., 2000) and its human homolog Toll-related receptor (TLR) (Medzhitov et al., 1997; Rock et al., 1998; Medzhitov and Janeway, 2000) both recognize the lipopolysaccharide (LPS) endotoxins of gram-negative bacteria via a pathway involving the destruction of the inhibitor of NF-κB (Cactus in *Drosophila*), releasing NF-κB (Dorsal and Dif in *Drosophila*) to enter the nucleus to initiate a program of gene expression. This involves activation of a variety of genes including those for the production of

John J. Marchalonis and Samuel F. Schluter, Department of Microbiology and Immunology, University of Arizona, College of Medicine, P.O. Box 24-5049, Tucson, AZ 85724. *G. Kerr Whitfield,* Department of Biochemistry, University of Arizona, College of Medicine, P.O. Box 24, Tucson, AZ 85724.

The Innate Immune Response to Infection
Ed. by S. H. E. Kaufmann, R. Medzhitov, and S. Gordon
©2004 ASM Press, Washington, D.C.

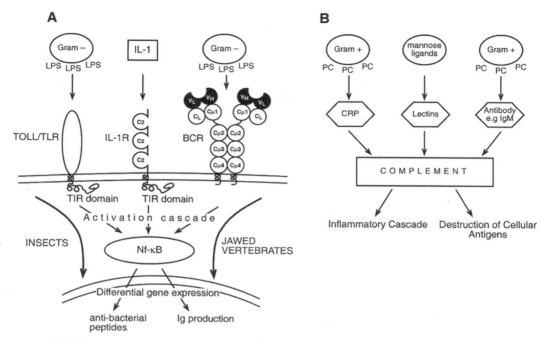

FIGURE 1 Overview of mechanisms of recognition and activation used in defense and differentiation by organisms ranging from insects to vertebrates. (A) Pathways of cell activation that are mediated by NF-κB. Signal pathways are activated by receptors anchored at the cell surface by transmembrane domains. NF-κB in the cytoplasm is induced to enter the nucleus and activate gene expression. The Toll and Toll-related receptors (Toll/TLR) and the B-cell receptor (BCR) recognize LPS on the surface of gram-negative bacteria (Gram-). IL-1R, which contains IgG C2-type domains, is activated by the cytokine IL-1. Toll/TLR and IL-1R have signaling domains in the cytoplasm termed TIR domains. The recognition unit of BCR is Ig and contains V and C1 domains. (B) Humoral defense pathways that rely on the activation of complement for the effector phase. C-reactive protein (CRP) and antibody recognize PC on gram-positive bacteria (Gram+).

antibacterial peptides in *Drosophila* (Imler and Hoffman, 2002) and multiple effects including immunoglobulin (Ig) synthesis and class switching as well as protection against apoptotic events (Ghosh et al., 1998) in mammals.

Naturally occurring IgM antibodies, as well as induced antibodies, also can recognize LPS epitopes and feed into the NF-κB activation and differentiation cascade with one result being production of Ig by B lymphocytes. Although antibodies are products of the combinatorial immune system, natural IgM antibodies can be considered receptors in "innate

recognition" because there is no selection by antigen; their V_H and V_L genes tend to have an unmutated germ line sequence, and the recognition capacity overarches that of the innate immune system (Harindranath et al., 1991; Coutinho et al., 1995; Robey et al., 2000, 2002; Marchalonis et al., 2002a).

Although the extracellular recognition units of the Toll receptor and the cytokine interleukin-1 receptor (IL-1R) are completely different, with the latter consisting of three Ig superfamily (IgSF) domains related to constant regions of the C2 type (Sims et al., 1989), the cytoplasmic signaling domains of both are homologous and are termed Toll-interleukin-resistant (TIR) domains. The Toll pathways of insects (Imler and Hoffman, 2002) and those of TLRs of mice and humans (Medzhitov and Janeway, 2000; Rehli, 2002) have been considered in detail by others. We focus here on evolutionary relationships among recognition or signaling elements.

Toll, Ig C2 domains, and the mechanisms of activation and differentiation are phylogenetically ancient, but the interjection of antibody to the system is relatively recent and correlates with the emergence of jawed vertebrates approximately 450 million years ago (Marchalonis et al., 1998b; DuPasquier and Flajnik, 1999; Litman et al., 1999; Laird et al., 2000). The recognition/effector system that keys upon complement is more recent in evolutionary emergence, with direct homologs of C3, C4, and C5 complement components recognizable in lower deuterostomes including echinoderms and tunicates, as well as agnathan and jawed vertebrates (Sunyer and Lambris, 1998). C-reactive protein (CRP), a member of the pentraxin family, is phylogenetically ancient and widely distributed (Tharia et al., 2002). The mannose-binding lectins (C lectins) are effective in complement fixation even in lower chordates, including tunicates (Sekine et al., 2001), and occur in groups as ancient as Cnidarians (Reidling et al., 2000). Interestingly, a specific subpopulation of natural IgM antibodies of vertebrates ranging from sharks to mammals (Marchalonis et al., 2001) can bind phosphorylcholine (PC), which is a major antigenic determinant on gram-positive bacteria as well as on a variety of metazoan parasites. Thus, pentraxins (Mold et al., 2002), appropriate lectins, and antibodies can fix complement, leading to the destruction of cellular antigens and also products via the generation of proteolytic breakdown that lead to the generation of an inflammatory cascade. In addition to the members of the IgSF, acute-phase proteins of the pentraxin family, Toll/TLR receptors, and NF-κB, we briefly consider other molecules involved in the recogni-

tion and interplay among cells of the innate immune system and lymphocytes of the adaptive or combinatorial system.

A general hypothesis that we propose based on the phylogenetic appearance of molecules and consideration of their sequence homologies is that the basis of the innate immune system is ancient with aspects present in all animal metazoans, and even in some plants, but that the adaptive or combinatorial system arose relatively late in evolution and is restricted to jawed vertebrates. The combinatorial immune system is defined by the presence of antigen-specific lymphocytes, bona fide Ig family (as opposed to superfamily) members (i.e., Igs and T-cell receptors), and major histocompatibility (MHC) molecules. There is a crucial need for recombinase-activating genes (RAGs) 1 and 2 to enable the segmental scrambling of germ line gene segments to occur with the result of patterned diversification of variable domains of TCRs and antibodies. In developing this model we need to consider several points. First, the genes specifying molecules of critical importance to both innate and adaptive immunity tend to occur in families containing many multiple elements within species. Thus, it is extremely difficult, if not impossible, to determine orthologous or directly lineal relationships across large phylogenetic distances. Second, it is unlikely that the original function of systems critical for innate immunity were originally of an "immunological" nature. For example, NF-κB, which is now known to protect against apoptosis in many systems, arose early in evolution, possibly to protect against oxidative damage (Ghosh et al., 1998; Bowie and O'Neill, 2000) as well as damage caused by ionizing radiation (Basu et al., 1998). The third key point is that these ancient systems were present at the time of emergence of deuterostomes and subsequently vertebrates and were co-opted by the combinatorial system in its rapid evolutionary emergence (Marchalonis and Schluter, 1998). The evolution of the systems underlying innate and adaptive immunity is a saga of co-option followed by coevolution with functions changing from general cellular protection (e.g., antioxidants) to ontogenetic development and finally to "immune" recognition and regulation.

METAZOAN PHYLOGENY: A TIME OF PARADIGM CHANGES

To understand the evolutionary relationships among living metazoans, and to infer whether certain genes are shared between groups of organisms based on ancestral relatedness or have arisen independently, it is essential to have an accurate scheme of phylogeny. Recently, longstanding concepts of phylogenetic relationships have been shaken because of the incorporation of molecular data including sequences of mitochondrial DNA (Spruyt et al., 1998; Adoutte et al., 2000) and selected proteins (Venkatech et al., 2001) as well as morphological (Giribet, 2002) and developmental (Davidson et al., 1995) information.

Figure 2 presents a simplified version of recent constructs of metazoan phylogeny. Earlier considerations of metazoan phylogeny often incorporated the erroneous suggestion of an Aristotelian hierarchy from extant lower species through more complex invertebrates leading to deuterostomes, chordates, vertebrates, and eventually to humans. This concept leads to the often-stated teleological argument that, because vertebrates are more complex than are "lower forms," they need more complex defense mechanisms. However, the new phylogeny makes it clear that this is not the case. Ancestral deuterostomes branched off from the ancestral protostomes before the two major branches of protostomes, namely, lophotrochozoans (annelids, platyhelminths, and mollusks) and ecdysozoans (arthropods and nematodes), emerged. Thus, gene families in insects or nematodes would not be found in deuterostomes and mollusks unless they were present in forms ancestral to all three groups. There are, of course, the less likely possibilities of horizontal gene transfer or evolutionary convergence. By contrast, the traditional phylogeny supports the prediction that such gene

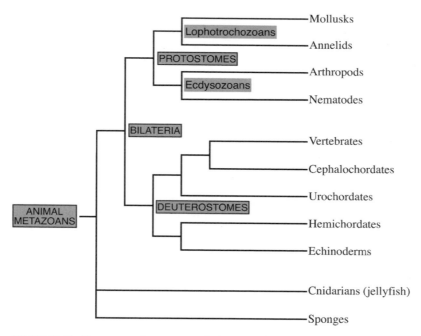

FIGURE 2 Summary of metazoan phylogeny. This scheme is based on recent molecular and morphological data.

families would indeed occur in all "higher" forms in the hierarchical scheme, particularly deuterostomes, unless deleted during speciation. Another key point is the realization that fungi are more closely related to animal metazoans than are plants (not shown in Fig. 2). The origins of the distinct classes of vertebrates within the deuterostome grouping are considered in detail below, pursuant to the origin and evolution of elements of the combinatorial or adaptive immune system. The availability of complete genome sequences of humans, teleost fish (zebrafish, *Danio rerio*; pufferfish, *Fugu rubripes*), the tunicate (*Ciona intestinalis*), the fruit fly (*Drosophila melanogaster*), the soil nematode (*Caenorhabditis elegans*), and various species of yeast (*Saccharomyces*) as well as plants (*Arabidopsis* and rice) offers a tremendous opportunity to ascertain the presence of homologous genes and gene segments across the spectrum of phylogenetic groupings. The definitive assignment of genes and families will eventually come from analyses of these and other genomes in progress.

In comparing sequences to determine whether homologous relationships exist, it is essential to consider several crucial points that have arisen in attempts to construct phylogenies of relevant multigene families, including Ig (Marchalonis, 1977; Ellison and Hood, 1983) and MHC domains (Flajnik and Kasahara, 2001; Kulski et al., 2002), superoxide dismutase (Fink and Scandalios, 2002), the IgSF (Williams and Barclay, 1988), the pentraxin and acute-phase protein family (Hughes, 1998), and the nuclear receptor superfamily (Owen and Zelent, 2000). First, analyses of multigene families unavoidably result in comparisons among paralagous members of the set, rather than directly lineal or orthologous genes. This stricture holds even for universally distributed proteins that are found in all living organisms and play a substantial role in immunoregulation in higher species. Martin and Burg (2002) have concluded that heat shock proteins cannot be used to construct reliable phylogenies because of the number of duplications and independent differentiation of members of this set

within species. The same consideration applies to superoxide dismutase, which is present in prokaryotes as well as eukaryotes, where distinctions are clear among the families found in plants as opposed to those in different groups of animals. A second point is that there is often an optimistic tendency to extrapolate homologous relationships based on weak overall quantitative measures of identity because a short stretch of peptide sequence or nucleotide identity may be apparent in molecules that largely show no evidence of homology. Klein (1998) defines a "twilight zone" where he considers it unreliable if overall identities are less than 20%.

An important consideration is the fact that many large proteins, including molecules incorporating domains of the IgSF, contain other unrelated sequences and domains that by themselves form characteristic functional motifs. By contrast, Igs and TCRs may contain short stretches of membrane-associated extra sequence, but do not form covalent associations with non-Ig domains. The membrane-associated leukemia inhibitory factors, for example, contain hemopoietin receptor SD100 domains, an IgSF domain, fibronectin type 3 domains, a transmembrane segment, and a box1/box2 cytoplasmic element (Gearing et al., 1991). Another example that is widely distributed among animal phyla is membrane-associated receptor tyrosine kinases (RTKs) that also contain Ig C2-like extracellular receptor domains in mammals (Masiakowski and Carroll, 1992), chondrichthian fish (Jennings et al., 1993), tunicates (J. J. Marchalonis, unpublished BLAST search, 2003), *C. elegans* (Popovici et al., 2002), and sponges (Pancer et al., 1996), but have C lectins as the extracellular recognition domain in the Cnidarian *Hydra vulgaris* (Reidling et al., 2000). Moreover, the protein tyrosine kinase domain itself is universal, occurring even in viruses. The products of RAGs, especially RAG1, and the vitamin D receptor (VDR) are good examples of large functional proteins containing multiple motifs. The former contains two characteristic DNA-binding segments that show different phylogenetic distributions as well as characteristic regions for DNA hydrolysis and transesterification (Marchalonis et al., 2003). The VDRs are ligand-specific transcription factors having a DNA-binding segment with wide phylogenetic distribution with the characteristic VDR protein molecule clearly present only in vertebrates, including lampreys (Whitfield et al., 2003). Consistent with these difficulties, investigators attempting to develop a coherent phylogeny for the members of the IgSF uniformly admit that it is difficult, if not impossible, to devise coherent phylogenetic trees, although it is possible to identify subsets within V- or C-like domains and predict a general scheme of emergence (Edelman, 1987; Halaby and Mornon, 1997; Smith and Xue, 1997; Teichmann and Chothia, 2000).

Figure 3 is a simplified "birth and death" scheme for the expansion of a putative ancestral gene into a family in one species, the differentiation via mutation of the individual genes, and their passage to a daughter species. Birth occurs via duplication and mutation. Death occurs via either deletion of individual genes or functional inactivation by mutations leading to the formation of inactive pseudogenes. The deletional process would result in an instant loss of the gene in question, whereas removal of inactive pseudogenes by neutral mutation would take more than 1 billion years to randomize a sequence to the point where recognizable homology is lost if the usual rate of approximately 10^{-9} substitutions per amino acid per year (Marchalonis et al., 2001) applies. A model of this nature can explain the phylogenetic distribution of genes encoding heat shock proteins, superoxide dismutase, pentraxins, and the nuclear receptor superfamily, as well as those of the IgSF and the restricted Ig family of jawed vertebrates.

INTERPLAY BETWEEN INNATE AND COMBINATORIAL IMMUNITY

PC

Bacteria are ancient entities arising in evolution more than 2 billion years ago. They exist as free-living organisms under a variety of environmental conditions as well as infectious and symbiotic agents in association with representatives of all eukaryotic phyla. The bacteria can be divided into two major groups, termed gram positive or gram negative, based

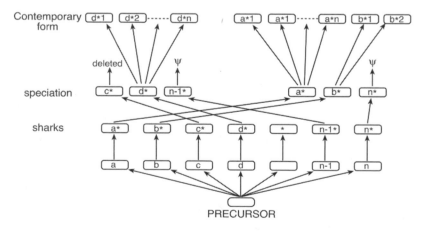

FIGURE 3 Birth and death scheme for the evolution of multigene families. Gene families are formed by gene duplication and mutation. Gene death occurs by mutation leading to pseudogenes (ψ) or by deletion from the genome. $\star$, derived from pervious precursor.

on the composition of their cell walls. PC was first discovered in the gram-positive bacterium *Streptococcus pneumoniae*, where it occurs in association with teichoic acid in the cell wall. The molecule occurs in a range of gram-positive bacteria as well as disease-causing eukaryotic organisms including the protozoans *Leishmania major* and *Trypanosoma cruzi*, a wide range of fungi, the trematode *Schistosoma mansoni*, and many varieties of nematodes (Harnett and Harnett, 1999). The recognition and destructive mechanisms generated by reaction against this ubiquitous epitope of parasitic organisms illustrate the interplay between innate and combinatorial immunity. Pentraxins such as CRP in mammals as well as their homologs in the horseshoe crab (Vasta et al., 1984) bind to PC. Jawed vertebrates from sharks to mammals (Marchalonis et al., 2001) have natural antibodies to this molecule. Recent studies indicate that the natural IgM antibodies of mice (Boes et al., 1998; Baumgarth et al., 2000; Ochsenbein and Zinkernagel, 2000; Shaw et al., 2000; Mold et al., 2002) as well as CRP (Mold et al., 2002) confer protection against infections by gram-positive bacteria because of the capacity of both recognition molecules to activate the complement system. Although jawed vertebrates have both recognition molecules, they are active under different conditions. The binding of CRP is Ca^{2+} dependent, whereas antibody binding is independent of the presence of this divalent cation. In our studies of natural serum components of sandbar sharks that bind PC in the absence of calcium, we isolated IgM antibodies that have restricted light chains with sequences similar to those of antibacterial antibodies of mice and the nurse shark (Marchalonis et al., 2001). The elasmobranch CRP homolog, like the CRP of mammals, requires the presence of Ca^{2+} for binding. The N-terminal sequence of the sandbar shark CRP, like that of another shark, the dogfish (Robey et al., 1983), was more similar to that of mammalian neuropentraxin than to the serum form of CRP. It is interesting that the CRP homologs of the horseshoe crab (Robey

and Liu, 1981) and the tunicate *Boltenia* (Davidson and Swalla, 2002) are also more closely related to neuropentraxins than to mammalian serum CRP. These results are consistent with the existence of the broad array of pentraxin-related molecules within individual species and throughout evolution, with the result that it is difficult to trace orthologous lines of particular gene descent to the great variety of metazoan species expressing representatives of this system (Hughes, 1998). However, there is substantial conservation of certain active segments of the molecules defined by short peptides to the extent that the CRPs of humans and the horseshoe crab share antigenic determinants (Ying et al., 1992) as well as an idiotypic determinant shared with the V_H segment of the murine PC-binding monoclonal antibody S107 (Vasta et al., 1984).

LPS

The second broad group of bacteria is the gram-negative group, of which *Salmonella* and *Escherichia coli* are well-studied members. The major distinguishing characteristic of this group is the outer wall layer made up of LPS, or endotoxin, that contains an outer carbohydrate core and an inner carbohydrate core that has lipid A associated with it (Chiller and Weigle, 1973). LPS exerts profound effects, stimulating macrophages in both vertebrates and invertebrates (Beck et al., 2002). It is also a B-cell mitogen, stimulating these lymphocytes to produce IgM antibodies (Izui et al., 1979). LPS interacts with clotting factors in the hemolymph of the horseshoe crab, *Limulus polyphemus*, to form instant gels (Levin and Bang, 1968). Three types of functionally active receptors for LPS have been characterized to date: the Toll family, insect hemolin, and antibodies. The system of molecules and genes that has received the greatest recent attention is that of the Toll family of *Drosophila* (Imler and Hoffman, 2002) and the homologous TLR family found in mammals (Rock et al., 1998). It is interesting that Toll was first discovered because of its involvement in embryological development, with its roles in resistance to microbial and fungal infections arising in subsequent studies. The developmental and induced protective pathway in *Drosophila* begins with an interaction of LPS or fungal determinants with cell surface-associated Toll that initiates a process of cell activation and differentiation mediated by molecules (DIF and Dorsal) that are homologous to the nuclear transcription factor NF-κB (Manfruelli et al., 1999). Toll homologs are widely distributed throughout phylogeny and form sets of multiple receptors with differing recognition properties within species, such as humans or fruit flies. The signaling pathway leading to NF-κB translocation to the nucleus entails interaction with the cytoplasmic domain of Toll, which is homologous to the cytoplasmic domain of the mammalian receptor for the cytokine IL-1R. However, the actual binding component of IL-1R is quite distinct from that of Toll, consisting of three IgSF C2 domains (Sims et al., 1989). There is a convergence of signaling mechanisms in that two clearly distinct types of recognition molecules operate in a parallel fashion involving the NF-κB system, which is itself widely distributed among animal and plant metazoans.

Insect hemolin, a soluble protein induced in insects by various stimuli, resembles the IL-1R molecule and neural cell adhesion molecules (NCAMs) in consisting of repeats of IgSF C2 domains (Sun et al., 1990; Su et al., 1998; Mendoza and Faye, 1999). Hemolin has been best studied in the giant silk moth, *Hyalophora cecropia*, and the tobacco hornworm, *Manduca sexta* (Yu and Kanost, 2002). The molecule has been reported to bind LPS directly. The third type of molecule known to bind specifically to LPS and to recognize different carbohydrate-defined subtypes is antibody. These types of antibodies can be induced in nude mice, which are deficient in T cells, by immunization with *E. coli* LPS (Marchalonis, 1974). The lack of input of T cells in this case suggests that the sequences of the V_H and V_L segments used in the antibodies are essentially germ line, with the antibodies falling into the category of "natural" antibodies. Recently, monoclonal

antibodies have been raised against LPS epitopes (Brooks et al., 2002, Haralambieva et al., 2002), indicating the capacity of specific recognition molecules of the combinatorial or adaptive immune system to bind the same molecules recognized by nonclonal members of the innate system. The central importance of molecules leading to the activation and translocation of NF-κB is emphasized because this transcription factor plays an essential role in the production of antibodies, and the presence of NF-κB homologs in insects (IκB equivalent to Cactus; NF-κB equivalent to Dorsal) is consistent with the wide phylogenetic distribution of this system that has been co-opted by the late-arriving immune system of jawed vertebrates.

MOLECULES OF "INNATE" IMMUNITY

Table 1 lists the distribution of molecules functioning in innate immunity, including collaboration between cells of the adaptive and innate systems, throughout phylogeny of animal metazoans. The taxonomic groups are organized in accordance with Fig. 2 above. The vertebrates are shown as a single phylum, although substantial differences occur between the jawless or agnathan vertebrates and the gnathostomes or jawed vertebrates. The examples cited are those in which unequivocal identification can be made based on either gene or protein sequence. BLAST searches to confirm identifications or extend possible families by homology were carried out by the procedure of Altschul et al. (1997) on the National Center for Biotechnology Information and Swiss Institute of Bioinformatics databases. The IgSF molecules are defined by limited sequence identity to Ig domains, generally 20% or less, coupled with indications of β-strand structures forming inner and outer β sheets suggestive of the Ig fold (Edmundson et al., 1975). However, the presence of Ig-like folds does not provide a direct indication of evolutionary relatedness. The best example of this is superoxide dismutase, an ancient widely distributed molecule involved in the preven-

TABLE 1 Distribution in phylogeny of molecules functioning in innate immunity[a]

Organisms	Pentraxin	NF-kB	Toll/TLR	Type C lectin	Galect.	Comp/a2M	RAG	Abs/TCR	MHC	IgSF	NRSF
Vertebrates	+	+	+	+	+	+	+	+	+	+	+
Cephalochordates (Amphioxus)			+			+	−	−	−	−	
Urochordates (tunicates)	+	+	+	+	+	+	−	−	−	+	+
Echinoderms		+	+	+		+	−	−	−	+	+
Mollusks (snail, oyster, squid)		+			+	+	−	−	−	+	
Annelids (earthworms, leeches)							−	−	−	+	
Arthropods (insects, crayfish)	+	+	+	+	+	+	−	−	−	+	+
Nematodes (C. elegans)	+	+	+	+	+	+	−	−	−	+	+
Cnidarians (jellyfish)											+
Sponges			+							+	−

[a]Abbreviations: Galect., galectin mannose-binding superfamily (S-type lectins); Comp/a2M, complement/a2M-macroglobulin superfamily; Abs/TCR, antibodies and T-cell receptors of the Ig family; NRSF, nuclear receptor superfamily.

tion of oxidative damage. This molecule has the Ig fold but lacks any sequence relatedness to Igs (Halaby and Mornon, 1997). Ig constant (C) domains consist of two β sheets forming a twisted sandwich, with the outer sheet comprising three β strands and the inner one constituted of four, for a total of seven β strands. The variable domain consists of nine β strands, usually with the extra two strands contributing to the second hypervariable segment (complementarity determining region [CDR2]). In the V domains, the four-stranded sheet is external, with the three-stranded sheet forming the internal contact surface for interaction with the C domain. With bona fide IgV and C domains (C1), the antigen recognition structures (with a few exceptions) consist of heterodimers with the loops separating the β strands, forming three CDRs in V_H and V_L structures. The β strands form a framework, and the inner β strands offer hydrophobic contact surfaces for dimerization. The C domains can undergo homophilic interaction with other C domains, a property that is useful in the giant muscle protein titin, or neuro-association molecules that form large strands for contraction and adhesion. Approximately 40% of proteins contain Ig-like domains (Doolittle, 1995).

A definitive characteristic of Ig-like domains are the presence of two cysteines forming an intrachain disulfide bond with a tryptophan (W) approximately 13 residues C terminal of the first cysteine. In three-dimensional folding, these two residues are approximately 2 Å apart, with the tryptophan protecting the disulfide bond. The length separating the C and W varies in variable domains from approximately 11 to 20 amino acids. In the constant domains, the C-W distance tends to be shorter (11 to 13 residues) and contains a characteristic phenylalanine-X-proline (FXP) in the center of the loop. The length between the sentinel tryptophan and the cysteine that closes the loop (residue 88 in V_L and 92 in V_H in the Kabat system) gives an indication of whether the molecule is a C type (either C1 or C2), intermediate (I), or V type. The distance is shortest for C domains, of greater length for I type, and longest for V domains because of the presence of the extra β strands and the loop comprising the second hypervariable region.

The next characteristic region of an Ig domain is a stretch of residues immediately N terminal to the cysteine that closes the internal disulfide bond. There tends to be a leucine (L) residue 16 amino acids N terminal to the cysteine, and the immediate sequence is generally tyrosine–tyrosine–cysteine (YYC) or tyrosine–X–cysteine (YXC). Because of the presence of Ig-like domains across such wide phylogenetic distances and the lack of strong identities, it is not feasible to derive exact cladograms or schemes of phylogenetic relatedness (Smith and Xue, 1997). Figure 4 is a composite scheme (Smith and Xue, 1997; Teichmann and Chothia, 2000) based on the conjecture that the I set was derived from the ancient ancestral homolog and it then gave rise to the Ig C2 set such as is found in the giant muscle-associated titin molecules. Ig C2 domains often occur in association with other protein domain motifs, particularly when they are expressed as cell surface receptors.

As mentioned above, the TIR domain of Toll and IL-1R is widely distributed in evolu-tion, with clear examples occurring in arthropods (Means et al., 2000) and mammals (Sims et al., 1989). A BLAST search of the recently reported genome of an ascidian, *Ciona*, indicated the presence of TIR at this phylogenetic level as well (J. J. Marchalonis, unpublished BLAST search, 2003). Receptor protein tyrosine kinases (RPTKs) have an intracellular tyrosine kinase domain that is widely distributed through living organisms, occurring in viruses, microbes, and probably all metazoans. The usual external recognition unit contains multiple copies of Ig C2 domains. These Ig C2-like domains show homologies to those of NCAMS and to the soluble hemolin and insulin-binding (Andersen et al., 2000) molecules of insects as well as to MDM (mollusk defense molecule) of snails (Hoek et al., 1996).

The RPTK molecule of the torpedo ray, a cartilaginous fish, is interesting because it has unequivocal homology to RPTKs of ascidians (J. J. Marchalonis, unpublished BLAST search, 2003), nematodes (Popovici et al., 2002), and higher vertebrates (Masiakowski and Carroll, 1992), although it contains an extra domain, a kringle, in addition to three Ig C2 domains and the intracellular tyrosine kinase domain. Ig C2-bearing RTKs are found even in sponges

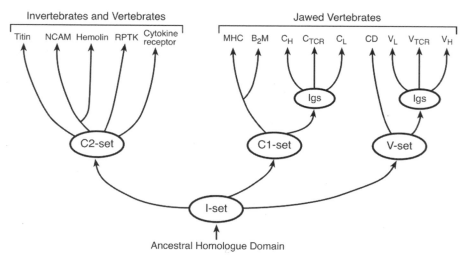

FIGURE 4 Formation and evolution of the IgSF domains. This scheme proposes that the I-type domain was the ancestral Ig domain type.

(Pancer et al., 1996), where one of the domains has properties of an I or V domain (Schacke et al., 1994; Blumbach et al., 1999). In addition, a family of soluble fibrinogen-related molecules produced by snails after parasitic infections contain an Ig-related domain (Adema et al., 1997).

Figure 5 illustrates the sequence comparisons around the cysteine in β-strand B (also termed 4-2) and the sentinel tryptophan found in β-strand C (also termed 3-1) and the intervening loop. This is a characteristic stretch of sequence that occurs in both C1 and C2 constant domains. The sequences from sandbar shark Cλ to nurse shark MHC class IIA are IgC1 domains, and the last three are IgC2 domains derived from moth hemolin, chick NCAM, and a *Ciona* domain identified by homology to the Ig C2 domains of the torpedo ray RTK. With the exception of the β₂-microglobulin (β2M) domains, which have a leucine (L) instead of the characteristic tryptophan (W), the cysteine and tryptophan molecules are universally conserved. Nonetheless, β2M molecules meet the strict statistical criteria for Ig C1 domains and fall within the MHC grouping in cladistic analysis (Marchalonis et al., 1998a, 1998b). As a first approximation, analysis of sequence within this critical stretch of the Ig C domain implies

clustering found in more detailed analysis, i.e., groupings of Cλs, Cκs, Cμs, and TCRCβ domains in evolution with lesser identities to TCRγ, MHC, and C2 domains. Notably, the similarity of TCRβs and Cλ sequences is apparent in this short stretch of sequence. The great diversity in evolution among the Ig C2-related domains is illustrated in the comparison of C2 segments of a moth, a vertebrate, and a tunicate in the last three sequences of Fig. 5.

The C1 and V sets are restricted to jawed vertebrates (Marchalonis et al., 1998b; DuPasquier and Flajnik, 1999; Litman et al., 1999). A recently described molecule from the amphioxus, a cephalochordate, contains domains that are possibly of a V or intermediate (I) nature as well as a putative chitin-binding segment (Cannon et al., 2002). There is considerable variation in these molecules, which the authors find consistent with these being recognition molecules in amphioxus. However, it is interesting to note that the segment between the first cysteine and the tryptophan (C–W) in C2 domains shows considerable variation from domain to domain within single multidomain molecules such as the multiple C2 domains in the titin molecule.

The pentraxins, also known as pentaxins, generally consist of a unit of approximately

	β strand 4-2(B)	loop	β strand 3-1 (C)	Matches with SbS Cλ
SbS Cλ	A T L V C L V S G F N P G A A E I E W T V D G S			24
Hu Cλ	A T L V C L I S D F Y P G A V T V A W K A D G S			15
Hu Cκ	A S V V C L L N N F Y P P E A K V Q W K V D N A			10
Bullfrog Cκ	A S T V C L V D K F Y P G G A Q V T W K G D N K			11
Goldfish CL	D A G V C L A S K G F P S D W S L S W K V D G S			9
Hu Cμ4	A T I T C L V T G F S P A D V F V E W M G R G E			10
SbS Cμ4	F Y L S C L V R G F S P R E I F V K W T V N D K			10
Hu TCRβ	A T L V C L A T G F F P D H V E L S W W V N G K			13
Chick TCRβ	A T L V C L A S G F F P D H L N L V W K V N G V			13
SbS TCRβ	A T V V C T V T D F Y P D N I R I F W L V D G K			12
SbS TCRγ	A L L T C L L T D F Y P E V I K V I W K I G G T			8
Hu TCRγ	G T Y L C L L E K F F P D V I K I H W E E K K S			8
Hu β2M	N F L M C Y V S G F H P S D I E V D L L K N G E			6
SbS β2M	N V L L C H A K D F T P P N F K L E L L E N G K			6
HLA-DQA	N T L I C L V D N I F P P V V N I T W S N G H S			7
HLA-DR2B	N L L V C S V S G F Y P A S I E V R W F R N G Q			11
NuShark IIA	N T L I C F A D G F Y P P H I T M K W R R N N E			8
Moth Hemolin	T V L E C I I E G N Q - Q G V K Y S W K K D G K			7
Chick NCAM	K F F L C Q V A G F A - K Y K D I S W F S P N G			4
Ciona (RTK)	V T L D C H A E G - I P E P - T L S W L R N G H			7

FIGURE 5 Comparative alignments of sequences around the crucial cysteine (C) and tryptophan (W) residues of Ig C1 domains (Igs, TCR, and MHC) and C2 domains of the NCAM group. The positions of the β strands and intervening loop are shown above the alignment. The number of residues identical with the sandbar shark λ light-chain sequence are shown on the right. Sandbar shark (SbS), human (Hu), bullfrog, goldfish, chicken (chick), nurse shark (NuShark), moth, and tunicate (Ciona) sequences were obtained from the databases at http://www.ncbi.nlm.nih.gov. The shark TCR and β2M sequences are from I. Jensen, S. F. Schluter, and J. J. Marchalonis (unpublished data).

200 amino acids that is clearly present in arthropods (Robey and Liu, 1981), in nematodes, in the tunicate *Boltenia* (Davidson and Swalla, 2002), and in all jawed vertebrates (Hughes, 1998). The *Boltenia* molecule is interesting because it is a large molecule of 477 amino acids that contains two CRP-like domains, as opposed to the closest homolog, namely, the serum amyloidlike protein (SAP) of *Limulus* or CRP of humans, which consists of one domain. The active form of the molecules tends to be pentamers in mammals and hexamers in the horseshoe crab (Marchalonis and Edelman, 1968). These molecules are noteworthy because they have the capacity to fix complement via the classical pathway (Gewurz et al., 1993), although their ancestral emergence appears to have preceded that of true complement components homologous to C3/4 and C5 in the lower chordates and cyclostomes (Hanley et al., 1992; Ishiguro et al., 1992; Hughes, 1994; Smith et al., 1998; Marino et al., 2002).

As described above, NF-κB is a key focal point in both innate and adaptive immune reactions, with the molecule itself being a phylogenetically ancient representative of the so-called Rel superfamily (Ghosh et al., 1998). NF-κB itself has a β-strand structure that is in many ways similar to that of Ig domains (Ghosh et al., 1995). In particular, it has a structure comparable to that formed by β-strand B of the Ig fold, which contains the N-terminal cysteine of the intrachain disulfide-bonded loop, and β-strand C, which contains the sentinel tryptophan. This segment shows clear homology in vertebrates, invertebrates, fungi, and plants, suggesting universality within metazoans of reactions mediated by this class of transcription factor (Staskawicz et al., 2001; Friedman and Hughes, 2002).

A phylogenetic tree of deuterostomes based on molecular data (Spruyt et al., 1998; Adoutte et al., 2000; Venkatech et al., 2001; Giribet, 2002; Whitfield et al., 2003; Schluter and Marchalonis, 2003) as well as paleontological considerations (Forey and Janvier, 1994; Valentine et al., 1999) is shown in Fig. 6. It has

been difficult to establish exact homologies of developmental and defense mechanisms based on histological observations, but recent developments, notably the determination of the complete genomes of three mammals (human, mouse, and rat) and teleost fish (pufferfish and zebrafish), as well as the recent publication of the draft genome of *Ciona intestinalis* (Dehal et al., 2002), enable a direct test of gene content of particular systems, including innate and adaptive immunity. Dehal et al. (2002) report that a systematic search of the *Ciona* genome failed to identify any of the crucial genes involved in adaptive immunity, such as Igs, TCRs, and MHC class I and II genes. We confirmed this negative result by a BLAST search of the *Ciona* database for possible homologs of sandbar shark β2M, TCRs γ and β, and Ig V and C genes of light and heavy chains, as well as the RAG1 gene, which is highly conserved in jawed vertebrates (Bernstein et al., 1996; Marchalonis et al., 1998a, 1998b). Dehal et al. suggested that they could not exclude the possibility that *Ciona* has highly divergent orthologs of several of these genes. However, we find this suggestion to be unlikely because the sequence homology of these molecules is so great between sharks and mammals (e.g., >60% overall for RAG1 and as much as 60% in the framework segments of V_H and V_L domains of certain Igs [Marchalonis et al., 1998a, 1998b]) that readily discernible homology should be retained in the tunicates unless a radical change in the rate of amino acid substitution occurred during the evolution of deuterostomes. Although few sequence data are available for the extant cyclostomes, exhaustive studies to identify proteins or genes homologous to definitive elements of the combinatorial (adaptive) immune system produced no positive results either in cyclostomes or in lower chordates. In addition, Dehal et al. (2002) made the striking discovery that *Ciona* contains orthologs for each of the 14 vertebrate proteosome genes, but none of the genes for immunoproteosome activity necessary for antigen processing. They conclude that *Ciona* lacks the antigen-presenting system for T cells

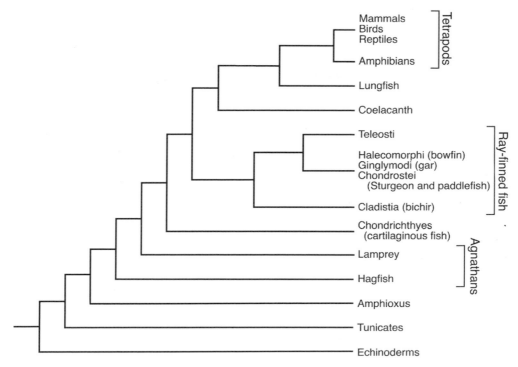

FIGURE 6 Phylogenetic tree of deuterostomes based on molecular data and paleontological considerations.

that is an essential component of the combinatorial immune system of all jawed vertebrates.

Cells morphologically resembling lymphocytes have been observed in tunicates (Warr et al., 1977), and events described as allograft rejection have been studied in detail (Saito et al., 1994; Rinkevich et al., 1998). The molecular evidence indicates that these phenomena are either parts of an ancient innate system or novel tunicate-specific responses, but are not related to the adaptive system of jawed vertebrates. Consistent with observations of others that complement components are found in cyclostomes (Hanley et al., 1992; Ishiguro et al., 1992), tunicates (Marino et al., 2002), and echinoderms (Smith, 2002), the *Ciona* genome contained possible complement genes including C1q-like and C6-like genes (Dehal et al., 2002). There are also three TLR genes and a variety of lectin genes. We found the *Ciona* database to be extremely useful in drawing

firmer, if not absolute, conclusions regarding the distribution of key molecules needed for combinatorial immunity (J. J. Marchalonis, unpublished BLAST search, 2003). The system provided appropriate positive findings as well as expected negative ones, so we take more confidence in the validity of the negative findings. For example, as expected from existing genetic analyses of protostomes and higher deuterostomes, *Ciona* contained DNA sequences specifying proteins significantly related to the TIR intracellular signal segment of Toll and TLR, Ig C2 domains detected by homology to the torpedo ray receptor tyrosine kinase, and the tyrosine kinase segment. By contrast, molecules homologous to RAG1 and RAG2 and Ig V and Ig C1 domains of mammals and sharks were not detectable in the *Ciona* database. The discrimination capacity was considerable in that, as we show in more detail below, the *Ciona* database contained molecules homologous to the so-called C3C4 "ring finger" type of zinc finger, but lacked the nonamer binding domain (NBD) that occurs only in RAG1 genes of jawed vertebrates, where it is involved in the recognition of the specific restriction signal sequences. Thus, the determination of the genome of one lower chordate supports the restriction of the combinatorial immune system to jawed vertebrates.

It appears that there is a major genetic discontinuity between the agnathan vertebrates, lampreys and hagfish, and the jawed vertebrates concerning the components of the combinatorial immune system. This conclusion is not due to something trivial such as difficulty in analysis of proteins or the DNA of these species using techniques appropriate in protostomes and jawed vertebrates. Numerous families of molecules relevant to recognition and regulation can be discerned in cyclostomes, with two of these also detected by means involving serology and protein chemistry as well as analysis of DNA or cDNA. These are complement components related to C3, C4, and C5 that have been isolated as proteins and characterized in terms of gene sequence, cell surface glycoprotein molecules related to the major anion transport (AE1 or band 3) of mammalian erythrocytes (Kay et al., 1995), VDRs (Whitfield et al., 2003) that are members of the nuclear receptor superfamily of ligand-specific transcription factors, and lectins homologous to human intelectin (Tsuji et al., 2001), an intestinal lectin binding to galactofuranosyl residues. In addition, lymphocyte-specific transcription factors such as SPI (Anderson et al., 2001; Mayer et al., 2002; Uinuk-Ool et al., 2002) and the cytokine IL-18 (Najakshin et al., 1999) have been detected in cyclostomes. When molecules homologous to those of higher vertebrates are found in lampreys, the percentage identity is essentially what one would expect according to usual rates of protein evolution, i.e., 1×10^{-9} to 3×10^{-9} substitutions per amino acid per year. For example, we have cloned a fragment of the lamprey AE1 homolog consisting of 160 amino acids that is approximately 60% identi-

cal to that of the human molecule in this region. The percentage amino acid identity between the human and lamprey Intelectins was 57%. Tsuji et al. (2001) reported homologies between the lamprey Intelectin, and an egg lectin of the clawed toad *Xenopus laevis* as well as a galactose-specific lectin of the ascidian *Halocynthia roretzi*. The *Ciona* genome database contained 20 scaffolds showing appreciable sequence identity to the lamprey Intelectin, with approximately 45% identity in the fibrinogen-related domain (residues 52 to 98) and 45% in the stretch of 130 amino acids from residues 130 to 259.

There is a member of the nuclear receptor superfamily that appears to be involved in at least two aspects of innate and/or combinatorial immunity. VDR, in addition to its well-known activity in calcium homeostasis (Haussler et al., 1998), is also involved in regulation of dendritic cells and T cells (Lemire, 2000; Griffin et al., 2001). Furthermore, VDR appears to be involved in recognition of certain xenobiotics and induction of cytochrome P450 enzymes to detoxify these potentially harmful compounds (Makishima et al., 2002). These actions are mediated by functional domains in VDRs that, as in other nuclear receptors, include a 66-residue DNA-binding domain containing two C4C4 zinc fingers and a longer (approximately 300 residues in humans) VDR ligand-binding domain (Haussler et al., 1998). Until recently, VDRs have been found only in vertebrates with bony skeletons. However, we recently cloned a VDR (Whitfield et al., 2003) from the lamprey *Petromyzon marinus* that is capable of binding vitamin D with high affinity and mediates transactivation of a reporter gene linked to a vitamin D response element from the human CYP3A4 gene (Goodwin et al., 1999). In addition, two VDR-like proteins are encoded in the recently assembled genome of the tunicate *Ciona intestinalis* (Dehal et al., 2002). A cladogram of representative VDRs is shown in Fig. 7 along with those putative nuclear receptors from the completed genomes of *Drosophila melanogaster* (Gelbart, 2003) and *C.*

elegans (Stein et al., 2001) that have the highest percent identity to VDRs. As can be seen from the computed percent identities of these VDRs and VDR-like proteins (Fig. 7, right side), there is a steady quantitative decline in identity as a function of time of ancestral divergences of the different animal groups. This is the expected pattern of a protein that has been retained and incrementally modified over the course of more than 500 million years of evolution. However, unlike the situation with respect to Ig V and C1 domains and RAG genes, detectable homology is retained for more than 700 million years separating ancestral protostomes and deuterostomes.

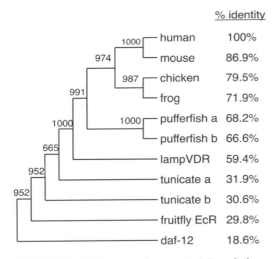

% identity

human	100%
mouse	86.9%
chicken	79.5%
frog	71.9%
pufferfish a	68.2%
pufferfish b	66.6%
lampVDR	59.4%
tunicate a	31.9%
tunicate b	30.6%
fruitfly EcR	29.8%
daf-12	18.6%

FIGURE 7 Cladogram of putative VDR orthologs. Chordate receptors were aligned, and percent identities with human VDR were computed with the BLAST alignment tool at http://www.ncbi.nlm.nih.gov/gorf/bl2.html. Alignment for fruit fly and nematode receptors was further refined in Clustal W. The lamprey sequence (lampVDR) is from Whitfield et al. (2003). Pufferfish and tunicate sequences are available from http://genome.jgi-psf.org/cgi-bin/searchGM2.cgi?db=ciona4 and from http://scrappy.fugu-sg.org/Fugu_rubripes. Other sequences were obtained from the databases at http://www.ncbi.nlm.nih.gov. Frog, *Xenopus laevis*; pufferfish, *Takafugu ruprides*; tunicate, *C. intestinalis*; fruit fly, *D. melanogaster* ecdysone receptor (EcR); daf-12, nematode (*C. elegans*) daf-12 protein. The latter two are the best matches for VDR in the fruit fly and nematode genomes.

THE ADAPTIVE OR COMBINATORIAL IMMUNE RESPONSE OF JAWED VERTEBRATES

Although the immune response of higher vertebrates has been termed adaptive, going back to the studies of Good and his associates in the late 1950s and early 1960s (Good and Papermaster, 1964), we prefer the term combinatorial because this nomenclature reflects the genetic mechanism involved in diversification. Furthermore, all defense mechanisms, including those of plants and invertebrates, by definition are "adaptive," so we stress the genetic mechanisms involved that are apparently restricted to gnathostomes. The combinatorial immune response appears to have emerged extremely rapidly in evolution about 450 million years ago, an event we have termed the "big bang." This was probably triggered as the result of the horizontal transfer of genes enabling site-specific recombination (Schatz et al., 1989; Oettinger et al., 1990; Marchalonis and Schluter, 1998; Schluter et al., 1999). Although there are many mechanisms of diversification of multiple sets of homologous genes, including, for example, the odorant receptors (Buck and Axel, 1991) and the pentraxins of horseshoe crabs (Tharia et al., 2002), the RAG genes provide a unique mechanism giving characteristic patterns of variability within the variable domains of Ig light and heavy chains and TCRs. Evidence supporting the concept of a big bang resulting from horizontal transfer of RAG gene precursors to an ancestral shark stems from the phylogenetic distribution of these molecules (Bernstein et al., 1996), the lack of introns within the coding segments of these molecules in sharks (Bernstein et al., 1996) and mammals (Oettinger et al., 1990; Hansen and McBlane, 2000), and the fact that RAG1/RAG2 constructs can be induced to act as transposases. The emergence of the combinatorial immune response was apparently accidental. It is reasonable to conclude that originally it was neither a defense mechanism nor a regulatory system, but its unparalleled capacity to generate recognition molecules (Marchalonis et al., 2002a) gave it the potential to function in regulation, maintenance of the integrity of the organism, and defense against foreign pathogens or deleterious mutant cells. The somatic combinatorial events gave a particular advantage in defense against pathogenic organisms or mutating cells because this system could respond in real time to ongoing modifications within the pathogens. Furthermore, in a parallel sense, the combinatorial system can respond to deleterious modifications in normal cells, such as the for-

mation of the senescent cell antigen (Kay, 1981) by defective erythrocytes, and initiate the removal of the damaged cells by antibody-dependent phagocytosis.

Following the patterns of co-option described above, the combinatorial system incorporated preexisting cellular and humoral mechanisms for activation and differentiation, including the fundamentally important NF-κB transcription factor pathway and the involvement of the universal heat shock proteins in

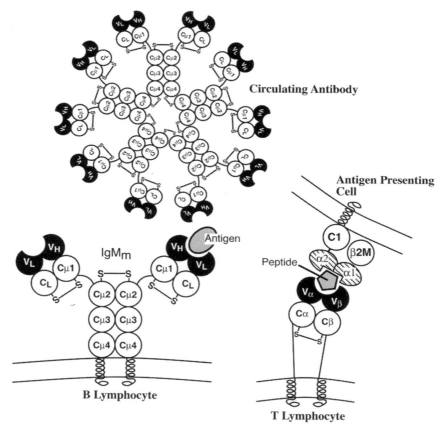

FIGURE 8 Representation of Ig recognition elements found in the combinatorial immune system of jawed vertebrates. Examples shown here are the IgM isotype and the α/β TCR. The membrane receptor on B lymphocytes consists of membrane-associated IgM monomer (IgM_m). The circulating form shown here is the pentamer. The antigen receptor on T lymphocytes is the α/β heterodimer depicted here recognizing peptide antigen presented by an MHC class I molecule on an antigen-presenting cell. All the variable (V) regions and constant (C) domains as well as the MHC C1 and the associated β2M are Ig C1 domains. The α1 and α2 MHC domains presenting peptides are unrelated to Igs. Adapted from Marchalonis and Schluter (1998) with permission.

presentation of antigen. Furthermore, antibodies joined CRPs and lectins in the capacity to activate the complement cascade. The repertoire of the combinatorial system as expressed at the two extremes of jawed vertebrates, sharks and humans, has the capacity to overarch the entire spectrum recognized by the ancient noncombinatorial molecules such as pentraxins, lectins, adhesion molecules, complement components, and the Toll/TLR recognition system. We have illustrated this above using the reaction to LPS of gram-negative organisms as well as gram-positive constituents such as PC and a variety of endogenous antigens.

The definitive elements of the combinatorial system are the cells of the lymphoid system, particularly lymphocytes and plasma cells, TCRs, and antibody recognition molecules, products of the MHC that present peptide antigens to TCRs (Fig. 8) and the RAG genes. Current data support the proposition that the RAG genes and Ig V and C domains occur only in jawed vertebrates. Although it is necessary to attain complete genomic sequence to

confirm this for cyclostomes, the lack of these genes in the lower chordate *C. intestinalis* buttresses the argument. Comparisons of RAG1 and RAG2 sequences and the overall organization of the RAGs show that this locus has been highly conserved during vertebrate evolution (Fig. 9). Shark RAG2 is 50% overall identical to the human molecule, and many sequence motifs are absolutely conserved in all vertebrate species studied. The shark RAG2 apparently has the same domain structure as the human molecule, consisting of a kelch region with sixfold symmetry resembling a turbine, an acidic hinge region, and a zinc finger domain. Residues identified in mutagenesis experiments as critical for activity in mammalian RAG2 molecules are conserved in the shark (Schluter and Marchalonis, 2003).

Thus, it appears that the ancestral vertebrate RAG2 had essentially the same structure and activity of the modern form. The same conclusions were obtained for RAG1, with the conservation even more striking. Overall, the shark and human proteins are 64% identical,

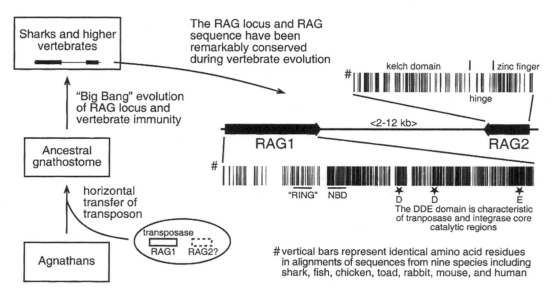

FIGURE 9 Schematic diagram summarizing the evolution and properties of the RAG genes. The genomic organization is shown in the boxes and line diagram, with the direction of transcription indicated by the arrows on the boxes. Domains identified in the proteins are indicated. "RING" is the ring zinc finger domain; NBD is the nonamer-binding domain. Adapted from Schluter and Marchalonis (2003) with permission.

but there is a gradient of identity within the molecule. RAG1 proteins consist of approximately 1,100 amino acids with the N-terminal residues from 1 to approximately 400 showing about 40% identity, but the remaining portion of the molecule shows approximately 80% identity among all vertebrate species (Bernstein et al., 1996). The molecule contains two DNA-binding segments, the zinc finger ring motif (Fig. 10), and the NBD (Fig. 11). The ring finger motif is ancient in emergence and widely distributed, being found in plants including *Arabidopsis*, in the yeast excision and repair enzymes RAD18 and RAD16, and in the ascidian *Ciona*. In addition to its presence in RAG1, ring is found in a large number of mammalian proteins, including breast cancer susceptibility-associated molecules. By contrast, the NBD is absolutely restricted to jawed vertebrates and shows greater than 80% identity in sequence comparisons ranging from shark to human. The genomic organization of the shark locus is essentially the same as that in all other jawed vertebrates, with RAG1 and RAG2 being in close juxtaposition and in the opposite transcriptional orientation. Shark RAGs do not contain introns within the coding regions. This lack of introns, when first observed in mouse RAGs, led Oettinger et al. (1990) to propose that they were of prokaryotic origin. We agree with this interpretation, although introns have been observed in the

coding regions of teleost RAGs (Hansen and Kaatari, 1995). We believe that this is a secondary development because phylogenetic schemes constructed with RAG2 sequences (Schluter and Marchalonis, 2003) as well as other markers (Venkatech et al., 2001) (Fig. 6) indicate that cartilaginous fishes are the basal vertebrates and that the ancestral teleosts diverged early from the ancestors of the tetrapods.

The system was essentially complete at the beginning, if extant cartilaginous fishes can be taken as representative of the original state, in that Ig family antibodies comprised of light chains and μ-like heavy chains are present (Marchalonis and Edelman, 1965), the full range of TCRs (α/β and γ/δ) are present (Rast et al., 1997), and both MHC class I and class II molecules (Bartl et al., 1997; Flajnik et al., 1999) plus the complete set of complement components (Dodds et al., 1998; Smith, 1998) occur. Hagfish and lampreys are clearly vertebrates. They possess cells resembling lymphocytes and plasma cells morphologically (Zapata et al., 1981; Mayer et al., 2002) and express complement components (Hanley et al., 1992; Ishiguro et al., 1992), some cell surface markers (Mayer et al., 2002) and transcription factors (Anderson et al., 2001; Uinuk-Ool et al., 2002) characteristic of lymphocytes, but lack Igs, TCRs, MHC products, and RAG genes. The first antibodies to appear in evolution are

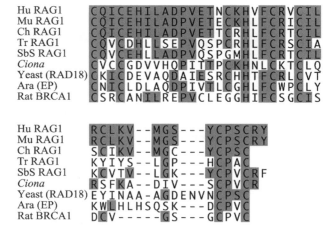

FIGURE 10 Phylogenetic distribution of the ring finger motif found in RAG1. Sequences were obtained from the databases at; http://www.ncbi.nlm.nih.gov. Human (Hu); mouse (Mu); chicken (Ch); trout (Tr); tunicate (Ciona); *Arabidopsis* (Ara); RAD, nucleotide excision repair protein; EP, C3HC4-type ring finger; BRCA, breast cancer.

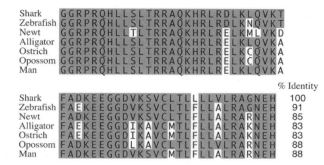

FIGURE 11 Phylogenetic distribution of the RAG1 NBD.

	% Identity
Shark	100
Zebrafish	91
Newt	85
Alligator	83
Ostrich	83
Opossom	88
Man	88

apparently homologous to mammalian IgM (Marchalonis, 1977). There is substantial evidence of conservation of V_H and V_L framework structure among antibodies and TCRs of all extant vertebrates. There is no convincing evidence to date of major affinity maturation in IgM of any species, although it is reasonable to propose that some increase in strength of binding or affinity would be selected by multiple immunizations correlated with cell proliferation and selection of antigen. Natural IgM antibodies, which are sometimes considered part of the innate system (Boes et al., 1998; Ochsenbein and Zinkernagel, 2000; Marchalonis et al., 2001; Rodman et al., 2001), have V_H and V_L sequences that are identical or closely similar to germ line sequences in species where these comparisons have been made (Harindranath et al., 1993; Coutinho et al., 1995; Robey et al., 2000). In all cases, the formation of CDR3 requires gene rearrangement involving the V segment, the joining (J) segment, and in some cases the diversity (D) segment. Although many members of the nonrearranging IgSF occur in mammals and other vertebrates (Colonna and Samaridis, 1995; Kubagawa et al., 1997; DuPasquier et al., 1999; Yoder et al., 2001; Moretta et al., 2002) as well as in diverse groups of invertebrates (see above), actual Ig family members occur only in the jawed vertebrates. Somewhat paradoxical results are obtained using molecular clock-type estimates based on the rate of mutation of Ig and TCR constant domains to calculate the time of origin of these molecules in evolution

(Marchalonis and Schluter, 1998; Marchalonis et al., 1998a). Based on a rate of 10^{-9} substitutions per amino acid per year, we estimated that Ig constant domains might have arisen approximately 1 billion years ago, a result predicting that bona fide C1 domains should be detectable in extant lower chordates as well as protostome invertebrates. However, analyses of the draft *Ciona* genome and the complete genome sequences of *Drosophila* and *Caenorhabditis* indicate that this cannot be the case. Based on available data, the constant domains of TCRs mutate approximately three times more rapidly than those of Ig light chains. If these rates are accurate, TCRs arose approximately 450 to 500 million years ago, a time that is consistent with current thinking regarding the time of origin of the jawed vertebrates. It may well be that representatives of the ancestral species expressing the original Ig family domains are extinct, so we will never be able to identify the exact ancestral molecules.

A large number of V and C sequences have been determined for Ig light and heavy chains and for a smaller number of sequences for TCR α, β, γ and δ chains for nonmammalian species including birds, reptiles, amphibians, teleost fish, and cartilaginous fish. Nearly all of the detailed information for these species has been obtained by the sequencing of germ line genes or cDNA copies, and there is little functional evidence regarding binding properties and the actual function of homologs in "lower" species. There have been no X-ray crystallographic analyses of nonmammalian Igs to date, but the clear sequence homologies, particularly in the frameworks, have enabled the use of characterized human Ig light- and heavy-chain domains as templates to construct three-dimensional models for light-chain (Schluter et al., 1989) and heavy-chain (Marchalonis et al., 1998a; Ramsland et al., 2001) variable domains of shark Igs. Figure 12 compares the sequence of sandbar shark λ-like light-chain clone 5.1 (Hohman et al., 1992) with the human λ light-chain Mcg, giving the positions of the β strands and structural characteristics of the loops involved in the binding of antigen in the variable domains. This shark Vλ shows a high degree of identity, approximately 60% in the frameworks, to that of the Vλ6 subset of humans and mice (Reidl et al., 1992; Yacine et al., 2002). This molecule represents the predominant light-chain family in carcharhine sharks. All cartilaginous fish to date appear to possess the same sets of light and heavy chains, but in different proportions. For example, molecules of this type are a minor subset in the horned shark, where they have

been termed type II light chains (Rast et al., 1994). The variable domains of the pre-B-cell receptor also resemble primitive λ chains in sequence in both the variable and the constant domains. Construction of three-dimensional models using Mcg as a template (Schluter et al., 1989) allows the conclusion that the three-dimensional structures of the Vλ and Cλ domains of sandbar shark light chains are similar to those of their mammalian homologs. The arrangement of the β strands in the Ig fold is strongly conserved here (and that we show below for TCRs), but the structures of the loops, particularly complex ones such as the CDR3 segments that are formed by interaction of V and J segments in light chains and by V, D, and J segments in heavy chains and TCR β chains, require crystallographic analysis of individual molecules to determine exact structures.

The predominant secreted form of antibody in sharks is IgM, which comprises up to 50% of total serum protein. Cladistic analysis shows that shark V_H families have an overall simi-

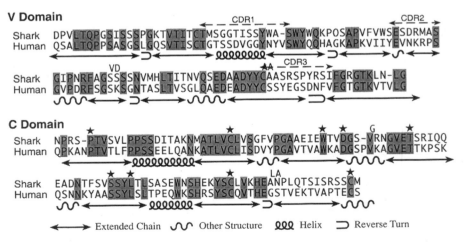

FIGURE 12 Comparative alignment of sandbar shark λ (cDNA clone 5.1) (Hohman et al., 1992) sequence with human λ light-chain Mcg (Vλ5) (Fett and Deutsch, 1974). The structural features depicted, including extended chain (β band), reverse turn, and other structures, are those of human λ light chain as determined by X-ray crystallography. Shortened structures are indicated by gaps and insertions are designated by placement of the residues above the corresponding segment. Identities between sequences are shaded. Residues conserved in all light chains are indicated by stars above the sequence. Adapted from Marchalonis et al. (2002b) with permission.

larity to the VH3 cluster of heavy chains of higher vertebrates (Bernstein et al., 1996; Greenberg et al., 1996; Schluter et al., 1997). Figure 13 shows an alignment of the VDJ sequence of two sandbar shark Vμ clones compared with that of a human VH3 molecule derived from a human monoclonal IgM autoantibody to TCRs (Robey et al., 2000). Three-dimensional models constructed based on these alignments support the hypothesis of strong conservation of three-dimensional structure of the Ig variable domain in evolution.

Cladistic studies of the relationship among Ig domains indicate that TCRs and light chains had a common ancestor early in evolution and that their divergence occurred following the ancestral divergence of variable domains of light chains and heavy chains (Marchalonis et al., 1998a). The functional relationship between TCRs and MHC antigens is a clear example of coevolution because the predominant type of TCRs in mice and humans, the α/β TCR, has evolved to recognize peptide antigens presented by MHC molecules. It is possible that the TCR originally resembled antibodies in recognizing three-dimensional shapes in the absence of presentation. This possibility is strengthened by the fact that the minor set of TCRs in these species, TCRγδ, can recognize a variety of antigens in the absence of MHC presentation

(Richards and Nelson, 2000). Ongoing studies with TCRs of the sandbar shark support the overall relatedness of Ig domains in evolution and the fundamental structural homology between TCR and Ig domains. In the comparison of V region sequences of human and shark λ light chains and TCR β and γ chains, blocks of substantial identity are obvious (Fig. 14). These occur especially at the end of the first framework (FR1 residues 15 to 23), the WYXQ sequence at the beginning of FR2 (residues 37 to 40), residues immediately N terminal to cysteine 88, a framework 3 that closes the internal S-S loop, and the characteristic FR4 motif FGXGT (residues 109 to 115) of the joining segment. This motif is found in light chains and TCRs. By contrast, heavy chains have the homologous JH (FR4) motif WGXGT. It is noteworthy that segments encoded by the J chain that are not themselves Ig are characteristic markers of complete Ig V domains (Schluter and Marchalonis, 1986), indicating that the molecules arose by RAG-mediated recombination.

EVOLUTIONARY CONCLUSIONS

Because we and others have recently presented evolutionary overviews of the vertebrate adaptive or combinatorial system in detail, we have stressed here the generality of recognition mechanisms, coupled with a commonality of

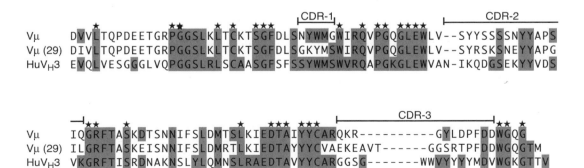

FIGURE 13 Comparative alignment of two sandbar shark Vμ (Shen et al., 1996) sequences with that of a human VH3 (HuV_H3) monoclonal IgM autoantibody (Robey et al., 2000). The CDR segments shown are those defined by Kabat et al. (1991) for human sequences. Residues shared with the human sequence are shaded. Universally conserved residues are denoted by a star. Adapted from Marchalonis et al. (2002b) with permission.

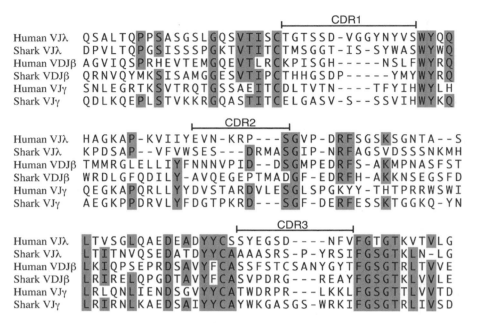

FIGURE 14 Comparative alignments of human VJλ (Mcg), TCR VDJβ (Yanagi et al., 1984), and TCR VJγ (Hochstenbach et al., 1988) and sandbar shark VJλ, TCR VDJβ, TCR VJγ. The shark TCR sequences are from Jensen, Schluter, and Marchalonis (unpublished data). The shading indicates positions with at least four matches. Adapted from Marchalonis et al. (2002b) with permission.

signaling mechanisms and with recent genomic advances to test hypotheses regarding the phylogenetic distribution of essential elements required by the combinatorial system. Intracellular signaling mechanisms, including TIR and protein tyrosine kinase, are apparently ancient in emergence and universal in distribution. Recognition molecules, including lectins and pentraxins, likewise are ancient in emergence and widely distributed. Representatives of the IgSF occur in all metazoans, where they function as adhesion domains in muscle-related proteins and cell adhesion factors as well as recognition domains for peptide-type hormones and microbial LPSs. These Ig domains tend to be of the Ig C2 type that has the capacity to form noncovalent dimers that function in cell-cell adhesion and ligand-specific activation in the Toll/TLR system. Bona fide Ig family V and C1 domains occur only in jawed vertebrates, as does the RAG1/RAG2 recombination system allowing

combinatorial diversification to occur. The recent availability of the draft genome of the tunicate *Ciona intestinalis* was a very useful data source to determine whether characteristic genes of innate or combinatorial immunity were restricted to protostomes or deuterostomes, or could be present in both. As expected, based on available genetic and functional data, this lower chordate had genes specifying proteins homologous to Ig C2 domains, tyrosine receptor protein kinases, various functional lectins, complement components, and a small set of possible cytokine receptors. However, it lacked the molecules crucial to the combinatorial immune system, namely, antibodies, TCRs, MHC products, and RAG1 and RAG2. It will be necessary to determine the genome sequence for lampreys to establish whether these genes are likewise totally absent in the extant cyclostomes that are considered to represent the most anciently arisen group of extant vertebrates. With the exception of the molecules defining the combinatorial or adaptive system, cyclostomes have molecules appropriate for their phylogenetic position with the percentage of sequence identity expected from the rates of divergence with the jawed vertebrates. These molecules include the major anion transport molecule of cell surfaces, AE1, complement components, and the VDR from the nuclear receptor superfamily. Overall, elements that function as parts of innate immunity are widely dispersed throughout the metazoans, with the commonalities described above, but with unique differences in individual groups or species as a consequence of separate evolution. The combinatorial system of jawed vertebrates is a relative latecomer, but it has co-opted existing mechanisms for recognition, cell activation, and cell/cell communication as well as presenting an ensemble of receptor specificities overarching that of the more ancient and invariant innate recognition units. The innate system, likewise, co-opted receptors and mechanisms used in differentiation and defense against general stresses such as oxidative damage by incorporating them into pattern recognition systems enabling defense against microbes and fungi as well as general reactions to stress. It is likely that in each individual species where co-option occurred, it was followed by a coevolution dependent on the stringency of the selective environment.

ACKNOWLEDGMENTS

This research was supported in part by grant MCB-022149 from the National Science Foundation to J.J.M. and by grant DK33351 from the National Institutes of Health to Mark Haussler. We thank Diana Humphreys for valuable assistance in the preparation of the manuscript.

REFERENCES

Adema, C. M., L. A. Hertel, R. D. Miller, and E. S. Loker. 1997. A family of fibrinogen-related proteins that precipitate parasite-derived molecules is produced by an invertebrate after infection. *Proc. Natl. Acad. Sci. USA* **94:**8691–8696.

Adoutte, A., G. Balavoine, N. Lartillot, O. Lespinet, B. Prud'homme, and R. De Rosa. 2000. The new animal phylogeny: reliability and implications. *Proc. Natl. Acad. Sci. USA* **97:**4453–4456.

Altschul, S. F., T. L. Madden, A. A. Schaffer, J. Zhang, Z. Zhang, W. Miller, and D. J. Lipman. 1997. Gapped BLAST and PSI-BLAST: a new generation of protein database search programs. *Nucleic Acids Res.* **25:**3389–3402.

Andersen, A. S., P. H. Hansen, L. Schaffer, and C. Kristensen. 2000. A new secreted insect protein belonging to the immunoglobulin superfamily binds insulin and related peptides and inhibits their activities. *J. Biol. Chem.* **275:**16948–16953.

Anderson, M. K., X. Sun, A. L. Miracle, G. W. Litman, and E. V. Rothenberg. 2001. Evolution of hematopoiesis: three members of the PU.1 transcription factor family in a cartilaginous fish, *Raja eglanteria. Proc. Natl. Acad. Sci. USA* **98:**553–558.

Bartl, S., M. A. Baish, M. J. Flajnik, and Y. Ohta. 1997. Identification of Class I genes in cartilaginous fish: the most ancient group of vertebrates displaying an adaptive immune response. *J. Immunol.* **159:**6097–6104.

Basu, S., K. R. Rosenzweig, M. Youmell, and B. D. Price. 1998. The DNA dependent protein kinase participates in the activation of NFκB following DNA damage. *Biochem. Biophys. Res. Commun.* **247:**79–83.

Baumgarth, N., O. Herman, G. Jager, L. Brown, L. Herzenberg, and J. Chen. 2000. B-1 and B-2 cell-derived immunoglobulin M antibodies are nonredundant components of the protective response to influenza virus infection. *J. Exp. Med.* **192:**271–280.

Beck, G., T. W. Ellis, G. S. Habicht, S. F. Schluter, and J. J. Marchalonis. 2002. Evolution of the acute phase response: iron release by echinoderm (Asteria forbesi) coelomocytes. *Dev. Comp. Immunol.* **26:**11–26.

Bernstein, R. M., S. F. Schluter, H. Bernstein, and J. J. Marchalonis. 1996. Primordial emergence of the recombination activating gene 1 (RAG1): sequence of the complete shark gene indicates homology to microbial integrases. *Proc. Natl. Acad. Sci. USA* **93:**9454–9459.

Blumbach, B., B. Diehl-Seifer, J. Seack, R. Steffen, I. M. Muller, and W. E. G. Muller. 1999. Cloning and expression of new receptors belonging to the immunoglobulin superfamily from the marine sponge *Geodia cydonium. Immunogenetics* **49:**751–763.

Boes, M., A. P. Prodeus, T. Schmidt, M. C. Carroll, and J. Chen. 1998. A critical role of natural immunoglobulin M in immediate defense against systemic bacterial infection. *J. Exp. Med.* **188:**2381–2386.

Bowie, A., and L. A. O'Neill. 2000. The interleukin-1 receptor/Toll-like receptor superfamily: signal generators for pro-inflammatory interleukins and microbial products. *J. Leukoc. Biol.* **67:**508–514.

Brooks, D. W., R. H. Robertson, C. L. Lutze-Wallace, and W. Pfahler. 2002. Monoclonal antibodies specific for Campylobacter fetus lipopolysaccharides. *Vet. Microbiol.* **87:**37–49.

Buck, L., and R. Axel. 1991. A novel multigene family may encode odorant receptors: a molecular basis for odor recognition. *Cell* **65**:175–187.

Cannon, J. P., R. N. Haire, and G. W. Litman. 2002. Identification of diversified genes that contain immunoglobulin-like variable regions in a protochordate. *Nat. Immunol.* **12**:1200–1207.

Chiller, J. M., and W. O. Weigle. 1973. Termination of tolerance to human gamma globulin in mice by antigen and bacterial lipopolysaccharide (endotoxin). *J. Exp. Med.* **137**:740–750.

Colonna, M., and J. Samaridis. 1995. Cloning of immunoglobulin superfamily members associated with HLA-C and HLA-B recognition by human natural killer cells. *Science* **269**:405–408.

Coutinho, A., M. Kazatchkine, and A. Avrameas. 1995. Natural autoantibodies. *Curr. Opin. Immunol.* **7**:812–818.

Davidson, B., and B. J. Swalla. 2002. A molecular analysis of ascidian metamorphosis reveals activation of an innate immune response. *Development* **129**:4739–4742.

Davidson, E. H., K. J. Peterson, and R. A. Camerson. 1995. Origin of bilaterian body plans: evolution of development regulatory mechanisms. *Science* **270**:1319–1325.

Dehal, P., Y. Satou, R. K. Campbell, J. Chapman, B. Degnan, A. De Tamaso, B. Davidson, A. Di Gregorio, M. Gelpke, D. M. Goodstein, N. Harafuji, K. E. M. Hastings, I. Ho, K. Hotta, W. Huang, T. Kawashima, P. Lemaire, D. Martinez, I. A. Meinertzhagen, S. Necula, M. Nonaka, N. Putnam, S. Rash, H. Saiga, M. Satake, A. Terry, et al. 2002. The draft genome of Ciona intestinalis: insights to chordate and vertebrate origins. *Science* **298**:2157–2167.

Dodds, A., S. Smith, R. Levine, and A. Willis. 1998. Isolation and initial characterization of complement components C3 and C4 of the nurse shark and the channel catfish. *Dev. Comp. Immunol.* **22**:207–216.

Doolittle, R. F. 1995. The multiplicity of domains in proteins. *Annu. Rev. Biochem.* **64**:287–314.

DuPasquier, L., and M. Flajnik. 1999. Origin and evolution of the vertebrate immune system, p. 605–650. *In* W. E. Paul (ed.), *Fundamental Immunology.* Lippincott-Raven, Philadelphia, Pa.

DuPasquier, L., M. Courtet, and I. Chretien. 1999. Duplication and MHC linkage of the CTX family of genes in Xenopus and in mammals. *Eur. J. Immunol.* **29**:1729–1739.

Edelman, G. 1987. CAMs and Igs: cell adhesion and the evolutionary origins of immunity. *Immunol. Rev.* **100**:11–45.

Edmundson, A. B., R. R. Ely, E. E. Abola, M. Schiffer, and N. Pagniotopoulos. 1975. Rotational allomerision and divergent evolution of domains in immunoglobulin light chains. *Biochemistry* **14**:3933–3936.

Ehrlich, P. 1900. On immunity with special references to cell life. *Proc. R. Soc. London* **66**:424–448.

Ellison, J., and L. Hood. 1983. Human antibody genes: evolutionary and molecular genetic perspectives. *Adv. Hum. Genet.* **13**:113–147.

Fett, J. W., and H. F. Deutsch. 1974. Primary structure of the Mcg lambda chain. *Biochemistry* **13**:4102–4114.

Fink, R. C., and J. G. Scandalios. 2002. Molecular evolution and structure-function relationships of the superoxide dismutase gene families in angiosperms and their relationship to other eucaryotic and procaryotic superoxide dismutases. *Arch. Biochem. Biophys.* **399**:19–36.

Flajnik, M. F., and M. Kasahara. 2001. Comparative genomics of the MHC: glimpses into the evolution of the adaptive immune system. *Immunity* **15**:351–356.

Flajnik, M., Y. Ohta, C. Namikawa-Yamada, and M. Nonaka. 1999. Insight into the primordial MHC from studies in ectothermic vertebrates. *Immunol. Rev.* **167**:59–67.

Forey, P., and P. Janvier. 1994. Evolution of the early vertebrates. *Am. Sci.* **82**:554–565.

Friedman, R., and A. Hughes. 2002. Molecular evolution of the NFκB signaling system. *EMBO J.* **11**:829–837.

Gearing, D. P., C. J. Thut, T. Vandenbos, S. D. Gimpel, P. B. Delaney, J. King, V. Price, D. Cosman, and M. P. Beckman. 1991. Leukemia inhibitory factor receptor is structurally related to the IL-6 signal transducer, gp130. *EMBO J.* **10**:2839–2848.

Gelbart, W. M. 2003. The FlyBase database of the Drosophila genome projects and community literature. *Nucleic Acids Res.* **30**:106–108.

Gewurz, H., S. C. Ying, H. Jiang, and T. F. Lint. 1993. Nonimmune activation of the classical complement pathway. *Behring Inst. Mitt.* **93**:138–147.

Ghosh, G., G. Van Duyne, S. Ghosh, and P. Sigler. 1995. Structure of NFκB p50 homodimer bound to a κB site. *Nature* **373**:303–310.

Ghosh, S., M. J. May, and E. B. Kopp. 1998. NFκB and REL proteins: evolutionarily conserved mediators of immune responses. *Annu. Rev. Immunol.* **16**:225–260.

Giribet, G. 2002. Current advances in the phylogenetic reconstruction of metazoan evolution. A new paradigm for the Cambrian explosion? *Mol. Phylogenet. Evol.* **24**:345–357.

Good, R. A., and B. W. Papermaster. 1964. Ontogeny and phylogeny of adaptive immunity. *Adv. Immunol.* **4**:1–115.

Goodwin, B., E. Hodgson, and C. Liddle. 1999. The orphan human pregnane X receptor mediates the transcriptional activation of CYP3A4 by rifampicin through a distal enhancer module. *Mol. Pharmacol.* **56**:1329–1339.

Greenberg, A. S., A. L. Hughes, J. Guo, D. Avila, E. C. McKinney, and M. F. Flajnik. 1996. A novel "chimeric" antibody class in cartilagenous fish: IgM may not be the primordial immunoglobulin. *Eur. J. Immunol.* **26:**1123–1129.

Griffin, M. D., W. Lutz, V. A. Phan, L. A. Bachman, D. J. McKean, and R. Kumar. 2001. Dendritic cell modulation by 1alpha,25 dihydroxyvitamin D3 and its analogs: a vitamin D receptor dependent pathway that promotes a persistent state of immaturity in vitro and in vivo. *Proc. Natl. Acad. Sci. USA* **98:**6800–6805.

Halaby, D. M., and J. P. E. Mornon. 1997. The immunoglobulin superfamily: an insight on its tissular, species and functional diversity. *J. Mol. Evol.* **46:**389–400.

Hanley, P., J. W. Hook, D. A. Raftos, A. A. Gooley, R. Trent, and R. L. Raison. 1992. Hagfish humoral defense protein exhibits structural and functional homology with mammalian complement components. *Proc. Natl. Acad. Sci. USA* **89:**7910–7914.

Hansen, J. D., and S. L. Kaatari. 1995. The recombination activation gene 1 (RAG1) of rainbow trout (*Oncorhynchus mykiss*): cloning, expression and phylogenetic analysis. *Immunogenetics* **42:**188–195.

Hansen, J. D., and J. F. McBlane. 2000. Recombination-activating genes, transposition, and the lymphoid-specific combinatorial immune system: a common evolutionary connection. *Curr. Top. Microbiol. Immunol.* **248:**111–135.

Haralambieva, I. H., I. D. Iankov, D. P. Petrov, I. V. Miadenov, and I. G. Mitov. 2002. Monoclonal antibody of IgG isotype against a cross-reactive lipopolysaccharide epitope of Chlamydia and Salmonella Re chemotype enhances infectivity in L-929 fibroblast cells. *FEMS Immunol. Med. Microbiol.* **33:**71–76.

Harindranath, N., I. Goldfarb, H. Ikematsu, S. Burastero, R. Wilder, A. Notkins, and P. Casali. 1991. Complete sequence of the genes encoding the VH and VL regions of low- and high-affinity monoclonal IgM and IgA1 rheumatoid factors produced by CD5+ B cells from a rheumatoid arthritis patient. *Int. Immunol.* **3:**865–875.

Harindranath, N., H. Ikematsu, A. L. Notkins, and P. Casali. 1993. Structure of the VH and VL segments of polyreactive and monoreactive human natural antibodies to HIV-1 and *Escherichia coli* β-galactosidase. *Int. Immunol.* **5:**1523–1533.

Harnett, W., and M. Harnett. 1999. Phosphorylcholine: friend or foe of the immune system. *Immunol. Today* **20:**125–129.

Haussler, M. R., G. K. Whitfield, C. A. Haussler, J.-C. Hsieh, P. D. Thompson, S. H. Selznick, D. C. Encinas, and P. W. Jurutka. 1998. The nuclear vitamin D receptor: biological and molecular regulatory properties revealed. *J. Bone Miner. Res.* **13:**325–349.

Hochstenbach, F., C. Parker, J. McLean, V. Gieselmann, H. Band, I. Bank, L. Chess, H.

Spits, J. L. Strominger, J. G. Seidman, et al. 1988. Characterization of a third form of the human T cell receptor gamma/delta. *J. Exp. Med.* **168:**761–776.

Hoek, R. M., A. B. Smit, J. M. Vink, M. de Jong-Brink, and W. P. M. Geraerts. 1996. A new Ig-superfamily member, molluscan defence molecule (MDM) from *Lymnaea stagnalis* is down-regulated during parasitosis. *Eur. J. Immunol.* **26:**939–944.

Hohman, V. S., S. F. Schluter, and J. J. Marchalonis. 1992. Complete sequence of a cDNA clone specifying sandbar shark immunoglobulin light chain: gene organization and implications for the evolution of light chains. *Proc. Natl. Acad. Sci. USA* **89:**276–280.

Hughes, A. L. 1994. Phylogeny of the C3/C4/C5 complement-component gene family indicates that C5 diverged first. *Mol. Biol. Evol.* **11:**417–425.

Hughes, A. L. 1998. Protein phylogenies provide evidence of a radical discontinuity between arthropod and vertebrate immune system. *Immunogenetics* **47:**283–296.

Imler, J., and J. Hoffman. 2002. Toll receptors in Drosophila: a family of molecules regulating development and immunity. *Curr. Top. Microbiol. Immunol.* **270:**63–79.

Ishiguro, H., K. Kobayashi, M. Suzuki, K. Titani, S. Tomonaga, and Y. Kurosawa. 1992. Isolation of a hagfish gene that encodes a complement component. *EMBO J.* **11:**829–837.

Izui, S., R. Eisenberg, and F. Dixon. 1979. IgM rheumatoid factors in mice injected with bacterial lipopolysaccharides. *J. Immunol.* **122:**2096–2102.

Jennings, C. G., S. M. Dyer, and S. J. Burden. 1993. Muscle-specific trk-related receptor with a kringle domain defines a distinct class of receptor tyrosine kinases. *Proc. Natl. Acad. Sci. USA* **90:**2895–2899.

Kabat, E., T. Wu, and H. Perry. 1991. *Sequences of Proteins of Immunological Interest.* NIH Pub. 91-3242. National Institutes of Health, Bethesda, Md.

Kay, M. 1981. Isolation of the phagocytosis-inducating IgG binding antigen on senescent somatic cells. *Nature* **289:**491–494.

Kay, M. M. B., C. Cover, S. F. Schluter, R. M. Bernstein, and J. J. Marchalonis. 1995. Band 3, the anion transporter, is conserved during evolution: implications for aging and vertebrate evolution. *Cell Mol. Biol.* **41:**833–842.

Klein, J. 1998. In an immunological twilight zone. *Proc. Natl. Acad. Sci. USA* **95:**11504–11505.

Kubagawa, H., P. D. Burrows, and M. D. Cooper. 1997. A novel pair of immunoglobulin-like receptors expressed by B cells and myeloid cells. *Proc. Natl. Acad. Sci. USA* **94:**5261–5266.

Kulski, J., T. Shiina, T. Anzai, S. Kohara, and H. Inoko. 2002. Comparative genomic analysis of the MHC: the evolution of class I duplication blocks, diversity and complexity from shark to man. *Immunol. Rev.* **190:**95–122.

Laird, D., A. De Tomaso, M. D. Cooper, and I. Weissman. 2000. 50 million years of chordate evolution: seeking the origins of adaptive immunity. *Proc. Natl. Acad. Sci. USA* **97**:6924–6926.

Lemaitre, B., M. Meister, S. Govind, P. Georgel, R. Steward, J. Reichhart, and J. Hoffman. 1995. Functional analysis and regulation of nuclear import of dorsal during the immune response in Drosophila. *EMBO J.* **14**:536–545.

Lemire, J. 2000. 1,25-Dihydroxyvitamin D hormone with immunomodulatory properties. *Z. Rheumatol.* **59**:24–27.

Levin, J., and F. Bang. 1968. Clottable protein in Limulus: its localization and kinetics of its coagulation by endotoxin. *Thromb. Diath. Haemorrh.* **31**:186–197.

Litman, G. W., M. K. Anderson, and J. P. Rast. 1999. Evolution of antigen binding receptors. *Annu. Rev. Immunol.* **17**:109–147.

Makishima, M., T. T. Lu, W. Xie, G. K. Whitfield, H. Domoto, R. M. Evans, M. R. Haussler, and D. J. Mangelsdorf. 2002. Vitamin D receptor as an intestinal bile acid sensor. *Science* **296**:1313–1316.

Manfruelli, P., J. Reichhart, R. Steward, J. Hoffman, and B. Lemaitre. 1999. A mosaic analysis in Drosophila fat body cells of the control of antimicrobial peptide genes by the Rel proteins Dorsal and DIF. *EMBO J.* **18**:3380–3391.

Marchalonis, J. J. 1974. Antibodies and surface immunoglobulins of immunized congenitally athymic (nu/nu) mice. *Aust. J. Exp. Biol. Med. Sci.* **52**:535–547.

Marchalonis, J. J. 1977. *Immunity in Evolution.* Harvard University Press, Cambridge, Mass.

Marchalonis, J. J., and G. M. Edelman. 1965. Phylogenetic origins of antibody structure. I. Multichain structure of immunoglobulins in the smooth dogfish, *Mustelus canis*. *J. Exp. Med.* **122**:601–618.

Marchalonis, J. J., and G. Edelman. 1968. Isolation and characterization of a natural hemagglutinin from Limulus polyphemus. *J. Mol. Biol.* **32**:453–465.

Marchalonis, J. J., and S. F. Schluter. 1998. A stochastic model for the rapid emergence of specific vertebrate immunity incorporating horizontal transfer of systems enabling duplication and combinatorial diversification. *J. Theor. Biol.* **193**:429–444.

Marchalonis, J. J., S. F. Schluter, R. M. Bernstein, and V. S. Hohman. 1998a. Antibodies of sharks: revolution and evolution. *Immunol. Rev.* **166**:103–122.

Marchalonis, J. J., S. F. Schluter, R. M. Bernstein, and A. B. Edmundson. 1998b. Phylogenetic emergence and molecular evolution of the immunoglobulin family. *Adv. Immunol.* **70**:417–506.

Marchalonis, J. J., M. K. Adelman, B. J. Zeitler, P. M. Sarazin, M. Jaqua, and S. F. Schluter. 2001. Evolutionary factors in the emergence of the combinatorial germline antibody repertoire. *Adv. Exp. Med. Biol.* **484**:13–30.

Marchalonis, J. J., S. V. Kaveri, L. D. Lacroix-Desmazes, and M. D. Kazatchkine. 2002a. Natural recognition repertoire and the evolutionary emergence of the combinatorial immune system. *FASEB J.* **16**:842–848.

Marchalonis, J. J., I. Jensen, and S. F. Schluter. 2002b. Structural, antigenic and evolutionary analyses of immunoglobulins and T cell receptors. *J. Mol. Recognit.* **15**:260–271.

Marchalonis, J. J., G. K. Whitfield, and S. F. Schluter. 2003. Rapid evolutionary emergence of the combinatorial recognition repertoire. *Integrat. Comp. Biol.* **43**:347–359.

Marino, R., Y. Kimura, R. De Santis, J. Lambris, and M. Pinto. 2002. Complement in urochordates: cloning and characterization of two C3-like genes in the ascidian Ciona intestinalis. *Immunogenetics* **53**:1055–1064.

Martin, A., and T. Burg. 2002. Perils of paralogy: using HSP70 genes for inferring organismal phylogenies. *Syst. Biol.* **51**:570–587.

Masiakowski, P., and R. Carroll. 1992. A novel family of cell surface receptors with tyrosine kinase-like domain. *J. Biol. Chem.* **267**:26181–26190.

Mayer, W. E., T. Uinuk-Ool, H. Tichy, L. Gartland, J. Klein, and M. D. Cooper. 2002. Isolation and characterization of lymphocyte like cells from a lamprey. *Proc. Natl. Acad. Sci. USA* **99**:14350–14355.

Means, T., D. Golenbock, and M. Fenton. 2000. Structure and function of Toll-like receptor proteins. *Life Sci.* **68**:241–258.

Medzhitov, R., and C. J. Janeway. 2000. The Toll receptor family and microbial recognition. *Trends Microbiol.* **8**:452–456.

Medzhitov, R., P. Preston-Hurlburt, and C. J. Janeway. 1997. A human homologue of the Drosophila Toll protein signals activation of adaptive immunity. *Nature* **388**:394–397.

Mendoza, H., and I. Faye. 1999. Phsyiological aspects of the immunoglobulin superfamily in invertebrates. *Dev. Comp. Immunol.* **23**:359–374.

Metchnikoff, E. 1905. *Immunity in Infective Diseases.* Cambridge University Press, Cambridge, United Kingdom.

Mold, C., P. Rodic-Polic, and T. Du Clos. 2002. Protection from Streptococcus pneumoniae infection by C-reactive protein and natural antibody requires complement but not Fc gamma receptors. *J. Immunol.* **168**:6375–6381.

Moretta, L., R. Biassoni, C. Bottino, C. Cantoni, D. Pende, M. C. Mingari, and A. Moretta. 2002. Human NK cells and their receptors. *Microbes Infect.* **4**:1539–1544.

Najakshin, A., L. Mechetine, B. Alabyev, and A. Taranin. 1999. Identification of an IL-8 homology in lamprey (Lampetra fluviatilis): early evolutionary divergence of chemokines. *Eur. J. Immunol.* **29**:373–389.

Ochsenbein, A., and R. M. Zinkernagel. 2000. Natural antibodies and complement link innate and acquired immunity. *Immunol. Today* **21**:624–630.

Oettinger, M. A., D. G. Schatz, C. Gorka, and D. Baltimore. 1990. RAG-1 and RAG-2, adjacent genes that synergistically activate V(D)J recombination. *Science* **248**:1517–1523.

Owen, G., and A. Zelent. 2000. Origins and evolutionary diversification of the nuclear receptor superfamily. *Cell. Mol. Life Sci.* **57**:809–827.

Pancer, Z., M. Kruse, H. Schacke, U. Scheffer, R. Steffen, P. Kovacs, and W. E. G. Muller. 1996. Polymorphism in the immunoglobulin-like domains of the receptor tyrosine kinase from the sponge *Geodia cydonium*. *Cell. Adhes. Commun.* **4**:327–339.

Popovici, C., D. Isnardon, D. Birnbaum, and R. Roubin. 2002. Caenorhabditis elegans receptors related to mammalian vascular endothelial growth factor receptors are expressed in neural cells. *Neurosci. Lett.* **329**:116–120.

Ramsland, P., A. Kaushik, J. J. Marchalonis, and A. Edmundson. 2001. On the incorporation of long CDR3s into V domains: implications for the structural evolution of the antibody combining site. *Exp. Clin. Immunogenetics* **18**:179–191.

Rast, J. P., M. K. Anderson, T. Ota, R. T. Litman, M. Margittal, M. J. Shamblott, and G. W. Litman. 1994. Immunoglobulin light chain class multiplicity and alternative organizational forms in early vertebrate phylogeny. *Immunogenetics* **40**:83–99.

Rast, J. P., M. K. Anderson, S. J. Strong, C. Luer, R. T. Litman, and G. W. Litman. 1997. α, β, γ, and δ T cell antigen receptor genes arose early in vertebrate phylogeny. *Immunity* **6**:1–11.

Rehli, M. 2002. Of mice and men: species variations of Toll-like receptor expression. *Trends Immunol.* **23**:375–378.

Reidl, L. S., C. M. Kinoshita, and L. A. Steiner. 1992. Wild mice express an Ig Vλ gene that differs from any Vλ in Balb/c but resembles a human Vλ subgroup. *J. Immunol.* **149**:471–480.

Reidling, J., M. A. Miller, and R. E. Stelle. 2000. Sweet Tooth, a novel receptor protein-tyrosine kinase with C-type lectin-like extracellular domains. *J. Biol. Chem.* **275**:10323–10330.

Richards, M. H., and J. L. Nelson. 2000. The evolution of vertebrate antigen receptors: a phylogenetic approach. *Mol. Biol. Evol.* **17**:146–155.

Rinkevich, B., I. Weissman, and A. DeTomaso. 1998. Transplantation of Fu-HC incompatible zooids in Botryllus schlosseri results in chimerism. *Biol. Bull.* **195**:98–106.

Robey, F. A., and T. Y. Liu. 1981. Limulin: a C-reactive protein from *Limulus polyphemus*. *J. Biol. Chem.* **256**:969–974.

Robey, F. A., T. Tanaka, and T. Y. Liu. 1983. Isolation and characterization of two major serum proteins from the dogfish, Mustelus canis, C-reactive protein and amyloid P component. *J. Biol. Chem.* **258**:3889–3894.

Robey, I. F., S. F. Schluter, D. E. Yocum, and J. J. Marchalonis. 2000. Production and characterization of monoclonal IgM autoantibodies specific for the T cell receptor. *J. Protein Chem.* **19**:9–21.

Robey, I. F., A. B. Edmundson, S. F. Schluter, D. E. Yocum, and J. J. Marchalonis. 2002. Specificity mapping of human anti-T cell receptor monoclonal natural antibodies: defining the properties of epitope recognition promiscuity. *FASEB J.* **16**:1642–1652.

Rock, F., G. T. Hardiman, J. C. Timons, R. Kastelein, and J. Bazan. 1998. A family of human receptors structurally related to Drosophila Toll. *Proc. Natl. Acad. Sci. USA* **95**:588–593.

Rodman, T. C., J. D. Lutton, S. Jiang, H. B. Al-Kouatly, and R. Winston. 2001. Circulating natural IgM antibodies and their corresponding human cord blood cell-derived Mabs specifically combat the Tat protein of HIV. *Exp. Hematol.* **29**:1004–1009.

Rutschmann, S., A. Jung, C. Hetru, J. Reichhart, J. Hoffman, and D. Ferrandon. 2000. The Rel protein DIF mediates the antifungal but not the antibacterial host defense in Drosophila. *Immunity* **12**:569–580.

Saito, Y., E. Hirose, and H. Watanabe. 1994. Allorecognition in compound ascidians. *Int. J. Dev. Biol.* **38**:237–247.

Schacke, H., B. Rinkevich, V. Gamulin, I. M. Muller, and W. E. G. Muller. 1994. Immunoglobulin-like domain is present in the extracellular part of the receptor tyrosine kinase from the marine sponge *Geodia cydonium*. *J. Mol. Recognit.* **7**:273–276.

Schatz, D., M. Oettinger, and D. Baltimore. 1989. The V(D)J recombination activating gene, RAG-1. *Cell* **59**:1035–1048.

Schluter, S. F., and J. J. Marchalonis. 1986. Antibodies to synthetic joining segment peptide of the T-cell receptor β chain: serological cross-reaction between products of T-cell receptor genes, antigen binding T-cell receptors and immunoglobulins. *Proc. Natl. Acad. Sci. USA* **83**:1872–1876.

Schluter, S. F., and J. J. Marchalonis. 2003. Cloning of shark RAG2 and characterization of the RAG1/RAG2 locus. *FASEB J.* **17**:470–472.

Schluter, S. F., C. J. Beischel, S. A. Martin, and J. J. Marchalonis. 1989. Sequence analysis of homogeneous peptides of shark immunoglobulin light chains by tandem mass spectrometry: correlation with gene sequence and homologies among variable and constant region peptides of sharks and mammals. *Mol. Immunol.* **27**:17–23.

Schluter, S. F., R. M. Bernstein, and J. J. Marchalonis. 1997. Molecular origins and evolution of immunoglobulin heavy-chain genes of jawed vertebrates. *Immunol. Today* **18**:543–549.

Schluter, S. F., R. M. Bernstein, H. Bernstein, and J. J. Marchalonis. 1999. "Big Bang" emergence of the combinatorial immune system. *Dev. Comp. Immunol.* **23**:107–111.

Sekine, H., A. Kenjo, K. Azumi, G. Ohi, M. Takahashi, R. Kasukawa, N. Ichikawa, M. Nakata, T. Mizuochi, M. Matsushit, Y. Endo, and T. Fujita. 2001. An ancient lectin-dependent complement system in an ascidian: novel lectin isolated from the plasma of the solitary asicidian, *Halocynthia roretzi*. *J. Immunol.* **167**:4504–4510.

Shaw, P. X., S. Horkko, M. K. Chang, L. K. Curtiss, W. Palinski, G. J. Silverman, and J. L. Witztum. 2000. Natural antibodies with the T15 idiotype may act in atherosclerosis, apoptotic clearance, and protective immunity. *J. Clin. Invest.* **105**: 1731–1740.

Shen, S. X., R. M. Bernstein, S. F. Schluter, and J. J. Marchalonis. 1996. Heavy-chain variable regions in carcharhine sharks: development of a comprehensive model for the evolution of VH domains among the gnathanstomes. *Immunol. Cell Biol.* **74**:357–364.

Sims, J. E., T. Z. Armel, D. P. Carrington, C. J. McMahan, J. M. Wignall, C. J. March, and S. K. Dower. 1989. Cloning the interleukin 1 receptor from human T cells. *Proc. Natl. Acad. Sci. USA* **86**:8946–8950.

Smith, D. K., and H. Xue. 1997. Sequence profiles of immunoglobulin and immunoglobulin-like domains. *J. Mol. Biol.* **274**:530–545.

Smith, L. C. 2002. Thioester function is conserved in SpC3, the sea urchin homologue of the complement component C3. *Dev. Comp. Immunol.* **26**:603–614.

Smith, L. C., C. S. Shih, and S. G. Dachenhausen. 1998. Coelomocytes express SpBf, a homologue of factor B, the second component in the sea urchin complement system. *J. Immunol.* **1616**:6784–6789.

Smith, S. 1998. Shark complement: an assessment. *Immunol. Rev.* **166**:67–78.

Spruyt, N., C. Delarbre, G. Gachelin, and V. Laudet. 1998. Complete sequence of the amphioxus (Branchiostoma lanceolatum) mitochondrial genome: relations to vertebrates. *Nucleic Acids Res.* **26**:3279–3285.

Staskawicz, B., M. B. Mudgett, J. Dangl, and J. Galan. 2001. Common and contrasting themes of plant and animal diseases. *Science* **292**:2285–2289.

Stein, L., P. Sternberg, R. Durbin, J. Thierry-Mieg, and J. Spieth. 2001. WormBase network access to the genome and biology of Caenorhabditis elegans. *Nucleic Acids Res.* **29**:82–86.

Su, X. D., L. N. Gastinel, D. E. Vaughn, I. Faye, P. Poon, and P. J. Bjorkman. 1998. Crystal structure of hemolin: a horseshoe shape with implications for homophilic adhesion. *Science* **281**:991–995.

Sun, S. C., I. Lindstrom, H. G. Boman, I. Faye, and O. Schmidt. 1990. Hemolin: an insect-immune protein belonging to the immunoglobulin superfamily. *Science* **250**:1729–1731.

Sunyer, J. O., and J. D. Lambris. 1998. Evolution and diversity of the complement system of poikilothermic vertebrates. *Immunol. Rev.* **166**:39–57.

Teichmann, S. A., and C. Chothia. 2000. Immunoglobulin superfamily proteins in *Caenorhabditis elegans*. *J. Mol. Biol.* **296**:1367–1383.

Tharia, H., A. Shrive, J. Mills, C. Arme, G. Williams, and T. Greenhough. 2002. Complete cDNA sequence of SAP-like pentraxin from Limulus polyphemus: implications for pentraxin evolution. *J. Mol. Biol.* **316**:583–597.

Tsuji, S., J. Uehori, M. Matsoumoto, Y. Suzuki, A. Matsuhisa, K. Toyoshima, and T. Seya. 2001. Human intelectin is a novel soluble lectin that recognizes galactofuranose in carbohydrate chains of bacterial cell wall. *J. Biol. Chem.* **276**:23456–23463.

Uinuk-Ool, T., W. E. Mayer, A. Sato, R. Dongak, M. D. Cooper, and J. Klein. 2002. Lamprey lymphocyte-like cells express homologs of genes involved in immunologically relevant activities of mammalian lymphocytes. *Proc. Natl. Acad. Sci. USA* **99**:14356–14361.

Valentine, J., D. Jablonski, and D. Erwin. 1999. Fossils, molecules and embryos: new perspectives on the Cambrian explosion. *Development* **126**:851–859.

Vasta, G. R., J. J. Marchalonis, and H. Kohler. 1984. Invertebrate recognition protein cross-reacts with an immunoglobulin idiotype. *J. Exp. Med.* **159**:1270–1276.

Venkatech, B., M. V. Erdmann, and S. Brenner. 2001. Molecular synapomorphies resolve evolutionary relationships of extant jawed vertebrates. *Proc. Natl. Acad. Sci. USA* **98**:11382–11387.

Warr, G., J. Decker, T. Mandel, D. DeLuca, R. Hudson, and J. J. Marchalonis. 1977. Lymphocyte-like cells of the tunicate, Pyura stolonifera: binding of lectins, morphological and functional studies. *Aust. J. Exp. Biol. Med. Sci.* **55**:151–164.

Whitfield, G. K., H. T. L. Dang, S. F. Schluter, R. M. Bernstein, T. Bunag, L. A. Manzon, G. Hsieh, C. Encinas-Dominguez, J. H. Youson, M. R. Haussler, and J. J. Marchalonis. 2003. Cloning of a functional Vitamin D receptor from the lamprey Petromyson marinus, an ancient vertebrate lacking calcified bones or teeth. *Endocrinology* **144**:2714–2716.

Williams, A. F., and A. N. Barclay. 1988. The immunoglobulin superfamily—domains for cell surface recognition. *Annu. Rev. Immunol.* **6**:381–405.

Yacine, M., Y. Amrani, M. Xavier, P. Cazenave, and S. Adrien. 2002. The Ig light chain restricted B6.kappa-lambda SEG mouse strain suggests that the IGL locus genomic organization is subject to constant evolution. *Immunogenetics* **54**:106–119.

Yanagi, Y., Y. Yoshikai, K. Leggett, S. P. Clark, I. Aleksander, and T. W. Mak. 1984. A human T cell-specific cDNA clone encodes a protein having extensive homology to immunoglobulin chains. *Nature* **308:**145–149.

Ying, S., J. Marchalonis, A. Gewurz, J. Siegel, H. Jiang, and H. Gewutz. 1992. Reactivity of anti-human C reactive protein (CRP) and serum amyloid P component (SAP) monoclonal antibodies with limulin and pentraxins of other species. *Immunology* **76:**324–330.

Yoder, J. A., M. G. Mueller, S. Wei, B. C. Corliss, D. M. Prather, T. Willis, R. T. Litman, J. V. Djeu, and G. W. Litman. 2001. Immune type receptor genes in zebrafish share genetic and functional properties with genes encoded by the mammalian leukocyte receptor cluster. *Proc. Natl. Acad. Sci. USA* **98:**6771–6776.

Yu, X. Q., and M. R. Kanost. 2002. Binding of hemolin to bacterial lipopolysaccharide and lipoteichoic acid. An immunoglobulin superfamily member from insects as a pattern recognition receptor. *Eur. J. Biochem.* **269:**1827–1834.

Zapata, A., C. Ardavin, R. Gomariz, and J. Leceta. 1981. Plasma cells in the ammocoete of Petromyzon marinus. *Cell Tissue Res.* **221:**203–208.

DROSOPHILA RESPONSES TO MICROBIAL INFECTION: AN OVERVIEW

Jules A. Hoffmann and Petros Ligoxygakis

2

Insect immunity started as a field of research more than a century ago, when Cuénot in Nancy, France (Cuénot, 1891), and Kowalevsky in St. Petersburg, Russia (Kowalevsky, 1892), analyzed the role of blood cells and phagocytic tissues in clearance of invading bacteria from the hemolymph (the insect analogue of mammalian blood). Serious impetus was given to the field in the 1920s by Metalnikow at the Pasteur Institute in Paris (Metalnikow, 1920) and by Paillot in Lyon, France (Paillot, 1921). The independent studies of the Pasteur group (which included Chorine, Toumanoff, and Zernoff, who had emigrated to Paris with Metalnikow) and of Paillot conclusively established that the injection of attenuated bacteria into lepidopteran larvae conferred protection against subsequent injections of normally lethal doses. These results were in agreement with a report by Glaser, published 2 years earlier (Glaser, 1918), stating that blood from grasshoppers presented antibacterial activity following injection of bacterial cultures. The studies of Metalnikow and Paillot extended over more than a decade and ended in 1933 in two partly contradictory reviews. Metalnikow insisted that the antibacterial defense of lepidopteran larvae was mainly sustained by cellular reactions (phagocytosis, giant cell formation, encapsulation) and, to a lesser extent, involved the secretion of bacteriolytic substances (Metalnikow, 1929). In contrast, Paillot emphasized the role of humoral soluble factors produced by the cells participating in the immune reaction (Paillot, 1933).

Almost half a century later these antimicrobial factors were indeed identified through the pioneering work of Hans Boman and associates in Stockholm (Steiner et al., 1981). During the early 1980s, these researchers isolated two families of novel antibacterial peptides, which they named cecropins and attacins, from immunized pupae of the attacid moth *Hyalophora cecropia*. The studies on antimicrobial peptide identification were rapidly extended to other insect species and eventually to *Drosophila*. During the past decade, the ease of genetic analysis has made the fruit fly an organism of choice for the study of innate host defense. In this chapter we concentrate on recent developments in this field of study.

Jules A. Hoffmann, Réponse Immunitaire et Développement chez les Insectes, Institut de Biologie Moléculaire et Cellulaire UPR9022 CNRS, 15 rue René Descartes 67084, Strasbourg, France. *Petros Ligoxygakis,* Genetics Unit, Department of Biochemistry, University of Oxford, South Parks Road, Oxford OX1 3QU, United Kingdom.

The Innate Immune Response to Infection
Ed. by S. H. E. Kaufmann, R. Medzhitov, and S. Gordon
©2004 ASM Press, Washington, D.C.

A GENERAL VIEW OF *DROSOPHILA* IMMUNE DEFENSES

Drosophila, like all insects, is very resistant to microbial infections, mounting a multifaceted reaction against invading non-self. Barrier epithelia serve as a first-line obstruction against microorganism entry. Epidermal surfaces such as the digestive and genital tracts, the trachea, and the Malpighian tubules all produce antimicrobial peptides that inhibit microbial growth (Ferrandon et al., 1998; Tzou et al., 2000). Those microorganisms invading the general body cavity (called the hemocoele; *Drosophila* lacks an organized blood vessel system) are countered by both humoral and cellular reactions. The humoral reactions involve the almost immediate induction of proteolytic cascades, which lead to localized melanization and blood coagulation (Ashida and Brey, 1995) and to the rapid synthesis of antimicrobial peptides by the fat body, the functional equivalent of the mammalian liver (Bulet et al., 1999; Hoffmann and Reichhart, 2002). The cellular reactions are mediated by *Drosophila* blood cells (hemocytes) and are best illustrated by phagocytosis or by capsule formation (in the case of larger invading microorganisms) (Lanot et al., 2001).

CELLULAR IMMUNITY

Drosophila blood cells (hemocytes) play a significant role in host defense. However, the molecular mechanisms underlying their function remain largely unknown. Three mature hemocyte types are found in circulation: plasmatocytes, crystal cells, and lamellocytes (for a review, see Rizki, 1984).

Plasmatocytes

Plasmatocytes exhibit strong phagocytic activity against microorganisms. At the onset of metamorphosis, they further differentiate into active macrophagelike cells and participate in tissue remodeling by ingesting apoptotic cells. The plasmatocyte lineage is comparable, both in terms of ultrastructure and of function, to the mammalian monocyte or macrophage lineage (Rizki, 1984). Plasmatocytes are present at all stages of development in *Drosophila* and represent the vast majority of the blood cells (>95%).

Phagocytosis involves the initial recognition of non-self by the binding of specific receptors in blood cells to target molecular structures. Recognition is followed by the eventual actin-dependent engulfment of phagocytosed material in phagosomes, where it is cleared by lysosomal enzymes, reactive oxygen species, and nitric oxide. To date, two recognition receptors have been identified through their abilities to mediate phagocytosis in *Drosophila* macrophagelike S2 cells, which express phagocytic properties similar to those of mammalian cells. The two *Drosophila* genes identified by this approach are those encoding the peptidoglycan recognition protein LC (PGRP-LC) and the *Drosophila* scavenger receptor class I (dSR-CI) (Ramet et al., 2001, 2002). Another way for blood cells to fight off invading microbes is to bind to molecules that have been deposited by the host on the invading microorganism, a process called opsonization. The *Drosophila* genome contains four candidate genes for such a function, which encode proteins significantly similar to the thiolester proteins of the complement $C3/\alpha_2$ macroglobulin superfamily (Lagueux et al., 2000). The *Anopheles* homologue of these was shown to serve as a complementlike opsonin and to promote phagocytosis of gram-negative bacteria (Levashina et al., 2001).

Crystal Cells

Crystal cells were initially identified for their large cytoplasmic crystalline inclusions (Rizki, 1984). The crystals were proposed to correspond to the enzymes and substrates responsible for humoral melanization (Rizki et al., 1980). They contain at least the precursor of the key enzyme in this process, namely, prophenoloxidase. It has been recently shown that the Notch signaling pathway plays an instructive role in the differentiation of crystal cells. *Notch* loss-of-function mutations result in decreased numbers of crystal cells. Conversely, overexpression of *Notch* provokes an overproliferation of crystal cells (Duvic et al., 2002).

Lamellocytes

The third hemocyte type is only occasionally encountered in healthy animals and is called the lamellocyte (Lanot et al., 2001; Rizki, 1984). Lamellocytes differentiate following infection of *Drosophila* larvae by parasitic wasps (Carton and Nappi, 1997). Because wasp eggs are too large to be phagocytosed, lamellocytes wrap around the invader to form a capsule. Encapsulation is accompanied by melanization, killing the parasite presumably by asphyxiation or through the local production of cytotoxic intermediates during melanin synthesis. Lamellocytes are large flat cells, with few cytoplasmic organelles, and have never been observed at the embryonic and adult stages. As in crystal cells, *Notch* plays a role in the proliferation of lamellocytes following parasitization. In contrast to the case of crystal cells, however, forced expression of *Notch* does not result in lamellocyte overproduction (Duvic et al., 2002).

PROTEOLYTIC CASCADES LEADING TO HEMOLYMPH-BORNE MELANIZATION

With an open circulatory system, invertebrates must have immediate defense reactions to entrap intruders and coagulation mechanisms to prevent plasma loss upon wounding. Infection-dependent melanization is the most immediate response following microbial challenge or septic injury and requires the activation of phenoloxidase (PO), which is an oxidoreductase that catalyzes the conversion of phenols to quinones. The quinones can be directly toxic to bacteria, fungi, and eucaryotic parasites and can also polymerize nonenzymatically to form melanotic capsules that surround parasites (Pye, 1974; Nappi et al., 1995; Nappi and Ottaviani, 2000). PO is present in the hemolymph as an inactive precursor, prophenoloxidase, that must be proteolytically activated by a serine protease.

This protease, which is the terminal component of a proteolytic cascade, has been identified in several insect species and has been called a prophenoloxidase-activating enzyme (PPAE) (Ashida and Brey, 1995; Chosa et al., 1997; Jiang et al., 1998).

Biochemical studies in crustaceans by Söderhäll and coworkers (for a review, see Söderhäll and Cerenius, 1998) and in the silkworm *Bombyx mori* by Ashida and collaborators (for a review, see Ashida and Brey, 1997) have established that this protease cascade can be initiated upon recognition of non-self molecular patterns such as β-1,3-glucans, peptidoglycans, lipopolysaccharides (LPSs), or aberrant tissue. Proteins that are able to bind such carbohydrates have been isolated from both insects and crustaceans. In these species the presence of serine protease inhibitors regulates this process by preventing excessive activation. Moreover, activated PO shows a tendency to form aggregates, which allows a tight control of the reaction's localization. This is essential, as a number of intermediate compounds during melanin synthesis are cytotoxic.

Recently, the identification of the blood serine protease inhibitor Spn27A provided genetic evidence toward the introduction of melanization into the larger picture of host defense regulation in *Drosophila* (De Gregorio et al., 2002a; Ligoxygakis et al., 2002a). Absence of this serpin in the hemolymph leads to a high rate of spontaneous melanization both in larvae and in adults and a constitutively elevated PO activity. In wild-type adult flies, Spn27A is depleted from the hemolymph during the melanization process (Ligoxygakis et al., 2002a). Moreover, a major player in the control of antimicrobial peptide gene expression, the Toll pathway, regulates this infection-dependent depletion. In Toll pathway mutants, serpin depletion and PO activation are blocked. Elimination of the serpin during melanization is most probably dependent on a protease. Infection-dependent secretion of this protease or of the factor that triggers its activation in the hemolymph is in need of NF-κB-mediated transcription and requires de novo protein synthesis (Ligoxygakis et al., 2002a).

Generally, serpins employ a suicide substrate strategy to interact with their cognate proteases. This interaction is largely directed by an exposed carboxyl-terminal reactive center loop which binds to the active site of the target protease, resulting in covalent linkage with the substrate. Sequence comparison of the reactive center loop of Spn27A with the PO cleavage site implies the same serine protease as the target, presumably a PPAE (Ligoxygakis et al., 2002a). Moreover, it has been biochemically shown that Spn27A interacts with the PPAEs of other insect species and that insect serpins highly homologous to Spn27A inhibit their respective PPAEs (De Gregorio et al., 2002a). Genome-wide studies have revealed that there are three to four PPAE candidate genes in the *Drosophila* genome, whose transcription is upregulated following septic injury (De Gregorio et al., 2001; Irving et al., 2001). Identification of this serpin's target protease in *Drosophila* is now one of the priorities because it will provide valuable insight into the activation of the melanization reaction and suggest ways of genetically manipulating the process. The significance of such information is underlined by the importance of melanization in insects such as the mosquito *Anopheles gambiae*, a vector of the most deadly malaria parasite *Plasmodium falciparum*. Genetically selected strains of this mosquito, refractory to malarial parasite development, were shown to encapsulate certain malarial parasites within a melanin sheath during their passage through the midgut, exhibiting in essence constitutive melanization that arrests invasion and leads to ultimate killing of the parasite (Christophides et al., 2002). Interestingly, there are three serpins that are highly homologous to Spn27A in the *Anopheles* genome (Christophides et al., 2002).

HUMORAL IMMUNITY

Inducible AMPs

The hallmark of the humoral response is the infection-induced synthesis in the fat body cells of several different families of potent antimi-

crobial peptides (AMPs) (Fig. 1). Seven of these families of AMPs have been characterized molecularly and/or biochemically (Bulet et al., 1999; Hoffmann and Reichhart, 2002). AMPs are secreted into the hemolymph, where their combined concentrations can reach over 300 μM in infected flies.

Analysis of the role of each AMP gene family in vivo is problematic because of the numerous AMPs present in the *Drosophila* genome as well as their presumed functional redundancy. Their importance, however, is underlined by the very low survival rates of flies which fail to express certain AMPs during an infection. In a recent study, overexpression of a particular AMP gene or a combination of AMPs was able to rescue this phenotype (Tzou et al., 2002). Although this result is suggestive of the contribution of AMPs to the systemic host defense, it must be noted that the concentrations achieved with the expression system used were probably far higher than the physiological ones.

The nature of the invading microorganism dictates, to some extent, which type of AMP will be produced (Bulet et al., 1999; Hoffmann and Reichhart, 2002). This specificity is best illustrated by the induction of *drosomycin* and *metchnikowin* following fungal or gram-positive bacterial infection. In contrast, gram-negative bacteria preferentially induce the expression of *diptericin*, *attacin*, *cecropin*, and *drocosin*. The discovery of distinct antimicrobial responses to different classes of microorganisms led to the hypothesis that different pathways regulate AMP gene expression.

Signaling Pathways Controlling Humoral Immune Defenses

In the early 1990s it was shown that the promoters of the AMP genes contained sequence motifs related to mammalian NF-κB response elements (Engstrom et al., 1993; Kappler et al., 1993; Meister et al., 1994). Experiments in transgenic flies established that these motifs are mandatory for inducibility following infection (Meister et al., 1994). At that time, studies on the dorsoventral axis formation in *Drosophila* early embryogenesis had established the signif-

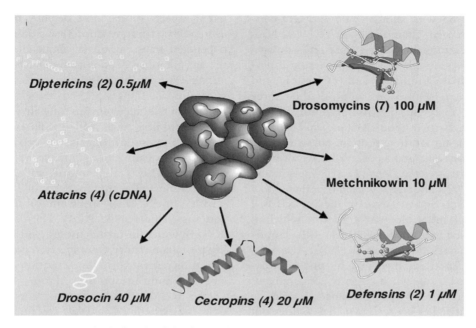

FIGURE 1 The hallmark of the humoral response is the synthesis and secretion into the hemolymph of several potent AMPs by fat body cells. Seven of these families of small cationic peptides have been biochemically and molecularly characterized and are presented here. The gene copy numbers are shown in parentheses followed by the maximum concentration that each peptide can reach after infection. Their main biological activities in physiological concentrations are anti-gram-negative for Diptericins, Attacins, Cecropins, and Drosocin; anti-gram-positive for Defensins; and antifungal for Drosomycins and Metchnikowin.

icant similarity between the Toll pathway-dependent nuclear translocation of the NF-κB–related transcription factor Dorsal and the activation of NF-κB in mammalian cells after immune challenge (for a review, see Belvin and Anderson, 1996). This analogy suggested a role for the Toll pathway in the immune induction of AMP genes and prompted a genetic analysis of Toll pathway mutants.

It was subsequently shown that induction of the antifungal peptide Drosomycin as well as resistance to fungal infections required an intact Toll receptor and several members of the pathway (Lemaitre et al., 1996). Parallel studies defined a locus coding for a then unknown gene referred to as *imd* (immune deficiency) as being essential for the induction of antibacterial AMPs and resistance to gram-negative sepsis (Lemaitre et al., 1995). These data therefore indicated that Toll and Imd were the two immune signaling pathways regulating the sys-

temic humoral defense in *Drosophila* and set the stage for further genetic analysis of the signal transduction events during a microbial infection.

The Toll Pathway and Resistance to Fungal or Gram-Positive Bacterial Infections. Toll is a transmembrane receptor with an extracellular domain containing leucine-rich repeats and an intracellular region showing considerable similarities with the corresponding part of the interleukin-1 receptor. The latter is generally referred to as the TIR (Toll–interleukin-1 receptor) domain (Imler and Hoffmann, 2001). Upon fungal or gram-positive bacterial infection, Toll recruits via its TIR region, the *Drosophila* homologue of myeloid differentiation marker 88, which in addition to its TIR domain contains a death domain (DD) (Tauszig-Delamasure et al., 2002; Horng and Medzhitov, 2001). Interaction between

DmMyD88 with another TIR and DD-containing protein Tube (Letsou et al., 1991) leads to the recruitment of yet a third DD-containing molecule with an additional serine-threonine kinase domain, Pelle (Shelton and Wasserman, 1993). Along with Toll, these three proteins represent the Toll receptor–adaptor complex formed upon signaling, and mutants altered in any of these proteins fail to respond to a fungal or a gram-positive bacterial infection (Lemaitre et al., 1996; Tauszig-Delamasure et al., 2002). The signal is then transduced to a latent transcription factor of the NF-κB Rel family of inducible transactivators, which is complexed with the *Drosophila* IκB homologue, Cactus (Geisler et al., 1992). Dissociation of Cactus is mediated by phosphorylation. The kinase, which targets Cactus, remains unknown. An obvious candidate would be Pelle, but it has been shown that it does not phosphorylate Cactus directly (Shen and Manley, 1998). The substrate of the Pelle kinase is still unidentified. Cactus is targeted for degradation, and the Rel protein is free to translocate to the nucleus and activate target genes. The *Drosophila* genome encodes three Rel proteins, each of which contains a DNA-binding domain and a Rel dimerization region. These proteins are Dorsal, which mediates Toll signaling during dorsoventral axis formation (Steward, 1987), Dorsal-related immunity factor (DIF) (Ip et al., 1993), and Relish (Dushay et al., 1996) (see Imd Pathway and Resistance to Gram-Negative Bacterial Infections, below). DIF is the major mediator of Toll signaling during fungal or gram-positive bacterial infections in adults (Rutschmann et al., 2000a). Dorsal is able to substitute for DIF in larvae, whereas DIF is able to rescue embryos lacking Dorsal (Manfruelli et al., 1999; Stein et al., 1998). Genome-wide analyses of *Drosophila* immune responses indicate that DIF activates a large number of genes at various time points (De Gregorio et al., 2002b; Boutros et al., 2002). Following septic injury, DIF translocates to the nucleus in 20 min (our unpublished observations). We assume that there are distinct waves of transcription concerning different aspects of the host defense, from the acute melanization reaction that requires DIF-dependent transcription (at about 40 min) to the antimicrobial peptide genes *drosomycin* and *metchnikowin* (at about 180 min) to a variety of late-induced transcriptional targets whose functional relevance remains to be investigated.

The finding that Toll mediates innate immune responses in flies stimulated research efforts investigating the existence of Toll-like receptors (TLRs) in mammals and humans. This culminated in the discovery of 10 TLRs, which sense a large spectrum of microbial patterns (Akira et al., 2001). They signal to NF-κB, which in turn activates genes encoding proinflammatory cytokines and costimulatory molecules involved in activation of adaptive immune responses. From the fly perspective, one of the key questions at that point was whether *Drosophila* Toll functions as a pattern recognition receptor (PRR) like its mammalian counterparts or is activated by the cytokinelike cysteine knot polypeptide Spaetzle (Spz) similarly to the embryonic system (Mizuguchi et al., 1998). During embryonic patterning, Spz is proteolytically cleaved by the sequential activation of three serine proteases required in the germ line, Gastrulation defective, Snake, and Easter (LeMosy et al., 1999). However, in null mutants of these proteases, challenge-induced activation of the Toll pathway is not affected, as illustrated by wild-type induction of the antifungal peptide Drosomycin (Lemaitre et al., 1996). Part of the answer came from mutations in the blood serine protease inhibitor (serpin), Spn43Ac. These mutations, initially isolated by Pascal Heitzler and coworkers, were called *necrotic* (*nec*) due to their lethal phenotype in early adulthood (Heitzler et al., 1993). Further studies showed that in *nec* mutants Spz is predominantly presented as a cleaved form and Drosomycin is constitutively expressed (Levashina et al., 1999). These results indicated that Toll activation is dependent on Spz, which is cleaved by a serpin-controlled proteolytic cascade. In conclusion, *Drosophila* Toll does not interact directly with microbial patterns, but Spz acts as its ligand, similarly to embryonic development. The Toll signaling pathway is summarized in Fig. 2.

The *nec* mutant phenotype is suppressed in a Spz or Toll loss-of-function background. This result gave the proof of concept for a genetic screen for suppressors of *nec*, the assumption being that a mutation in the target protease would suppress constitutive activation of the Toll pathway. Persephone (Psh), the first serine protease, which triggers Toll signaling following immune challenge, was isolated (Ligoxygakis et al., 2002b). When challenged with fungi, *psh* mutants exhibit a severely reduced level of *drosomycin* transcription compared with wild-type flies. Moreover, these flies are highly susceptible to fungal infections, behaving in this respect as Toll pathway mutants. Interestingly, *psh* flies showed a wild-type pattern of

survival and wild-type levels of *drosomycin* induction after immune challenge by gram-positive bacteria. These data pointed to distinct proteases or proteolytic cascades, which activate the Toll pathway following fungal versus gram-positive bacterial infection (Fig. 2).

In addition to Toll, the *Drosophila* genome contains eight related genes encoding transmembrane receptors (Tauszig et al., 2000). Their diverse and dynamic patterns of expression during embryogenesis suggest roles in development (Kambris et al., 2002), while their leucine-rich repeats could mediate homophilic interactions in adhesion-based signaling as documented for Toll and 18Wheeler (Keith and Gay, 1990; Eldon et al., 1994). Finally, it is relevant to note that the adaptor protein DmMyD88 interacts specifically with Toll but does not bind most of the other members of

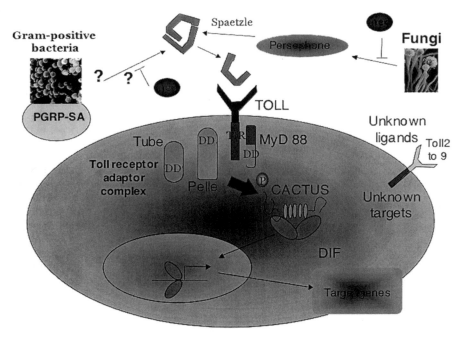

FIGURE 2 Present view of Toll-dependent induction of immune genes following fungal or gram-positive bacterial infection. One of the sensors of gram-positive infection is a circulating recognition protein, PGRP-SA. The recognition receptor(s) for fungi is not yet known. Conversely, it is not clear how PGRP-SA signals to Spz and whether *nec* plays a role in inhibiting activation of the proteolytic cascade triggered by gram-positive bacteria as in the one for fungi. Finally, the signaling pathways and the ligands of other *Drosophila* Tolls remain to be identified.

the family (Tauszig-Delamasure et al., 2002), which in turn are not able to activate *drosomycin* in a cell culture assay (Tauszig et al., 2000). These results lead us to question whether, in addition to Toll, the other eight Tolls are involved at all in the *Drosophila* host defense.

In the context of the valuable cross talk between the studies on the *Drosophila* host defense and on mammalian innate immunity, it is relevant that we realize that we may not fully equate Toll signaling with that of the TLRs. The data available for *Drosophila* indicate that Toll is not activated by direct interaction with microbial ligands, but rather more responds to the cleavage product of the cytokine Spz. Cleavage of Spz in turn depends on a proteolytic amplification cascade, which is triggered when upstream proteins interact with microbial patterns in the hemolymph (or in the extracellular matrix). Discrimination of infectious organisms that activate Toll (i.e.,

fungal and gram-positive bacterial infections) occurs at this upstream level (see below). This is in stark contrast with the situation described for the TLR family, whose members appear to directly interact with and discriminate between distinct microbial patterns.

Imd Pathway and Resistance to Gram-Negative Bacterial Infections. The Imd pathway governs defenses against gram-negative bacteria by controlling the induction of a number of genes, including most of those encoding the antibacterial peptides (Fig. 3). Induction of these AMP genes is mediated by the NF-kB-like protein Relish, which like the mammalian NF-kB compound proteins p100 and p105, is composed of a DNA-binding Rel homology domain and an inhibitory ankyrin repeat region (Stoven et al., 2000). Activation of Relish requires a signal-induced endoproteolytic cleavage, which frees the Rel transactivating region from the inhibitory domain,

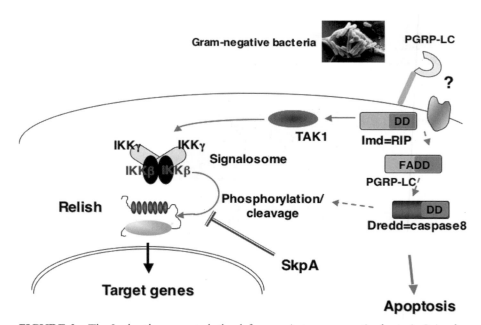

FIGURE 3 The Imd pathway controls the defense against gram-negative bacteria. It is relevant here to note that the receptor is still unknown. The putative transmembrane PGRP-LC does not qualify as one but rather is more of a part of an extensive receptor–adaptor complex (see also text).

allowing the nuclear translocation of the Rel homology domain. Relish cleavage generates a cytoplasmic Cactus-like carboxyl-terminal peptide. The Imd pathway controls Relish activation, rendering flies highly susceptible to gram-negative bacterial infections (Dushay et al., 1996; Stoven et al., 2000). By using genetic screens for mutations with similar phenotypes, considerable progress has been made in recent years toward the understanding of events that link Relish phosphorylation and cleavage to gram-negative bacterial infection.

It is now understood that the Imd pathway shares similarities with the tumor necrosis factor receptor-1 pathway in mammals (for a review, see Locksley et al., 2001). *imd* encodes a protein with significant sequence identity to the DD kinase of mammalian receptor interacting protein, which interacts with tumor necrosis factor receptor-1 (Georgel et al., 2001). In mammals, the receptor interacting protein plays a role both in NF-κB activation and apoptosis (Locksley et al., 2001). The *Drosophila* Fas-associated DD (dFADD)–containing protein acts downstream of *imd*; the two proteins interact through their DDs (Naitza et al., 2002). FADD possibly links Imd to the caspase-8 homologue DREDD (Leulier et al., 2000), which may be required for the cleavage of Relish (Stoven et al., 2000). This hypothesis is derived from the presence of a potential cleavage site in the Relish linker domain, suggesting processing by a caspase protease, and from the fact that in *dredd* mutants Relish is no longer cleaved (Stoven et al., 2000). The current hypothesis is that Imd, dFADD, and DREDD constitute a part of an extensive receptor–adaptor complex, which detects gram-negative infection. Mutants with alterations in any of these genes fail to induce Diptericin when challenged with gram-negative bacteria and are highly prone to this kind of infection. Cleavage of Relish is proteasome independent but requires the *Drosophila* equivalent of the IKK signalosome. This is composed of two proteins with structural similarities to mammalian IKKγ and IKKβ, encoded by the genes *kenny* and *immune response deficient*

5 (*ird5*), respectively (Rutschmann et al., 2000b; Lu et al., 2001). Mutants altered in both of these components are sensitive to gram-negative bacterial infection but resist gram-positive or fungal infections like wild-type flies. Studies with cell cultures further showed that the *Drosophila* signalosome equivalent is activated in response to LPSs and that this activation results in phosphorylation and cleavage of Relish (Silverman et al., 2000). It has been proposed that the gene *dTAK1* (transforming growth factor-β activating kinase 1), encoding a mitogen-activated protein 3 kinase with homology to mammalian *TAK1*, directly activates the fly IKK signalosome. Because *dTAK1* functions downstream of *imd* and upstream of the signalosome, this kinase is a good candidate for the direct triggering of the signalosome in response to infection (Vidal et al., 2001). Although activation of Relish is proteasome independent, genetic studies indicate that the proteasome negatively regulates the Imd pathway by degrading Relish. Mutations in the *SkpA* gene specifically upregulate the antibacterial peptide gene *diptericin* in unchallenged flies whereas the antifungal peptide gene *drosomycin* remains unaffected (Khush et al., 2002). *SkpA* encodes a homologue of the yeast and mammalian Skp1 proteins that are components of the Skp1/Cullin/F-box protein (SCF)-E3 ubiquitin ligases (Karin and Ben-Neriah, 2000). Inhibition of this SCF complex in cultured cells increases the steady-state levels of both the full-length and the processed forms of Relish, containing only the Rel homology domain (Khush et al., 2002).

At present one of the major unanswered questions concerning the Imd pathway is the nature of the receptor sensing gram-negative sepsis. It is unclear whether it is a bona fide pattern recognition receptor or it responds to infection through activation of a proteolytic cascade. The recently isolated putative transmembrane PGRP-LC (see below) (Ramet et al., 2002; Gottar et al., 2002; Choe et al., 2002) does not qualify as the receptor of the Imd pathway. Null mutants for *PGRP-LC* are less affected both in terms of diptericin expression and their rates of survival following bacterial infection than loss-of-function mutants for intracellular components of the Imd pathway (Gottar et al., 2002). This indicates that there should be additional PRRs that sense infection by gram-negative bacteria. Moreover, the absence of an intracytoplasmic signaling domain suggests that PGRP-LC is a possible coreceptor of the putative Imd pathway receptor complex.

Recognition of Non-Self in *Drosophila*. Genetic screens and an RNAi-based screen in macrophagelike cultured cells have recently identified PRRs in *Drosophila*. The three *Drosophila* PRRs identified by these approaches are PGRP-SA, PGRP-LC, and dSR-CI (Ramet et al., 2002; Gottar et al., 2002; Choe et al., 2002; Michel et al., 2001). PGRP-SA and PGRP-LC belong to a group of evolutionarily conserved proteins, which received their designation in reference to their initial discovery as gram-positive interacting proteins. The *Drosophila* family of PGRP molecules have either a short form (PGRP-S) and are secreted or a long form and are presumed to be transmembrane (PGRP-L) (Werner et al., 2000).

PGRP-SA was isolated as a sensor of gram-positive infection in *Drosophila* (Michel et al., 2001) (Fig. 2). A mutation in this gene abolishes Toll-dependent activation of the response to this type of infection. As a result, flies carrying such a mutation have severely reduced survival rates following gram-positive bacterial challenge. PGRP-SA circulates in the blood; the transfer of hemolymph from wild-type to mutant flies could rescue the phenotype of these mutants.

PGRP-LC was identified as a receptor for gram-negative sepsis (Ramet et al., 2002; Gottar et al., 2002; Choe et al., 2002) (Fig. 3). In *PGRP-LC* mutants, activation of immune responses following infection by gram-negative bacteria is severely impaired, and flies die soon after they are infected. Conversely, overexpression of *PGRP-LC* induces activation of the antibacterial peptide diptericin, generally used as a transcriptional readout of the Imd

pathway (Gottar et al., 2002; Choe et al., 2002). Furthermore, cells depleted of *PGRP-LC* RNA are less able to phagocytose after infection with *Escherichia coli* and are not responsive to LPSs (Ramet et al., 2002).

The dSR-CI was identified in an RNAi-based screen for PRRs in the *Drosophila* S2 macrophagelike cell line (Ramet et al., 2001). It belongs to scavenger receptors, an expanding family of proteins with the ability to bind a broad range of polyanionic ligands. dSR-CI was found to bind both gram-negative (*E. coli*) and gram-positive (*Staphylococcus aureus*) bacteria. RNA interference of dSR-CI transcripts results in a 20 to 30% reduction of the phagocytic capacity of *Drosophila* S2 cells. There are three additional members of the *Drosophila* class C SRs: dSR-CII, dSR-CIII, and dSR-CIV. CIII and CIV appear to be secreted, whereas CII is predicted to be a transmembrane protein.

Another family of putative PRRs is the gram-negative binding recognition proteins (GNBPs) (Lee et al., 1996). At least one of the three *Drosophila* GNBPs, GNBP-1, recognizes common immune elicitors, such as LPS and β-1,3-glucan. When its expression is blocked in cell culture, NF-κB-mediated immune gene expression is severely reduced (Kim et al., 2000). It has been observed previously that *Bombyx* GNBP exclusively binds gram-negative bacteria (Lee et al., 1996). In the case of *Anopheles* GNBP, the binding specificity is unknown, but the *Anopheles* GNBP mRNA is more responsive to gram-positive bacteria than to gram-negative bacteria, and yeast is ineffective as an inducer (Dimopoulos et al., 1997). These results suggest that different members of the GNBP family may have different specificities for the recognition of diverse pathogens, leaving open the possibility that *Drosophila* GNBP-2 and GNBP-3 have different pattern recognition characteristics than GNBP-1 and may serve in the recognition of different microbial pathogens.

Recent studies monitoring transcriptional expression profiles in a genome-wide manner have identified several hundreds of genes responsive to infection (Boutros et al., 2002; De Gregorio et al., 2002b, 2001; Irving et al., 2001). The discerned patterns, albeit very dynamic, show a strong correlation with the published data. These patterns can be dissected into distinct temporal responses, revealing possible links between pathway activation and temporal organization of the response. The Toll and Imd pathways are the major players in regulating these defenses (Boutros et al., 2002; De Gregorio et al., 2002b). In addition, a role for the JNK and JAK-STAT signaling pathways is suggested because they contribute to the expression of microbial challenge-induced genes (Boutros et al., 2002). Among the responsive genes are many small peptides of unknown function that may represent new effector molecules with antimicrobial activity (Boutros et al., 2002; De Gregorio et al., 2001; Irving et al., 2001).

Comparison of the data sets obtained in these studies with results from similar studies in other model systems will help identify networks of genes involved in innate immunity and characterize their function, ultimately leading to models that would reflect the in vivo complexity of signaling.

REFERENCES

Akira, S., K. Takeda, and T. Kaisho. 2001. Toll-like receptors: critical proteins linking innate and acquired immunity. *Nat. Immunol.* **2:**675–708.

Ashida, M., and P. T. Brey. 1995. Role of the integument in insect defense: prophenoloxidase cascade in the cuticular matrix. *Proc. Natl. Acad. Sci. USA* **92:**10698–10702.

Ashida, M., and P. Brey. 1997. Recent advances in research on the insect prophenoloxidase cascade, p. 133–172. *In* P. T. Brey and D. Hultmark (ed.), *Molecular Mechanisms of Immune Responses in Insects.* Chapman & Hall, London, United Kingdom.

Belvin, M. P., and K. V. Anderson. 1996. A conserved signalling pathway: the *Drosophila* Toll-dorsal pathway. *Annu. Rev. Cell Dev. Biol.* **12:**393–416.

Boutros, M., H. Agaisse, and N. Perrimon. 2002. Sequential activation of signalling pathways during innate immunity in *Drosophila. Dev. Cell* **3:**711–722.

Bulet, P., C. Hetru, J.-L. Dimarcq, and D. Hoffmann. 1999. Antimicrobial peptides in insects; structure and function. *Dev. Comp. Immunol.* **23:**329–344.

Carton, Y., and A. J. Nappi. 1997. *Drosophila* cellular immunity against parasitoids. *Parasitol. Today* **13:**218–227.

Choe, K.-M., T. Werner, S. Stoven, D. Hultmark, and K. V. Anderson. 2002. Requirement for a peptidoglycan recognition protein PGRP in Relish activation and Antibacterial immune responses in *Drosophila. Science* **296:**359–361.

Chosa, N., T. Fukumitsu, K. Fujimoto, and E. Ohnishi. 1997. Activation of prophenoloxydase A1 by an activating enzyme in *Drosophila melanogaster. Insect Biochem. Mol. Biol.* **27:**61–68.

Christophides, G. K., et al. 2002. Immunity-related genes and gene families in *Anopheles gambiae*: a comparative genomic analysis. *Science* **298:**159–165.

Cuénot, L. 1891. Etudes sur le sang et les glandes lymphatiques dans la serie animale. *Arch. Zool. Gen.* **2:**13–90.

De Gregorio, E., P. T. Spellman, G. M. Rubin, and B. Lemaitre. 2001. Genome-wide analysis of the *Drosophila* immune response by using oligonucleotide microarrays. *Proc. Natl. Acad. Sci. USA* **98:**12590–12595.

De Gregorio, E., S.-J. Han, W.-J. Lee, M.-J. Baek, T. Osaki, S. I. Kawabata, B. L. Lee, S. Iwanaga, B. Lemaitre, and P. T. Brey. 2002a. An immune-responsive Serpin regulates the melanization cascade in *Drosophila. Dev. Cell.* **3:**581–592.

De Gregorio, E., P. T. Spellman, P. Tzou, G. M. Rubin, and B. Lemaitre. 2002b. The Toll and Imd pathways are the major regulators of immune response in *Drosophila. EMBO J.* **21:**2568–2579.

Dimopoulos, G., A. Richman, H. M. Muller, and F. C. Kafatos. 1997. Molecular immune responses of the mosquito Anopheles gambiae to bacteria and malaria parasites. *Proc. Natl. Acad. Sci. USA* **94:**11508–11511.

Dushay, M. S., B. Asling, and D. Hultmark. 1996. Origins of immunity: Relish, a compound Rel-like gene in the antibacterial defence of *Drosophila. Proc. Natl. Acad. Sci. USA* **93:**10343–10347.

Duvic, B., J. A. Hoffmann, M. Meister, and J. Royet. 2002. Notch signaling controls lineage specification during Drosophila larval hematopoiesis. *Curr. Biol.* **12:**1923–1927.

Eldon, E., S. Kooyer, D. D'Evelyn, M. Duman, P. Lawinger, J. Botas, and H. Bellen. 1994. The *Drosophila 18wheeler* is required for morphogenesis and has striking similarities to *Toll. Development* **120:**885–899.

Engstrom, Y., L. Kadalayil, S.-C. Sun, C. Samakovlis, and D. Hultmark. 1993. KappaB-like motifs regulate the induction of immune genes in *Drosophila. J. Mol. Biol.* **232:**327–333.

Ferrandon, D., A. C. Jung, M. Criqui, B. Lemaitre, S. Uttenweiler-Joseph, L. Michaut, J. Reichhart, and J. A. Hoffmann. 1998. A drosomycin-GFP reporter transgene reveals a local immune response in Drosophila that is not dependent on the Toll pathway. *EMBO J.* **17**:1217–1227.

Geisler, R., A. Bergmann, Y. Hiromi, and C. Nusslein-Volhard. 1992. *Cactus*, a gene involved in dorsoventral pattern formation of *Drosophila*, is related to the IκB gene family of vertebrates. *Cell* **71**:613–621.

Georgel, P., S. Naitza, C. Kappler, D. Ferrandon, D. Zachary, C. Swimmer, C. Kopczynski, G. Duyk, J. M. Reichhart, and J. A. Hoffmann. 2001. *Drosophila* Immune Deficiency (Imd) is a Death Domain protein that activates the antibacterial defence and can promote apoptosis. *Dev. Cell* **1**:503–514.

Glaser, G. W. 1918. On the existence of immunity principles in Insects. *Psyche* (Boston, Mass.) **25**:38–46.

Gottar, M., V. Gobert, T. Michel, M. Belvin, G. Duyk, J. A. Hoffmann, D. Ferrandon, and J. Royet. 2002. The *Drosophila* immune response against Gram negative bacteria is mediated by a peptidoglycan recognition protein. *Nature* **416**:640–644.

Heitzler, P., D. Coulson, M. T. Saenz-Robles, M. Ashburner, J. Roote, P. Simpson, and D. Gubb. 1993. Genetic and cytogenetic analysis of the 43A-E region containing the segment polarity gene *costa* and the cellular polarity genes *prickle* and *spiny-legs* in *Drosophila melanogaster*. *Genetics* **135**:105–115.

Hoffmann, J. A., and J.-M. Reichhart. 2002. *Drosophila* innate immunity: an evolutionary perspective. *Nat. Immunol.* **3**:121–125.

Horng, T., and R. Medzhitov. 2001. *Drosophila* Myd88 is an adapter in the Toll signalling pathway. *Proc. Natl. Acad. Sci. USA* **98**:12654–12658.

Imler, J.-L., and J. A. Hoffmann. 2001. Toll receptors in innate immunity. *Trends Cell Biol.* **11**:304–311.

Ip, Y. T., M. Reach, Y. Engstrom, L. Kadalayil, H. Cai, S. Gonzalez-Crespo, K. Tatei, and M. Levine. 1993. Dif, a dorsal-related gene that mediates an immune response in *Drosophila*. *Cell* **75**:753–763.

Irving, P., L. Troxler, T. S. Heuer, M. Belvin, C. Kopczynski, J.-M. Reichhart, J. A. Hoffmann, and C. Hetru. 2001. A genome-wide analysis of immune responses in *Drosophila*. *Proc. Natl. Acad. Sci. USA* **98**:15119–15124.

Jiang, H., Y. Wang, and M. R. Kanost. 1998. Pro-Phenoloxydase activating proteinase from an insect, *Manduca sexta*: a bacteria-inducible protein similar to *Drosophila* Easter. *Proc. Natl. Acad. Sci. USA* **95**:12220–12225.

Kambris, Z., J. A. Hoffmann, J.-L. Imler, and M. Capovilla. 2002. Tissue and stage-specific expression of the Tolls in *Drosophila* embryos. *Mech. Dev.* **22**:311–317.

Kappler, C., M. Meister, M. Lagueux, E. Gateff, J. A. Hoffmann, and J. M. Reichhart. 1993. Insect immunity: two 17-bp repeats nesting a kappaB-related sequence confer inducibility to the diptericin gene

and bind a polypeptide in bacteria-challenged *Drosophila*. *EMBO J.* **12**:1561–1568.

Karin, M., and Y. Ben-Neriah. 2000. Phosphorylation meets ubiquitination: the control of NF-κB activity. *Annu. Rev. Immunol.* **18**:621–663.

Keith, F. J., and N. J. Gay. 1990. The *Drosophila* membrane receptor Toll can function to promote cellular adhesion. *EMBO J.* **9**:4299–4306.

Khush, R. S., W. D. Cornwell, J. N. Uram, and B. Lemaitre. 2002. A ubiquitin-proteasome pathway represses the Drosophila immune deficiency signaling cascade. *Curr. Biol.* **20**:1728–1737.

Kim, Y. S., J. H. Ryu, S. J. Han, K. H. Choi, K. B. Nam, I. H. Jang, B. Lemaitre, P. T. Brey, and W. J. Lee. 2000. Gram-negative bacteria-binding protein, a pattern recognition receptor for lipopolysaccharide and beta-1, 3-glucan that mediates the signaling for the induction of innate immune genes in *Drosophila melanogaster* cells. *J. Biol. Chem.* **275**:32721–32727.

Kowalevsky, A. 1892. Sur les organes excréteurs chez les Arthropodes terrestres. *Congr. Int. Zool.* (Moscow) **1**:187–205.

Lagueux, M., E. Perrodou, E. A. Levashina, M. Capovilla, and J. A. Hoffmann. 2000. Constitutive expression of a complement-like protein in Toll and JAK gain of function mutants of *Drosophila*. *Proc. Natl. Acad. Sci. USA* **97**:11427–11432.

Lanot, R., D. Zachary, F. Holder, and M. Meister. 2001. Post-embryonic hematopoiesis in *Drosophila*. *Dev. Biol.* **230**:243–257.

Lee, W. J., J. D. Lee, V. V. Kravchenko, R. J. Ulevich, and P. T. Brey. 1996. Purification and molecular cloning of an inducible Gram-negative bacteria-binding protein from the silkworm *Bombyx mori*. *Proc. Natl. Acad. Sci. USA* **93**:7888–7893.

Lemaitre, B., E. Kromer-Metzger, L. Michaut, E. Nicolas, M. Meister, P. Georgel, J. M. Reichhart, and J. A. Hoffmann. 1995. A recessive mutation, *immune deficiency* (*imd*), defines two distinct control pathways in the *Drosophila* host defence. *Proc. Natl. Acad. Sci. USA* **92**:9465–9469.

Lemaitre, B., E. Nicolas, L. Michaut, J.-M. Reichhart, and J. A. Hoffmann. 1996. The dorsoventral regulatory gene cassette *spaetzle/Toll/cactus* controls the potent antifungal response in *Drosophila* adults. *Cell* **86**:973–983.

LeMosy, E. K., C. C. Hong, and C. Hashimoto. 1999. Signal transduction by a protease cascade. *Trends Cell Biol.* **9**:102–107.

Letsou, A., S. Alexander, K. Orth, and S. A. Wasserman. 1991. Genetic and molecular characterisation of *tube*, a *Drosophila* gene maternally required for embryonic dorsoventral polarity. *Proc. Natl. Acad. Sci. USA* **88**:810–814.

Leulier, F., A. Rodriguez, R. S. Khush, J. M. Abrams, and B. Lemaitre. 2000. The *Drosophila* caspase Dredd is required to resist Gram-negative bacterial infection. *EMBO Rep.* **1**:353–358.

Levashina, E. A., E. Langley, C. Green, D. Gubb, M. Ashburner, J. A. Hoffmann, and J. M. Reichhart. 1999. Constitutive activation of Toll-mediated antifungal defence in serpin-deficient *Drosophila. Science* **285**:1917–1919.

Levashina, E. A., L. F. Moita, S. Blandin, G. Vriend, M. Lagueux, and F. C. Kafatos. 2001. Conserved role of a complement-like protein in phagocytosis revealed by dsRNA knockout in cultured cells of the mosquito *Anopheles gambiae. Cell* **104**:709–718.

Ligoxygakis, P., N. Pelte, C. Ji, V. Leclerc, B. Duvic, M. Belvin, H. Jiang, J. A. Hoffmann, and J.-M. Reichhart. 2002a. A serpin mutant links Toll activation to melanization in the host defense of Drosophila. *EMBO J.* **21**:6330–6337.

Ligoxygakis, P., N. Pelte, J. A. Hoffmann, and J.-M. Reichhart. 2002b. Activation of *Drosophila* Toll during fungal infection by a novel blood serine protease. *Science* **297**:114–117.

Locksley, R. M., N. Killeen, and M. J. Lenardo. 2001. The TNF and TNF receptor superfamilies: integrating mammalian biology. *Cell* **104**:487–501.

Lu, Y., L. Wu, and K. V. Anderson. 2001. The antibacterial arm of the *Drosophila* innate immune response requires an IκB kinase. *Genes Dev.* **15**:104–110.

Manfruelli, P., J.-M. Reichhart, R. Steward, J. A. Hoffmann, and B. Lemaitre. 1999. A mosaic analysis in *Drosophila* fat body cells of the control of antimicrobial peptide genes by the Rel proteins Dorsal and DIF. *EMBO J.* **18**:3380–3391.

Meister, M., A. Braun, C. Kappler, J.-M. Reichhart, and J. A. Hoffmann. 1994. Insect immunity: a transgenic analysis in *Drosophila* defines several functional domains in the diptericin promoter. *EMBO J.* **14**:5958–5966.

Metalnikow, S. 1920. L'immunité chez les Insectes. *CR. Acad. Sci. Paris* **171**:757–834.

Metalnikow, S. 1929. Immunité d'adaptation et immunité de defense. *CR. Soc. Biol.* **101**:34–67.

Michel, T., J.-M. Reichhart, J. A. Hoffmann, and J. Royet. 2001. *Drosophila* Toll is activated by Gram-positive bacteria via a circulating peptidoglycan recognition protein. *Nature* **414**:756–759.

Mizuguchi, K., J. S. Parker, T. L. Blundel, and N. G. Gay. 1998. Getting knotted: a model for the structure and function of Spaetzle. *Trends Biochem. Sci.* **23**: 239–242.

Naitza, S., C. Rosse, C. Kappler, P. Georgel, M. Belvin, D. Gubb, J. Camonis, J. A. Hoffmann, and J. M. Reichhart. 2002. The *Drosophila* immune defence against Gram-negative infection requires the death domain protein FADD. *Immunity* **17**:576–591.

Nappi, A. J., and E. Ottaviani. 2000. Cytotoxicity and cytotoxic molecules in invertebrates. *Bioessays* **22**: 469–480.

Nappi, A. J., E. Vass, F. Frey, and Y. Carton. 1995. Superoxide anion generation in *Drosophila* during melanotic encapsulation of parasites. *Eur. J. Cell Biol.* **68**:450–456.

Paillot, A. 1921. Méchanisme de l'immunité humorale chez les Insectes. *CR. Acad. Sci. Paris* **172**:397–416.

Paillot, A. 1933. *L'Infection chez les insectes (immunité et symbiose)*. Editions G. Patissier, Trévoux, France.

Pye, A. E. 1974. Microbial activation of prophenoloxidase from immune insect larvae. *Nature* **251**: 610–613.

Ramet, M., A. Pearson, P. Manfruelli, X. Li, H. Koziel, V. Gobel, E. Chung, M. Krieger, and R. A. Ezekowitz. 2001. Drosophila scavenger receptor CI is a pattern recognition receptor for bacteria. *Immunity* **15**:1027–1038.

Ramet, M., P. Manfruelli, A. Pearson, B. Mathey-Prevot, and R. A. Ezekowitz. 2002. Functional genomic analysis of phagocytosis and identification of a Drosophila receptor for E. coli. *Nature* **416**:644–648.

Rizki, T. M. 1984. The cellular defense system of *Drosophila melanogaster*, p. 579–604. *In* R. C. King and H. Akai (ed.), *Insect Ultrastructure*, vol. 2. Plenum, New York, N.Y.

Rizki, T. M., R. M. Rizki, and E. H. Grell. 1980. A mutant affecting the crystal cells in *Drosophila melanogaster. Roux Arch. Dev. Biol.* **188**:91–99.

Rutschmann, S., A. C. Jung, C. Hetru, J. M. Reichhart, J. A. Hoffmann, and D. Ferrandon. 2000a. The Rel protein DIF mediates the antifungal but not the antibacterial host defence in *Drosophila. Immunity* **12**:569–580.

Rutschmann, S., A. C. Jung, R. Zhou, N. Silverman, J. A. Hoffmann, and D. Ferrandon. 2000b. Role of the *Drosophila* IKKγ in a Toll-independent antibacterial immune response. *Nat. Immunol.* **1**:342–347.

Shelton, C. A., and S. A. Wasserman. 1993. *Pelle* encodes a protein kinase required to establish dorsoventral polarity in the *Drosophila* embryo. *Cell* **72**:515–525.

Shen, B., and J. L. Manley. 1998. Phosphorylation modulates direct interactions between the Toll receptor, Pelle kinase and Tube. *Development* **125**:4719–4728.

Silverman, N., R. Zhou, S. Stoven, N. Pandey, D. Hultmark, and T. Maniatis. 2000. A *Drosophila* IκB kinase complex required for Relish cleavage and antibacterial immunity. *Genes Dev.* **14**:2461–2471.

Söderhäll, K., and L. Cerenius. 1998. Role of the prophenoloxidase-activating system in invertebrate immunity. *Curr. Opin. Immunol.* **10**:23–28.

Stein, D., J. S. Goltz, J. Jurcsak, and L. Stevens. 1998. The Dorsal-related immunity factor (Dif) can define the dorsal-ventral axis of polarity in the Drosophila embryo. *Development* **11**:2159–2169.

Steiner, H., D. Hultmark, A. Engström, H. Bennich, and H. G. Boman. 1981. Sequence and specificity of two antibacterial proteins involved in insect immunity. *Nature* **292**:246–248.

Steward, R. 1987. Dorsal, an embryonic polarity gene in *Drosophila* is homologous to the vertebrate proto-oncogene, *c-rel*. *Science* **238**:692–694.

Stoven, S., I. Ando, L. Kadalayil, Y. Engstrom, and D. Hultmark. 2000. Activation of the NF-κB factor Relish by rapid endoproteolytic cleavage. *EMBO Rep.* **1**:347–352.

Tauszig, S., E. Jouanguy, J. A. Hoffmann, and J.-L. Imler. 2000. Toll-related receptors and the control of antimicrobial expression in *Drosophila*. *Proc. Natl. Acad. Sci. USA* **97**:10520–10525.

Tauszig-Delamasure, S., H. Bilak, M. Capovilla, J. A. Hoffmann, and J.-L. Imler. 2002. *Drosophila MyD88* is required for the response to fungal and Gram-positive bacterial infections. *Nat. Immunol.* **3**: 91–97.

Tzou, P., S. Ohresser, D. Ferrandon, M. Capovilla, J. M. Reichhart, B. Lemaitre, J. A. Hoffmann, and J. L. Imler. 2000. Tissue-specific inducible expression of antimicrobial peptide genes in Drosophila surface epithelia. *Immunity* **13**:737–748.

Tzou, P., J. M. Reichhart, and B. Lemaitre. 2002. Constitutive expression of a single antimicrobial peptide can restore wild-type resistance to infection in immunodeficient Drosophila mutants. *Proc. Natl. Acad. Sci USA* **99**:2152–2157.

Vidal, S., R. S. Khush, F. Leulier, P. Tzou, M. Nakamura, and B. Lemaitre. 2001. Mutations in the *Drosophila dTAK1* gene reveal a conserved function for MAPKKKs in the control of rel/NF-κB dependent innate immune responses. *Genes Dev.* **15**: 1900–1912.

Werner, T., G. Liu, D. Kang, S. Ekengren, H. Steiner, and D. Hultmark. 2000. A family of peptidoglycan recognition proteins in the fruit fly *Drosophila melanogaster*. *Proc. Natl. Acad. Sci. USA* **97**: 13772–13776.

MAMMALIAN CELLS

NEUTROPHILS: THE POWER WITHIN

Taco W. Kuijpers and Dirk Roos

3

Neutrophils form the major type of leukocytes in peripheral blood, with counts ranging from 40 to 70% of the leukocytes under normal conditions. Neutrophils are also called polymorphonuclear (PMN) leukocytes or "granulocytes," but strictly speaking this last name is a designation that includes neutrophilic granulocytes (neutrophils), eosinophilic granulocytes (eosinophils), and basophilic granulocytes (basophils). This nomenclature is derived from the differences in color between the many granular structures in the cytoplasm of these cells from standard hematoxylin-eosin staining procedures. Neutrophilic granulocytes protect the human body against bacterial and fungal infections. For this purpose, neutrophils are equipped with a machinery to sense the site of an infection, to crawl toward the invading microorganisms, and to ingest and kill them (Malech and Nauseef, 1997). Thus, for proper functioning of this line of defense, sufficient neutrophils must be generated and released from the bone marrow, and these cells must be capable of executing a large number of different functions. However, because the neutrophil products are also potentially harmful to the host tissue, many safeguards exist to prevent such unwanted side effects.

DEVELOPMENT

Neutrophils mature in the bone marrow in about 2 weeks, a process in which the myeloid-specific growth factors granulocyte colony-stimulating factor (G-CSF) and granulocyte monocyte CSF (GM-CSF) play an important role (Fig. 1). In the first half of this 2-week period, the neutrophil precursor cells undergo five divisions and differentiate from myeloblasts through promyelocytes to neutrophilic myelocytes. Myeloblasts are cells with a large nucleus relative to the surrounding cytoplasm, which contains no or few granules. In the promyelocyte stage, the so-called azurophil granules are formed, and the specific granules are formed in the myelocytic stage. Because cell divisions still occur after azurophil granule formation has stopped, these granules are distributed over the daughter cells and are complemented with specific granules actively formed during the myelocytic stage. The final ratio of azurophil to specific granules is about 1:2. Later stages of neutrophil differentiation

Taco W. Kuijpers, Emma Children's Hospital, Academic Medical Centre, University of Amsterdam, Amsterdam, The Netherlands. *Dirk Roos,* Sanquin Research at CLB, and Landsteiner Laboratory, Academic Medical Center, University of Amsterdam, Amsterdam, The Netherlands.

The Innate Immune Response to Infection
Ed. by S. H. E. Kaufmann, R. Medzhitov, and S. Gordon
©2004 ASM Press, Washington, D.C.

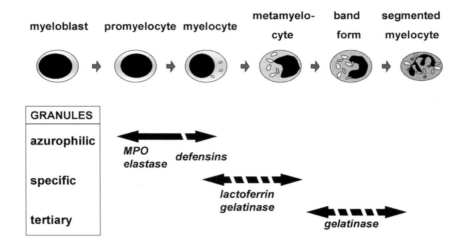

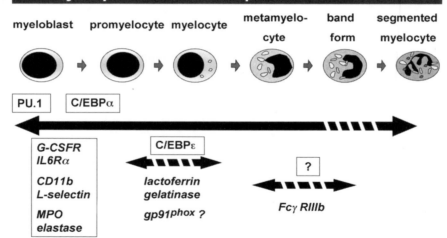

FIGURE 1 Neutrophil life span and stages of maturation. (Top) Schematic representation of the maturation of the myeloid lineage and the formation of granular structures during neutrophil development. In the promyelocyte stage, the azurophil granules (in light gray) are formed, whereas the specific granules (in medium gray) are formed in the myelocytic stage. Later, the tertiary granules and secretory granules (in dark gray) are generated. The stages of differentiation during which the various granules and their content are being formed are indicated by the arrows and main proteins underneath. (Bottom) Transcription factors involved in the synthesis and expression of key molecules and structures for neutrophil development and function. PU.1 and C/EBPα are important for expression of the G-CSFR and the α chain of the IL-6R, adhesion molecules such as CD62L (L-selectin) and CD11b (α chain of β_2 integrin CD11b/CD18 or Mac-1/CR3), and the main azurophil granular proteins MPO and serine proteases such as elastase. C/EBPε is important for the expression of the specific granules and their contents, and for the main membrane-associated β subunit of the NADPH oxidase system gp91^{phox}. The transcription factor(s) involved in the expression of one of the most abundantly expressed surface molecules on neutrophils, i.e., FcγRIIIb, remains to be identified.

comprise metamyelocytes, band forms, and segmented cells. As the names indicate, these stages are characterized by the typical appearance of the neutrophil nucleus. Divisions do not take place during this period.

About 60% of all nucleated cells in the bone marrow belong to the myeloid series. During myelopoiesis, which includes the development of granulocytic and monocytic lineages, transcription factors from several families are active, including AML1/CBF beta, C/EBP, Ets, c-Myb, HOX, and MZF-1 (Fig. 1). Few of these factors are expressed exclusively in myeloid cells; instead it appears that they cooperatively regulate transcription of myeloid-specific genes. These factors can be held responsible—in some way or another—for certain phenotypic aberrations when deficient in mice or humans (Anderson et al., 1999; Lekstrom-Himes et al., 1999; Zhang et al., 1998).

The bone marrow comprises a reserve pool of mature neutrophils of about 20 times the number of neutrophils in the circulation. Under normal conditions, these cells are released into the blood 2 days after completion of their maturation.

It is not known exactly which factors cause egress of blood cells from the bone marrow under normal conditions. It is believed that both MMP9 and elastase play an important role in the egress of CD34$^+$ stem cells as well as mature neutrophils from the bone marrow environment. During infections, neutrophils are released sooner, together with band forms (up to 10^{12} per day in adults instead of the usual 10^{11} per day). The appearance of immature neutrophils in the blood is reflected by a decreased chemotactic responsiveness of these cells. In the circulation, about half of the neutrophils are in a marginated pool of cells sequestered in postcapillary venules. This pool is released when epinephrine is generated by exercise or injected intravenously. Neutrophils circulate for only 6 to 10 h; thereafter, they move to the tissues, where they remain active for about 2 to 6 days, depending on the clinical conditions (longer under circumstances of inflammation). Part of the neutrophils will disappear in the gut but very little is known about other sites of neutrophil apoptosis and destruction by tissue macrophages.

Normally, less than 2% of all neutrophils in the body are circulating in the blood. In case the number of neutrophils in the peripheral blood is strongly reduced for unknown reasons (neutropenia) and/or a lack of releasability from the bone marrow by G-CSF or corticosteroids has been found, bone marrow examination and myeloid cell culture may be needed to assess the production, maturation, and differentiation of the bone marrow pool of neutrophils. A helpful alternative in evaluating the total body mass of neutrophils is the plasma level of a neutrophil-specific protein, such as Fcγ receptor (FcγR) type IIIb (FcγRIIIb, one of the opsonin receptors involved in phagocytosis and microbicidal activity) (Huizinga et al., 1994). This protein is released from the plasma membrane during neutrophil activation or apoptosis in the tissues and probably diffuses back into the bloodstream passively or by lymph flow.

Defects in neutrophil production or release from the bone marrow are diagnosed more often and more easily than qualitative (functional) phagocytic defects. However, functional defects may also accompany neutropenia. Such functional defects are seen in severe chronic neutropenia (SCN) as well as in the more complex and syndromal forms of neutropenia such as Shwachman syndrome or the metabolic disease glycogen storage disease (GSD) type 1b (non-a) (Kuijpers, 2002). Several causes of neutropenia can be diagnosed (Table 1). Treatment consists of antibiotic prophylaxis to support the patients in reducing colonization with commensals and with particular pathogens and/or G-CSF administration in a 3-week regimen. Final cure of the underlying disease can be reached only by allogeneic bone marrow transplantation, a definite but potentially fatal procedure that is performed only in the case of insufficient benefits from intensified supportive care measures.

TABLE 1 Neutropenia: quantitative defects, pathomechanism, and inheritance

Category	Type	Inheritance[a]	Gene defect (chrom.)
Immune mediated	Neonatal alloimmune neutropenia		
	Benign neutropenia of childhood		
	Autoimmune neutropenia (in association with SLE, JCA, etc.)		Multigenic
(Toxicity)	Drug-related neutropenia		
Congenital	Reticular dysgenesis	Sporadic/AR	
	Kostmann syndrome (classical KS)	AR	
	G-CSFR defect	AD	GCSFR (1p34.3)
	SCN	Sporadic/AD	ELA2 (19p13.3)
	Cyclic neutropenia	AD	ELA2 (19p13.3)
Syndrome associated	Shwachman-Diamond syndrome	AR	SBDS (7q11)
	Fanconi anemia (groups A to E)	AR	Multiple
	Dyskeratosis congenita	X linked (AR)	DKC1 (Xq28)
	Chediak-Higashi syndrome	AR	LYST (1q43)
	Griscelli syndrome	AR	MYO5A (15q21), other
	Cartilage hair hypoplasia	AR	CHH (9p13)
	Hyper-IgM syndrome (X linked)	X linked	XHIM (Xq26.3)
	Autoimmune lymphoproliferative syndrome	AD/sporadic	APT1 (10q24)
	Barth syndrome	X linked	G4.5 (Xq28)
	GSD-1b	AR	G6PT (11q23.3)
	Organic aciduria	AR	Multiple

[a]AR, autosomal recessive; AD, autosomal dominant.

GROWTH FACTOR RECEPTORS AND NEUTROPHILS

G-CSF (or GM-CSF) exerts a dual effect: induction of myeloid development through an increase in the number of CFU and a boost in their survival potential throughout its stages of differentiation. The effect of G-CSF is transmitted to the myeloid cell through the G-CSF receptor (G-CSFR). G-CSF and G-CSFR knockout mice show a similar phenotype of neutropenia, with decreased numbers of hematopoietic progenitor cells in the bone marrow, reduced expansion and terminal differentiation of these progenitors into mature neutrophils, and increased apoptosis of the neutrophils that do mature. A maturational arrest does not occur in these mice (Liu et al., 1996).

To date, a germ line mutation in the G-CSFR has been identified in only one child with congenital neutropenia. Instead, somatic mutations have been regularly observed in patients with SCN. Most of these SCN patients suffer from a neutropenia of <200 neutrophils per µl from birth onward. Mutations in the G-CSFR can be found but are not congenital; instead, they can be acquired over time. A hot spot of such mutations lies in an intracellular domain stretching over 45 amino acids. These mutations result in premature stop codons that cause deletion of the C terminus of the G-CSFR. Although expression levels of the receptor remain unperturbed, the distal maturation signals are now lacking, leaving the proliferative signaling route via the membrane-proximal part of the cytoplasmic tail of the G-CSFR intact (Dong et al., 1997). Mutations in G-CSFR indicate a more dismal course of the disease, with an increased risk for acute myeloid leukemia of about 2% annually (Zeidler et al., 2000).

In contrast to the sporadic cases of congenital SCN with a permanent form of neutropenia, human cyclic neutropenia (CN) is an autosomal dominant disease in which neutrophil production from the bone marrow oscillates with 21-day periodicity. The number of circulating neutrophils varies over time between almost normal and zero. The locus for CN was mapped by positional cloning to chromosome 19p13.3 and was identified as the *ELA2* gene encoding neutrophil elastase, the most prominent serine protease of neutrophil and monocyte granules (Dale et al., 2000). Subsequent studies showed that the same *ELA2* gene was also somatically mutated in >80% of SCN patients. Both normal and abnormal transcripts are expressed. The heterozygous single-base substitutions in CN and SCN are encountered throughout the molecule and can be found in SCN as well as in CN patients (Dale et al., 2000).

Neutrophil elastase is normally synthesized in the myeloblasts as an inactive proenzyme but is packaged in the azurophil granules in its active form. Because mice with heterozygous or homozygous *ELA2* deletions do not show neutropenia (Belaaouaj et al., 1998), gain-of-function mutations have been proposed to explain both the neutropenia and the autosomal dominant inheritance (in SCN) (Dale et al., 2000). Whether the enhanced apoptosis observed in SCN and CN progenitor cells is the result of these gain-of-function mutations, leakiness of the granular compartments, or aberrant routing of the proenzyme is as yet unknown. As to how mutated elastase and premature apoptosis lead to the clocklike timing of hematopoiesis in CN or cause a more permanent neutropenia is as yet a complete mystery.

CHEMOTAXIS AND CELL ACTIVATION

Leukocytes are able to recognize concentration differences in a gradient of chemotaxins and to direct their movement toward the source of these agents, i.e., toward the inflammatory site. This is again a very complicated process, the details of which are largely unknown (Bokoch, 1996; Murdoch and Finn, 2000). Probably the occupation of a threshold difference in the number of chemotaxin receptors on one side of the cell induces the cytoskeletal rearrangements needed for movement. As described in more detail below (see Neutrophil Adhesion and Extravasation), adhesion molecules (such as the β_2 integrins on neutrophils) are essential for the connections with the tissue cells or with the extracellular matrix proteins that must be formed at the front of the moving neutrophils and broken at the rear end (Kuijpers et al., 1992; Springer, 1994). Moreover, for continued sensing of the chemotaxin gradient, the chemotaxin receptors on the neutrophil must be freed from their ligand for repeated usage. This occurs through internalization of the ligand-receptor complex, intracellular disruption of the connection, and reappearance of the free receptor on the leukocyte surface.

Many of the chemotaxins involved in granulocyte movement are small proteins of about 60 to 100 amino acids, very homologous in structure, known as the chemokine superfamily. This family of leukocyte activators consists of over 30 different chemotactic molecules. Most chemokines can be classified into α (CXC) and β (CC) chemokines, distinguished by the presence or absence of a single amino acid between the first two of four conserved cysteines. The γ (single C) and δ (CX$_3$C) classes of chemokines have only recently been coined, each with as yet one member (lymphotactin and fractalkine or neurotactin, respectively). As exemplified by interleukin-8 (IL-8), the first CXC member described, most CXC chemokines activate neutrophils, whereas the CC chemokines act toward various lymphocyte subsets, monocytes, and eosinophils and basophils. The chemokines are produced by host cells in response to inflammation, injury, hypoxia, or other forms of stress.

In addition, chemotactic peptides are released by infecting microorganisms (e.g., formyl-methionyl-leucyl-phenylalanine [fMLP]) and the host complement system (the split product of activated C5 [C5a]). Lipid mediators, such as leukotriene B$_4$ and the platelet-activating factor, are also strong chemoattractants. For each of these agents, specific receptors on the granulocyte exist. These receptors as well as those for the chemokines belong to the seven-span super-family of integral membrane proteins with seven transmembrane domains. Ligand specificity is created by differences in the extracellular domains. The intracellular domains interact with various trimeric guanidine triphosphate-binding proteins, thus enabling a link with intricate signal transduction pathways leading to a wide range of functional responses, the complexity of which is still largely unclear.

Neutrophils from G-CSFR knockout mice demonstrate a disturbed chemotactic activity toward various chemotactic factors—e.g., chemokines (IL-8 or its analogues) and chemotactic peptides (fMLP or C5a)—in the presence of a normal expression of chemotaxin receptors (Betsuyaku et al., 1999). Also, G-CSF-induced neutrophils of patients with SCN are functionally defective in chemotaxis (Kasper et al., 2000). Although it has been suggested that G-CSF may already negatively influence the chemotactic responsiveness due to the accelerated bone marrow transit time of myeloid cells and the resulting relative immaturity of circulating neutrophils, we have not observed any decreased chemotaxis of neutrophils derived from patients using G-CSF for other reasons than congenital neutropenia. We thus believe that the neutrophil defect in chemotaxis observed with SCN may very well be inherent to the neutrophils generated in these specific (G-CSF-treated) patients. A defect in chemotaxis by neutrophils with a disturbed *GCSFR* or *ELA2* gene cannot be easily reconciled with the function of either of these molecules per se. One explanation may be their increased susceptibility to cell death signals perturbing the intracellular machinery for movement (although still morphologically normal upon isolation), as indicated by the rapid decay in functionality (Dransfield et al., 1995). Alternatively, the machinery required for motility may be affected in some way by either of the above-mentioned gene defects. Small GTPases

of the Rho family, in particular Rac-2 in neutrophils (Ambruso et al., 2000), have been shown to be crucial in the signaling leading to cytoskeletal remodeling and cellular motility. In SCN, a change in the ratio of expression between small GTPases and their regulatory proteins has been described, which is a more probable cause of the chemotaxis defect observed in the G-CSF-induced neutrophils (Kasper et al., 2000). However, the underlying cause of this disturbed ratio is still unknown.

NEUTROPHIL ADHESION AND EXTRAVASATION

After egress of neutrophils from the bone marrow to the circulation, the neutrophils adhere to the vascular lining and move into the tissues by squeezing in between two adjacent endothelial cells without disturbing the endothelial cell layer. This process is called diapedesis. Because of its lobulated nucleus, the neutrophil, with its diameter of 10 to 12 μm, is very flexible, which facilitates its passage through pores down to 1 μm. The processes of adhesion of neutrophils to endothelial cells and subsequent diapedesis take place at postcapillary venules. Extravasation is a multistep process involving adhesion molecules and activating agents that act as (pro-) inflammatory mediators.

The adhesion molecules dominating the picture of leukocyte traffic consist of members of the selectin and integrin family, as well as their respective ligands (Fig. 2). The first step consists of the initial contact between endothelial cells and neutrophils marginated by the fluid flow of the blood. The margination allows a reversible interaction between these two cell types mediated by selectin molecules. The vascular lining becomes activated within the local environment of an inflammatory tissue reaction and begins to express the adhesion molecules E selectin (CD62E) or P selectin (CD62P). The low-avidity interaction of these selectins with their ligands on the neutrophils forces the neutrophils to slow down and make a rolling movement along the vessel wall. Rolling enables the neutrophil to then make a more stable contact (cell spread-

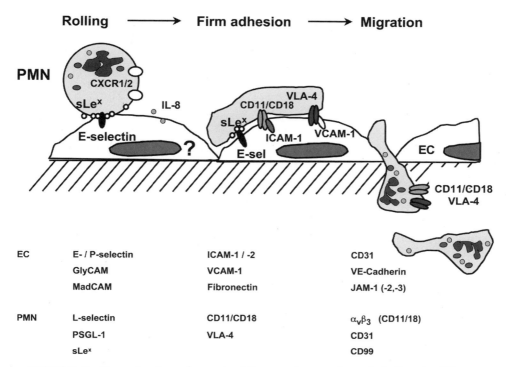

FIGURE 2 Transmigration of a neutrophil across the vascular endothelium in different steps. The steps are believed to take place in consecutive order, in which different adhesion molecules take part. The first selectin-driven rolling is followed by integrin-mediated firm adhesion. Final transmigration of phagocytes proceeds partly by integrin-mediated processes and several adhesion molecules of the Ig-like supergene family among which are ICAMs, VCAM, CD31/PECAM-1 (platelet-endothelial cellular adhesion molecule), and the recently described junctional adhesion molecule-1 (JAM-1) on endothelial cells. The relative contributions of these various molecules as active receptors and passive ligands may differ for neutrophils, eosinophils, basophils, or monocytes to migrate through monolayers of endothelial or epithelial cells. VLA, very late antigen; EC, endothelial cell; PSGL-1, P-selectin-glycoprotein ligand-1.

ing) through the interaction of integrin molecules on the neutrophil surface with accessory molecules such as intercellular adhesion molecule 1 (ICAM-1) on endothelial cells. For this interaction, the integrin molecules must first be activated (see below). The activating signals consist of binding of the above-mentioned chemotaxins to neutrophil surface receptors and of the cross-linking of the selectin ligands on the surface of neutrophils. The chemotaxins can be derived from the endothelial cells or from underlying tissues and can be exposed on the luminal side of the endothelial cells or diffusing from in between the cells (Kuijpers et al., 1992). Once the rolling neutrophils have come to a stop, they can respond to the gradi-

ent of chemotaxins, which then guides the firmly adhering cells from the bloodstream into the adjacent site of inflammation.

In contrast to the low-avidity binding of neutrophils to selectins, the second and third steps of firm adhesion and subsequent locomotion depend on changes in binding avidity of the integrin receptors on the leukocytes for adhesion and locomotion. These adhesion molecules consist of heterodimeric structures of an α chain covalently associated with a β chain. One particular β chain may associate with one of the various α chains. As a consequence, several integrin receptor subfamilies exist. The β_2 integrin receptor subfamily is expressed only on leukocytes and comprises four different heterodimeric proteins, each of which contains a different α subunit, i.e., $\alpha_L\beta_2$ (LFA-1; CD11a/CD18), $\alpha_M\beta_2$ (CR3; CD11b/ CD18), $\alpha_X\beta_2$ (gp150,95; CD11c/ CD18), and $\alpha_D\beta_2$ (CD11d/CD18) (Chamaillard et al., 2003).

Neutrophils express the β_2 integrins, especially CR3 (CD11b/CD18), at very high levels and strongly depend on their presence and function, whereas the other leukocytic cell types also express alternative integrin receptors (e.g., β_1 integrins) for adhesion and additional functions related to adhesive properties. These β_1 integrins, some of which are also present on neutrophils, are mainly involved in binding to extracellular matrix proteins, whereas β_2 integrins have a special function in cell-to-cell contact (Loike et al., 1999). At the molecular level, the integrins normally exist in a low-avidity binding state, which will hardly bind their ligand or counterreceptor. Upon cellular activation, the integrins on leukocytes undergo intramolecular changes in conformation and then recognize and bind their ligand with high (shear-resistant) avidity. Switching from low- to high-avidity binding states (and vice versa) of these integrins allows the cell to migrate.

During the process of diapedesis through the endothelial cell layer, homotypic interaction between CD31 molecules on leukocytes and endothelial cells is thought to promote the integrin-mediated extravasation. Additional molecules involved in the final step of transmigration have been recently identified as CD99 and a group of so-called junctional adhesion molecules (Aurrand-Lions et al., 2002). It is unclear whether alternative adhesion molecules exist with a similar propagating role in integrin-dependent migration of leukocytes into the extravascular space. Other binding molecules and mechanisms play an additional role in the case of epithelial cell linings, such as different types of cadherins that are important in the opening of tight junctions, as well as CD47—also known as the integrin-associated protein—functioning as an integrator of transepithelial movement (Liu et al., 2002).

SENSING DANGER SIGNALS: PATTERN RECOGNITION

Recently, a family of receptor proteins, the Toll-like receptors (TLRs), has been identified in mammals (Akira et al., 2001). TLRs mediate cellular responses to a large array of microbial ligands. Apart from exogenous danger signals, and also endogenous proteins, such as heat shock proteins exposed actively or diffusing from injured tissue, are candidate TLR ligands. At present, 10 different human TLR proteins have been cloned.

TLR2 is the receptor for a variety of microbial ligands, including bacterial lipoproteins, lipopeptides, lipoteichoic acid (LTA), and peptidoglycans (PGNs) from gram-positive bacteria, mycobacterial ara-lipoarabinomannan, and yeast zymosan. The TLR2-mediated bacterial recognition or "sensing" participates in the elimination of invading bacteria, regardless of its possible cooperation with TLR1 or TLR6 (Ozinsky et al., 2000). The cooperation of various TLRs may add greater specificity or a broader range of ligand recognition capacity to the TLR proteins as well as enhance their signal transduction capacity (Fig. 3). TLR10 shows homology to TLR6, making it also a likely candidate for cooperation with TLR2 (Akira et al., 2001).

TLR4 is a receptor for gram-negative bacteria-derived endotoxin or lipopolysaccharide (LPS). This has been demonstrated in both mouse and human cells (Poltorak et al., 1998). A point mutation in the C3H/HeJ mouse *tlr4* gene is responsible for the resistance of these mice to LPS. The confusion over whether TLR2, TLR4, or both function as primary LPS receptors arose because commercial preparations of *Escherichia coli*-derived LPS contain a phenol-extractable TLR2-stimulating component, perhaps a lipopeptide, which stimulates cells via TLR2. When this component was removed by exhaustive phenol extraction of the LPS, the remaining activity was mediated by TLR4 (Hirschfeld et al., 2000). Moreover, it has become clear that LPSs from other bacterial strains (e.g., from *Porphyromonas gingivalis* or *Bacteroides fragilis*) indeed preferentially trigger via TLR2 instead of TLR4 (Netea et al., 2002).

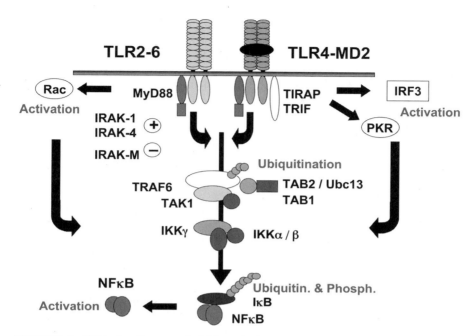

FIGURE 3 TLR signaling cascade. TLRs, which recognize pathogen-associated molecular patterns, and members of the proinflammatory IL-1R family, share homologies in their cytoplasmic domains called Toll/IL-1R/plant R gene homology (TIR) domains. Human TLR4 and TLR2 recognize LPS or LTA and bacterial PGNs, respectively. Intracellular signaling mechanisms mediated by TIRs are similar, with MyD88 and tumor receptor-associated factor 6 (TRAF6) having critical roles. Ubiquitination through transforming growth factor beta-activated kinase-1 (TAK1) and TAK-binding protein (TABs) activates TRAF6 to form the platform required for TAK1-mediated activation of inhibitor of NF-κB kinase (IKK). This complex consists of three enzymatic subunits (IKKα and -β) and a stabilizing subunit (NEMO or IKKγ) and acts as a serine kinase inhibitor of NF-κB (IκB). Signal transduction between MyD88 and TRAF6 is known to involve the serine-threonine kinase IRAK-1 and homologous proteins, IRAK-2, -4, and IRAK-M(yeloid). IRAK-4 is essential for responsiveness to viral and bacterial challenges, whereas IRAK-M downregulates the IRAK-mediated activation in phagocytes and dendritic cells. In contrast to the activation through ubiquitination of TRAF6, the phosphorylation and ubiquitination of IκB lead to its proteasome-mediated breakdown after release of a now activated, dimerized NF-κB. Although MyD88-mediated responses are the main way for TLR signaling, TLR4-associated TIR-containing adaptor protein (TIRAP) can bypass MyD88 by direct activation of a double-stranded RNA-dependent protein kinase (PKR) and/or the cytosolic transcription factor interferon regulatory factor-3 (IRF-3). Both pathways lead to NF-κB activation, increased gene transcription, and early release of inflammatory factors such as beta interferon by the innate immune system. In a similar way, TLR2 is able to activate the small GTPases Rac-1 and Rac-2, involved in cytoskeletal rearrangement and the generation of motile strength and contraction for movement, phagocytosis, degranulation, and NADPH oxidase activation.

Another important receptor for microbial ligands is CD14. CD14 is a glycosyl-phosphatidylinositol-anchored protein expressed at high levels on the surface of circulating monocytes (Ingalls et al., 1999). CD14 has also been detected in neutrophils, where it primarily resides within granules. A soluble form of CD14 is present in serum. Membrane and soluble CD14 proteins function as coreceptors for microbial ligands, including LPS, zymosan, PGN, and ara-lipoarabinomannan. It is believed that CD14 cooperates with TLR4 (Ingalls et al., 1999). Finally, Miyake and colleagues have identified an extracellular protein,

MD-2, that binds TLR4 and enhances LPS-induced NF-κB activation in cells expressing TLR4 (Shimazu et al., 1999). Although it remains to be confirmed, MD-2 may directly bind LPS.

Neutrophils express TLR2, TLR4, and CD14 at relatively low levels (in addition to TLR1 and TLR6) when compared with monocytes and macrophages (Kurt-Jones et al., 2002). Basophils express TLR2 and TLR4 but not CD14, whereas eosinophils express none of these proteins. Individual variation in expression levels may exist for as yet unknown reasons. GM-CSF (but not G-CSF) induces increased expression of TLR2 in many but not all individuals. Visintin et al. (2001) noted that TLR1 and TLR4 levels may also be highly variable between donors, with estimates of monocyte TLR4 surface expression ranging from 400 to 3,200 molecules per cell and levels of TLR1 ranging from 0 to 5,400 molecules per cell. The concentration of LPS required to activated neutrophils is about 100- to 1,000-fold higher than that needed for monocytes. After monocyte depletion by negative magnetic selection, neutrophil responses to LPS are heavily dependent on the presence of a very low level of monocytes (Sabroe et al., 2002). Thus, it still remains to be determined to what extent neutrophil TLRs may actually react to LPS itself. The localization of the neutrophil-expressed TLRs over the various granular compartments varies, as we have found for TLR1, -2, -4, and -6 (unpublished). Neutrophils have not yet been shown to express any of the other TLRs.

In sum, we can state that cellular responses to recognition patterns in microbial molecules are dependent on the total repertoire of TLRs and additional sensing receptors displayed on a cell, on necessary cofactors, and on the levels of these receptors and cofactors present.

TLR Signaling

Most TLR family members have a conserved intracellular signaling motif, the so-called TIR domain. This signaling motif, which is also found in the intracellular domain of the IL-1 (IL-1R), is responsible for NF-κB activation and translocation after TLR or IL-1R engagement and is an essential signaling pathway for IL-β and tumor necrosis factor alpha (TNF-α) secretion (Kawai et al., 1999). Activation of most TLRs leads to recruitment of myeloid differentiation marker 88 (MyD88), which contains an intracellular signaling domain and a death domain (Thornberry and Lazebnik, 1998). MyD88 interacts with various IL-1R-associated kinases (IRAKs), leading to the initiation of a signal transduction cascade culminating in nuclear translocation of NF-κB family members and altered gene expression (Fig. 3). In addition to MyD88-mediated signaling, TLR2 has been shown to also interact with the Rac-1 GTPase, thereby initiating a signaling cascade that also results in NF-κB translocation and possibly other nontranscriptional cellular responses (Arbibe et al., 2000). There are four homologous IRAKs that determine the signaling cascade. Apart from the initially identified IRAK-1 and -2, it is clear now that IRAK-M prevents dissociation of activating IRAK-1 and IRAK-4 from MyD88 and subsequent formation of IRAK-TRAF6 complexes. IRAK-M$^{-/-}$ cells exhibit increased cytokine production upon TLR/IL-1 stimulation, as well as increased inflammatory responses in mice to bacterial infection. Thus, IRAK-M regulates TLR signaling and innate immune homeostasis, in which IRAK-4 has emerged as a dominant and nonredundant signaling candidate, whereas in myeloid cells IRAK-M prevents signaling through this pathway (Kobayashi et al., 2002; Suzuki et al., 2002).

Recently, a novel protein containing a TIR domain and designated TIRAP/MAL (MyD88-adaptor-like protein) has been identified (Fitzgerald et al., 2001; Horng et al., 2001). Upon overexpression in 293 cells, this TIR domain-containing adaptor protein (TIRAP) leads to the activation of NF-κB and TIRAP association with TLR4 and double-strand RNA-dependent protein kinase (PKR) (Horng et al., 2001). The importance of whether TIRAP/

MAL activates NF-κB via IRAK-2, but not via IRAK-1, by forming heterodimers with MyD88 (Fitzgerald et al., 2001) remains unclear. Although both reports suggest the participation of TIRAP/MAL in MyD88 (and IRAK)-independent signaling, further investigation, such as an analysis of knockout mice, is needed to clarify the role this protein plays in this pathway.

Any More Sense?

Cytosolic NOD1 and NOD2 proteins have recently been reported to act as intracellular receptors for bacterial PGNs, i.e., a unique diaminopimelate-containing *N*-acetylglu-cosamine-*N*-acetylmuramic acid (GlcNAc-MurNAc) tripeptide motif found in gram-negative bacterial PGN and a bacterial muramyldipeptide MurNAc-L-Ala-DisoGln PGN motif common to all bacteria, respectively (Chamaillard et al., 2003; Girardin et al., 2003a, 2003b; Inohara et al., 2003). It was also reported that a dominant-negative form of NOD1 blocked the activation of NF-κB induced by microinjection of (impure) LPS or by infection with *Shigella flexneri*, implying that cytoplasmic bacterial products were detected by NOD proteins. Under physiologic conditions, NOD1 is expressed by multiple tissues (Inohara et al., 1999), whereas NOD2 proteins are predominantly expressed by monocytes and macrophages or cytokine-activated intestinal epithelial cells (Gutierrez et al., 2002; Ogura et al., 2001b). These molecules have recently been linked to a subgroup of familial autoinflammatory disease entities such as Crohn's disease and Blau's syndrome by mutations in NOD2 (Hugot et al., 2001; Miceli-Richard et al., 2001; Ogura et al., 2001a). The roles of the NOD proteins are discussed in more detail below.

The occurrence of a pro- or an anti-inflammatory reaction as well as the switch from a pro- into an anti-inflammatory reaction will not only be dictated by the number of phagocytic cells involved but also at the molecular level. Activating receptors expressed on neutrophils and monocytes infiltrating into human tissues infected with bacteria (but not inflammatory lesions per se) have been identified as TREM-1 and TREM-2 (Bouchon et al., 2001; Daws et al., 2001). These molecules are upregulated on neutrophils by bacteria or their products (e.g., *Pseudomonas aeruginosa, Staphylococcus aureus*, LTA, LPS) (Daws et al., 2001), and probably interact with an as yet unknown ligand, either a changed self-ligand or pathogen-derived products, as another pattern recognition receptor. The TREM genes are localized on chromosome 6p, as are the genes of other activating and sensing receptors with a single immunoglobulin (Ig)-like domain on cells of the innate immune system (e.g., CD83, NKp30, and NKp44) (Ravetch and Lanier, 2000; Young and Uhrberg, 2002).

Neutrophils express a myeloid-specific Ig superfamily member, CD200R, which senses the environment to restrain its tissue-damaging activity via association with the SH2-containing inositol phosphatase (SHIP), consistent with a role in downregulation of myeloid activity (Barclay et al., 2002). For this action, neutrophils have to engage CD200, a glycoprotein exposed by many opposing tissue cells. This scenario is reminiscent of the signals perceived by cells of the adaptive immune system, as well as natural killer (NK) cells and monocytes and macrophages. Such surface molecules in humans are known as the killer Ig-like receptors, Ig-like transcripts, and signal regulatory proteins (SIRPs).

These receptor families share many properties by generally containing two to three Ig-like domains, and both inhibitory and activating members exist. Their ligands, where known, are self-ligands expressed on the cell surface. Thus, killer Ig-like receptors and at least two Ig-like transcripts are known to recognize different antigens of the HLA class I of proteins, whereas SIRP1α binds CD47 (integrin-associated protein) on hematopoietic cells (Oldenborg et al., 2000; Young and Uhrberg, 2002). The activating members of these families stimulate cells by associating to membrane adaptor molecules with cytoplasmic immunoreceptor tyrosine-based activation motifs (ITAM), as also found in the activating FcγRs (see Phagocytosis and Microbicidal Activity, below). The tyrosine phosphorylation of these molecules permits binding and activation of tyrosine kinases such as Syk and ZAP-70 (Ravetch and Lanier, 2000; Young and Uhrberg, 2002). Studies in CD200 knockout mice have further indicated that an exaggerated innate immune response can result in unforeseen damage, either autoinflammatory or pathogen driven (Barclay et al., 2002). The extent to which many of the responses tested are the result of excessive macrophage or neutrophil reactivity and delayed resolution of the inflammatory response is as yet unclear. Also, the molecular regulation of expression of CD200 and its in vitro functions are described in more detail below.

PHAGOCYTOSIS AND MICROBICIDAL ACTIVITY

Neutrophils operate in concert with antibodies and complement factors, so-called opsonins. Microorganisms covered with these proteins are bound to neutrophils through specific opsonin receptors on the plasma membrane. Antibodies bind with their Fab regions to microbial antigens. In this way, the Fc regions of these antibodies are closely packed together on the microbial surface. This spatial arrangement enhances complement activation, thus leading to binding of C3b and C3bi to the microorganisms and subsequent binding of the microbes to the neutrophil complement receptor type 1 (CR1) and CR3, respectively. On the other hand, the proximity of the antibody Fc regions also promotes direct binding of the opsonized microorganisms to the Fc receptors on the neutrophils.

FcγRs are glycoproteins that function in the immune response through their ability to bind the Fc portion of immunoglobulin G (IgG). There are three main classes: FcγRI, FcγRII, and FcγRIII. Each has its characteristic IgG binding avidity, expression profile among hematopoietic cells, and functional properties. Further complexity arises from the fact that each FcγR is encoded by various genes and that these genes are subject to alternative splicing. For example, FcγRII is encoded by three genes (FCGR2A, FCGR2B, and FCGR2C), resulting in at least six protein isoforms, generated by alternative mRNA splicing (Ravetch and Bolland, 2001).

The FcRs can functionally be divided into activating and inhibitory receptors (Fig. 4). The activation results from the interaction of FcRs containing a so-called ITAM with immune complexes or cytotoxic autoantibodies, which initiates and propagates an inflammatory response. The cytoplasmic ITAM consists of two copies of the sequence YxxL (Y, tyrosine; L, leucine; x, any amino acid). Within this motif, the tyrosines are phosphorylated after receptor cross-linking, and the integrity of these conserved sequences is required for efficient phagocytosis. The ITAM is present in the cytoplasmic tail of FcγRIIa and in the γ chains associated with FcγRI and FcγRIIIa; the ζ chain associated with FcγRIIIa contains even three copies of this motif (see Fig. 4). In vitro, the activating pathway initiated by phosphorylation of these receptors can be interrupted by coligation to FcγRIIb. The FcγRIIb1 and -b2 cytoplasmic regions (65 and 46 amino acids, respectively) are generated by differential mRNA splicing, giving rise to a 19-amino-acid insert into the intracellular tail of FcγRIIb1. Both FcγRIIb receptors, FcγRIIb1 and FcγRIIb2, contain only one copy of the cytoplasmic YxxL sequence and—instead of transmitting an activating signal—now transduce inhibitory signals. These FcRs also contain a so-called immunoreceptor tyrosine-based inhibitory motif (ITIM) consisting of the ITYSLL sequence in both FcγRIIb isoforms. The present knowledge on how these negative signals are generated and transduced in B cells is scarce and often contradictory, but, on the whole, suggests the involvement of intracellular protein tyrosine phosphatases (i.e., SHP-1, SHP-2) and inositol-5 phosphatase (i.e., SHIP), probably by direct association (Bruhns et al., 2000; Pearse et al., 1999; Ravetch and Bolland, 2001).

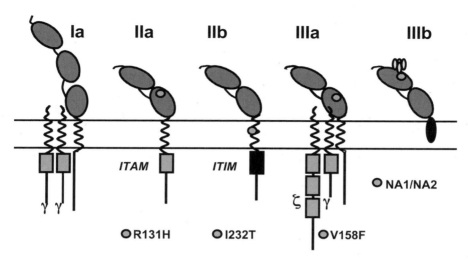

FIGURE 4   FcγRs, polymorphic variants, and associated signaling molecules. The allelic frequencies among the FcγRs behave as susceptibility markers between certain patient groups and control cohorts, or as disease-modifying markers within certain patient cohorts with respect to the symptoms or course of the disease. In the macrophage-specific FcγRIa, no allelic variation has until now been described. In FcγRIIa and FcγIIIa, several allelic variations have been defined. The FcγRIIa-131R/R genotype is associated with a higher binding capacity and affinity for IgG2 by all phagocytes and NK cells, in contrast to its opposite, the homozygous FcγRIIa-131H/H genotype. The inhibitory FcγRIIb contains a polymorphic site in the transmembrane domain. Questions regarding the physiological meaning and functional impact of this polymorphism remain to be answered. The FcγRIIIa-176V/F genotype variation adds considerable complexity to disease outcome and interpretation. These latter two receptors are expressed on macrophages and NK cells. The neutrophil-specific antigens NA1 and NA2 are located on lipid-anchored FcγRIIIb. NA1 and NA2 forms of FcγRIIIb differ by four amino acids and the corresponding genes by five nucleotides. A direct functional consequence has not been firmly established. Variations in all these FcγR polymorphic gene frequencies are encountered among ethnic groups. Altered forms of these genes may thus create clinical variation in case of IgG-dependent inflammatory and/or infectious disease among the various races, as do the different individual genetic backgrounds.

Most likely, three types of FcγRs are present on resting neutrophils: the activating FcγRIIa and FcγRIIIb and the inhibitory FcγRIIb. Only after activation of neutrophils by interferons or growth factors is an additional activating FcγR expressed, i.e., FcγRI, which binds monomeric IgG with high affinity. In contrast, the constitutively expressed FcγRIIa and FcγRIIIb bind monomeric IgG only with low avidity, but can efficiently bind immune complexes containing multiple IgG molecules.

A polymorphism in FcRγRIIa defines the intrinsic ability to recognize the four IgG sub-classes. IgG2 antibodies, often formed against microbial carbohydrate structures, react only with the so-called L131 type of FcγRIIa (with a leucine at amino acid position 131). Individuals with this isotype are better protected against infections with certain microorganisms than individuals with the R131 type of FcγRIIa (arginine at position 131). FcγRIII has two variants, a transmembrane form (FcγRIIIa) expressed on macrophages and NK cells and a neutrophil-specific form (FcγRIIIb) linked to the plasma membrane by a lipid anchor, which allows very rapid redistribution and early localization of opsonized material. Although there is a polymorphism in FcγRIIIb (NA1/NA2, depending on differences in glycosylation), its effect on clinical outcome is as yet not as clear as in the case of FcγRIIa (Oldenborg et al., 2000). There is also a polymorphic site present in the transmembrane domain of the inhibitory FcγRIIb, of which the meaning in terms of function is largely unclear. This site has been associated with clinical severity in a study of Japanese systemic lupus erythematosus patients (Kyogoku et al., 2002). In contrast to all other transmembrane FcγR members, the FcγRIIIb on neutrophils can be rapidly shed from the membrane during functional activation or during the process of programmed cell death (apoptosis) in the tissues. As mentioned above, the presence of soluble FcγRIIIb in plasma in combination with its relatively long half-life renders this molecule a prime candidate for the estimation of total neutrophil mass (Huizinga et al., 1994).

Binding of opsonized material to neutrophil surface receptors leads to concentration of such receptors around the area of contact. Subsequently, the cell extends pseudopods that engulf the particle. By consecutive receptor binding, these pseudopods fit tightly around the particle and finally fuse with each other to form a closed membrane vesicle (phagosome) around the particle, within the neutrophil. Neutrophils may overeat in infected areas and die from congestion. Macroscopically, this is manifested as pus formation. Apart from phagocytosis, receptor binding also starts two other processes, the generation of reactive oxygen compounds and the release of granule contents (degranulation). Both reactions are localized events in that they are restricted to the release of microbicidal products into the phagosome. However, the secretion of these products begins before the phagosome is closed (Fig. 5), and some of the oxygen compounds and granule enzymes may thus escape into the extracellular environment of the neutrophils (Weiss, 1989). Moreover, neutrophils adhering to opsonized material that is too large to be ingested (e.g., immune complexes deposited along basement membranes) may secrete these products in large quantities into the extracellular space, with serious consequences for the surrounding tissue (Weiss, 1989). The components required for granule traffic and membrane fusion are starting to become unraveled. Although not restricted to the innate immune system, defects in such processes may also result in clinical defects, such as those observed in the Chediak-Higashi syndrome with giant granules in the granulocytes and—as a consequence of a degranulation defect—serious neutrophil chemotaxis and killing defects.

Degranulation does not occur in resting neutrophils. Only during phagocytosis or adherence of neutrophils to large substrates do intracellular signaling events induce the fusion of granules with the plasma membrane. Neutrophils contain at least two different types of granule. The azurophil granules resemble the lysosomes in other cell types in that they contain acid hydrolases, with a low pH optimum. Moreover, these granules also contain myeloperoxidase (MPO) and a number of serine proteinases. In addition, the azurophil granules also contain large amounts of defensins, small peptides with a broad range of bactericidal activity, and bactericidal permeability-increasing protein, a very potent antibiotic against gram-negative bacteria. Lysozyme, an enzyme that hydrolyzes certain PGNs of gram-positive bacteria, is present in the azurophil as well as in the specific granules of neutrophils. Proteins exclusively found in the specific granules comprise lactoferrin, an iron-binding and therefore bacteriostatic protein, vitamin B_{12}-binding protein, and the metalloproteinases collagenase and gelatinase. The latter two enzymes help the neutrophil traverse into tissue compartments. Finally, neutrophils also contain so-called secretory vesicles, which actively exchange their membrane-bound receptors and enzymes with the plasma membrane.

Simultaneous with degranulation, a membrane-bound oxidase enzyme complex located in the membrane of secretory vesicles and specific granules is activated to generate reactive oxygen compounds needed in the killing

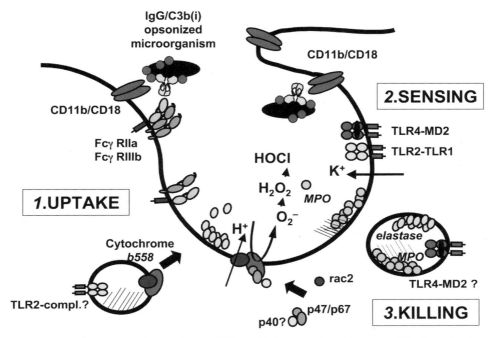

FIGURE 5 Recognition, uptake, and killing of microorganisms by neutrophils. Opsonized microorganisms bind with Fc regions of IgG antibodies to FcγRs and with C3b/C3bi fragments to CR1 and CR3 on the surface of the neutrophils. As a result, the microorganisms are engulfed by the neutrophils and taken up into an intracellular phagosome. Neutrophil granules fuse with the phagosome membrane and deposit their contents into the phagosome. A membrane-bound oxidase is activated and starts to generate superoxide (O_2^-) also into the phagosome. The superoxide is spontaneously converted into hydrogen peroxide (H_2O_2), which reacts with MPO released by the granules to yield additional toxic oxygen compounds. Sensing and triggering through TLRs and other sensing molecules take place at the outer plasma membrane and at the membrane of the phagolysosome.

process (Fig. 5). This NADPH oxidase complex is composed of several subunits in the plasma membrane (cytochrome b_{558} subunits p22-*phox* and gp91-*phox*) and a number of activity-regulating proteins in the cytoplasm (p40-*phox*, p47-*phox*, and p67-*phox*) (Roos and Curnutte, 1999). Phagocytes at rest do not generate superoxide. Only after opsonin and ligand binding to cell surface receptors is the active NADPH oxidase assembled to generate superoxide (O_2^-) in phagocytes. Superoxide spontaneously dismutates into hydrogen peroxide (H_2O_2), which may then react with chloride ions to form hypochlorous acid (HOCl) in a reaction catalyzed by MPO. This

enzyme is an abundant constituent of neutrophil azurophil granules and is released upon cell activation into the phagosome and into the extracellular space. HOCl is very toxic for a broad range of microorganisms but is rather short-lived. However, it can react with primary and secondary amines and thus give rise to N-chloramines, some of which are very stable microbicidal agents. Under normal phagocytosing conditions, neutrophils convert more than 75% of their superoxide into hypochlorous acid and N-chloramines and thus create a highly toxic environment within the phagosomes and in the cell surroundings (Weiss, 1989). The interaction between protease activity and NADPH oxidase activity has been indicated by recent studies on the immediate changes after microbial uptake in the phagolysosome (Reeves et al., 2002). The generation of O_2^- in the phagosome not only leads to influx of protons in the phagosome, for charge compensation, but also to the influx of potassium. This last process induces the release of proteases from the negatively charged proteoglycan matrix of the azurophil granules that have fused with the phagosome (Fig. 5).

NEUTROPHIL APOPTOSIS: PROGRAMMED CELL DEATH AS A DEFAULT ROUTE

When released from the bone marrow, neutrophils have a short life span and rapidly undergo spontaneous apoptosis within hours in the extravascular tissues. Survival of both the immature myeloid progenitor cells and mature PMN leukocytes can be extended by delaying apoptosis through the action of a wide variety of agents, including G-CSF and GM-CSF (Adams and Cory, 1998; Brach et al., 1992; Van den Berg et al., 2001). Neutrophils are predisposed to cell death by apoptosis. Apoptosis prevents the cytotoxic contents from the neutrophil granules from being released into the surrounding tissues and facilitates the elimination of cells by tissue macrophages. The exact molecular mechanisms underlying apoptosis are unknown, although members of the Bcl-2 protein family and caspases have been shown to be involved in neutrophils (Hengartner, 2000; Moulding et al., 1998; Thornberry and Lazebnik, 1998).

Recent work has demonstrated that these two groups of proteins are intimately connected at the level of mitochondria: the Bcl-2 homologues govern the activity of caspases by exerting their effect through the regulation of the mitochondrial function (Maianski et al., 2002). Proapoptotic Bcl-2 proteins, such as Bax, redistribute from the cytosol to the mitochondria to disturb the mitochondrial membrane integrity by forming channels, which facilitates the subsequent release of cytochrome c and the activation of Apaf-1 and downstream caspases. The antiapoptotic protein Bcl-2 is believed to mediate—at least partially—its effect through the inhibition of Bax redistribution and activity. The family of caspase proteases executes the cleavage of specific targets, which finally leads to cell disassembly and death. Among these proteases, caspase-3 stands out for the large number of substrates that it destroys, including nuclear proteins, cytoplasmic structures, and cytoskeletal elements. The potential of granulocytes to perform certain functional tasks is changed dramatically by these events.

Regarding the role of Bcl-2 proteins in the process of neutrophil apoptosis, one should realize that mature PMN leukocytes were until recently considered to possess no or only few rudimentary mitochondria, which do not play a role in the active life of the cell. We have shown that freshly isolated neutrophils do contain a large number of mitochondria with a characteristic elongated shape, although their functional capacities are still unclear. As previously reported, in vitro aging of neutrophils is accompanied by a progressive loss of functions, such as adherence, chemotaxis, phagocytosis, and the generation of reactive oxygen species (Dransfield et al., 1995). Our own findings in this respect have further indicated that the loss of neutrophil function upon aging is not just a consequence of apoptosis but may precede some early hallmarks of this process. When externalization of phosphatidylserine (PS) lipids to the outer leaflet of the plasma membrane was taken as an early event in the execution phase of apoptosis, about one-third of viable aged neutrophils had already lost the ability to migrate, produce H_2O_2, and phagocytose small particles. Even more cells no longer phagocytose big particles (unpublished). Thus, functional deterioration is a process independent of cell death and often precedes the earliest events of apoptosis. Neutrophils undergoing spontaneous apoptosis in culture dramatically downregulate expression of FcγRIIIb, CD62L, and the seven-span receptors fMLP and CXCR2. In contrast, the reduction in CXCR1 expression is only modest, and CXCR4, which is undetectable on fresh cells, is even upregulated on early apoptotic cells that expose PS (Nagase et al., 2002). Downregulation of chemoattractant receptors on aging and apoptotic neutrophils will likely have dramatic consequences for the trafficking of these cells in vivo. This might reflect mechanisms to prevent the exit of functionally incompetent neutrophils from the circulation and to prevent the exit of these cells from the site of inflammation. The relevance of CXCR4 de novo expression on apoptotic neutrophils remains to be clarified.

In this respect it should be acknowledged that the functional capacity of aging neutrophils can indeed be rescued by both G–CSF and GM–CSF, but at a differential level of efficacy and side effects, rendering G–CSF the growth factor to be preferred for therapeutic use.

Apart from some rare examples of intramedullary apoptosis of myeloid (progenitor) cells in myelodysplasia or Shwachman syndrome, mature circulating neutrophils do not expose PS. Neither in autoimmune neutropenias nor in inflammatory conditions of neutropenia as met during septicemia or severe pneumonia are the neutrophils in the bloodstream engaged in a premature process of cell death. To date, we have observed only in GSD type 1b (GSD1b) that the circulating mature neutrophils are undergoing premature apoptosis (Kuijpers et al., 2003). GSD1b is caused by inherited defects of the glucose-6-phosphate transporter, accompanied by neutropenia and/or neutrophil dysfunction (in chemotaxis, O_2^- generation, and Ca^{2+} mobilization). We now believe that the neutrophil functions in GSD1b may be reduced considerably if not completely by the premature aging of the differentiated neutrophils.

Clearance of Apoptotic Bodies

The impact of PS exposure can only be speculated. Enhanced elimination of not yet fully differentiated myeloid cells by macrophages via the PS receptor most likely occurs in concert with CD14, deposited mannose-binding lectin, and/or complement fragments (Ogura et al., 2001a; Savill and Fadok, 2000). In some of the neutropenic syndromes this is assumed to occur in the environment of the bone marrow prior to neutrophil egress. As demonstrated in our study on GSD1b, the noneliminated neutrophils can be observed in the circulation as the early-apoptotic Annexin-V$^+$ neutrophils that outnumber the late-apoptotic neutrophils with clustered mitochondria and condensed nuclei (Kuijpers et al., 2003). These late-apoptotic neutrophilic bodies are likely to be removed more rapidly than the early-apoptotic cells because of auxiliary binding proteins or receptors in addition to PS on the plasma membrane. Splenomegaly in GSD1b may become apparent only when the spleen is suddenly overloaded by increased clearance of apoptotic cells during infections and/or exaggerated bone marrow production. In case of severe neutropenia, in vivo G–CSF administration may affect splenic size by extramedullary hematopoiesis, sometimes complicated by clinical hypersplenism requiring dose reduction or splenectomy.

Under normal circumstances, neutrophils will be mainly eliminated in the extravascular space. Macrophages and—most likely—tissue cells such as fibroblasts will cooperatively be involved in this process. PS exposure is believed to be insufficient for this process, and additional molecules must be exposed or bound to the surface of apoptotic neutrophils for proper recognition. Because of the large surface area, the disposal of neutrophils in the intestinal tract may also be an important way to both protect the mucosal lining and at the same time discard these potentially harmful cells from the body.

Inflammation or Apoptosis: Yin and Yang?

The above-mentioned NODs, which had been proclaimed—but not proven—to act as intracellular LPS receptors but instead recognize muramylpeptidic PGNs, belong to the so-called nucleotide-binding site and leucine-rich repeat (NBS/LRR) family of proteins. These family members are believed to be critical signaling components regulating at different levels the activation of NF-κB, cytokine processing, and apoptosis. Each family member contains an N-terminal protein–protein interaction domain that mediates assembly with a signaling partner. Nod1 (CARD4), Nod2 (CARD15), and Ipaf/Clan (CARD12) have an N-terminal caspase recruitment domain (CARD) in common with some molecules of the caspase family (human caspase-1, -4, and -5) involved in processing the proforms of IL-1 and IL-18, as well as apoptotic protease-activating factor-1 (APAF-1)-induced clustering of and cytochrome *c*-mediated activation of caspase-9. Together these proteins form a complex in the cell called an apoptosome (Fig. 6A). APAF-1 has, however, a long WD-40 repeat domain instead of the more flexible LRR domains and does not formally belong to the NBS/LRR family of proteins.

Instead of CARD, members of the NBS/LRR family may contain a PYRIN domain, designated after the protein pyrin that is genetically mutated in a fever syndrome known as familial Mediterranean fever (FMF). Because of the structural similarity with APAF-1, Bertin's group has named these members PYPAF1 to -8 (Fiorentino et al., 2002; Harton et al., 2002; Hlaing et al., 2001; Martinon et al., 2002; Shiohara et al., 2002; Wang et al., 2002). PYPAF-1, -5, and -7 are highly expressed in PMN leukocytes; others are more ubiquitously expressed. Furthermore, PYPAF-4 (also called PAN2) has an inhibitory role in NF-κB activation, thus preventing the positive effects of some of the other PYPAFs (Fiorentino et al., 2002). The classical protein called pyrin by itself, and mutated in FMF, may regulate the inflammasome in a negative way (Dowds et al., 2003). Hybrid molecules such as ASC (apoptosis-related speck-like protein) and CARD7 (also known as DEFCAP) have both an N-terminal PYRIN and a C-terminal CARD domain and may function as a docking or adaptor protein,

linking PYRIN-PYRIN domains as well as conveying CARD-CARD interactions (Hlaing et al., 2001; Shiohara et al., 2002). The interactions between these protein domains constitute molecular structures, such as the so-called inflammasome (Martinon et al., 2002), a molecular platform for some of the above-mentioned cellular functions (Fig. 6B). An alternative molecular mechanism underlying procaspase-1 processing involves interaction between the CARD domains of caspase-1 and a serine-threonine kinase RIP2. RIP2 can interact with TRAF6 (see Fig. 4) or Nod1 (and Nod2). The consequence of these CARD interactions is that Nod1 enhances procaspase-1 oligomerization and processing, thus enhancing caspase-1-induced IL-1β secretion. Two CARD-containing inhibitors of caspase-1 have been identified as Pseudo-ICE and ICEBERG. Both proteins closely resemble caspase-1 in its prodomain, bind to both caspase-1 and RIP2, and prevent further active processing (Green and Melino, 2001).

Many of these NBS/LRR family members are predominantly or even selectively expressed in neutrophils and/or monocytes. The mechanism or ligands—either extracellular or intracellular—that activate these proteins to function as an inflammasome are as yet unclear. These protein platforms may play a role in switching from an initially proinflammatory reaction to an anti-inflammatory response by programmed cell death required for the resolution of inflammation, as suggested by the clinical features of the group of inherited fever and autoinflammatory syndromes that have been genetically characterized to date (Aganna et al., 2002; Dodé et al., 2002; Feldmann et al., 2002; Hoffman et al., 2001; Hugot et al., 2001; Miceli-Richard et al., 2001; Ogura et al., 2001a; French FMF Consortium, 1997; International FMF Consortium, 1997). Although speculative, defects in these tightly organized switches in the innate neutrophil response may result in overexaggerated reactivity and collateral damage as observed during sepsis or severe tissue damage.

CONCLUDING REMARKS

In the first phase of inflammatory responses or other forms of stress, chemotaxins such as C5a, lipid mediators, and so-called chemokines are produced. The secretion of chemokines can be firmly induced by the proinflammatory cytokines derived from tissue macrophages and T cells, such as TNF-α, IL-1β and gamma interferon, or by bacterial products such as fMLP, LPS, LTA and PGNs.

The cellular composition and duration of an inflammatory response may differ among the different inflammatory reactions (e.g., bacterial versus parasitic infection, allergy, delayed-

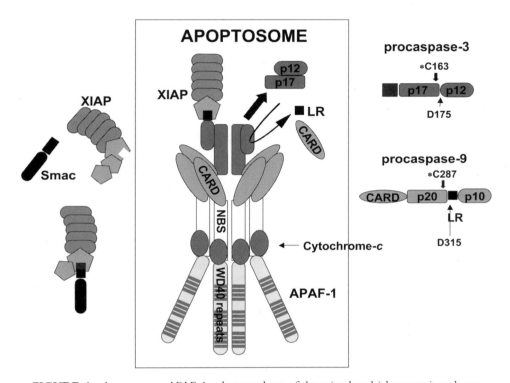

FIGURE 6 Apoptosome. APAF-1, a key regulator of the mitochondrial apoptosis pathway, contains three functional regions: an N-terminal CARD that can bind to procaspase-9; a CED-4-like region enabling self-oligomerization; and a regulatory C terminus with so-called WD-40 repeats masking the CARD and CED-4 region. During apoptosis, cytochrome *c* is released from the mitochondrial intermembranous space and, together with dATP, can relieve the inhibitory action of the WD-40 repeats to enable the oligomerization of APAF-1 and the subsequent recruitment and activation of procaspase-9 in a so-called apoptosome. Catalytically active processed caspase-9 or inactive unprocessed caspase-9 initially binds to the APAF-1 apoptosome and recruits caspase-3 via an interaction between the active-site cysteine (C287) in caspase-9 and a critical aspartate (D175) in caspase-3. XIAP, an X-linked member of the inhibitor of apoptosis protein family, is normally present in the cytosol but directly interacts with the "active" apoptosome to associate with oligomerized and processed caspase-9 and thus indirectly as well as directly influences the activation of caspase-3. Progression of apoptosis depends on (i) simultaneous release of Smac/DIABLO from the mitochondria into the cytosol, competing XIAP away from its association with processed caspase-9, thereby allowing caspase-9 to activate caspase; and (ii) caspase-3 cleavage of the XIAP-binding linker region (LR), resulting in the progression of inevitable apoptosis through further activating steps and cleavage of intracellular substrates. (*Continued next page*)

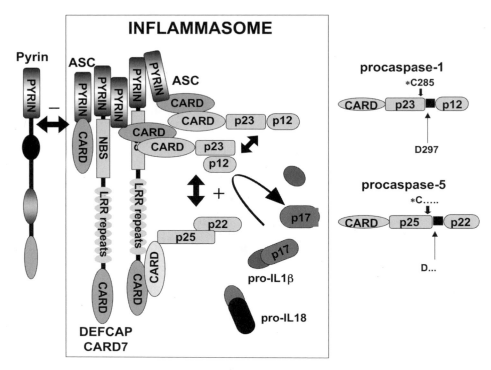

FIGURE 6 *(continued)* Inflammasome(s). Generation of IL-1β and IL-18 via cleavage of its proform requires the activity of an interleukin-converting enzyme (ICE), also known as the CARD-containing caspase-1. The precise mechanism involved in the activation of the proinflammatory caspases remains elusive, but the available data suggest that a high-molecular-weight caspase-activating complex comprises caspase-1, caspase-5, apoptosis-signaling complex (ASC or Pycard), and CARD7 (NALP1 or DEFCAP), both PYRIN and CARD domain-containing proteins sharing structural homology with the cytosolic NODs (NOD-1 and -2). This protein platform (inflammasome) in the cytosol of phagocytes is able to induce pro-IL-1β maturation through the proximity-driven cross-activation of inflammatory caspases, induced by inflammatory triggers such as LPS. The p45 precursor form of caspase-1 (which contains four cleavage sites) is activated, leading to formation of protein subunits (p10 and p20) that are flanked by Asp-X bonds. It is most conceivable that the proenzyme is activated autocatalytically. The active site of caspase-1 at Cys-285 can cleave the 31-kDa precursor protein pro-IL-1β at Asp116-Ala117, whereby it creates the 17.5-kDa mature, biologically active cytokine. Among the rapidly expanding families of proteins containing either or both of these domains, the PYRIN as well as the CARD domain can create interactions between different family members. The classical protein called pyrin by itself, and mutated in FMF (see text), may regulate the inflammasome negatively. Thus, the function of these large complexes depends on the ability of additional CARD or PYRIN domain-containing proteins to regulate the degree of activation. The CARD-containing caspase-9 is thought to propagate a death signal by triggering other caspase activation in response to cytochrome *c*-mediated events, such as the additional caspases (caspase-2, -3, -6, -7, -8, and -10), in which caspase-3 is required for the activation of the four other caspases (-2, -6, -8, and -10) in a feedback amplification loop. In contrast, the CARD-containing caspase-1, -4, and -5 fail to be activated under the same conditions and seem restricted to the inflammatory loop of cytokine release and proinflammatory activity.

type hypersensitivity reaction). The process of recruitment is complex and still incompletely understood. Once recruited, the neutrophils have a wide range of toxic mechanisms to fight any invading microorganism, as described. These mechanisms are strongly regulated and delicately controlled because an overexcessive or premature induction of the toxic activities may result in the inactivation of protease inhibitors and activation of several cascades of activating substances (e.g., the coagulation, the fibrinolytic, and the complement systems). As a consequence, bacteremia may progress to septic shock and disseminated intravascular coagulation, a community-acquired pneumonia may develop into acute or adult respiratory distress syndrome, and hypoxia or reperfusion injury can lead to fatal circulatory collapse.

In conclusion, neutrophils are very useful but also very dangerous tools to protect the host from bacterial and fungal infections.

REFERENCES

Adams, M. J., and S. Cory. 1998. The Bcl-2 protein family: arbiters of cell survival. *Science* **281:**1322–1326.

Aganna, E., F. Martinon, P. N. Hawkins, J. B. Ross, D. C. Swan, D. R. Booth, H. J. Lachmann, R. Gaudet, P. Woo, C. Feighery, F. E. Cotter, M. Thome, G. A. Hitman, J. Tschopp, and M. F. McDermott. 2002. Association of mutations in the NALP3/CIAS1/PYPAF1 gene with a broad phenotype including recurrent fever, cold sensitivity, sensorineural deafness, and AA amyloidosis. *Arthritis Rheum.* **46:**2445–2452.

Akira, S., K. Takeda, and T. Kaisho. 2001. Toll-like receptors: critical proteins linking innate and acquired immunity. *Nat. Immunol.* **2:**675–680.

Ambruso, D. R., C. Knall, A. N. Abell, J. Panepinto, A. Kurkchubasche, G. Thurman, C. Gonzalez-Aller, A. Hiester, M. de Boer, R. J. Harbeck, R. Oyer, G. L. Johnson, and D. Roos. 2000. Human neutrophil immunodeficiency syndrome is associated with an inhibitory Rac2 mutation. *Proc. Natl. Acad. Sci. USA* **97:**4654–4659.

Anderson, K. L., K. A. Smith, H. Perkin, G. Hermanson, C. G. Anderson, D. J. Jolly, R. A. Maki, and B. E. Torbett. 1999. PU.1 and the granulocyte- and macrophage colony-stimulating factor receptors play distinct roles in late-stage myeloid cell differentiation. *Blood* **94:**2310–2318.

Arbibe, L., J. P. Mira, N. Teusch, L. Kline, M. Guha, N. Mackman, P. J. Godowski, R. J.

Ulevitch, and U. G. Knaus. 2000. Toll-like receptor 2-mediated NF-kappa B activation requires a Rac1-dependent pathway. *Nat. Immunol.* **1:**533–540.

Aurrand-Lions, M., C. Johnson-Leger, and B. Imhof. 2002. The last molecular fortress in leukocyte trans-endothelial migration. *Nat. Immunol.* **3:**116–118.

Barclay, A. N., G. J. Wright, G. Brooke, and M. H. Brown. 2002. CD200 and membrane protein interactions in the control of myeloid cells. *Trends Immunol.* **23:**285–290.

Belaaouaj, A., R. McCarthy, M. Baumann, Z. Gao, T. J. Ley, S. N. Abraham, and S. D. Shapiro. 1998. Mice lacking neutrophil elastase reveal impaired host defense against gram negative bacterial sepsis. *Nat. Med.* **4:**615–618.

Betsuyaku, T., F. Liu, R. M. Senior, J. S. Haug, E. J. Brown, S. L. Jones, K. Matsushima, and D. C. Link. 1999. A functional granulocyte colony-stimulating factor receptor is required for normal chemoattractant-induced neutrophil activation. *J. Clin. Invest.* **103:**825–832.

Bokoch, G. M. 1996. Chemoattractant signalling and leukocyte activation. *Blood* **86:**1649–1660.

Bouchon, A., F. Facchetti, M. A. Welgand, and M. Colonna. 2001. TREM-1 amplifies inflammation and is a crucial mediator of septic shock. *Nature* **410:**1103–1107.

Brach, M. A., S. deVos, H. J. Gruss, and F. Herrmann. 1992. Prolongation of survival of human polymorphonuclear neutrophils by granulocyte-macrophage colony-stimulating factor is caused by inhibition of programmed cell death. *Blood* **80:**2920–2924.

Bruhns, P., F. Vely, O. Malbec, W. H. Fridman, E. Vivier, and M. Daeron. 2000. Insufficient phosphorylation prevents FcγRIIB from recruiting the SH2 domain-containing protein tyrosine phosphatase SHP-1. *J. Biol. Chem.* **275:**37357–37364.

Chamaillard, M., M. Hashimoto, Y. Horie, J. Masumoto, S. Qiu, L. Saab, Y. Ogura, A. Kawasaki, K. Fukase, S. Kusumoto, M. A. Valvano, S. J. Foster, T. W. Mak, G. Nunez, and N. Inohara. 2003. An essential role for NOD1 in host recognition of bacterial peptidoglycan containing diaminopimelic acid. *Nat. Immunol.* **4:**702–707.

Dale, D. C., R. E. Person, A. A. Boylard, A. G. Aprikyan, C. Bos, M. A. Bonilla, L. A. Boxer, G. Kanourakis, C. Zeidler, K. Welte, K. F. Benson, and M. Horwitz. 2000. Mutations in the gene encoding neutrophil elastase in congenital and cyclic neutropenia. *Blood* **96:**2317–2322.

Daws, M. R., L. L. Lanier, W. R. Seaman, and J. C. Ryan. 2001. Cloning and characterization of a novel mouse myeloid DAP12-associated receptor family. *Eur. J. Immunol.* **31:**783–791.

Dodé, C., N. Le Du, L. Cuisset, F. Letourneur, J. M. Berthelot, G. Vaudour, A. Meyrier, R. A.

Watts, D. G. Scott, A. Nicholls, B. Granel, C. Frances, F. Garcier, P. Edery, S. Boulinguez, J. P. Domergues, M. Delpech, and G. Grateau. 2002. New mutations of CIAS1 that are responsible for Muckle-Wells syndrome and familial cold urticaria: a novel mutation underlies both syndromes. *Am. J. Hum. Genet.* **70**:1498–1506.

Dong, F., D. C. Dale, M. A. Bonilla, M. Freedman, A. A. Fasth, H. J. Neijens, J. Palmblad, G. L. Briars, G. Carlsson, A. J. Veerman, K. Welte, B. Lowenberg, and I. P. Touw. 1997. Mutations in the granulocyte colony-stimulating factor receptor gene in patients with severe congenital neutropenia. *Leukemia* **11**:120–125.

Dowds, T. A., J. Masumoto, F. F. Chen, Y. Ogura, N. Inohara, and G. Nunez. 2003. Regulation of cryopyrin/Pypaf1 signaling by pyrin, the familial Mediterranean fever gene product. *Biochem. Biophys. Res. Commun.* **302**:575–580.

Dransfield, I., S. C. Stocks, and C. Haslett. 1995. Regulation of cell adhesion molecule expression and function associated with neutrophil apoptosis. *Blood* **85**:3264–3273.

Feldmann, J., A. Prieur, P. Quartier, P. Berquin, E. Cortis, D. Teillac-Hamel, A. Fischer, and G. de Saint Basile. 2002. Chronic infantile neurological cutaneous and articular syndrome is caused by mutations in CIAS1, a gene highly expressed in polymorphonuclear cells and chondrocytes. *Am. J. Hum. Genet.* **70**:198–203.

Fiorentino, L., C. Stehlik, V. Oliveira, M. E. Ariza, A. Godzik, and J. C. Reed. 2002. A novel PAAD-containing protein that modulates NF-kappa B induction by cytokines tumor necrosis factor-alpha and interleukin-1beta. *J. Biol. Chem.* **277**:35333–35340.

Fitzgerald, K. A., E. M. Palsson-McDermott, A. G. Bowie, C. A. Jefferies, A. S. Mansell, G. Brady, E. Brint, A. Dunne, P. Gray, M. T. Harte, D. McMurray, D. E. Smith, J. E. Sims, T. A. Bird, and L. A. O'Neill. 2001. Mal (MyD88-adapter-like) is required for Toll-like receptor-4 signal transduction. *Nature* **413**:78–83.

French FMF Consortium. 1997. A candidate gene for familial Mediterranean fever. *Nat. Genet.* **17**:25–31.

Girardin, S. E., I. G. Boneca, L. A. Carneiro, A. Antignac, M. Jehanno, J. Viala, K. Tedin, M. K. Taha, A. Labigne, U. Zathringer, A. J. Coyle, P. S. DiStefano, J. Bertin, P. J. Sansonetti, and D. J. Philpott. 2003a. Nod1 detects a unique muropeptide from gram-negative bacterial peptidoglycan. *Science* **300**:1584–1587.

Girardin, S. E., I. G. Boneca, J. Viala, M. Chamaillard, A. Labigne, G. Thomas, D. J. Philpott, and P. J. Sansonetti. 2003b. Nod2 is a general sensor of peptidoglycan through muramyl dipeptide (MDP) detection. *J. Biol. Chem.* **278**:8869–8872.

Green, D. R., and G. Melino. 2001. ICE heats up. *Cell Death Differ.* **8**:549–550.

Gutierrez, O., C. Pipaon, N. Inohara, A. Fontalba, Y. Ogura, F. Prosper, G. Nunez, and J. L. Fernandez-Luna. 2002. Induction of Nod2 in myelomonocytic and intestinal epithelial cells via nuclear factor-kappa B activation. *J. Biol. Chem.* **277**:41701–41705.

Harton, J. A., M. W. Linhoff, J. Zhang, and J. P. Ting. 2002. CATERPILLER: a large family of mammalian genes containing CARD, pyrin, nucleotide-binding, and leucine-rich repeat domains. *J. Immunol.* **169**:4088–4093.

Hengartner, M. O. 2000. The biochemistry of apoptosis. *Nature* **407**:770–776.

Hirschfeld, M., Y. Ma, J. H. Weis, S. N. Vogel, and J. J. Weis. 2000. Cutting edge: repurification of lipopolysaccharide eliminates signaling through both human and murine toll-like receptor 2. *J. Immunol.* **165**:618–622.

Hlaing, T., R. F. Guo, K. A. Dilley, J. M. Loussia, T. A. Morrish, M. M. Shi, C. Vincenz, and P. A. Ward. 2001. Molecular cloning and characterization of DEFCAP-L and -S, two isoforms of a novel member of the mammalian Ced-4 family of apoptosis proteins. *J. Biol. Chem.* **276**:9230–9238.

Hoffman, H. M., J. L. Mueller, D. H. Broide, A. A. Wanderer, and R. D. Kolodner. 2001. Mutation of a new gene encoding a putative pyrin-like protein causes familial cold autoinflammatory syndrome and Muckle-Wells syndrome. *Nat. Genet.* **29**:301–305.

Horng, T., G. M. Barton, and R. Medzhitov. 2001. TIRAP: an adapter molecule in the Toll signaling pathway. *Nat. Immunol.* **2**:835–841.

Hugot, J. P., M. Chamaillard, H. Zouali, S. Lesage, J. P. Cezard, J. Belaiche, S. Almer, C. Tysk, C. A. O'Morain, M. Gassull, V. Binder, Y. Finkel, A. Cortot, R. Modigliani, P. Laurent-Puig, C. Gower-Rousseau, J. Macry, J. F. Colombel, M. M. Sahbatou, and G. Thomas. 2001. Association of NOD2 leucine-rich repeat variants with susceptibility to Crohn's disease. *Nature* **411**:599–603.

Huizinga, T. W., M. de Haas, M. H. van Oers, M. Kleijer, H. Vile, P. A. van der Wouw, A. Moulijn, H. van Weezel, D. Roos, and A. E. von dem Borne. 1994. The plasma concentration of soluble Fc-gamma RIII is related to production of neutrophils. *Br. J. Haematol.* **87**:459–463.

Ingalls, R. R., H. Heine, E. Lien, A. Yoshimura, and D. Golenbock. 1999. Lipopolysaccharide recognition, CD14, and lipopolysaccharide receptors. *Infect. Dis. Clin. North Am.* **13**:341–353.

Inohara, N., T. Koseki, L. del Peso, Y. Hu, C. Yee, S. Chen, R. Carrio, J. Merino, D. Liu, J. Ni, and G. Nunez. 1999. Nod1, an Apaf-1-like activator of caspase-9 and nuclear factor kB. *J. Biol. Chem.* **274:** 14560–14567.

Inohara, N., Y. Ogura, A. Fontalba, O. Gutierrez, F. Pons, J. Crespo, K. Fukase, S. Inamura, S. Kusumoto, M. Hashimoto, S. J. Foster, A. P. Moran, J. L. Fernandez-Luna, and G. Nunez. 2003. Host recognition of bacterial muramyl dipeptide mediated through NOD2. Implications for Crohn's disease. *J. Biol. Chem.* **278:**5509–5512.

International FMF Consortium. 1997. Ancient missense mutations in a new member of the RoRet gene family are likely to cause familial Mediterranean fever. *Cell* **90:**797–807.

Kasper, B., N. Tidow, D. Grothues, and K. Welte. 2000. Differential expression and regulation of GTPases (RhoA and Rac2) and GDIs (LyGDI and RhoGDI) in neutrophils from patients with severe congenital neutropenia. *Blood* **95:**2947–2953.

Kawai, T., O. Adachi, T. Ogawa, K. Takeda, and S. Akira. 1999. Unresponsiveness of MyD88 deficient mice to endotoxin. *Immunity* **11:**115–122.

Kobayashi, K., L. D. Hernandez, J. E. Galan, C. A. Janeway, Jr., R. Medzhitov, and R. A. Flavell. 2002. IRAK-M is a negative regulator of Toll-like receptor signaling. *Cell* **110:**191–202.

Kuijpers, T. W. 2002. Clinical symptoms and neutropenia: the balance of neutrophil development, functional activity, and cell death. *Eur. J. Pediatr.* **161:**S75–S82.

Kuijpers, T. W., B. C. Hakkert, M. H. Hart, and D. Roos. 1992. Neutrophil migration across monolayers of cytokine-prestimulated endothelial cells: a role for platelet-activating factor and IL-8. *J. Cell Biol.* **117:**565–572.

Kuijpers, T. W., N. A. Maianski, A. T. Tool, G. P. Smit, J. P. Rake, D. Roos, and G. Visser. 2003. The presence of apoptotic neutrophils in the circulation of patients with Glycogen Storage Disease type 1b (GSD1b). *Blood* **101:**5021–5024.

Kurt-Jones, E. A., L. Mandell, C. Whitney, A. Padgett, K. Gosselin, P. E. Newburger, and R. W. Finberg. 2002. Role of toll-like receptor 2 (TLR2) in neutrophil activation: GM-CSF enhances TLR2 expression and TLR2-mediated interleukin 8 responses in neutrophils. *Blood* **100:**1860–1868.

Kyogoku, C., H. M. Dijstelbloem, N. Tsuchiya, Y. Hatta, H. Kato, A. Yamaguchi, T. Fukazawa, M. D. Jansen, H. Hashimoto, J. G. van de Winkel, C. G. Kallenberg, and K. Tokunaga. 2002. Fcgamma receptor gene polymorphisms in Japanese patients with systemic lupus erythematosus: contribution of FCGR2B to genetic susceptibility. *Arthritis Rheum.* **46:**1242–1254.

Lekstrom-Himes, J. A., S. E. Dorman, P. Kopar, S. M. Holland, and J. I. Gallin. 1999. Neutrophil-specific granule deficiency results from a novel mutation with loss of function of the transcription factor CCAAT/enhancer binding protein epsilon. *J. Exp. Med.* **189:**1847–1852.

Liu, F., H. F. Wu, R. Wesselschmidt, T. Kornaga, and D. C. Link. 1996. Impaired production and increased apoptosis of neutrophils in granulocyte colony-stimulating factor receptor-deficient mice. *Immunity* **5:**491–501.

Liu, Y., H. J. Buhring, K. Zen, S. L. Burts, F. J. Schnell, I. R. Williams, and C. A. Parkos. 2002. Signal regulatory protein (SIRPα), a cellular ligand for CD47, regulates neutrophil transmigration. *J. Biol. Chem.* **277:**10028–10036.

Loike, J. D., L. Cao, S. Budhu, E. E. Marcantonio, J. El Khoury, S. Hoffman, T. A. Yednock, and S. C. Silverstein. 1999. Differential regulation of beta 1 integrins by chemoattractants regulates neutrophil migration through fibrin. *J. Cell Biol.* **144:**1047–1056.

Maianski, N. A., F. P. Mul, J. D. van Buul, D. Roos, and T. W. Kuijpers. 2002. Granulocyte Colony-Stimulating factor (G-CSF) inhibits in neutrophils the mitochondria-dependent activation of Caspase-3. *Blood* **99:**672–679.

Malech, H. L., and W. M. Nauseef. 1997. Primary inherited defects in neutrophil function: etiology and treatment. *Semin. Hematol.* **34:**279–290.

Martinon, F., K. Burns, and J. Tschopp. 2002. The inflammasome: a molecular platform triggering activation of inflammatory caspases and processing of proIL-beta. *Mol. Cell* **10:**417–426.

Miceli-Richard, C., S. Lesage, M. Rybojad, A. M. Prieur, S. Manouvrier-Hanu, R. Hafner, M. Chamaillard, H. Zouali, G. Thomas, and J. P. Hugot. 2001. CARD15 mutations in Blau syndrome. *Nat. Genet.* **29:**19–20.

Moulding, D. A., J. A. Quayle, C. A. Hart, and S. W. Edwards. 1998. Mcl-1 expression in human neutrophils: regulation by cytokines and correlation with cell survival. *Blood* **92:**2495–2502.

Murdoch, C., and A. Finn. 2000. Chemokine receptors and their role in inflammation and infectious diseases. *Blood* **95:**3032–3043.

Nagase, H., M. Miyamasu, M. Yamaguchi, M. Imanishi, N. H. Tsuno, K. Matsushima, K. Yamamoto, Y. Morita, and K. Hirai. 2002. Cytokine-mediated regulation of CXCR4 expression in human neutrophils. *J. Leukoc. Biol.* **71:**711–717.

Netea, M. G., M. van Deuren, B. J. Kullberg, J. M. Cavaillon, and J. W. van der Meer. 2002. Does the shape of lipid A determine the interaction of LPS with Toll-like receptors? *Trends Immunol.* **23:**135–139.

Ogden, C. A., A. deCathelineau, P. R. Hoffmann, D. Bratton, B. Ghebrehiwet, V. A. Fadok, and P. M. Henson. 2001. C1q and mannose binding lectin engagement of cell surface calreticulin and CD91 initiates macropinocytosis and uptake of apoptotic cells. *J. Exp. Med.* **194:**781–795.

Ogura, Y., D. K. Bonen, N. Inohara, D. L. Nicolae, F. F. Chen, R. Ramos, H. Britton, T. Moran, R. Karaliuskas, R. H. Duerr, J. P. Achkar,

S. R. Brant, T. M. Bayless, B. S. Kirschner, S. B. Hanauer, G. Nunez, and J. H. Cho. 2001a. A frameshift mutation in NOD2 associated with susceptibility to Crohn's disease. *Nature* **411:**603–606.

Ogura, Y., N. Inohara, A. Benito, F. F. Chen, S. Yamaoka, and G. Nunez. 2001b. Nod2, a Nod1/Apaf-1 family member that is restricted to monocytes and activates NF-kB. *J. Biol. Chem.* **276:**4812–4818.

Oldenborg, P. A., A. Zheleznyak, Y. F. Fang, C. F. Lagenaur, H. D. Gresham, and F. P. Lindberg. 2000. Role of CD47 as a marker of self on red blood cells. *Science* **288:**2051–2054.

Ozinsky, A., D. M. Underhill, J. D. Fontenot, A. M. Hajjar, K. D. Smith, C. B. Wilson, L. Schroeder, and A. Aderem. 2000. The repertoire for pattern recognition of pathogens by the innate immune system is defined by cooperation between toll-like receptors. *Proc. Natl. Acad. Sci. USA* **97:**13766–13771.

Pearse, R. N., T. Kawabe, S. Bolland, R. Guinamard, T. Kurosaki, and J. V. Ravetch. 1999. SHIP recruitment attenuates Fc gamma RIIB-induced B cell apoptosis. *Immunity* **10:**753–760.

Poltorak, A., X. He, I. Smirnova, M. Y. Liu, C. V. Huffel, X. Du, D. Birdwell, E. Alejos, M. Silva, C. Galanos, M. Freudenberg, P. Ricciardi-Castagnol, B. Layton, and B. Beutler. 1998. Defective LPS signaling in C3H/HeJ and C57BL/10ScCr mice: mutations in Tlr4 gene. *Science* **282:**2085–2088.

Ravetch, J. V., and S. Bolland. 2001. IgG Fc receptors. *Annu. Rev. Immunol.* **19:**275–290.

Ravetch, J. V., and L. L. Lanier. 2000. Immune inhibitory receptors. *Science* **290:**84–89.

Reeves, E. P., H. Lu, H. L. Jacobs, C. G. Messina, S. Bolsover, G. Gabella, E. O. Potma, A. Warley, J. Roes, and A. W. Segal. 2002. Killing activity of neutrophils is mediated through activation of proteases by K+ flux. *Nature* **416:**291–297.

Roos, D., and J. T. Curnutte. 1999. Chronic granulomatous disease, p. 353–374. *In* H. D. Ochs, C. I. E. Smith, and J. M. Puck (ed.), *Primary Immunodeficiency Diseases. A Molecular and Genetic Approach.* Oxford University Press, New York, N.Y.

Sabroe, I., E. C. Jones, L. R. Usher, M. K. Whyte, and S. K. Dower. 2002. Toll-like receptor (TLR)2 and TLR4 in human peripheral blood granulocytes: a critical role for monocytes in leukocyte lipopolysaccharide responses. *J. Immunol.* **168:**4701–4710.

Savill, J., and V. Fadok. 2000. Corpse clearance defines the meaning of cell death. *Nature* **407:**784–788.

Shimazu, R., S. Akashi, H. Ogata, Y. Nagai, K. Fukudome, K. Miyake, and M. Kimoto. 1999. MD-2, a molecule that confers lipopolysaccharide responsiveness on Toll-like receptor 4. *J. Exp. Med.* **189:**1777–1782.

Shiohara, M., S. Taniguchi, J. Masumoto, K. Yasui, K. Koike, A. Komiyama, and J. Sagara. 2002. ASC, which is composed of a PYD and a CARD, is up-regulated by inflammation and apoptosis in human neutrophils. *Biochem. Biophys. Res. Commun.* **293:**1314–1318.

Springer, T. A. 1994. Traffic signals for lymphocyte recirculation and leukocyte emigration: the multistep paradigm. *Cell* **76:**301–314.

Suzuki, N., S. Suzuki, G. S. Duncan, D. G. Millar, T. Wada, C. Mirtsos, H. Takada, A. Wakeham, A. Itie, S. Li, J. M. Penninger, H. Wesche, P. S. Ohashi, T. W. Mak, and W. C. Yeh. 2002. Severe impairment of interleukin-1 and Toll-like receptor signalling in mice lacking IRAK-4. *Nature* **416:**750–756.

Thornberry, N. A., and Y. Lazebnik. 1998. Caspases: enemies within. *Science* **281:**1312–1316.

Van den Berg, J. M., S. Weyer, J. J. Weening, D. Roos, and T. W. Kuijpers. 2001. Divergent effects of tumor necrosis factor alpha on apoptosis of human neutrophils. *J. Leukoc. Biol.* **69:**467–473.

Visintin, A., A. Mazzoni, J. H. Spitzer, D. H. Wyllie, S. K. Dower, and D. M. Segal. 2001. Regulation of toll-like receptors in human monocytes and dendritic cells. *J. Immunol.* **166:**249–255.

Wang, L., G. A. Manji, J. M. Grenier, A. Al-Garawi, S. Merriam, J. M. Lora, B. J. Geddes, M. Briskin, P. S. DiStefano, and J. Bertin. 2002. PYPAF7, a novel PYRIN-containing Apaf1-like protein that regulates activation of NF-kappa B and caspase-1-dependent cytokine processing. *J. Biol. Chem.* **277:**29874–29880.

Weiss, S. J. 1989. Tissue destruction by neutrophils. *N. Engl. J. Med.* **320:**365–376.

Young, N. T., and M. Uhrberg. 2002. KIR expression shapes cytotoxic repertoires: a developmental program of survival. *Trends Immunol.* **23:**71–75.

Zeidler, C., L. A. Boxer, D. C. Dale, M. Freedman, S. Kinsey, and K. Welte. 2000. Management of Kostmann syndrome in the G-CSF era. *Br. J. Hematol.* **109:**490–495.

Zhang, P., A. Iwama, M. W. Datta, G. J. Darlington, D. C. Link, and D. G. Tenen. 1998. Upregulation of interleukin 6 and granulocyte colony-stimulating factor receptors by transcription factor CCAAT enhancer binding protein alpha (C/EBP alpha) is critical for granulopoiesis. *J. Exp. Med.* **188:**1173–1184.

THE BIOLOGY OF MACROPHAGES

R. Tedjo Sasmono and David A. Hume

4

Macrophages are much more than the big eaters implied by their name. Metchnikoff (1893) was the first person to use the term "macrophage" to describe a large cell able to take up microorganisms (Tauber and Chernyak, 1991). Asschoff (1924) later assigned these cells to the reticuloendothelial system (RES), which included reticular cells, endothelial cells, fibroblasts, histiocytes, and monocytes (Auger and Ross, 1992). The RES term was replaced by the term mononuclear phagocytes system (MPS) when it was recognized that a subset of these RES cells derive from bone marrow precursors (van Furth et al., 1972). The MPS family of cells comprises bone marrow progenitor cells, promonocytes, peripheral blood monocytes, and tissue macrophages.

Macrophages are part of the innate immune system, recognizing, engulfing, and destroying many potential pathogens including bacteria, pathogenic protozoa, fungi, and helminths. Macrophages can also recognize syngeneic tumor cells and some virus-infected cells as well as normal cells undergoing programmed cell death (apoptosis) (Auger and Ross, 1992;

Henson et al., 2001). Aside from their roles in primary innate immunity, macrophages function as regulator and effector cells in both humoral and cell-mediated immune responses (Morrissette et al., 1999). Upon phagocytosis, macrophages degrade proteins and process the antigens for presentation on major histocompatibility complex (MHC) molecules, where T cells can recognize the substances as "foreign" (Unanue and Allen, 1986; Underhill et al., 1999). When activated in an immune response, macrophages acquire microbicidal and tumoricidal activities involving reactive-oxygen species and reactive-nitrogen metabolites (Adam and Hamilton, 1984; Fang and Vazquez-Torres, 2002; Nathan and Hibbs, 1991).

The destructive potential of macrophages and their ability to secrete regulators of the function of neighboring cells contribute to many aspects of homeostasis. For example, within the bone marrow and spleen, macrophages engulf expelled nuclei of mature red cells and contribute to the control of hematopoiesis by their secretion of a wide range of cytokines and also by a contact-mediated mechanism (Crocker and Milon, 1992; Sadahira and Mori, 1999). During embryonic development, macrophages play an important role in scavenging dying cells and clearing

R. Tedjo Sasmono and David A. Hume, Institute for Molecular Bioscience, The University of Queensland, St. Lucia Q4072, Australia.

The Innate Immune Response to Infection
Ed. by S. H. E. Kaufmann, R. Medzhitov, and S. Gordon
©2004 ASM Press, Washington, D.C.

areas of programmed cell death and thereby contribute to organogenesis (Hopkinson-Woolley et al., 1994; Lichanska and Hume, 2000). These functions are maintained in the adult, where the macrophage lineage is intimately involved in wound healing, tissue repair, and bone remodeling (Morrissette et al., 1999; Opdenakker and Van Damme, 1992; Shapiro et al., 1991; Wilson, 1997). Macrophages are also important in many aspects of homeostasis, for example, in the metabolism of cholesterol (de Villiers et al., 1998).

The diversity of functions of macrophages provides a link between innate and acquired immunity and the numerous physiological changes that contribute to host defense. Conversely, dysregulated macrophage function causes much of the pathology of infectious, inflammatory, and malignant diseases. In this chapter, we consider the origins, differentiation, and functions of macrophages throughout the body. We place particular emphasis on the mouse as an experimental model.

MACROPHAGE DIFFERENTIATION

The cells of the MPS are derived from pluripotent hematopoietic stem cells in bone marrow that further differentiate into monoblasts, promonocytes, and monocytes and mature to become tissue macrophages (van Furth et al., 1972). Optimal proliferation and differentiation of mononuclear phagocytes from pluripotent progenitors require the presence of a combination of polypeptide growth factors. These include macrophage colony-stimulating factor (M-CSF or CSF-1), granulocyte-macrophage colony-stimulating factor (GM-CSF), interleukin-6 (IL-6), IL-3, stem cell factor, IL-1, leukemia inhibitory factor, and gamma interferon (IFN-γ) (Lee, 1992; Metcalf, 1989, 1997; Wiktor-Jedrzejczak and Gordon, 1996). Of these, CSF-1 is the only factor that is absolutely required for macrophage differentiation and proliferation in vivo; and as the sole added factor, CSF-1 can also direct macrophage differentiation from bone marrow progenitors in vitro (Cecchini et al., 1994; Hume and Gordon,

1983b; Hume et al., 1988; Stanley et al., 1997; Tushinski et al., 1982).

Homozygous mutation of the CSF-1 gene in the osteopetrotic ($Csf1^{op}/Csf1^{op}$) mice (Wiktor-Jedrzejczak et al., 1990; Yoshida et al., 1990) produces viable mice in which bone resorption is impaired, causing defective formation of marrow cavity (osteopetrosis). This deficiency is due to a reduced number of multinucleated osteoclasts, which are formed from common progenitors to macrophages. $Csf1^{op}/Csf1^{op}$ mice are also deficient in macrophage numbers in most tissues. Some populations are unaffected, such as bone marrow monocytes and macrophages in lymph nodes and thymus (Cecchini et al., 1994), suggesting that CSF-1-independent macrophage populations exist (Cecchini et al., 1994; Felix et al., 1990; Umeda et al., 1996; Wiktor-Jedrzejczak et al., 1990; Wiktor-Jedrzejczak and Gordon, 1996; Yoshida et al., 1990). Perhaps reflecting the importance of macrophages in development, $Csf1^{op}/Csf1^{op}$ mice also have developmental defects of the nervous and reproductive systems (Cohen et al., 1999; Michaelson et al., 1996; Naito et al., 1991). The osteopetrotic phenotype and macrophage/osteoclast deficiency in these mice spontaneously recover with age, probably because of the actions of Flt-3 ligand and/or the vascular endothelial growth factor (VEGF-A) (Niida et al., 1999), which can act on macrophages through the *fms*-like receptor tyrosine kinases Flt-1 (Neufeld et al., 1999) and Flt-3 (Lean et al., 2001). Mice with a targeted disruption of CSF-1 receptor encoded by the c-*fms* proto-oncogene ($Csf1r^-/Csf1r^-$) have been described (Dai et al., 2002).

The phenotypic features of these mice clearly recapitulate the CSF-1 mutant mice in that they have an osteopetrotic phenotype, mononuclear phagocyte deficiency, and reproductive defects (Dai et al., 2002). The effect of the c-*fms* mutation appeared to be more severe than the CSF-1 mutation in $Csf1^{op}/Csf1^{op}$ mice, but contributions of genetic background are likely. There is anecdotal evidence (unpublished, and J. W. Pollard, personal communication) that the CSF-1 mutation cannot be bred onto certain inbred mouse genetic backgrounds, which presumably differ in their ability to produce compensatory growth factors such as VEGF-A or the Flt-3 ligand. Whatever the subtleties, the phenotype of the c-*fms*-deficient mouse demonstrates that CSF-1 action is indeed mediated through binding to its receptor encoded by the c-*fms* gene and that this growth factor and its receptor are absolutely required for normal macrophage development (Dai et al., 2002).

MACROPHAGE DIFFERENTIATION MARKERS

Macrophages in tissues share a number of features outlined in Table 1. The study of mononuclear phagocyte biology in vivo was expedited by the advent of monoclonal antibodies that recognize some of the macrophage-restricted molecules above, as well as surface proteins of an unknown function. These are not reviewed in detail here; their applications in the mouse have been discussed in detail elsewhere (Gordon, 1999; Leenen et al., 1994; McKnight and Gordon, 1998b). In the mouse, the F4/80 antigen remains one of the most useful macrophage markers. The F4/80 antibody recognizes a member of a family of genes that includes human epidermal growth factor (EGF) module-containing mucinlike hormone

TABLE 1 Common features of macrophages

Tissue location (adjacent to basement membranes of epithelial and endothelial cells)
Ramified or stellate appearance
Characteristic ultrastructure by electron microscopy
High levels of lysosomal enzymes and other lysosomal proteins
Novel ectoenzymes and cytoplasmic enzymes (e.g., nonspecific esterase)
Adhesion to plastic
High phagocytic and endocytic activities
Specific surface receptors
    Fc and complement receptors
    Pattern recognition receptors (including CD14, Toll-like receptors, scavenger receptors, lectins)
    Regulatory receptors (e.g., CSF-1, GM-CSF, etc.)

receptor 1 and human CD97 (McKnight and Gordon, 1998a). Members of the EGF-TM7 family are characterized by a variable number of NH_2-terminal EGF domains and seven transmembrane-spanning hydrophobic regions, resembling the G-protein-coupled peptide hormone receptor family. The intervening years since the description of F4/80 have not revealed a clear function. The knockout mouse has no clear phenotype (McKnight and Gordon, 1998a), but this could be related to the presence of a related gene with overlapping expression (Caminschi et al., 2001). Clues as to function may come from CD97, for which a cellular ligand (CD55) has been identified (McKnight and Gordon, 1998a).

F4/80 antigen is present on the cell surface of a family of cells that includes all well-defined members of the MPS in the mouse. A unique advantage of the F4/80 antibody was that it bound to an epitope that was resistant to glutaraldehyde fixation and paraffin embedding. For this reason, it was possible to produce high-quality images from perfusion-fixed mouse tissues. The full impact of these images was not evident at the time because they could not be reproduced in print. A large collection of them has been scanned and deposited in a database at www.imb.uq.edu.au/groups/hume/tissuesDB3.html, together with annotation and some comments about possible functions of the macrophages in particular locations.

Most macrophage markers are actually also expressed in other hematopoietic and non-hematopoietic cell types, albeit at lower levels, or are expressed only in certain conditions and thereby define macrophage subsets. Even the F4/80 antibody fails to detect a macrophage population in the marginal zone of lymphoid organs and lung macrophages (Hume and Gordon, 1983b). It is greatly reduced in a subset of inflammatory peritoneal macrophages and diminished in other activated macrophages (Chan et al., 1998; Hirsch and Gordon, 1982). Osteoclasts, a close relative of macrophages, do not express F4/80 (Gordon, 1995). Among alternatives, Mac-1 (CD11b), another widely employed macrophage marker, is also expressed in natural killer (NK) cells, granulocytes, and subsets of B and T lymphocytes (Lai et al., 1998). Mac-1 is absent in Kupffer cells and expressed at very low levels in alveolar macrophages (Dorger et al., 2001; Flotte et al., 1983). The macrophage mannose receptor is expressed only in macrophage subsets and is also highly expressed in endothelial cells (Takahashi et al., 1998), whereas CD14 is also expressed by neutrophils (Greaves and Gordon, 2002).

Given the key role of CSF-1 in macrophage proliferation, differentiation, survival, and development, we considered that c-*fms* might be applied as a definitive marker of macrophage lineage. This gene has been widely used in macrophage detection and localization and provides a marker of the earliest events in macrophage development, including the development of embryonic phagocytes (Herbomel et al., 2001; Hume et al., 1995; Lichanska et al., 1999). We have defined the key *cis*-acting elements required for tissue-specific expression of the c-*fms* gene. As it must be, given the requirement for CSF-1 in macrophage differentiation, the rearrangement of the chromatin assembly of the c-*fms* locus is one of the earliest events in commitment of bone marrow progenitors to the macrophage lineage (Tagoh et al., 2002). We produced a line of mice in which the c-*fms* promoter directs expression of the enhanced green fluorescent protein (EGFP) to cells of the macrophage lineage (Sasmono et al., 2003). The *MacGreen* mice provide a unique model system in which the family of mononuclear phagocytes can be studied. The expression of the EGFP transgene closely resembles that of the F4/80 antigen, but extends to F4/80-negative populations of macrophages. Color Plate 1 shows a selection of examples of the expression of the EGFP transgene in organs of the mouse, highlighting the numbers, locations, and characteristic morphology of the cells of the MPS.

ONTOGENY OF MACROPHAGES

Primitive hematopoiesis in vertebrate embryos occurs first in blood islands in the yolk sac (Moore and Metcalf, 1970). The definitive hematopoiesis first occurs in the fetal liver (Moore and Metcalf, 1970). The embryonic liver, which is formed at 9.5 days postconception (dpc) in the mouse, is colonized by progenitor cells in two waves of migration. The first is from the yolk sac at 9.5 to 10.0 dpc and the second is from the aorta-gonad-mesonephros (AGM) area at 10.0 to 10.5 dpc. In the liver, they form mixed populations, although only the progenitor cells from the AGM are able to contribute to definite blood cells (reviewed by Dzierzak et al., 1998; Lichanska and Hume, 2000; Yoder, 2001).

Embryonic phagocytes appear in the yolk sac and embryo proper before the formation of blood circulations and the occurrence of hepatic hematopoiesis. Using c-*fms* as a marker, macrophagelike cells were detected simultaneously in the yolk sac and the mouse embryo at 9.5 dpc (Hume et al., 1995; Lichanska et al., 1999). In the yolk sac, they were detected as isolated individual cells with no apparent association with blood islands (Hume et al., 1995; Lichanska et al., 1999). Later in development, embryonic phagocytes were distributed throughout the embryo and might constitute 5 to 10% of total cells at 11.5 to 12.5 dpc (Lichanska et al., 1999). These cells are particularly concentrated in sites where apoptosis and intensive tissue turnover occur such as in the interdigital area in the developing footplates and in the brain (Hume et al., 1995; Lichanska et al., 1999; Lichanska and Hume, 2000). Cells positive for macrophage markers could also be detected in developing organs and tissues such as in the spleen, thymus, lung, kidney, heart, muscles, branchial arches, epidermis, limbs, and eyes (reviewed by Lichanska and Hume, 2000). Similarly, EGFP-positive cells in the *MacGreen* mouse embryos could also be observed in those areas (Sasmono et al., 2003). A striking model system for studying the ontogeny of early phagocytes is the zebrafish, where they can be monitored with live imaging. The cells emerge well before the formation of blood circulation, differentiate in the yolk sac, and eventually spread over the head of the embryo (Herbomel et al., 1999). Invasion of embryonic macrophages into embryonic tissues requires the expression of c-*fms*. In the c-*fms*-deficient *panther* mutant of zebrafish, embryonic phagocytes differentiate and behave normally in the yolk sac, but then fail to invade embryonic tissues. CSF-1 expressed by the target tissues apparently attracts embryonic macrophages to colonize them (Herbomel et al., 2001). There is evidence that embryonic phagocytes represent a quite distinct pathway. For a start, the macrophage-specific transcription factor PU.1 is not required for their appearance, whereas a mutation in this gene severely compromises hematopoiesis in the liver (Lichanska et al., 1999). Second, the temporal and spatial patterns of expression of macrophage markers such as F4/80 antigen, S100A8, S100A9, and lysozyme (Lichanska et al., 1999) suggested that embryonic phagocytes differ in their differentiation pathway and marker gene expression from macrophages produced via classic hematopoietic progenitors in the liver. Finally, embryonic phagocytes may retain a proliferative potential once they have differentiated (Herbomel et al., 2001; Lichanska and Hume, 2000). These observations leave open the question of whether embryonic phagocytes are retained in adults or are completely replaced by classical monocyte-derived cells later in development.

MACROPHAGE HETEROGENEITY

The purpose of defining a cell lineage such as the MPS is to permit predictions about biological function based on detection of that cell type in a particular location. When we detect large numbers of F4/80-positive or c-*fms* EGFP-positive cells in a lesion, we presume that they will be capable of secreting inflammatory cytokines and eliciting a certain kind of tissue damage. Such predictions are based on an underlying assumption that there is a level of consistency to the ways that sets of genes are coexpressed to define a transcriptional phenotype. We and others have addressed that question by examining comprehensive gene expression profiles of isolated mouse macrophage populations (Ravasi et al., 2002; Rosenberger et al., 2000; Wardrop et al.,

2002). In collaboration with the RIKEN Genome Sciences Center in Japan, we compared the expression profiles of isolated mouse macrophages with the published profile of genes expressed in 49 mouse tissues (Bono et al., 2002; Miki et al., 2001). Full details of this analysis and the raw data have been presented elsewhere (Wells et al., 2003b) and are loaded on our website at www.imb.uq.edu.au/ groups/hume. The most important conclusion from this study for definition of the MPS is that macrophages segregated to a separate branch on a Stanford Gene Tree analysis, related to hematopoietic tissues such as spleen (which contain numerous macrophages) but clearly distinct in their expression profile. Among the genes that are macrophage specific or at least highly enriched are all of the components of the phagocytic apparatus including the lysosomal hydrolases and many predicted membrane proteins of known and unknown function. In collaboration with RIKEN, we have undertaken large-scale expressed sequence tray profiling of mouse macrophages. These studies reveal that macrophages are a remarkably complex source of mRNA and express numerous novel genes (Wells et al., 2003b).

The other conclusion is that the cells we call macrophages can exhibit a very broad range of gene expression steady states. We examined the response of macrophages to the archetypal microbial regulator of their gene expression, lipopolysaccharide (LPS). In a separate review, we assembled a list of more than 500 genes that are known to be induced by LPS in macrophages from a survey of the literature (Hume et al., 2002). These genes provided a historical validated set for the array analysis. Others have already shown that the set of inducible genes in macrophages is quite distinct and only partly overlapping, if one compares stimuli such as virus, bacterial, or yeast challenge (Sweet and Hume, 1996). The documented set of stimuli can alter macrophage gene expression numbers into the hundreds and is beyond the scope of this chapter. We can presume that each elicits its own unique pattern. In addition, there are combinatorial effects, of which the archetype is the combined response of macrophages to T-cell products (e.g., IFN-γ) and LPS (Ehrt et al., 2001). Even other microbial products that act via other Toll-like receptors, closely related to the LPS-signaling component *Tlr4*, have additive and distinct effects on macrophage gene expression (Hume et al., 2001) and can be affected in quite opposite directions by agonists such as CSF-1 (Sweet et al., 2002).

The phenotypic plasticity of macrophages that can be generated in vitro presumably underlies the wide range of phenotypes observed in vivo. Resident tissue macrophages discussed below adapt to their local environment to perform specific functions. Almost any local disturbance of tissue normality, be it infection, normal cell turnover or wounding, immune response, or malignancy, causes rapid recruitment of macrophages. Recruited macrophages exhibit many phenotypic differences from resident tissue macrophages. The generic term "macrophage activation" is commonly used to describe this process, but the nature of an activated macrophage population depends on both the nature of the recruiting stimulus and the location. A PubMed search on "macrophage activation AND review" generates thousands of articles, each dealing with a specific disease focus or etiological agent in a particular organ. Broadly speaking, there has been a focus in the literature on a dichotomy between the cells recruited by a sterile stimulus (the macrophages associated with wound repair and regeneration and also foreign-body responses) and the cells recruited by immunological stimuli. The latter are commonly called activated macrophages and ascribed a greater destructive potential than resident or "elicited" cells (Gordon, 1995). With the availability of better markers and more comprehensive analyses, these definitions are less useful, and it becomes more relevant to rigorously link the definition of the population phenotype to the inducing stimulus and the location. Every macrophage population is likely to be different. An interesting side issue is the extent to which resident and recruited macrophages can

be said to have differentiated in the sense that they become less plastic with time in a specific location. Resident macrophages certainly can become activated. For example, activation of microglial cells in particular is regarded as a significant event in many brain diseases (Barron, 1995; Kreutzberg, 1996; Thomas, 1999; Williams et al., 2001). A related issue is what happens to recruited macrophages once the recruiting stimulus has been resolved (which is the point of the infiltration). Many of the macrophages certainly die in situ. Apoptotic cells are themselves a major stimulus to macrophage recruitment (Messmer and Pfeilschifter, 2000; Savill and Fadok, 2000), but this is a process aimed at resolution and regeneration and a part of normal tissue homeostasis. Resident macrophages in defined locations are probably themselves replaced by being engulfed by their replacement. Inflammatory cells enter draining lymphatics to acquire new functions as antigen-presenting cells, or perhaps to die and be eliminated there. To our knowledge, there is no evidence of recycling into the circulation and/or reacquisition of a monocytelike phenotype.

To add one additional layer of complexity, the set of inducible genes observed in mouse macrophages with a defined agonist such as LPS is influenced by genetic background, and cDNA microarrays are starting to give an insight into the full extent of this variation. In a published study, we compared BALB/c and SJL mice, which differ, among other things, at the Bcg locus that controls susceptibility to intracellular pathogens (Wardrop et al., 2002). Others have also observed global differences in gene regulatory profiles in macrophages from different strains and have linked them to genetic tendencies to generate Th1- or Th2-dominated T-cell-mediated immune responses. They have even gone so far as to coin the terms M1 and M2 responses for macrophages (Mills et al., 2000). Our own microarray studies of a wider range of strains suggest that each has its own unique LPS-inducible gene expression profile, including an idiosyncratic set of genes for which there is no detectable expression

(Wells et al., 2003a). This kind of functional polymorphism is actually not so surprising, given the diversity in immunoglobulin, T-cell receptor, MHC, and NK cell receptor genes. A functional innate immune system is required only when a pathogen challenges. By definition, a successful pathogen evades the innate immune system, and mammalian hosts are under strong selection pressure to deal with the full diversity of possible pathogen evasion strategies.

TRANSCRIPTION FACTORS THAT CONTROL MACROPHAGE DEVELOPMENT AND FUNCTION

The regulation of functions of the macrophages requires expression of macrophage-specific genes, which, in turn, is likely to involve a number of lineage-specific transcription factors. Many such factors are shared with closely related cell types, particularly neutrophils and B cells. There have been a number of recent reviews of macrophage-specific transcription (Friedman, 2002; Himes and Hume, in press; Lenny et al., 1997; Tenen et al., 1997; Valledor et al., 1998; Xie et al., 2001), so we do not deal with this topic in detail.

Transcription factors that control macrophage development can be grouped based on the differentiation stages they mainly involve. Several transcription factors are required for macrophage development because they regulate the differentiation of myeloid cells (such as PU.1 and AML-1) or are important for the survival of stem cells and/or pluripotent myeloid precursors (GATA-2, SCL, and c-Myb). Another group of transcription factors regulates the expression of functionally important genes, but they are not absolutely required for macrophage development. These include NF-M/C/EBPα, HOXB7, and c-Myc, which regulate intermediate stages of myeloid differentiation, and C/EBPβ, EGR-1, IRF-1, NF-Y, and some Jun/Fos and Stat proteins, which control macrophage maturation (reviewed by Valledor et al., 1998).

PU.1, a member of the Ets transcription factor family, has been described as a master regulator of myeloid genes (Tenen et al., 1997).

This transcription factor is expressed at highest levels in myeloid and B cells, but not in T cells (Chen et al., 1995; Klemsz et al., 1990). Although it acts as a transcriptional activator in B cells, in macrophages PU.1 may act as a transcriptional activator or repressor depending on the context of the DNA sequence its binds to (Ross et al., 1994). PU.1 cooperates with other transcription factors to regulate gene expressions (Nagulapalli et al., 1995; Ross et al., 1998). PU.1 regulates the expression of immunoglobulin genes, receptors for phagocytosis and growth, other cell surface molecules, and many other macrophage-specific genes (Lloberas et al., 1999). The importance of PU.1 for normal hematopoiesis is clearly demonstrated by the deficiency in myelopoiesis in PU.1 null mice (McKercher et al., 1996; Scott et al., 1994). As noted above, PU.1 might not be essential for the development of early embryonic macrophages, because PU.1 mRNA could not be detected in all embryonic phagocytes (Lichanska et al., 1999). The c-*fms* gene promoter contains several PU.1 binding sites upstream of the multiple transcription sites (Ross et al., 1998); because this promoter lacks the initiator (*Inr*) sequences, PU.1 may recruit general transcription factors to initiate transcription (Ross et al., 1998; Xie et al., 2001). Ross et al. (1998) demonstrated that PU.1 sites alone could act as a macrophage-specific minimal promoter.

The AML-1 transcription factor, a member of the core binding factor family, recognizes the DNA target TGTGGT and is required for the transcriptional activity of several enhancers and promoters, including those for myeloid-specific myeloperoxidase, neutrophil elastase, defensin (NP-3) (Lenny et al., 1997), and human c-*fms* (Zhang et al., 1996). In vivo, this transcription factor requires interaction with additional factors to fully activate the promoters and enhancers. Direct interactions between AML-1B and Ets-1 and between AML-1B and C/EBPα have been demonstrated in vitro (Lenny et al., 1997).

The promoters of many myeloid-specific genes contain the CAAT/enhancer binding protein (C/EBP) consensus binding sites and are targets for transcriptional regulation by C/EBP family members. These include the genes for myeloperoxidase, neutrophil elastase, and a number of myeloid CSF receptors, i.e., G-CSF, CSF-1 (c-fms), and GM-CSF (Lenny et al., 1997; Tenen et al., 1997). As well as PU.1 and AML-1, C/EBP can interact with a number of transcription factors, including PU.1, NF-κB, and Rel proteins, members of the CREB/ATF family, Sp1, RB, and members of the fos/jun zipper family (reviewed by Tenen et al., 1997). In the human c-fms promoter, C/EBPα binds to CCAAT elements and interacts with AML-1 to activate transcription (Zhang et al., 1996). In the mouse, neither of these sites is perfectly conserved and, instead, AML-1 acts primarily through intronic enhancer elements (S. R. Himes and D. A. Hume et al., unpublished). However, C/EBPβ (NF-IL6) does bind to the mouse c-fms promoter and strongly activates transcription (Xie et al., 2002).

Another transcription factor that is important for myeloid proliferation and differentiation is c-Myb (Friedman, 2002). In cooperation with Ets-2, Myb transcriptionally regulates the expression of CD13/aminopeptidase N (Shapiro, 1995). On the c-fms promoter, Myb acted as a repressor and blocked the action of Ets-1 and Ets-2 (Reddy et al., 1994). In keeping with this effect, c-myb expression declines as macrophages differentiate. Myb also regulates the transcription of several genes, including the CD34 gene, mim-1, c-myc, cdc2, the CD4, lysozyme, and T-cell receptor genes, and c-myb itself (Lenny et al., 1997; Valledor et al., 1998). Myb can interact with AML-1 and can synergize with C/EBP to transactivate the neutrophil elastase promoter (Hernandez-Munain et al., 1996; Oelgeschlager et al., 1996).

Several studies have identified another transcription factor family involved in macrophage differentiation. The microphthalmia transcription factor (Mitf) family member TFEC was coexpressed with other known MiT family members (Mitf, TFE3, TFEB) in murine macrophages (Rehli et al., 1999). The occurrence of osteopetrosis in mice with Mitf mutations indicates that there is a relationship between Mitf and osteoclast and macrophage differentiation (Hodgkinson et al., 1993; Rehli et al., 1999).

TISSUE-SPECIFIC MACROPHAGE POPULATIONS

Mononuclear phagocyte development in an adult animal occurs in the bone marrow and passes through the following steps: pluripotent stem cell, committed stem cell, monoblast, promonocyte, monocyte (bone marrow), monocyte (peripheral blood), and finally macrophage (tissues) (van Furth et al., 1972). Monoblasts are the most immature recognizable mononuclear phagocyte cells (van der Meer et al., 1985). According to kinetic studies in the mouse, monoblast division gives rise to two promonocytes. In turn, division of promonocytes generates monocytes, so there is at least a fourfold increase in cell number during progression of monoblasts to monocytes (van Furth, 1992). In normal conditions, monoblasts and promonocytes are not detected in peripheral blood (Takahashi et al., 1996). Monocyte differentiation in the bone marrow proceeds rapidly. In mice, the cell cycle time of monoblasts is 11.9 h, whereas that of monocytes is 16.2 h (Takahashi et al., 1996). After maturation, monocytes enter the blood circulation within 24 h and distribute throughout the body (van Furth, 1992). It has been generally accepted that monocytes have no proliferative capacity after maturation (Takahashi et al., 1996), but subpopulations of human monocytes have been shown to proliferate in response to CSF-1 (Moss and Hamilton, 2000), and there is ongoing debate about the local proliferative activity of tissue macrophages.

Blood Monocytes

Blood monocytes already possess migratory, chemotactic, pinocytic, and phagocytic activities, as well as receptors for immunoglobulin G (IgG) Fc domains (FcR) and iC3b complement (Fearon, 1983; McKenzie and Schreiber,

1998). Under steady-state conditions, only small numbers of monocytes traverse the endothelial lining of the blood vessels, mainly to maintain the number of resident macrophage populations (van Furth, 1998). In disease state or tissue injury, a variety of cytokines and chemoattractants can modulate monocyte adhesion to endothelial cells and subsequent transendothelial migration. This process involves a wide variety of adhesion molecules and ligands, particularly members of the integrin and selectin families, that are expressed on monocyte and endothelial cell surfaces (Muller, 2001; van Furth, 1998).

Peritoneal Macrophages

Peritoneal macrophages are the most studied primary macrophages in mice because they are easily isolated by peritoneal lavage. It has been suggested that they are either nonadherent or weakly adherent in situ. This phenomenon has been correlated with the low level of expression of class A scavenger receptors (Kim et al., 1997), which mediate Ca^{2+}-independent adhesion in vitro. Soon after injection of an irritant of any kind, the resident macrophages adhere to the peritoneal lining, and there is a major influx of inflammatory cells. The inflammatory phenotype of these cells depends on the nature of the stimulus (Gordon et al., 1995; Hamilton et al., 1999). Although they are widely studied, the physiological importance of peritoneal macrophages is debatable, and the peritoneal environment, with a very low oxygen tension, is quite unusual. For the remainder of this chapter, we focus on the characteristics and function of major tissue macrophage populations, highlighting some of their physiological as well as their immunological roles.

Kupffer Cells

Kupffer cells are resident macrophages in the liver. They reside in the lumen of hepatic sinusoids and are anchored to the endothelium by long cytoplasmic processes. These cells probably represent the largest macrophage population in the body (Hashimoto et al., 1996;

Laskin et al., 2001). Kupffer cells contribute to the clearance of red cells and apoptotic cells and basically all foreign particulate and materials from the portal circulation, primarily by means of phagocytosis (Dini et al., 2002; Gordon et al., 1995). Although Kupffer cells are commonly considered as a single population in the liver, heterogeneity exists and seems to be related to the blood supply. Kupffer cells are more abundant in the periphery of liver lobules than centrilobular regions (Hume et al., 1984c). The periportal Kupffer cells are larger and more mature, possess greater lysosomal enzyme activities, and are more phagocytic than cells in the centrilobular area (Bouwens et al., 1992; Laskin et al., 2001; Sleyster and Knook, 1982). A range of studies indicate that Kupffer cells have a unique cell surface marker profile (Auger and Ross, 1992; Flotte et al., 1983; Hume and Gordon, 1985; van Oosten et al., 2001), perhaps reflecting their unique chronic exposure to LPS and other microbial components in the portal blood entering the liver.

Splenic Macrophages

Splenic macrophages are also a heterogeneous population of cells. The spleen receives a rich blood supply via the splenic artery and is drained by the splenic vein into the hepatic portal system. The splenic macrophages are an important component of the innate immune system, as evidenced by the incidence of septicemia following splenectomy (Altamura et al., 2001). Histologically, the spleen contains discrete white nodules, the so-called white pulp, embedded in red matrix called the red pulp. The white pulp consists of lymphoid aggregations, whereas the red pulp, making up the bulk of the organ, is a highly vascular tissue (Wheater et al., 1987). Between the two is the so-called marginal zone (Carol et al., 1999). Each site has distinct types of macrophages: the red pulp macrophages, the marginal zone macrophages, the periarteriolar lymphoid sheath macrophages, and the marginal metallophilic macrophages, all of which possess different characteristics. Macrophages in the red pulp have a function in hematopoiesis and phagocytosis, whereas the marginal-zone macrophage population is known to be active in trapping particles in the blood and clearance of excess antigens (Gordon, 1995). These sinus-lining phagocytes resemble liver Kupffer cells in morphology, as well as the expression of F4/80 antigen and receptors for IgG (Nusrat et al., 1988). The marginal-zone cells lack F4/80 (Hume et al., 1983b), but selectively express a quite distinct set of receptors involved in recognition of microorganisms or immune-opsonized particles (Morse et al., 2001; Takahashi et al., 1996; van der Laan et al., 1999). A final population of mononuclear phagocytes, the so-called interdigitating cells or splenic dendritic cells (DCs), reside within the T-cell areas. The biology of these cells is considered separately below.

Pulmonary Macrophages

Pulmonary macrophages can be divided into three populations that interact with quite different environments: alveolar macrophages, interstitial macrophages, and intravascular macrophages. Each has distinct patterns of gene expression and function (Laskin et al., 2001; Lohmann-Matthes et al., 1994). With their location at the interphase between air and lung tissues, alveolar macrophages represent the first line of defense against inhaled or aspirated microbes that enter the lung, and they are very actively phagocytic and equipped to kill microorganisms (Lohmann-Matthes et al., 1994). Within the lung stroma, substantial numbers of macrophages can be detected, although difficulties in isolation and lack of surface markers have constrained their phenotypic characterization. These interstitial macrophages, compared to alveolar cells, have been found to be smaller, more uniform, and considerably less phagocytic (Johansson et al., 1997; Laskin et al., 2001).

Two mechanisms apparently contribute to recruitment of pulmonary macrophages: chemotactic attraction of monocytes from the lung blood pool and local replication in the lung (Fels and Cohn, 1986; Lohmann-Matthes

et al., 1994). Monocytes pass from the interstitium into alveoli, and alveolar macrophages themselves proliferate in vitro in response to CSFs (Chen et al., 1988; Golde et al., 1974; Maus et al., 2002; van Furth and Sluiter, 1986). Local proliferation of pulmonary macrophages has been described (Evans et al., 1987; Pforte et al., 1993; Tarling and Coggle, 1982). In addition to the alveolar and interstitial macrophages, the other macrophage population in the lung is the pulmonary intravascular macrophages. These poorly studied cells are mature phagocytes that are found adhering to capillary endothelial cells within the lungs of certain animal species such as ruminants, horses, and cats, but not in humans and rodents (Brain et al., 1999). In these species, they play a major role in the phagocytosis of circulating particles such as red blood cells, bacteria, and immune complexes (Geiser, 2002).

Pleural Macrophages

Other thoracic macrophages of relevance to pulmonary defense and some lung disease processes are the pleural macrophages resident in the pleural space and macrophages present in regional lymph nodes that receive lymphatic drainage from the lung (Lehnert, 1992). Pleural macrophages are functionally and phenotypically different from alveolar macrophages and are more similar to peritoneal macrophages in regard to histochemical properties and expression of membrane antigens. They are probably involved in cell-mediated immune responses within the pleural space (Dorger et al., 2001; Gjomarkaj et al., 1999).

Microglia

Microglia are the resident macrophage population in the normal healthy adult nervous system (Perry, 1994). These cells represent about 10% of the adult brain cell population (Alliot et al., 1999). There are two different forms of microglial cells that differ both in phenotype and in morphology: amoeboid microglia, which exist transiently in the developing and diseased brain and are the most mobile form of microglia, and ramified microglia, which predominate in normal and healthy brain tissue (Kaur et al., 2001).

Microglia form the first line of defense against injury to the central nervous system. These cells are rapidly activated in a variety of pathological conditions and proliferate vigorously (Klein et al., 1997). Immature amoeboid microglia have been known to phagocytose dying cells and their processes and also secrete cytokines that promote gliogenesis and angiogenesis (Perry, 1994). They function in removal of degenerating neurons and their processes during normal development (Hume et al., 1983a; Perry, 1994). Ramified microglia assist in the immune surveillance of the nervous system (Kreutzberg, 1996) and appear to provide trophic support for the adjacent neuronal and nonneuronal cells (Chamak et al., 1994). Microglia actively phagocytose amyloid-β plaques in Alzheimer's disease, and this activity is enhanced by the overexpression of c-*fms* (Mitrasinovic and Murphy, 2002).

Macrophages of the Gastrointestinal Mucosa

The macrophages of the gastrointestinal mucosa are not commonly recognized as being one of the largest macrophage populations in the body (Lee et al., 1985). Macrophages resident in the gastrointestinal tract constitute about 10 to 20% of mononuclear cells in lamina propria (Hume et al., 1987; Pavli and Doe, 1992). Although they are mostly restricted to the lamina propria, these cells are occasionally observed within the epithelium (Soesatyo et al., 1990). One function of intestinal macrophages is the disposal of apoptotic epithelial cells and the regulation of mucosal epithelial renewal (Nagashima et al., 1996). Like Kupffer cells in the liver, intestinal macrophages are exposed chronically to microbial products, yet they are not constitutively activated. The interaction of macrophages with bacteria is thought to involve CD14, LPS, and the LPS-binding protein receptor (Ulevitch and Tobias, 1995) and CD89 and the IgA1 and IgA2 receptor (Morton et al., 1996). Intestinal lamina propria macrophages are devoid of both of these

molecules, which may explain their insensitivity to intestinal lumenal contents (Smith et al., 2001). CD14-expressing cells are detected in the intestinal lamina propria, but are thought to derive from the recently recruited monocytes (Grimm et al., 1995). Aside from the lack of CD14, intestinal macrophages have a quite distinctive complement of other surface markers compared with macrophages in other sites (Pavli et al., 1990; Rogler et al., 1998; Soesatyo et al., 1990).

Endocrine Macrophages

Endocrine macrophage populations have been described in the adrenal gland, pituitary gland, thyroid, parathyroid and islets of Langerhans and pineal glands, and in the testis and ovary (Hume et al., 1984a). In the adrenal gland, macrophages were more numerous in the cortical reticularis and zona glomerulosa, whereas only a few cells were observed in zona fasciculata and in the adrenal medulla (Hume et al., 1984a; Schober et al., 1998). This distribution pattern suggests region-specific functions. Abundant cell death in the cortical zone apparently accounts for the high density of macrophages in this region (Schober et al., 1998). Macrophages in the adrenal cortex may have a function related to the steroidogenic activity of one of their secreted products, IL-1α (O'Connell et al., 1994). In the medulla, macrophages are usually found in close contact with the chromaffin cells. Chromaffin cells, the catecholamine hormone noradrenaline and adrenaline secretor (Wheater et al., 1987), express a wide range of growth factor receptors. Macrophage-derived cytokines may signal toward these cells (Schober et al., 1998). Indeed, paracrine signaling between macrophages and bovine adrenal chromaffin cells has been demonstrated (Currie et al., 2000).

In the pineal gland, it has been suggested that the macrophages and microglia are active phagocytes that are also probably involved in the immunoregulatory function in the gland (Kaur et al., 1997). In other endocrine organs, macrophages are present in the islets of Langerhans in the pancreas and in the thyroid and parathyroid glands. As in other endocrine organs such as the testis and ovary, these populations of macrophages may contribute to the control of hormone production (Hume et al., 1984a).

Macrophages are found throughout the reproductive tracts of both males and females (Hume et al., 1984a) and have been proposed to act as regulators of fertility at several levels. Mice with a mutation in the CSF-1 gene, which affects the number of macrophages and hormonal regulation of the reproductive system, have a defect in their reproduction (Cohen et al., 1999). In the male reproductive system, macrophages are mainly found in the testis interstitium among the Ledyig cells, the testosterone-producing cells. They can also be found in the cauda and caput epididymis, prostate, seminal vesicles, and vas deferens (Pollard et al., 1997). After the Leydig cell, testicular macrophages represent the largest cell population resident in the testis interstitium, with the density comparable to that of the Kupffer cells in the liver (Hedger, 1997). About 20 to 25% of cells in the interstitium are macrophages, but no macrophages could be detected within the seminiferous tubule (Cohen et al., 1999; Hume et al., 1984a). Circulating monocytes are the major source of testicular macrophages (Mendis-Handagama et al., 1987), but local proliferation may also occur (Gaytan et al., 1995). Macrophages in the testis interstitium interact intimately with Leydig cells. Microvilli of the Leydig cells are apparently inserted within coated vesicles on the macrophage surface. This interaction suggests that macrophages play some roles in regulating steroidogenesis (Cohen et al., 1999). Indeed, testicular macrophages produce 25-hydroxycholesterol, a substrate that can be converted to testosterone by the neighboring Leydig cells (Lukyanenko et al., 2001; Nes et al., 2000). Apart from a role in steroidogenesis, macrophages may also have a spermiophage activity leading to infertility in several human syndromes. This suggestion was based on the increased number of macrophages in the basement membrane and in the lumen of seminiferous tubules in pathological conditions (Frungieri et al., 2002), a phenomenon that has never been observed before in other healthy mammals (Cohen et al., 1999). In terms of immunological function, testicular macrophages secrete a novel subset of important inflammatory cytokines (Kern et al., 1995) that may contribute to the immunologically privileged or immunosuppressive environment of the testis (Cohen et al., 1999; Gerdprasert et al., 2002).

Ovarian Macrophages

In the female reproductive system, macrophages are abundant in the ovary and corpora lutea; in the cervix, endometrium, and myometrium of the uterus; and in the oviduct fimbriae (Cohen et al., 1999; Hume et al., 1984a, 1984c). Ovarian macrophages are mainly found in the interstitium, being excluded from the germ cell compartment, except in atretic follicles where macrophages are recruited for the destruction of defunct follicle (Cohen et al., 1999). Just before ovulation, macrophages are abundant in the theca layer of the follicles, suggesting an active role for these cells in tissue remodeling during the ovulatory process (Brannstrom et al., 1994). Ovarian macrophages are central to both the formation and the destruction of the corpus luteum. Infiltrating in significant numbers following follicle rupture, they have been proposed to participate in luteogenesis and regulation of luteal cell steroidogenesis (Gaytan et al., 1998; Pate and Landis Keyes, 2001). Conversely, the numbers in the corpus luteum increase markedly during luteolysis, and the macrophages actively ingest dying cells (Gaytan et al., 1998; Kasuya, 1997; Pate and Landis Keyes, 2001). Like testicular macrophages, ovarian macrophages secrete a range of cytokines (Itoh et al., 1999) that may mediate many of their actions on other ovarian cells.

Uterine Macrophages

Uterine macrophages (Mackler et al., 2000) are found throughout the endometrium during pregnancy, as well as in stroma and connective tissues around the muscles in the myometrium. In the mouse, the number of uterine macrophages increases as pregnancy progresses, reaching a peak after the midpoint of gestation. As pregnancy nears conclusion, their number decreases, particularly in the endometrium. This has been associated with the decrease of inducible nitric oxide synthase production that leads to the promotion of vasodilatation and uterine smooth muscle relaxation. At the same time, a stable population is maintained in the myometrium (Mackler et al., 2000). From this it has been hypothesized that withdrawal of these cells may participate in an escape from contractile inhibition at term (Mackler et al., 2000). After parturition, macrophage numbers increase in the uterus. This may enable participation in wound healing, tissue repair, and the restoration of the uterus to the nonpregnant state, ready for the subsequent cycle (Mackler et al., 2000).

Kidney Macrophages

Kidney macrophages have not been considered a major resident population, and much of the study of mononuclear phagocytes in this organ focuses on renal inflammatory diseases. There are actually numerous interstitial macrophages in the kidney, especially in the medulla, but their presence is obscured by their spreading pattern, which extends lengthwise along the tubules (Hume and Gordon, 1983a). Although less numerous in the cortex, macrophages have been observed to be always found in close proximity to the macula densa and the afferent and efferent arterioles of the glomerular capillary bed (Hume and Gordon, 1983a). Kidney macrophages express CSF-1 and its receptor (c-*fms*) (Hemmerlein et al., 2000), and the deficiency of these two molecules severely depletes the number of macrophages (Cecchini et al., 1994; Dai et al., 2002). The kidney mesangial cells, cells of endothelial origin, have been considered to be phagocytic and may express CSF-1 and its receptor (c-*fms*) (Mori et al., 1990; Watanabe et al., 2001), but they lack most other macrophage markers (Hume and Gordon,

1983a). Large numbers of macrophages infiltrate the renal parenchyma in all types of renal damage (Kipari and Hughes, 2002; Nikolic-Paterson and Atkins, 2001). Tubulointerstitial macrophage accumulation has been described to be related to the degree of renal dysfunction (Nikolic-Paterson and Atkins, 2001). Interstitial inflammatory macrophages induce both tubular injury and tubular cell apoptosis (Tesch et al., 1999). Macrophages may cause renal cell death directly via a range of secretory products (Kipari and Hughes, 2002). Indirectly, accumulation of macrophages may alter vascular supply to the epithelium, leading to hypoxia and apoptosis (Kipari and Hughes, 2002). Conversely, there is recent evidence that the inhibition of macrophage infiltration in a transgenic mouse caused a paradoxical increase in the severity of renal injury in experimental nephritis (Erwig et al., 2001), suggesting a protective or regulatory role of macrophages in glomerular inflammation.

Synovial Macrophages

Synovial macrophages are of particular interest because the joints are affected by some of the most widespread and debilitating inflammatory diseases affecting humans. The type A synovial cells (macrophages) interdigitate with the type B cells (fibroblasts) in the synovial membrane (Athanasou, 1995; Hume et al., 1984b). In normal conditions, the predominant cell type in the synovium is the type B cells, whereas in rheumatoid conditions, the synovium lining type A cell number is greatly increased (Athanasou, 1995). Synovial macrophages are mainly derived from circulating monocytes (Athanasou, 1995). In some circumstances, they may differentiate into osteoclastlike cells and become involved in bone resorption (Chang et al., 1992).

Osteoclasts

Osteoclasts are multinucleated giant cells that reside on endosteal bone surfaces and the periosteal surface beneath the periosteum and are actively involved in bone resorption. Mononuclear osteoclasts share a common progenitor with macrophages, and fusion of these cells generates multinucleated osteoclasts (Udagawa et al., 1990). Hence, the osteoclast lineage has been considered as a part of the mononuclear phagocyte system (Cecchini et al., 1997). Osteoclast production is CSF-1 dependent, as demonstrated in *Csf1op/Csf1op* mice that lack mature and functional osteoclasts, thus resulting in an osteopetrotic phenotype (Wiktor-Jedrzejczak et al., 1990; Yoshida et al., 1990). During osteoclastogenesis, c-*fms* mRNA is expressed in osteoclast precursor cells at late stages and is subsequently followed by expression of the receptor activator of nuclear factor B (RANK), which determines the fate of these cells to become osteoclasts in the presence of RANK ligand (Arai et al., 1999; Teitelbaum, 2000). Mature osteoclasts express c-*fms* (Hofstetter et al., 1992; Kawakami et al., 1999), and CSF-1 can acutely regulate osteoclastic bone resorption (Edwards et al., 1998). Osteoclast precursors and mature osteoclasts do not express F4/80 (Hume et al., 1984b). However, there is a substantial F4/80-positive macrophage population lining all bone surfaces (Hume et al., 1984b), and their likely function in bone resorption has largely been ignored.

DCs

DCs are considered the principal accessory cells of the vertebrate immune system (Banchereau and Steinman, 1998; Mellman and Steinman, 2001). They are defined functionally by their ability to take up a diverse array of antigens such as foreign cells and microorganisms, process them into short antigenic peptides, load the peptides onto major MHC molecules, and then deliver the resulting complexes to the cell surface (Mellman et al., 1998; Steinman et al., 1999). These complexes will then serve as a ligand for an antigen-specific T-cell receptor that eventually initiates primary immune responses (Mellman and Steinman, 2001; Mellman et al., 1998; Steinman et al., 1999). During development, DC maturation correlates with their functional repertoire. Immature DCs are very effective in antigen

uptake and processing but are unable to prime T cells, whereas mature DCs have a diminished capacity to take up antigens but are very effective at stimulating T cells (Mellman and Steinman, 2001). Most DCs found in the body are derived from myeloid precursors, leading to the term "myeloid DC" (Steinman and Inaba, 1999). However, a subset of DCs display lymphoid markers and are referred to as "lymphoid DC" (Shortman and Liu, 2002). Myeloid DCs take up antigens in the periphery and migrate to the lymphoid organs to initiate immunity, whereas lymphoid DCs are found in the thymic medulla and lymph node T-cell area and are responsible for immunotolerance (Steinman and Inaba, 1999). Myeloid and lymphoid DCs may also have different cytokine activators (Shortman and Liu, 2002; Steinman and Inaba, 1999). Nevertheless, in the *MacGreen* mice, all identifiable DC populations express the EGFP transgene, which is absent from T cells and B cells.

DCs that reside in the epidermis, the Langerhans cells (LCs), are considered as immature antigen-presenting DCs (Mellman and Steinman, 2001; Steinman and Inaba, 1999). They are phagocytic, but are unable to present antigen. Upon encountering an infectious agent, they migrate to the lymph node, where their capacity to present antigens and activate T cells matures (Mellman et al., 1998; Morrissette et al., 1999). On the basis of the expression of CD8(low) and CD11b, some have placed this cell population in between myeloid and lymphoid DCs (Shortman and Liu, 2002). There is a debate that has generated more heat than light as to whether DCs and LCs should be included in the mononuclear phagocyte system. In the original definitions of DCs, the cells were very poorly endocytic, but the emerging model now has phagocyte-acquiring DC-like activities. A hallmark of DCs is the expression of high levels of class II MHC antigens, but the vast majority of tissue "macrophages" in the mouse, except those of the liver, peritoneum, and red pulp of spleen, express class II MHC antigens (Hume, 1985). The observation that development and differentiation of DCs and LCs were not compromised in CSF-1-deficient mice encouraged the view that their ontogeny was distinct (Takahashi et al., 1992; Witmer-Pack et al., 1993); however, in the recently character-ized CSF-1R (c-*fms*) knockout mice, the num-ber of LCs was significantly decreased (Dai et al., 2002). What is certainly the case is that DC-like cells can be generated in culture from puri-fied human peripheral blood monocytes (Romani et al., 1994, 1996; Sallusto and Lanza-vecchia, 1994) and from bone marrow progen-itors that express c-*fms* and can also give rise to macrophages and osteoclasts (Miyamoto et al., 2001; Zhang et al., 1998). In our view, it remains questionable whether there is any real basis for a clear dichotomy between DCs and the other mononuclear phagocyte cell types. There appears to be a continuum of cellular phenotypes that invites classification at the ex-tremes, but lacks a clear distinguishing bound-ary. DCs appear no more different from other mononuclear cells than microglia are from Kupffer cells.

Thymus is a primary lymphoid organ in which the classical macrophage and DC-like phenotypes coexist, probably in the same compartments. In this organ, massive imma-ture thymocyte cell death occurs and the thy-mocytes are rapidly ingested by macrophages (Feng et al., 2002; Surh and Sprent, 1994). There is an intimate relationship between macrophages and lymphocytes in that thymic macrophages in both cortex and medulla have lymphocytes bound to their surfaces and some exhibit evidence of lymphocyte internaliza-tion (Samms et al., 2001; Wood, 1985).

CONCLUSION AND FUTURE DIRECTIONS

Mononuclear phagocytes are present in every organ in the body as a major cell population. There is clearly substantial phenotypic plastic-ity. With the combined availability of complete genome and transcriptome sequences, gene expression array technology, and markers allowing purification of tissue macrophages, the future will provide an opportunity to fully characterize the different tissue macrophage populations and the diversity of mononuclear phagocytes attracted to different disease sites in vivo. Such information will provide an ever-increasing insight into their precise role in innate immunity. The ability of the blood monocyte to take on so many different pheno-typic states suggests a more provocative view—that they may be able to act as a kind of mobile stem cell giving rise to many other cell types. Some of the evidence for this view has been presented elsewhere (Hume et al., 2002). The availability of macrophage-specific transgenes, and transgenic approaches to lineage tracing, will provide new opportunities to explore the true function of this family of cells.

REFERENCES

Adam, D. O., and T. A. Hamilton. 1984. The cell biology of macrophage activation. *Annu. Rev. Immunol.* **2:**283–318.

Alliot, F., I. Godin, and B. Pessac. 1999. Microglia derive from progenitors, originating from the yolk sac, and which proliferate in the brain. *Brain Res. Dev. Brain Res.* **117:**145–152.

Altamura, M., L. Caradonna, L. Amati, N. M. Pellegrino, G. Urgesi, and S. Miniello. 2001. Splenectomy and sepsis: the role of the spleen in the immune-mediated bacterial clearance. *Immuno-pharmacol. Immunotoxicol.* **23:**153–161.

Arai, F., T. Miyamoto, O. Ohneda, T. Inada, T. Sudo, K. Brasel, T. Miyata, D. M. Anderson, and T. Suda. 1999. Commitment and differentiation of osteoclast precursor cells by the sequential expression of c-Fms and receptor activator of nuclear factor kappaB (RANK) receptors. *J. Exp. Med.* **190:**1741–1754.

Athanasou, N. A. 1995. Synovial macrophages. *Ann. Rheum. Dis.* **54:**392–394.

Auger, M. J., and J. A. Ross. 1992. The biology of the macrophage, p. 1–57. *In* C. E. Lewis and J. O. McGee (ed.), *The Macrophage.* Oxford University Press, Oxford, United Kingdom.

Banchereau, J., and R. M. Steinman. 1998. Dendritic cells and the control of immunity. *Nature* **392:**245–252.

Barron, K. D. 1995. The microglial cell. A historical review. *J. Neurol. Sci.* **134**(Suppl.)**:**57–68.

Bono, H., T. Kasukawa, Y. Hayashizaki, and Y. Okazaki. 2002. READ: RIKEN Expression Array Database. *Nucleic Acids Res.* **30:**211–213.

Bouwens, L., P. De Bleser, K. Vanderkerken, B. Geerts, and E. Wisse. 1992. Liver cell heterogeneity: functions of non-parenchymal cells. *Enzyme* **46:**155–168.

Brain, J. D., R. M. Molina, M. M. DeCamp, and A. E. Warner. 1999. Pulmonary intravascular macrophages: their contribution to the mononuclear phagocyte system in 13 species. *Am. J. Physiol.* **276:**L146–L154.

Brannstrom, M., V. Pascoe, R. J. Norman, and N. McClure. 1994. Localization of leukocyte subsets in the follicle wall and in the corpus luteum throughout the human menstrual cycle. *Fertil. Steril.* **61:**488–495.

Caminschi, I., L. M. Lucas, M. A. O'Keeffe, H. Hochrein, Y. Laabi, F. Kontgen, A. M. Lew, K. Shortman, and M. D. Wright. 2001. Molecular cloning of F4/80-like-receptor, a seven-span membrane protein expressed differentially by dendritic cell and monocyte-macrophage subpopulations. *J. Immunol.* **167:**3570–3576.

Carol, M., C. Pelegri, A. Franch, J. Garcia-Valero, C. Castellote, and M. Castell. 1999. An image analysis strategy to determine the distribution of cell types in spleen sections. *Acta Histochem.* **101:**281–291.

Cecchini, M. G., M. G. Dominguez, S. Mocci, A. Wetterwald, R. Felix, H. Fleisch, O. Chisholm, W. Hofstetter, J. W. Pollard, and E. R. Stanley. 1994. Role of colony stimulating factor-1 in the establishment and regulation of tissue macrophages during postnatal development of the mouse. *Development* **120:**1357–1372.

Cecchini, M. G., W. Hofstetter, J. Halasy, A. Wetterwald, and R. Felix. 1997. Role of CSF-1 in bone and bone marrow development. *Mol. Reprod. Dev.* **46:**75–83.

Chamak, B., V. Morandi, and M. Mallat. 1994. Brain macrophages stimulate neurite growth and regeneration by secreting thrombospondin. *J. Neurosci. Res.* **38:**221–233.

Chan, J., P. J. Leenen, I. Bertoncello, S. I. Nishikawa, and J. A. Hamilton. 1998. Macrophage lineage cells in inflammation: characterization by colony-stimulating factor-1 (CSF-1) receptor (c-Fms), ER-MP58, and ER-MP20 (Ly-6C) expression. *Blood* **92:**1423–1431.

Chang, J. S., J. M. Quinn, A. Demaziere, C. J. Bulstrode, M. J. Francis, R. B. Duthie, and N. A. Athanasou. 1992. Bone resorption by cells isolated from rheumatoid synovium. *Ann. Rheum. Dis.* **51:**1223–1229.

Chen, B. D., M. Mueller, and T. H. Chou. 1988. Role of granulocyte/macrophage colony-stimulating factor in the regulation of murine alveolar macrophage proliferation and differentiation. *J. Immunol.* **141:**139–144.

Chen, H. M., P. Zhang, M. T. Voso, S. Hohaus, D. A. Gonzalez, C. K. Glass, D. E. Zhang, and D. G. Tenen. 1995. Neutrophils and monocytes express high levels of PU.1 (Spi-1) but not Spi-B. *Blood* **85:**2918–2928.

Cohen, P. E., K. Nishimura, L. Zhu, and J. W. Pollard. 1999. Macrophages: important accessory cells for reproductive function. *J. Leukoc. Biol.* **66:**765–772.

Crocker, P. R., and G. Milon. 1992. Macrophages in the control of hematopoiesis, p. 115–156. *In* C. E. Lewis and J. O. D. McGee (ed.), *The Natural Immune System. The Macrophage.* IRL Press, Oxford, United Kingdom.

Currie, K. P., Z. Zhou, and A. P. Fox. 2000. Evidence for paracrine signaling between macrophages and bovine adrenal chromaffin cell Ca(2+) channels. *J. Neurophysiol.* **83:**280–287.

Dai, X. M., G. R. Ryan, A. J. Hapel, M. G. Dominguez, R. G. Russell, S. Kapp, V. Sylvestre, and E. R. Stanley. 2002. Targeted disruption of the mouse colony-stimulating factor 1 receptor gene results in osteopetrosis, mononuclear phagocyte deficiency, increased primitive progenitor cell frequencies, and reproductive defects. *Blood* **99:**111–120.

de Villiers, W. J., J. D. Smith, M. Miyata, H. M. Dansky, E. Darley, and S. Gordon. 1998. Macrophage phenotype in mice deficient in both macrophage-colony-stimulating factor (op) and apolipoprotein E. *Arterioscler. Thromb. Vasc. Biol.* **18:**631–640.

Dini, L., P. Pagliara, and E. C. Carla. 2002. Phagocytosis of apoptotic cells by liver: a morphological study. *Microsc. Res. Tech.* **57:**530–540.

Dorger, M., S. Munzing, A. M. Allmeling, K. Messmer, and F. Krombach. 2001. Phenotypic and functional differences between rat alveolar, pleural, and peritoneal macrophages. *Exp. Lung Res.* **27:**65–76.

Dzierzak, E., A. Medvinsky, and M. de Bruijn. 1998. Qualitative and quantitative aspects of haematopoietic cell development in the mammalian embryo. *Immunol Today* **19:**228–236.

Edwards, M., U. Sarma, and A. M. Flanagan. 1998. Macrophage colony-stimulating factor increases bone resorption by osteoclasts disaggregated from human fetal long bones. *Bone* **22:**325–329.

Ehrt, S., D. Schnappinger, S. Bekiranov, J. Drenkow, S. Shi, T. R. Gingeras, T. Gaasterland, G. Schoolnik, and C. Nathan. 2001. Reprogramming of the macrophage transcriptome in response to interferon-gamma and Mycobacterium tuberculosis: signaling roles of nitric oxide synthase-2 and phagocyte oxidase. *J. Exp. Med.* **194:**1123–1140.

Erwig, L. P., D. C. Kluth, and A. J. Rees. 2001. Macrophages in renal inflammation. *Curr. Opin. Nephrol. Hypertens.* **10:**341–347.

Evans, M. J., M. P. Sherman, L. A. Campbell, and S. G. Shami. 1987. Proliferation of pulmonary alveolar macrophages during postnatal development of rabbit lungs. *Am. Rev. Respir. Dis.* **136:**384–387.

Fang, F. C., and A. Vazquez-Torres. 2002. Nitric oxide production by human macrophages: there's NO doubt about it. *Am. J. Physiol. Lung Cell. Mol. Physiol.* **282:**L941–L943.

Fearon, D. T. 1983. The human C3b receptor. *Springer Semin. Immunopathol.* **6**:159–172.

Felix, R., M. G. Cecchini, W. Hofstetter, P. R. Elford, A. Stutzer, and H. Fleisch. 1990. Impairment of macrophage colony-stimulating factor production and lack of resident bone marrow macrophages in the osteopetrotic op/op mouse. *J. Bone Miner. Res.* **5**:781–789.

Fels, A. O., and Z. A. Cohn. 1986. The alveolar macrophage. *J. Appl. Physiol.* **60**:353–369.

Feng, J. M., J. S. Wu, A. T. Campagnoni, and W. F. Chen. 2002. Nonspecific esterase released from thymic macrophages accumulates in the apoptotic thymocytes: an indication for this enzyme participating in the clearance of apoptotic thymocytes. *Eur. J. Immunol.* **32**:1386–1392.

Flotte, T. J., T. A. Springer, and G. J. Thorbecke. 1983. Dendritic cell and macrophage staining by monoclonal antibodies in tissue sections and epidermal sheets. *Am. J. Pathol.* **111**:112–124.

Friedman, A. D. 2002. Transcriptional regulation of granulocyte and monocyte development. *Oncogene* **21**:3377–3390.

Frungieri, M. B., R. S. Calandra, L. Lustig, V. Meineke, F. M. Kohn, H. J. Vogt, and A. Mayerhofer. 2002. Number, distribution pattern, and identification of macrophages in the testes of infertile men. *Fertil. Steril.* **78**:298–306.

Gaytan, F., J. L. Romero, C. Morales, C. Reymundo, C. Bellido, and E. Aguilar. 1995. Response of testicular macrophages to EDS-induced Leydig cell death. *Andrologia* **27**:259–265.

Gaytan, F., C. Morales, L. Garcia-Pardo, C. Reymundo, C. Bellido, and J. E. Sanchez-Criado. 1998. Macrophages, cell proliferation, and cell death in the human menstrual corpus luteum. *Biol. Reprod.* **59**:417–425.

Geiser, M. 2002. Morphological aspects of particle uptake by lung phagocytes. *Microsc. Res. Tech.* **57**:512–522.

Gerdprasert, O., M. K. O'Bryan, J. A. Muir, A. M. Caldwell, S. Schlatt, D. M. De Kretser, and M. P. Hedger. 2002. The response of testicular leukocytes to lipopolysaccharide-induced inflammation: further evidence for heterogeneity of the testicular macrophage population. *Cell Tissue Res.* **308**:277–285.

Gjomarkaj, M., E. Pace, M. Melis, M. Spatafora, M. Profita, A. M. Vignola, G. Bonsignore, and G. B. Toews. 1999. Phenotypic and functional characterization of normal rat pleural macrophages in comparison with autologous peritoneal and alveolar macrophages. *Am. J. Respir. Cell Mol. Biol.* **20**:135–142.

Golde, D. W., L. A. Byers, and T. N. Finley. 1974. Proliferative capacity of human alveolar macrophage. *Nature* **247**:373–375.

Gordon, S. 1995. The macrophage. *Bioessays* **17**:977–986.

Gordon, S. 1999. Macrophage-restricted molecules: role in differentiation and activation. *Immunol. Lett.* **65**:5–8.

Gordon, S., S. Clarke, D. Greaves, and A. Doyle. 1995. Molecular immunobiology of macrophages: recent progress. *Curr. Opin. Immunol.* **7**:24–33.

Greaves, D. R., and S. Gordon. 2002. Macrophage-specific gene expression: current paradigms and future challenges. *Int. J. Hematol.* **76**:6–15.

Grimm, M. C., P. Pavli, E. Van de Pol, and W. F. Doe. 1995. Evidence for a CD14+ population of monocytes in inflammatory bowel disease mucosa—implications for pathogenesis. *Clin. Exp. Immunol.* **100**:291–297.

Hamilton, T. A., Y. Ohmori, J. M. Tebo, and R. Kishore. 1999. Regulation of macrophage gene expression by pro- and anti-inflammatory cytokines. *Pathobiology* **67**:241–244.

Hashimoto, S., M. Yamada, N. Yanai, T. Kawashima, and K. Motoyoshi. 1996. Phenotypic change and proliferation of murine Kupffer cells by colony-stimulating factors. *J. Interferon. Cytokine Res.* **16**:237–243.

Hedger, M. P. 1997. Testicular leukocytes: what are they doing? *Rev. Reprod.* **2**:38–47.

Hemmerlein, B., A. Markus, M. Wehner, A. Kugler, F. Zschunke, and H. J. Radzum. 2000. Expression of acute and late-stage inflammatory antigens, c-fms, CSF-1, and human monocytic serine esterase 1, in tumor-associated macrophages of renal cell carcinomas. *Cancer Immunol. Immunother.* **49**:485–492.

Henson, P. M., D. L. Bratton, and V. A. Fadok. 2001. Apoptotic cell removal. *Curr. Biol.* **11**:R795–R805.

Herbomel, P., B. Thisse, and C. Thisse. 1999. Ontogeny and behaviour of early macrophages in the zebrafish embryo. *Development* **126**:3735–3745.

Herbomel, P., B. Thisse, and C. Thisse. 2001. Zebrafish early macrophages colonize cephalic mesenchyme and developing brain, retina, and epidermis through a M-CSF receptor-dependent invasive process. *Dev. Biol.* **238**:274–288.

Hernandez-Munain, C., P. Lauzurica, and M. S. Krangel. 1996. Regulation of T cell receptor delta gene rearrangement by c-Myb. *J. Exp. Med.* **183**:289–293.

Himes, S. R., and D. A. Hume. Transcription factors that regulate macrophage development and function. *In Handbook of Experimental Pharmacology. Pharmacology of Macrophages.* Springer-Verlag, New York, N.Y., in press.

Hirsch, S., and S. Gordon. 1982. The use and limitation of monoclonal antibodies against mononuclear phagocytes. *Immunobiology* **161**:298–307.

Hodgkinson, C. A., K. J. Moore, A. Nakayama, E. Steingrimsson, N. G. Copeland, N. A. Jenkins, and H. Arnheiter. 1993. Mutations at the mouse microphthalmia locus are associated with defects in a gene encoding a novel basic-helix-loop-helix-zipper protein. *Cell* **74**:395–404.

Hofstetter, W., A. Wetterwald, M. C. Cecchini, R. Felix, H. Fleisch, and C. Mueller. 1992. Detection of transcripts for the receptor for macrophage colony-stimulating factor, c-fms, in murine osteoclasts. *Proc. Natl. Acad. Sci. USA* **89**:9637–9641.

Hopkinson-Woolley, J., D. Hughes, S. Gordon, and P. Martin. 1994. Macrophage recruitment during limb development and wound healing in the embryonic and foetal mouse. *J. Cell Sci.* **107**:1159–1167.

Hume, D. A. 1985. Immunohistochemical analysis of murine mononuclear phagocytes that express class II major histocompatibility antigens. *Immunobiology* **170**:381–389.

Hume, D. A., and S. Gordon. 1983a. Mononuclear phagocyte system of the mouse defined by immunohistochemical localization of antigen F4/80. Identification of resident macrophages in renal medullary and cortical interstitium and the juxtaglomerular complex. *J. Exp. Med.* **157**:1704–1709.

Hume, D. A., and S. Gordon. 1983b. Optimal conditions for proliferation of bone marrow–derived mouse macrophages in culture: the roles of CSF-1, serum, Ca2+, and adherence. *J. Cell. Physiol.* **117**:189–194.

Hume, D. A., and S. Gordon. 1985. The mononuclear phagocytes system of the mouse defined by immunohistochemical localisation of antigen F4/80, p. 9–17. *In* R. van Furth (ed.), *Mononuclear Phagocytes: Characteristic, Physiology and Function.* Martinus Nijhoff Publisher, Boston, Mass.

Hume, D. A., V. H. Perry, and S. Gordon. 1983a. Immunohistochemical localization of a macrophage-specific antigen in developing mouse retina: phagocytosis of dying neurons and differentiation of microglial cells to form a regular array in the plexiform layers. *J. Cell Biol.* **97**:253–257.

Hume, D. A., A. P. Robinson, G. G. MacPherson, and S. Gordon. 1983b. The mononuclear phagocyte system of the mouse defined by immunohistochemical localization of antigen F4/80. Relationship between macrophages, Langerhans cells, reticular cells, and dendritic cells in lymphoid and hematopoietic organs. *J. Exp. Med.* **158**:1522–1536.

Hume, D. A., D. Halpin, H. Charlton, and S. Gordon. 1984a. The mononuclear phagocyte system of the mouse defined by immunohistochemical localization of antigen F4/80: macrophages of endocrine organs. *Proc. Natl. Acad. Sci. USA* **81**:4174–4177.

Hume, D. A., J. F. Loutit, and S. Gordon. 1984b. The mononuclear phagocyte system of the mouse defined by immunohistochemical localization of antigen F4/80: macrophages of bone and associated connective tissue. *J. Cell Sci.* **66**:189–194.

Hume, D. A., V. H. Perry, and S. Gordon. 1984c. The mononuclear phagocyte system of the mouse

defined by immunohistochemical localisation of antigen F4/80: macrophages associated with epithelia. *Anat. Rec.* **210**:503–512.

Hume, D. A., W. Allan, P. G. Hogan, and W. F. Doe. 1987. Immunohistochemical characterisation of macrophages in human liver and gastrointestinal tract: expression of CD4, HLA-DR, OKM1, and the mature macrophage marker 25F9 in normal and diseased tissue. *J. Leukoc. Biol.* **42**:474–484.

Hume, D. A., P. Pavli, R. E. Donahue, and I. J. Fidler. 1988. The effect of human recombinant macrophage colony-stimulating factor (CSF-1) on the murine mononuclear phagocyte system in vivo. *J. Immunol.* **141**:3405–3409.

Hume, D. A., S. J. Monkley, and B. J. Wainwright. 1995. Detection of c-fms protooncogene in early mouse embryos by whole mount in situ hybridization indicates roles for macrophages in tissue remodelling. *Br. J. Haematol.* **90**:939–942.

Hume, D. A., D. M. Underhill, M. J. Sweet, A. O. Ozinsky, F. Y. Liew, and A. Aderem. 2001. Macrophages exposed continuously to lipopolysaccharide and other agonists that act via toll-like receptors exhibit a sustained and additive activation state. *BMC Immunol.* **2**:11.

Hume, D. A., I. L. Ross, S. R. Himes, R. T. Sasmono, C. A. Wells, and T. Ravasi. 2002. The mononuclear phagocyte system revisited. *J. Leukoc. Biol.* **72**:621–627.

Itoh, M., A. Yano, X. Li, K. Miyamoto, and Y. Takeuchi. 1999. Limited uptake of foreign materials by resident macrophages in murine ovarian tissues. *J. Reprod. Immunol.* **43**:55–66.

Johansson, A., M. Lundborg, C. M. Skold, J. Lundahl, G. Tornling, A. Eklund, and P. Camner. 1997. Functional, morphological, and phenotypical differences between rat alveolar and interstitial macrophages. *Am. J. Respir. Cell Mol. Biol.* **16**:582–588.

Kasuya, K. 1997. Elimination of apoptotic granulosa cells by intact granulosa cells and macrophages in atretic mature follicles of the guinea pig ovary. *Arch. Histol. Cytol.* **60**:175–184.

Kaur, C., C. H. Wu, and E. A. Ling. 1997. Immunohistochemical and tracer studies of macrophages/microglia in the pineal gland of postnatal rats. *J. Pineal Res.* **22**:137–144.

Kaur, C., A. J. Hao, C. H. Wu, and E. A. Ling. 2001. Origin of microglia. *Microsc. Res. Tech.* **54**:2–9.

Kawakami, M., S. Kuroda, K. Yamashita, C. A. Yoshida, K. Nakagawa, and K. Takada. 1999. Expression of CSF-1 receptor on TRAP-positive multinuclear cells around the erupting molars in rats. *J. Craniofac. Genet. Dev. Biol.* **19**:213–220.

Kern, S., S. A. Robertson, V. J. Mau, and S. Maddocks. 1995. Cytokine secretion by macrophages in the rat testis. *Biol. Reprod.* **53**:1407–1416.

Kim, J. G., C. Keshava, A. A. Murphy, R. E. Pitas, and S. Parthasarathy. 1997. Fresh mouse peritoneal macrophages have low scavenger receptor activity. *J. Lipid Res.* **38:**2207–2215.

Kipari, T., and J. Hughes. 2002. Macrophage-mediated renal cell death. *Kidney Int.* **61:**760–761.

Klein, M. A., J. C. Moller, L. L. Jones, H. Bluethmann, G. W. Kreutzberg, and G. Raivich. 1997. Impaired neuroglial activation in interleukin-6 deficient mice. *Glia* **19:**227–233.

Klemsz, M. J., S. R. McKercher, A. Celada, C. Van Beveren, and R. A. Maki. 1990. The macrophage and B cell-specific transcription factor PU.1 is related to the ets oncogene. *Cell* **61:**113–124.

Kreutzberg, G. W. 1996. Microglia: a sensor for pathological events in the CNS. *Trends Neurosci.* **19:**312–318.

Lai, L., N. Alaverdi, L. Maltais, and H. C. Morse III. 1998. Mouse cell surface antigens: nomenclature and immunophenotyping. *J. Immunol.* **160:**3861–3868.

Laskin, D. L., B. Weinberger, and J. D. Laskin. 2001. Functional heterogeneity in liver and lung macrophages. *J. Leukoc. Biol.* **70:**163–170.

Lean, J. M., K. Fuller, and T. J. Chambers. 2001. FLT3 ligand can substitute for macrophage colony-stimulating factor in support of osteoclast differentiation and function. *Blood* **98:**2707–2713.

Lee, F. D. 1992. The role of interleukin-6 in development. *Dev. Biol.* **151:**331–338.

Lee, S. H., P. M. Starkey, and S. Gordon. 1985. Quantitative analysis of total macrophage content in adult mouse tissues. Immunochemical studies with monoclonal antibody F4/80. *J. Exp. Med.* **161:**475–489.

Leenen, P. J., M. F. de Bruijn, J. S. Voerman, P. A. Campbell, and W. van Ewijk. 1994. Markers of mouse macrophage development detected by monoclonal antibodies. *J. Immunol. Methods* **174:**5–19.

Lehnert, B. E. 1992. Pulmonary and thoracic macrophage subpopulations and clearance of particles from the lung. *Environ. Health Perspect.* **97:**17–46.

Lenny, N., J. J. Westendorf, and S. W. Hiebert. 1997. Transcriptional regulation during myelopoiesis. *Mol. Biol. Rep.* **24:**157–168.

Lichanska, A. M., and D. A. Hume. 2000. Origins and functions of phagocytes in the embryo. *Exp. Hematol.* **28:**601–611.

Lichanska, A. M., C. M. Browne, G. W. Henkel, K. M. Murphy, M. C. Ostrowski, S. R. McKercher, R. A. Maki, and D. A. Hume. 1999. Differentiation of the mononuclear phagocyte system during mouse embryogenesis: the role of transcription factor PU.1. *Blood* **94:**127–138.

Lloberas, J., C. Soler, and A. Celada. 1999. The key role of PU.1/SPI-1 in B cells, myeloid cells and macrophages. *Immunol. Today* **20:**184–189.

Lohmann-Matthes, M. L., C. Steinmuller, and G. Franke-Ullmann. 1994. Pulmonary macrophages. *Eur. Respir. J.* **7:**1678–1689.

Lukyanenko, Y. O., J. J. Chen, and J. C. Hutson. 2001. Production of 25-hydroxycholesterol by testicu-lar macrophages and its effects on Leydig cells. *Biol. Reprod.* **64:**790–796.

Mackler, A. M., L. M. Green, P. J. McMillan, and S. M. Yellon. 2000. Distribution and activation of uterine mononuclear phagocytes in peripartum endometrium and myometrium of the mouse. *Biol. Reprod.* **62:**1193–1200.

Maus, U., J. Huwe, L. Ermert, M. Ermert, W. Seeger, and J. Lohmeyer. 2002. Molecular pathways of monocyte emigration into the alveolar air space of intact mice. *Am. J. Respir. Crit. Care Med.* **165:**95–100.

McKenzie, S. E., and A. D. Schreiber. 1998. Fc gamma receptors in phagocytes. *Curr. Opin. Hematol.* **5:**16–21.

McKercher, S. R., B. E. Torbett, K. L. Anderson, G. W. Henkel, D. J. Vestal, H. Baribault, M. Klemsz, A. J. Feeney, G. E. Wu, C. J. Paige, and R. A. Maki. 1996. Targeted disruption of the PU.1 gene results in multiple hematopoietic abnormalities. *EMBO J.* **15:**5647–5658.

McKnight, A. J., and S. Gordon. 1998a. The EGF-TM7 family: unusual structures at the leukocyte surface. *J. Leukoc. Biol.* **63:**271–280.

McKnight, A. J., and S. Gordon. 1998b. Membrane molecules as differentiation antigens of murine macrophages. *Adv. Immunol.* **68:**271–314.

Mellman, I., and R. M. Steinman. 2001. Dendritic cells: specialized and regulated antigen processing machines. *Cell* **106:**255–258.

Mellman, I., S. J. Turley, and R. M. Steinman. 1998. Antigen processing for amateurs and professionals. *Trends Cell Biol.* **8:**231–237.

Mendis-Handagama, S. M., G. P. Risbridger, and D. M. de Kretser. 1987. Morphometric analysis of the components of the neonatal and the adult rat testis interstitium. *Int. J. Androl.* **10:**525–534.

Messmer, U. K., and J. Pfeilschifter. 2000. New insights into the mechanism for clearance of apoptotic cells. *Bioessays* **22:**878–881.

Metcalf, D. 1989. The molecular control of cell division, differentiation commitment and maturation in haemopoietic cells. *Nature* **339:**27–30.

Metcalf, D. 1997. The molecular control of granulocytes and macrophages. *CIBA Found. Symp.* **204:**40–50.

Michaelson, M. D., P. L. Bieri, M. F. Mehler, H. Xu, J. C. Arezzo, J. W. Pollard, and J. A. Kessler. 1996. CSF-1 deficiency in mice results in abnormal brain development. *Development* **122:**2661–2672.

Miki, R., K. Kadota, H. Bono, Y. Mizuno, Y. Tomaru, P. Carninci, M. Itoh, K. Shibata, J. Kawai, H. Konno, S. Watanabe, K. Sato, Y. Tokusumi, N. Kikuchi, Y. Ishii, Y. Hamaguchi, I. Nishizuka, H. Goto, H. Nitanda, S. Satomi, A. Yoshiki, M. Kusakabe, J. L. DeRisi, M. B. Eisen, V. R. Iyer, P. O. Brown, M. Muramatsu, H. Shimada, Y. Okazaki, and Y. Hayashizaki. 2001. Delineating developmental and metabolic pathways in vivo by expression profiling using the RIKEN set of 18,816 full-length enriched mouse cDNA arrays. *Proc. Natl. Acad. Sci. USA* **98**:2199–2204.

Mills, C. D., K. Kincaid, J. M. Alt, M. J. Heilman, and A. M. Hill. 2000. M-1/M-2 macrophages and the Th1/Th2 paradigm. *J. Immunol.* **164**:6166–6173.

Mitrasinovic, O. M., and G. M. Murphy, Jr. 2002. Accelerated phagocytosis of amyloid-beta by mouse and human microglia overexpressing the macrophage colony-stimulating factor receptor. *J. Biol. Chem.* **277**: 29889–29896.

Miyamoto, T., O. Ohneda, F. Arai, K. Iwamoto, S. Okada, K. Takagi, D. M. Anderson, and T. Suda. 2001. Bifurcation of osteoclasts and dendritic cells from common progenitors. *Blood* **98**:2544–2554.

Moore, M. A., and D. Metcalf. 1970. Ontogeny of the haemopoietic system: yolk sac origin of in vivo and in vitro colony forming cells in the developing mouse embryo. *Br. J. Haematol.* **18**:279–296.

Mori, T., A. Bartocci, J. Satriano, A. Zuckerman, R. Stanley, A. Santiago, and D. Schlondorff. 1990. Mouse mesangial cells produce colony-stimulating factor-1 (CSF-1) and express the CSF-1 receptor. *J. Immunol.* **144**:4697–4702.

Morrissette, N., E. Gold, and A. Aderem. 1999. The macrophage—a cell for all seasons. *Trends Cell Biol.* **9**:199–201.

Morse, H. C., III, J. F. Kearney, P. G. Isaacson, M. Carroll, T. N. Fredrickson, and E. S. Jaffe. 2001. Cells of the marginal zone—origins, function and neoplasia. *Leukoc. Res.* **25**:169–178.

Morton, H. C., M. van Egmond, and J. G. van de Winkel. 1996. Structure and function of human IgA Fc receptors (Fc alpha R). *Crit. Rev. Immunol.* **16**:423–440.

Moss, S. T., and J. A. Hamilton. 2000. Proliferation of a subpopulation of human peripheral blood monocytes in the presence of colony stimulating factors may contribute to the inflammatory process in diseases such as rheumatoid arthritis. *Immunobiology* **202**:18–25.

Muller, W. A. 2001. New mechanisms and pathways for monocyte recruitment. *J. Exp. Med.* **194**:F47–F51.

Nagashima, R., K. Maeda, Y. Imai, and T. Takahashi. 1996. Lamina propria macrophages in the human gastrointestinal mucosa: their distribution, immunohistological phenotype, and function. *J. Histochem. Cytochem.* **44**:721–731.

Nagulapalli, S., J. M. Pongubala, and M. L. Atchison. 1995. Multiple proteins physically interact with PU.1. Transcriptional synergy with NF-IL6 beta (C/EBP delta, CRP3). *J. Immunol.* **155**:4330–4338.

Naito, M., S. Hayashi, H. Yoshida, S. Nishikawa, L. D. Shultz, and K. Takahashi. 1991. Abnormal differentiation of tissue macrophage populations in 'osteopetrosis' (op) mice defective in the production of macrophage colony-stimulating factor. *Am. J. Pathol.* **139**:657–667.

Nathan, C. F., and J. B. Hibbs, Jr. 1991. Role of nitric oxide synthesis in macrophage antimicrobial activity. *Curr. Opin. Immunol.* **3**:65–70.

Nes, W. D., Y. O. Lukyanenko, Z. H. Jia, S. Quideau, W. N. Howald, T. K. Pratum, R. R. West, and J. C. Hutson. 2000. Identification of the lipophilic factor produced by macrophages that stimulates steroidogenesis. *Endocrinology* **141**:953–958.

Neufeld, G., T. Cohen, S. Gengrinovitch, and Z. Poltorak. 1999. Vascular endothelial growth factor (VEGF) and its receptors. *FASEB J.* **13**:9–22.

Niida, S., M. Kaku, H. Amano, H. Yoshida, H. Kataoka, S. Nishikawa, K. Tanne, N. Maeda, and H. Kodama. 1999. Vascular endothelial growth factor can substitute for macrophage colony-stimulating factor in the support of osteoclastic bone resorption. *J. Exp. Med.* **190**:293–298.

Nikolic-Paterson, D. J., and R. C. Atkins. 2001. The role of macrophages in glomerulonephritis. *Nephrol. Dial. Transplant.* **16**:3–7.

Nusrat, A. R., S. D. Wright, A. A. Aderem, R. M. Steinman, and Z. A. Cohn. 1988. Properties of isolated red pulp macrophages from mouse spleen. *J. Exp. Med.* **168**:1505–1510.

O'Connell, N. A., A. Kumar, K. Chatzipanteli, A. Mohan, R. K. Agarwal, C. Head, S. R. Bornstein, A. B. Abou-Samra, and A. R. Gwosdow. 1994. Interleukin-1 regulates corticosterone secretion from the rat adrenal gland through a catecholamine-dependent and prostaglandin E2-independent mechanism. *Endocrinology* **135**:460–467.

Oelgeschlager, M., I. Nuchprayoon, B. Luscher, and A. D. Friedman. 1996. C/EBP, c-Myb, and PU.1 cooperate to regulate the neutrophil elastase promoter. *Mol. Cell. Biol.* **16**:4717–4725.

Opdenakker, G., and J. Van Damme. 1992. Cytokines and proteases in invasive processes: molecular similarities between inflammation and cancer. *Cytokine* **4**:251–258.

Pate, J. L., and P. Landis Keyes. 2001. Immune cells in the corpus luteum: friends or foes? *Reproduction* **122**:665–676.

Pavli, P., and W. F. Doe. 1992. Intestinal macrophages, p. 177–188. *In* R. P. McDermott and W. F. Stenson (ed.), *Inflammatory Bowel Diseases.* Elsevier, New York, N.Y.

Pavli, P., C. E. Woodhams, W. F. Doe, and D. A. Hume. 1990. Isolation and characterization of antigen-presenting dendritic cells from the mouse intestinal lamina propria. *Immunology* **70**:40–47.

Perry, V. H. 1994. *Macrophages and the Nervous System.* R.G. Landes Company, Georgetown, Tex.

Pforte, A., C. Gerth, A. Voss, B. Beer, K. Haussinger, U. Jutting, G. Burger, and H. W. Ziegler-Heitbrock. 1993. Proliferating alveolar macrophages in BAL and lung function changes in interstitial lung disease. *Eur. Respir. J.* **6:**951–955.

Pollard, J. W., M. G. Dominguez, S. Mocci, P. E. Cohen, and E. R. Stanley. 1997. Effect of the colony-stimulating factor-1 null mutation, osteopetrotic (csfm(op)), on the distribution of macrophages in the male mouse reproductive tract. *Biol. Reprod.* **56:**1290–1300.

Ravasi, T., C. Wells, A. Forest, D. M. Underhill, B. J. Wainwright, A. Aderem, S. Grimmond, and D. A. Hume. 2002. Generation of diversity in the innate immune system: macrophage heterogeneity arises from gene-autonomous transcriptional probability of individual inducible genes. *J. Immunol.* **168:**44–50.

Reddy, M. A., B. S. Yang, X. Yue, C. J. Barnett, I. L. Ross, M. J. Sweet, D. A. Hume, and M. C. Ostrowski. 1994. Opposing actions of c-ets/PU.1 and c-myb protooncogene products in regulating the macrophage-specific promoters of the human and mouse colony-stimulating factor-1 receptor (c-fms) genes. *J. Exp. Med.* **180:**2309–2319.

Rehli, M., A. Lichanska, A. I. Cassady, M. C. Ostrowski, and D. A. Hume. 1999. TFEC is a macrophage-restricted member of the microphthalmia-TFE subfamily of basic helix-loop-helix leucine zipper transcription factors. *J. Immunol.* **162:** 1559–1565.

Rogler, G., M. Hausmann, D. Vogl, E. Aschenbrenner, T. Andus, W. Falk, R. Andreesen, J. Scholmerich, and V. Gross. 1998. Isolation and phenotypic characterization of colonic macrophages. *Clin. Exp. Immunol.* **112:**205–215.

Romani, N., S. Gruner, D. Brang, E. Kampgen, A. Lenz, B. Trockenbacher, G. Konwalinka, P. O. Fritsch, R. M. Steinman, and G. Schuler. 1994. Proliferating dendritic cell progenitors in human blood. *J. Exp. Med.* **180:**83–93.

Romani, N., D. Reider, M. Heuer, S. Ebner, E. Kampgen, B. Eibl, D. Niederwieser, and G. Schuler. 1996. Generation of mature dendritic cells from human blood. An improved method with special regard to clinical applicability. *J. Immunol. Methods* **196:**137–151.

Rosenberger, C. M., M. G. Scott, M. R. Gold, R. E. Hancock, and B. B. Finlay. 2000. *Salmonella typhimurium* infection and lipopolysaccharide stimulation induce similar changes in macrophage gene expression. *J. Immunol.* **164:**5894–5904.

Ross, I. L., T. L. Dunn, X. Yue, S. Roy, C. J. Barnett, and D. A. Hume. 1994. Comparison of the expression and function of the transcription factor PU.1 (Spi-1 proto-oncogene) between murine macrophages and B lymphocytes. *Oncogene* **9:**121–132.

Ross, I. L., X. Yue, M. C. Ostrowski, and D. A. Hume. 1998. Interaction between PU.1 and another Ets family transcription factor promotes macrophage-

specific Basal transcription initiation. *J. Biol. Chem.* **273:**6662–6669.

Sadahira, Y., and M. Mori. 1999. Role of the macrophage in erythropoiesis. *Pathol. Int.* **49:**841–848.

Sallusto, F., and A. Lanzavecchia. 1994. Efficient presentation of soluble antigen by cultured human dendritic cells is maintained by granulocyte/macrophage colony-stimulating factor plus interleukin 4 and downregulated by tumor necrosis factor alpha. *J. Exp. Med.* **179:**1109–1118.

Samms, M., M. Martinez, S. Fousse, M. Pezzano, and J. C. Guyden. 2001. Circulating macrophages as well as developing thymocytes are enclosed within thymic nurse cells. *Cell. Immunol.* **212:**16–23.

Sasmono, R. T., D. Oceandy, J. W. Pollard, W. Tong, P. Pavli, B. J. Wainwright, M. C. Ostrowski, S. R. Himes, and D. A. Hume. 2003. A macrophage colony-stimulating factor receptor (CSF-1R)-green fluorescent protein transgene is expressed throughout the mononuclear phagocyte system of the mouse. *Blood* **101:**1155–1163.

Savill, J., and V. Fadok. 2000. Corpse clearance defines the meaning of cell death. *Nature* **407:**784–788.

Schober, A., K. Huber, J. Fey, and K. Unsicker. 1998. Distinct populations of macrophages in the adult rat adrenal gland: a subpopulation with neurotrophin-4-like immunoreactivity. *Cell Tissue Res.* **291:**365–373.

Scott, E. W., M. C. Simon, J. Anastasi, and H. Singh. 1994. Requirement of transcription factor PU.1 in the development of multiple hematopoietic lineages. *Science* **265:**1573–1577.

Shapiro, L. H. 1995. Myb and Ets proteins cooperate to transactivate an early myeloid gene. *J. Biol. Chem.* **270:**8763–8771.

Shapiro, S., E. Campbell, R. Senior, and H. Welgus. 1991. Proteinases secreted by human mononuclear phagocytes. *J. Rheumatol.* **27**(Suppl.)**:**95–98.

Shortman, K., and Y. J. Liu. 2002. Mouse and human dendritic cell subtypes. *Nat. Rev. Immunol.* **2:**151–161.

Sleyster, E. C., and D. L. Knook. 1982. Relation between localization and function of rat liver Kupffer cells. *Lab. Invest.* **47:**484–490.

Smith, P. D., L. E. Smythies, M. Mosteller-Barnum, D. A. Sibley, M. W. Russell, M. Merger, M. T. Sellers, J. M. Orenstein, T. Shimada, M. F. Graham, and H. Kubagawa. 2001. Intestinal macrophages lack CD14 and CD89 and consequently are down-regulated for LPS- and IgA-mediated activities. *J. Immunol.* **167:**2651–2656.

Soesatyo, M., J. Biewenga, G. Kraal, and T. Sminia. 1990. The localization of macrophage subsets and dendritic cells in the gastrointestinal tract of the mouse with special reference to the presence of high endothelial venules. An immuno- and enzyme-histochemical study. *Cell Tissue Res.* **259:**587–593.

Stanley, E. R., K. L. Berg, D. B. Einstein, P. S. Lee, F. J. Pixley, Y. Wang, and Y. G. Yeung. 1997. Biology and action of colony-stimulating factor-1. *Mol. Reprod. Dev.* **46:**4–10.

Steinman, R. M., and K. Inaba. 1999. Myeloid dendritic cells. *J. Leukoc. Biol.* **66:**205–208.

Steinman, R. M., K. Inaba, S. Turley, P. Pierre, and I. Mellman. 1999. Antigen capture, processing, and presentation by dendritic cells: recent cell biological studies. *Hum. Immunol.* **60:**562–567.

Surh, C. D., and J. Sprent. 1994. T-cell apoptosis detected in situ during positive and negative selection in the thymus. *Nature* **372:**100–103.

Sweet, M. J., and D. A. Hume. 1996. Endotoxin signal transduction in macrophages. *J. Leukoc. Biol.* **60:** 8–26.

Sweet, M. J., C. C. Campbell, D. P. Sester, D. Xu, R. C. McDonald, K. J. Stacey, D. A. Hume, and F. Y. Liew. 2002. Colony-stimulating factor-1 suppresses responses to CpG DNA and expression of toll-like receptor 9 but enhances responses to lipopolysaccharide in murine macrophages. *J. Immunol.* **168:**392–399.

Tagoh, H., R. Himes, D. Clarke, P. J. Leenen, A. D. Riggs, D. Hume, and C. Bonifer. 2002. Transcription factor complex formation and chromatin fine structure alterations at the murine c-fms (CSF-1 receptor) locus during maturation of myeloid precursor cells. *Genes Dev.* **16:**1721–1737.

Takahashi, K., M. Naito, and L. D. Shultz. 1992. Differentiation of epidermal Langerhans cells in macrophage colony-stimulating-factor-deficient mice homozygous for the osteopetrosis (op) mutation. *J. Invest. Dermatol.* **99:**46S–47S.

Takahashi, K., M. Naito, and M. Takeya. 1996. Development and heterogeneity of macrophages and their related cells through their differentiation pathways. *Pathol. Int.* **46:**473–485.

Takahashi, K., M. J. Donovan, R. A. Rogers, and R. A. Ezekowitz. 1998. Distribution of murine mannose receptor expression from early embryogenesis through to adulthood. *Cell Tissue Res.* **292:**311–323.

Tarling, J. D., and J. E. Coggle. 1982. Evidence for the pulmonary origin of alveolar macrophages. *Cell Tissue Kinet.* **15:**577–584.

Tauber, A. I., and L. Chernyak. 1991. *Metchnikoff and the Origins of Immunology: From Metaphor to Theory.* Oxford University Press, New York, N.Y.

Teitelbaum, S. L. 2000. Bone resorption by osteoclasts. *Science* **289:**1504–1508.

Tenen, D. G., R. Hromas, J. D. Licht, and D. E. Zhang. 1997. Transcription factors, normal myeloid development, and leukemia. *Blood* **90:**489–519.

Tesch, G. H., A. Schwarting, K. Kinoshita, H. Y. Lan, B. J. Rollins, and V. R. Kelley. 1999. Monocyte chemoattractant protein-1 promotes macrophage-mediated tubular injury, but not glomerular injury, in nephrotoxic serum nephritis. *J. Clin. Invest.* **103:**73–80.

Thomas, W. E. 1999. Brain macrophages: on the role of pericytes and perivascular cells. *Brain Res. Rev.* **31:**42–57.

Tushinski, R. J., I. T. Oliver, L. J. Guilbert, P. W. Tynan, J. R. Warner, and E. R. Stanley. 1982. Survival of mononuclear phagocytes depends on a lineage-specific growth factor that the differentiated cells selectively destroy. *Cell* **28:**71–81.

Udagawa, N., N. Takahashi, T. Akatsu, H. Tanaka, T. Sasaki, T. Nishihara, T. Koga, T. J. Martin, and T. Suda. 1990. Origin of osteoclasts: mature monocytes and macrophages are capable of differentiating into osteoclasts under a suitable microenvironment prepared by bone marrow-derived stromal cells. *Proc. Natl. Acad. Sci. USA* **87:**7260–7264.

Ulevitch, R. J., and P. S. Tobias. 1995. Receptor-dependent mechanisms of cell stimulation by bacterial endotoxin. *Annu. Rev. Immunol.* **13:**437–457.

Umeda, S., K. Takahashi, L. D. Shultz, M. Naito, and K. Takagi. 1996. Effects of macrophage colony-stimulating factor on macrophages and their related cell populations in the osteopetrosis mouse defective in production of functional macrophage colony-stimulating factor protein. *Am. J. Pathol.* **149:**559–574.

Unanue, E. R., and P. M. Allen. 1986. Biochemistry and biology of antigen presentation by macrophages. *Cell. Immunol.* **99:**3–6.

Underhill, D. M., M. Bassetti, A. Rudensky, and A. Aderem. 1999. Dynamic interactions of macrophages with T cells during antigen presentation. *J. Exp. Med.* **190:**1909–1914.

Valledor, A. F., F. E. Borras, M. Cullell-Young, and A. Celada. 1998. Transcription factors that regulate monocyte/macrophage differentiation. *J. Leukoc. Biol.* **63:**405–417.

van der Laan, L. J., E. A. Dopp, R. Haworth, T. Pikkarainen, M. Kangas, O. Elomaa, C. D. Dijkstra, S. Gordon, K. Tryggvason, and G. Kraal. 1999. Regulation and functional involvement of macrophage scavenger receptor MARCO in clearance of bacteria in vivo. *J. Immunol.* **162:**939–947.

van der Meer, J. W. M., J. S. van de Gevel, R. de Water, L. A. Ginsel, C. H. Wouters, W. T. Daems, and R. van Furth. 1985. Proliferation and differentiation of mononuclear phagocytes in vitro, p. 243–254. *In* R. van Furth (ed.), *Mononuclear Phagocytes: Characteristic, Physiology, and Function.* Martinus Nijhoff, Dordrecht, The Netherlands.

van Furth, R. 1992. Production and migration of monocytes and kinetics of macrophages, p. 3–12. *In* R. van Furth (ed.) *Mononuclear Phagocytes: Biology of Monocytes and Macrophages.* Kluwer Academic Publisher, Amsterdam, The Netherlands.

van Furth, R. 1998. Human monocytes and cyto-kines. *Res. Immunol.* **149:**719–720.

van Furth, R., and W. Sluiter. 1986. Distribution of blood monocytes between a marginating and a circulating pool. *J. Exp. Med.* **163:**474–479.

van Furth, R., Z. Cohn, J. Hirsh, J. Humprey, W. Spector, and H. Langevoort. 1972. The mononuclear phagocyte system: a new classification of macrophages, monocytes and their precursors. *Bull. W. H. O.* **46:**845–852.

van Oosten, M., E. S. van Amersfoort, T. J. van Berkel, and J. Kuiper. 2001. Scavenger receptor-like receptors for the binding of lipopolysaccharide and lipoteichoic acid to liver endothelial and Kupffer cells. *J. Endotoxin Res.* **7:**381–384.

Wardrop, S. L., C. Wells, T. Ravasi, D. A. Hume, and D. R. Richardson. 2002. Induction of Nramp2 in activated mouse macrophages is dissociated from regulation of the Nramp1, classical inflammatory genes, and genes involved in iron metabolism. *J. Leukoc. Biol.* **71:**99–106.

Watanabe, S., A. Yoshimura, K. Inui, N. Yokota, Y. Liu, Y. Sugenoya, H. Morita, and T. Ideura. 2001. Acquisition of the monocyte/macrophage phenotype in human mesangial cells. *J. Lab. Clin. Med.* **138:**193–199.

Wells, C. A., T. Ravasi, G. J. Faulkner, P. Carninci, Y. Okazaki, Y. Hayashizaki, M. Sweet, B. J. Wainwright, and D. A. Hume. 2003a. Genetic control of the innate immune response. *BMC Immunol.* **4:**5.

Wells, C. A., T. Ravasi, R. Sultana, K. Yagi, P. Carninci, H. Bono, G. Faulkner, Y. Okazaki, J. Quackenbush, D. A. Hume, and P. A. Lyons. 2003b. Continued discovery of transcriptional units expressed in cells of the mouse mononuclear phagocyte lineage. *Genome Res.* **13:**1360–1365.

Wheater, P. R., H. G. Burkitt, and V. G. Daniels. 1987. *Functional Histology: A Text and Colour Atlas,* 2nd ed. Churchill Livingstone, London, United Kingdom.

Wiktor-Jedrzejczak, W., and S. Gordon. 1996. Cytokine regulation of the macrophage (M phi) system studied using the colony stimulating factor-1-deficient op/op mouse. *Physiol. Rev.* **76:**927–947.

Wiktor-Jedrzejczak, W., A. Bartocci, A. W. Ferrante, Jr., A. Ahmed-Ansari, K. W. Sell, J. W. Pollard, and E. R. Stanley. 1990. Total absence of colony-stimulating factor 1 in the macrophage-deficient osteopetrotic (op/op) mouse. *Proc. Natl. Acad. Sci. USA* **87:**4828–4832.

Williams, K., X. Alvarez, and A. A. Lackner. 2001. Central nervous system perivascular cells are immunoregulatory cells that connect the CNS with the peripheral immune system. *Glia* **36:**156–164.

Wilson, K. 1997. Wound healing: the role of macrophages. *Nurs. Crit. Care* **2:**291–296.

Witmer-Pack, M. D., D. A. Hughes, G. Schuler, L. Lawson, A. McWilliam, K. Inaba, R. M. Steinman, and S. Gordon. 1993. Identification of macrophages and dendritic cells in the osteopetrotic (op/op) mouse. *J. Cell Sci.* **104:**1021–1029.

Wood, G. W. 1985. Macrophages in the thymus. *Surv. Immunol. Res.* **4:**179–191.

Xie, Y., C. Chen, and D. A. Hume. 2001. Transcriptional regulation of c-fms gene expression. *Cell Biochem. Biophys.* **34:**1–16.

Xie, Y., C. Chen, M. A. Stevenson, D. A. Hume, P. E. Auron, and S. K. Calderwood. 2002. NF-IL6 and HSF1 have mutually antagonistic effects on transcription in monocytic cells. *Biochem. Biophys. Res. Commun.* **291:**1071–1080.

Yoder, M. C. 2001. Introduction: spatial origin of murine hematopoietic stem cells. *Blood* **98:**3–5.

Yoshida, H., S. Hayashi, T. Kunisada, M. Ogawa, S. Nishikawa, H. Okamura, T. Sudo, and L. D. Shultz. 1990. The murine mutation osteopetrosis is in the coding region of the macrophage colony stimulating factor gene. *Nature* **345:**442–444.

Zhang, D. E., C. J. Hetherington, S. Meyers, K. L. Rhoades, C. J. Larson, H. M. Chen, S. W. Hiebert, and D. G. Tenen. 1996. CCAAT enhancer-binding protein (C/EBP) and AML1 (CBF alpha2) synergistically activate the macrophage colony-stimulating factor receptor promoter. *Mol. Cell. Biol.* **16:**1231–1240.

Zhang, Y., A. Harada, J. B. Wang, Y. Y. Zhang, S. Hashimoto, M. Naito, and K. Matsushima. 1998. Bifurcated dendritic cell differentiation in vitro from murine lineage phenotype-negative c-kit+ bone marrow hematopoietic progenitor cells. *Blood* **92:**118–128.

THE REGULATORY ROLE OF DENDRITIC CELLS IN THE INNATE IMMUNE RESPONSE

F. Granucci, S. Feau, I. Zanoni, G. Raimondi, N. Pavelka,
C. Vizzardelli, and P. Ricciardi-Castagnoli

5

DENDRITIC CELL ORIGIN AND FUNCTION

In 1868, P. Langerhans described, for the first time, skin dendritic cells (DCs) that he named Langerhans cells (LCs). Their function was mysterious but their morphology was clearly "dendritic." About 100 years later, Steinman and Cohn assigned to these intriguing DCs a specific accessory function in the immune system (Steinman, 1991). It took an additional 30 years to fully reveal the unique role of DCs in that they regulate both innate and adaptive immunity, depending on the local microenvironment and on their ability to interact and respond to infectious agents (Steinman and Nussenzweig, 2002; Ricciardi-Castagnoli and Granucci, 2002). Because of their functional plasticity, different DC effector functions have been described that largely depend on the tissue origin and location, the microbial environment, and the presence or absence of tissue inflammation (Banchereau et al., 2000).

Cells of the DC lineage are continuously produced; they arise from bone marrow hematopoietic stem cells as myeloid progenitors and seed all organism tissues. Although rare (they represent less than 1% in every tissue), they are ubiquitously distributed in lymphoid and nonlymphoid tissues; together with macrophages, they recognize pathogens and regulate the inflammatory processes. This last property is not yet fully integrated into the current literature because of the intuitive view that, because DCs initiate the adaptive immune response, they should promote, rather than reduce, inflammatory responses. Global transcriptional analyses of DC responses point to the potential of DCs to control inflammatory responses rather than to promote them (Ricciardi-Castagnoli and Granucci, 2002).

Multipotent lineage-restricted progenitor cells can be identified in the bone marrow, based on the expression of cell surface markers such as c-kit and CD34 but are negative for Lin, Sca-1, and IL7Ra and express a low level of Fcγ receptor (FcγR) (Akashi et al., 2000). In the mouse, these common myeloid progenitor cells can give rise to DC precursors (Traver et al., 2000) as well as to precursors for granulocyte and macrophage and erythroid and megakaryocyte lineages.

DC lineage-specific markers are still missing, and it has been difficult to distinguish DC progenitors from other myeloid progenitors

F. Granucci, S. Feau, I. Zanoni, G. Raimondi, N. Pavelka, C. Vizzardelli, and P. Ricciardi-Castagnoli, University of Milano-Bicocca, Department of Biotechnology and Bioscience, 20126 Milan, Italy.

The Innate Immune Response to Infection
Ed. by S. H. E. Kaufmann, R. Medzhitov, and S. Gordon
©2004 ASM Press, Washington, D.C.

such as the granulocytes and macrophage precursors. The lack of molecular markers defining specific checkpoints in the myeloid differentiation pathway and the inability to clone these cells have hampered a detailed analysis of the DC lineage. Nevertheless, at least three transcription factors regulating hematopoietic development of DCs have been described; they are PU.1, RelB, and Ikaros. The transcription factor PU.1 is expressed in bone marrow-derived DCs (Anderson et al., 2000) and seems to be essential for the development of a myeloid-derived DC subset; indeed, PU.1-deficient mice lack most DC subsets (Guerriero et al., 2000). The transcription factor RelB belongs to the NF-κB/Rel family, and the translocation of the RelB protein from the cytoplasm to the nucleus has been correlated with DC activation (Hofer et al., 2001). Moreover, RelB-deficient mice have impaired functions and a reduced number of spleen DCs (Weih et al., 1995). Ikaros proteins have a dual role: in addition to their role as transcriptional activators, they have a role in chromatin remodeling and histone deacetylation when associated with other cell proteins that control hematopoietic development (Kim et al., 1999), including DC-specific lineage. In fact, deletion of the Ikaros DNA-binding domain from the mouse germ line generates a mutation with dominant-negative effects ($DN^{-/-}$) that results in DC depletion. Surprisingly, in this case, but also in the RelB-deficient mice, LCs are untouched (Wu et al., 1997), suggesting that the mechanisms controlling the development of skin DCs do not require either Ikaros or RelB.

DCs IN THE TISSUES

Epithelium-Associated DCs

DCs are strategically located in mucosal tissues that represent pathogen entry routes, where they continuously monitor the environment through the uptake of pathogens. Variations among tissue distribution and differences in phenotypic and functional expression indicate the existence of heterogeneous populations of DCs with diverse abilities to recognize infectious agents and to regulate inflammatory responses.

The Skin DC. LCs are the DCs that typically populate squamous epithelia including the skin, the conjunctiva, and the oral, respiratory, and genital mucosae. LCs differ from other DCs in the presence of a unique intracellular organelle, known as the Birbeck granule, and in the presence of distinct markers (Girolomoni et al., 2001).

In the skin, LCs are localized in the basal and suprabasal layers of the epidermis, where they form a dense network that represents the first hematopoietic barrier to the external pathogens. In noninflamed conditions, resident adult LCs are maintained by a renewable population of progenitors, present in the skin after birth (Merad et al., 2002). This is in contrast with other mucosal tissues (e.g., gut and airways) where DCs are continuously replaced by bone marrow-derived circulating progenitors. The inability of circulating LC progenitors to seed noninflamed skin has been demonstrated with two different experimental models. In these experiments, LCs were not replaced by donor cells in lethally irradiated mice that had received syngeneic bone marrow transplants, in contrast to DCs from most other tissues (Merad et al., 2002). Moreover, in parabiotic mice that share a blood circulation but have separate organs, no mixing of LCs has been observed. However, in the adult skin, circulating LC progenitor recruitment could be observed when the skin was treated by inflammatory stimuli, such as UV light. In this case, circulating LC progenitors, seeding the inflamed skin, were replacing the loss of resident LCs (Merad et al., 2002). This recruitment is based on the production by the inflamed epithelial cells of the chemokine monocyte chemoattractant protein 1 (MCP-1), a ligand for CCR2 that is expressed on migratory bloodborne LC progenitors (Sato et al., 2000; Vanbervliet et al., 2002). During the embryonic life, seeding of the skin with LC precursors takes place, most likely from the fetal liver, which contains such progenitors (Merad et al.,

2002). This early seeding is independent of MCP-1 because CCR2$^{-/-}$ mice have normal skin LCs. Soon after birth, LCs become autonomous, and in the absence of inflammation, a self-turnover of resident cells, which does not require the migration of bone marrow-derived progenitors, is established.

In common with other DCs, LCs residing in steady-state tissues are in an "immature" functional state in which their primary task is to sense the environment for infectious non-self signals and to capture, process, and transduce these signals. Interstitial DCs and LCs express distinct receptors for antigen uptake. In particular, LCs express Fcγ and Fcε receptors, the DEC-205 multilectin (in mice), and Langerin (in humans and mice), whereas human DCs possess the macrophage mannose receptor and DC-SIGN. LCs are the only DCs expressing Langerin, which routes extracellular multi-mannosylated ligands through Birbeck's granules to major histocompatibility complex (MHC) class II negative compartments (Valladeau et al., 2000). In contrast, interstitial DCs, but not LCs, express several isoforms of the type II lectin asialoglycoprotein receptor, which localizes to early endosomes and intersects with the MHC class II positive pathway. Therefore, LCs and DCs can exploit different receptors for antigen uptake and access to distinct antigen-processing pathways. When LCs become activated, this process triggers their migration from the epidermis to regional lymph nodes and the acquisition of potent T-cell-stimulating capacities.

Transforming growth factor β (TGF-β) is now recognized as an essential factor for the development of both mouse and human LCs: *tgfb1* null mice are devoid of LCs, and TGF-β drives the differentiation of monocyte and CD34$^+$ precursors into LCs. Of note, both TGF-β and ligation of E-cadherin, an adhesion molecule that retains LCs in the epidermis by establishing homotypic interactions with keratinocytes, inhibit LC maturation (Girolomoni et al., 2001).

LCs have been among the earliest and most investigated DCs in both humans and animals and are still providing important clues for understanding the role of DCs in the immune system.

The Gut DC. In the gut, DCs have been found in Peyer's patches (PPs) forming a dense layer of cells in the subepithelial dome (Ruedl and Hubele, 1997) beneath the follicle epithelium (Kelsall and Strober, 1996; Iwasaki and Kelsall, 2000) in close contact with M cells and in the lamina propria, where they are distributed along the entire intestinal epithelium (Maric et al., 1996). DCs have been shown to take up bacteria across the mucosal epithelium (Rescigno et al., 2001). This result was quite surprising, as the intestinal mucosa has always been considered almost inaccessible to microbes because of the presence of a brush border on the luminal cell surface and the belt of tight junctions (TJs) between epithelial cells. Thus, entry of pathogens was believed to occur mainly through the specialized M cells, which lack an organized brush border. Nevertheless, it has been shown that bacterial strains deficient in invasion genes (such as the SPI1$^{-/-}$ *Salmonella typhimurium* strain) are still able to reach the spleen following oral administration (Kohbata et al., 1986), suggesting an M-cell-independent pathway. This M-cell-independent pathway has been recently elucidated (Rescigno et al., 2001). Indeed, DCs are able to open the TJs between epithelial cells, send dendrites outside of the epithelium, and sample bacteria directly in the gut lumen. The molecular mechanism that allows the preservation of the integrity of the epithelial barrier is based on the expression and modulation by DCs of TJ proteins, such as occludin, claudin 1, Zonula occludens 1, and the junctional adhesion molecule. Occludin is constitutively expressed in immature DCs, but becomes downregulated upon microbial stimuli; this may be sufficient to loosen the epithelial TJ, a destabilization that is followed by the rapid formation of new junctions between the epithelium and the infiltrating DCs, thus preserving the integrity of the epithelial barrier.

A dual role of gut DCs can be foreseen. In physiological steady-state conditions, the lamina propria resident DC population may have regulatory functions maintaining DC homeostasis and eliciting an anti-inflammatory cytokine production. In contrast, during inflammation, it has been clearly shown that DCs, expressing the chemokine receptor CCR6, are recruited from the blood through a chemokine gradient, mostly based on macrophage inflammatory protein-3α (MIP-3α) expression by epithelial cells (Tanaka et al., 1999). The responsiveness of mucosal DC populations to inflammatory stimuli, in particular their rapid kinetics of recruitment that surprisingly is equivalent to that of neutrophils, underscores their relevance as antigen sentinels and regulators at the mucosal sites. Indeed, in pathological conditions, such as in Crohn's disease, a good deal of recent evidence suggests that the failure of a physiological innate immune response could degenerate into an autoimmune response. In fact, more than 15% of the patients with Crohn's disease bear mutations in the NOD2 gene (Hugot et al., 2001; Ogura et al., 2001), a member of a new family of cytosolic proteins that regulate host response to pathogens through NF-κB signaling (Inohara and Nunez, 2002) and that is primarily expressed in myeloid cells of the gut. Surprisingly, this is the first time that a single specific gene mutation has been linked to a human autoimmune disease. In gut myeloid cells, products of the NOD2 gene family are normally involved in sensing the enteric bacterial flora and, most likely, in dampening the inflammatory responses. Thus, the genetic defect may very well result in a deregulated cytokine production, which ultimately manifests itself with an overreactive adaptive immune response (Inohara and Nunez, 2002).

The Pulmonary DC. As already mentioned for gut and skin DCs, the role of pulmonary DCs is very complex and depends on the context and form in which antigen is acquired. The respiratory mucosa interfaces broadly with the environmental antigens that continuously challenge the immune system. Pulmonary DCs play a critical role in sampling antigens and in discriminating between pathogenic versus innocuous inhaled antigens. The peripheral immune system has evolved mechanisms to maintain a state of active hyporesponsiveness to innocuous antigens. It has been recently shown that pulmonary DCs from mice exposed to soluble proteins such as ovalbumin, in the absence of inflammation, produced a high concentration of interleukin-10 (IL-10); moreover, the adoptive transfer (in mice exposed to these soluble antigens) of these DCs (but not of IL-10$^{-/-}$ DCs) induced antigen-specific unresponsiveness in recipient mice (Akbari et al., 2001). These results indicate that, in the lungs, IL-10 production by DCs is critical for the induction of specific hyporeactivity, similar to what has been observed in intestine PP DCs (Iwasaki and Kelsall, 1999). On the other hand, if mice are exposed to antigens under conditions that result in airway hyperactivity, a vigorous inflammatory response is induced and no IL-10 production is detected.

The IL-10-producing DCs induce the secretion, in naive CD4 T cells, of IL-4 and a high concentration of IL-10, but not gamma interferon. IL-10 is associated with regulatory T cells (Tr1) that mediate a form of "tolerance" characterized by low proliferative capacity, low IL-2, high IL-10, and the ability to suppress inflammatory responses and to downregulate pathological antigen-specific immune responses in vivo (Groux et al., 1997). It is likely that IL-10-producing DCs, either from the gut or from the lungs, may induce the differentiation of Tr1 cells that preferentially develop at mucosal sites and are associated with IL-10 production.

In the absence of inflammation, innocuous antigens that are continuously encountered in the lungs by DCs induce antigen-specific unresponsiveness. However, in situations where DC regulation of innate responses is impaired (e.g., allergic individuals), Th2-biased inflammatory responses causing asthma can be observed (Wills-Karp, 1999). During inflammatory responses to a broad spectrum of stimuli, DCs are recruited into the airway epithelium (McWilliam et al., 1996), and it has been postulated that rapid DC recruitment could be a hallmark of acute inflammatory responses at mucosal sites (McWilliam et al., 1994).

Lymphoid-Associated DCs

In addition to the mucosal sites, DCs are also strategically located in lymphoid tissues where pathogens can be easily brought and concentrated. It is not fully understood if DCs from spleen and lymph nodes differ from DCs associated with the mucosal sites. Nevertheless, it is believed that, in lymphoid tissues, DCs have a "mature" phenotype (Banchereau and Steinman, 1998). This is associated with reduced endocytic and phagocytic capacities (see below), enhanced production of inflammatory cytokines and chemokines, and acquisition of migratory functions allowing antigen-loaded DCs to migrate from the marginal zones where they are located to the T-cell areas. Mature DCs acquire high cell surface MHC and costimulatory protein expression and have the ability to prime antigen-specific CD8[+] and CD4[+] T-cell responses (Ridge et al., 1998; Ingulli et al., 1997). In addition, they are programmed for apoptotic cell death (Winzler et al., 1997; De Smedt et al., 1996). Signals inducing this DC priming leading to maturation are represented by microorganisms and bacterial cell products. Although these stimuli are generally considered equivalent factors in inducing mouse and human DC maturation, there is increasing evidence that diverse types of immune responses may originate from DCs primed with different stimuli (Rescigno et al., 1999; Cella et al., 1999; Granucci et al., 2001a; d'Ostiani et al., 2000).

In the lymphoid organs, DCs have the unique opportunity to encounter and present antigens to the rare unprimed antigen-specific T cells. Naive T-cell priming requires sustained T-cell receptor (TCR) stimulation that is achieved by the formation of the so-called "immunological synapse" (Grakoui et al., 1999), a specialized molecular organization at

the contact region between DCs and T cells. The synapse is a concentric structure with a central supramolecular activation cluster enriched in TCRs and costimulatory molecules such as CD2 and CD28, which interact, respectively, with peptide-MHC complexes, CD58 (or CD48), and CD80 (or CD86), surrounded by a peripheral ring enriched in lymphocyte function-associated antigen 1 (LFA-1) integrin. The formation of supramolecular aggregates allows the costimulation and the sustained low-affinity interaction between TCRs and specific peptide-MHC complexes. The very high efficiency of DCs as antigen-presenting cells is not due to a DC-specific molecule but rather to (i) the high level of expression of cell membrane costimulatory proteins, (ii) the efficient antigen-processing machinery, and (iii) the secretion of cytokines. DCs acquire all these properties during the maturation process (Steinman, 2000).

We have recently shown that DCs are able to produce IL-2 on bacterial encounter (Granucci et al., 2001b). Thus, this cytokine could represent an additional relevant molecule conferring DCs the unique T-cell-stimulatory capacity. Moreover, IL-2 is a cytokine able to sustain also B and NK cell growth, and, during the late phases of antigen-specific T-cell responses, it contributes to the maintenance of T-cell homeostasis by promoting activation-induced cell death of effector T lymphocytes. Given the key regulatory role exerted by IL-2 in the immune system, it is not surprising that IL-2-deficient mice show a generalized immune system deregulation leading to autoimmunity and inflammatory colitis-like disease (Schimpl et al., 2002). The new finding that DCs can produce IL-2 may explain how DCs control innate and initiate adaptive immunity. Only microbial stimuli, but not inflammatory cytokines, are able to induce IL-2 secretion by DCs (Granucci et al., 2003), indicating that DCs can distinguish between the actual presence of an infection and a cytokine-mediated inflammatory process. DC-derived IL-2 may be particularly relevant to induce T-cell proliferation when the general avidity of the system (frequency of responder antigen-specific T cells, affinity for MHC-peptide complexes, frequency of particular MHC-peptide complexes at the cell surface) is low, as happens in vivo during immune responses to microorganisms.

DCs AND THE INNATE IMMUNE RESPONSE

DC Innate Antigen Receptor Repertoire and Phagocytosis

DC Antigen Receptor Repertoire. Interaction of DCs with pathogens seems to involve different classes of receptors that form the innate antigen receptor repertoire of DCs.

The Toll-like receptor (TLR) family (Aderem and Ulevitch, 2000) is responsible for DC maturation by transducing signaling pathways that lead to NF-κB and/or stress-induced kinase activation (Rescigno et al., 1998a); the second functional class of innate receptors expressed by DCs includes phagocytic receptors, such as the Scavenger receptors, and mediates bacterial internalization (Rescigno et al., 2002).

The *Drosophila* Toll protein, first described as a developmental protein, is required for antifungal immune responses in the adult fly (Lemaitre et al., 1996). Ten mammalian homologs of Toll have been described (for a review, see Akira et al., 2001, and Medzhitov and Janeway, 1997), and the microbial compounds able to activate cellular responses mediated by TLR2, -3, -4, -5, and -9 have been identified (Bendelac and Medzhitov, 2002). In particular, TLR2 is mainly involved in responses to microbial products from gram-positive bacteria (peptidoglycans or lipoproteins) as well as from yeast (Hirschfeld et al., 1999; Yoshimura et al., 1999; Underhill et al., 1999). By contrast, TLR4 mediates the interaction with gram-negative bacteria by transducing the signals derived from lipopolysaccharide (LPS) (Poltorak et al., 1998; Takeuchi et al., 1999; Qureshi et al., 1999). The engagement of TLR4 induces nuclear translocation of the nuclear factor-κB (NF-κB) transcription factor [71] by activation of an adaptor protein (myeloid differentiation marker 88) and a serine/threonine kinase. Mutations of the *tlr4* gene in C57BL/10ScCr or C3H/HeJ mice impede LPS signal transduction, and these mice become resistant to endotoxin yet highly susceptible to gram-negative infection (Poltorak et al., 1998).

Indeed, DC maturation induced by LPS or bacteria is mediated by NF-κB, and inhibition of NF-κB blocks phenotypical maturation of DCs (Hofer et al., 2001; Rescigno et al., 1998a). Three out of five members of the NF-κB family are rapidly recruited after DC activation (30 min), whereas RelB is translocated into the nucleus only 4 h after bacterial encounter, suggesting a role for this member in late events of DC maturation. Interestingly, activation of DCs by LPS promotes survival of the cells in a growth-arrested state after deprivation of growth factors (Rescigno et al., 1998a). This response is dependent on mitogen-activated protein kinases of the extracellular signal-related kinase (ERK) family, but the antiapoptotic mediators still need to be identified.

DCs express a moderate level of FcRs that is not modulated during maturation. DCs also express the Mac-1 molecule (CD11b/CD18; αMβ2 integrin), which is the CR3 complement receptor used for the phagocytosis of complement-coated bacteria. As with FcRs, the surface expression of Mac-1 molecules is not changed during activation of DCs. This is in contrast to monocytes and neutrophils that strongly upregulate Mac-1 expression during differentiation and in the presence of inflammatory stimuli. In addition to its role in receptor-mediated internalization, the Mac-1 molecule also mediates adhesion and chemotaxis (Anderson et al., 1986). Mac-1 is stored in intracellular vesicles, which are rapidly mobilized to the cell surface in response to chemoattractants (Miller et al., 1987).

Mannose receptors are believed to be expressed by DCs because internalization and presentation of mannosylated proteins are very efficient in DCs (Tan et al., 1997). The high mannan content in the bacterial oligosaccharide cell envelope in both gram-positive and gram-negative bacteria ensures efficient molecular recognition. Therefore, it is likely that bacteria use the mannose receptor pathway for internalization.

DCs and Phagocytosis. Despite several early reports on the uptake of particulate material and cells by DCs (Austyn, 1996), the phagocytic capacity of DCs has long been denied. One reason for this was the technical difficulty of growing DCs in their immature state. Only in this past decade has it become possible to grow and maintain in vitro homogeneous immature DCs (Winzler et al., 1997). Indeed, several studies have shown that DCs can not only internalize latex and zymosan beads (Inaba et al., 1993; Reis e Sousa et al., 1993; Austyn et al., 1994; Matsuno et al., 1996), but also apoptotic bodies (Parr et al., 1991) as well as microbes such as *Mycobacterium tuberculosis* BCG (bacillus Calmette-Guérin) (Inaba et al., 1993; Henderson et al., 1997), *Saccharomyces cerevisiae, Corynebacterium parvum, Staphylococcus aureus* (Reis e Sousa et al., 1993), *Leishmania* spp. (Blank et al., 1993), and *Borrelia burgdorferi* (Filgueira et al., 1996). The ability of DCs to phagocytose particulates or bacteria is greatest in immature DCs, whereas this capacity is reduced, but not abolished, in mature DCs (Henderson et al., 1997).

To be internalized, bacteria have to first be attached to phagocytosis-promoting receptors. This may take place either by a direct interaction between microbial adhesins and phagocytic receptors (nonopsonic uptake) or indirectly by opsonins, for example, antibody or complement. These act as bridging molecules between the microbial surface and the opsonin receptors of the phagocytes (opsonic uptake). The fusion (zipper model) of the phagosome to form a discrete vacuole is probably under the control of specific fusogenic proteins, which have still not been identified. Upon attachment, DCs engulf the bacterium by actively surrounding it with pseudopodia (Fig. 1). This process is started intrinsically when phagocytosis-promoting receptors of the Fc type are involved, but in the case of complement-type receptors, it is dependent on complementary signals. The movement of the pseudopodia in activated DCs involves actin-binding proteins, and it can be blocked by the drug cytochalasin D, which stops the polymerization of actin and inhibits phagocytosis. The rearrangement of the cytoskeleton is associated with DC motility (Winzler et al., 1997). Once

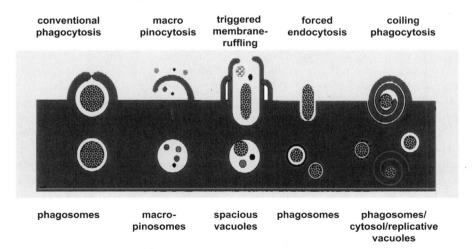

| conventional phagocytosis | macro pinocytosis | triggered membrane-ruffling | forced endocytosis | coiling phagocytosis |

| phagosomes | macro-pinosomes | spacious vacuoles | phagosomes | phagosomes/cytosol/replicative vacuoles |

FIGURE 1 Model of conventional and unconventional mechanisms of bacterial uptake.

a bacterium has been fully internalized in the phagosome, fusion of the phagosome with other intracellular vacuoles or granules takes place. Processing of bacterial molecules for antigen presentation occurs in lysosomes following their fusion with phagosomes. This process may take several hours, as antigen presentation of bacterial antigens is not observed earlier than 6 h following infection. In addition to the conventional zipper-type phagocytosis, DCs may use a number of other unconventional uptake mechanisms such as macropinocytosis and coiling phagocytosis (Rittig et al., 1994, 1996).

DC Antigen Processing and Cytokine Production

The phagocytic vacuole containing the bacteria normally fuses with a second type of vacuole, the lysosome, giving rise to a hybrid vacuole termed the phagolysosome. Model antigens expressed in recombinant gram-positive and gram-negative bacteria are processed and can be presented on both MHC I and II molecules (Rescigno et al., 1998b; Svensson et al., 1997; Corinti et al., 1999). Unlike macrophages, this exogenous pathway of MHC I presentation is TAP dependent (Rescigno et al., 1998b). This implies that exogenous bacterial antigens introduced by phagocytosis are directed into the classical pathway of MHC I presentation. Indeed, transport of whole bacterial proteins from phagolysosome to the cytosol takes place after phagocytosis of bacteria, as also shown with immune complex internalization (Rodriguez et al., 1999). The capacity of DCs to present bacterial antigens with very high efficiency on both MHC I and II molecules can be exploited to induce strong and long-lasting immunity toward bacteria as well as nominal antigens of interest. Several examples of partial protective immune responses achieved by injecting in vivo DCs loaded with microbes have been described for *Chlamydia trachomatis* (Su et al., 1998), *B. burgdorferi* (Mbow et al., 1997), and *Mycobacterium tuberculosis* (Demangel et al., 1999).

A few hours after bacterial infection, DCs synthesize a number of cytokines and chemokines (Granucci et al., 2001a, 2001b). Biologically active p70 IL-12 is produced by myeloid mouse DCs only in a very small amount after bacterial encounter, as compared with human monocyte-derived DCs (Corinti et al., 1999). Tumor necrosis factor alpha (TNF-α) and IL-6 are readily detected in DCs infected with either gram-positive or gram-negative bacteria. It is likely that the phenotypical and functional maturation, which occurs in DCs within 24 h of bacterial uptake, is the result of cytokine amplification during this response. Nevertheless, DC activation by TNF-α alone does not mimic the phenotypical maturation observed after bacterial infection. This is consistent with the finding that the pattern of genes induced after activation of DCs by TNF-α and LPS is very different and that the number of genes regulated during either LPS or bacterial activation is highly diverse (Granucci et al., 2001a). Indeed, maturation obtained by encounter with whole bacteria is quantitatively and qualitatively more pronounced, indicating the induction of several transducing pathways, likely via receptors, which recognize distinct bacterial components.

Treatment of DCs with bacteria resulted in a clear modification of cell surface DC activation markers. Consistent with acquisition of costimulatory activity during maturation is the upregulation of CD86 and CD40 molecules. The upregulation of these molecules has also been observed with *M. tuberculosis* BCG (Thurnher et al., 1997) and *M. tuberculosis* (Henderson et al., 1997), but it was not observed following the use of inert latex beads of various sizes. The upregulation of the costimulatory molecules and the coordinated translocation of MHC molecules at the cell surface are essential molecular events for the subsequent antigen presentation and activation of both CD4$^+$ and CD8$^+$ T cells. The internalization of bacteria is also associated with increased stability of MHC class I and class II peptide complexes. Indeed, the half-lives of MHC class II and class I peptide complexes change from 10 to 20 h and from 3 to 9 h, respectively. This has important consequences for T-cell induction because it increases the chances of DCs to encounter antigen-specific T cells in the draining lymph nodes (Rescigno et al., 1998b).

DC Interaction with NK Cells

Natural killer (NK) cells are cells of the innate immune system that exert their functions against virally infected or tumor cells. NK cell activity is primed during the early phases of an immune response, a few hours after infection. A key role of DCs in NK cell activation has been recently described for mice and humans (Moretta, 2002): DCs have been shown to prime NK cell cytolytic activity (Ferlazzo et al., 2002; Piccioli et al., 2002; Gerosa et al., 2002). This process requires cell-to-cell contact and is independent of IL-12 and IL-2 (Gerosa et al., 2002). DCs and NK cell cross talk is bidirectional because IL-2-activated NK cells induce immature DC activation, in terms of upregulation of costimulatory and MHC molecules and inflammatory cytokine production. NK-mediated DC activation also requires cell-to-cell contact and cytokine mediators such as TNF-α (Gerosa et al., 2002). Immature DCs can prime NK cell activity provided that they are cultured in the presence of IL-4 but not if they are propagated with the granulocyte-monocyte colony-stimulating factor only (Fernandez et al., 1999). Potential sources of IL-4 in vivo, during the early innate phase of the immune response, are NK T cells, basophiles, and mast cells, which have been recently shown to play a critical role in innate immunity during bacterial infections (Wedemeyer et al., 2000; Galli et al., 1999; Henz et al., 2001). Moreover, basophiles and mast cells also produce large amounts of TNF-α after bacterial and parasite interaction, and TNF-α is able to confer to DCs the ability to activate NK cells (Fernandez et al., 1999).

In addition to these new mechanisms recently described for NK cell priming, a classical method to activate NK cells in vitro is to culture the cells in the presence of IL-2. How-ever, IL-2-mediated NK cell activation has never been considered a possible event in vivo during immunocompetent responses because it was commonly believed that IL-2 was exclusively produced by T cells during the late phases of the immune response when the peak of gamma interferon production by activated NK cells was already exhausted (Biron et al., 1999). Nevertheless, as it has been shown that DCs are able to make IL-2 early after infection, the prediction is that DC-derived IL-2 could be involved in NK cell activation. In agreement with this hypothesis, we have recently found that bone marrow-derived DCs, cultured with the granulocyte-monocyte colony-stimulating factor only, become NK cell activators following interaction with microbial stimuli (F. Granucci, I. Zanoni, N. Pavelka and P. Ricciardi-Castagnoli, manuscript in preparation), whereas if DCs are propagated in the presence of IL-4, the efficiency of DC-mediated NK cell activation strongly depends on IL-2 (in vitro and in vivo) rather than on cell-to-cell contact. These observations suggest two possible pathways of NK cell priming by DCs, the first dependent on IL-4 and the second dependent on microbial stimuli and IL-2 (Fig. 2). Thus, an appropriate cytokine milieu can prime DCs to become competent for NK cell activation, independently from the presence of microbial stimuli and IL-2. Alternatively, following microbial encounter, DCs may acquire the ability to activate NK cells with the requirement of an IL-2-dependent process.

HOW INNATE AND ADAPTIVE IMMUNE RESPONSES ARE LINKED

Many of the bacteria that enter the body by oral or airway routes do not survive the inhospitable microenvironments that they encounter. Still, some microorganisms have evolved mechanisms to subvert this first line of defense and infect the host. Thus, mammals have developed second lines of defenses, consisting of innate and adaptive immune responses, to protect themselves from infectious microorganisms. The innate response is phylogenetically

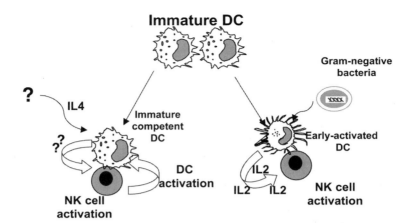

FIGURE 2 Two possible pathways of DC-mediated NK cell activation. According to the IL-4 pathway, immature DCs in the presence of IL-4 become competent NK cell activators. This process is bidirectional and requires cell-to-cell contact and soluble factors. According to the IL-2 pathway, early-microbial-activated DCs, IL-2 producers, acquire the ability to stimulate NK cells. This process depends on IL-2 and membrane proteins.

more ancient and, for a long time, it has been considered to be broadly directed to microorganisms. However, with the discovery of TLRs, involved in recognition of patterns characteristic of groups of microorganisms, the role of the innate immune system as a discriminating system has been reevaluated. Indeed, there is increasing evidence that the induction of different types of effector adaptive responses is dictated by the innate immune system after recognition of particular groups of pathogens (Medzhitov and Janeway, 1997). The central role of DCs in the induction of adaptive immune responses toward infectious agents has been extensively described (Steinman, 1991; Banchereau and Steinman, 1998), but recently a new role of DCs as a link between the innate and the adaptive immune responses has been proposed (Ricciardi-Castagnoli and Granucci, 2002) (Fig. 3). DCs are indeed widely distributed, especially in tissues that interface with the external environment, such as the skin, the gut, and the lungs, where they can perform a sentinel function for incoming pathogens and have the capacity to recruit and activate cells of the innate immune system (Rescigno et al., 1999; Sallusto et al., 1998; Fernandez et al., 1999). Uptake of pathogens induces a state of activation, which leads to the migration of the antigen-loaded DCs to the T-cell area of lymphoid organs where the antigen-specific cells of the adaptive immune response can be alerted. Thus, understanding the interaction of pathogens with DCs, and the early molecular events resulting from this interaction, should shed some light on the mechanisms of initiation of the immune response to infectious agents and on aspects of the pathogenicity and persistence of certain bacteria.

The recent explosion of interest in the study of the interaction between DCs and pathogens, both in vitro and in vivo, may provide an answer in the next few years to many key questions regarding how an immune response to infectious agents is induced and how to intervene when potentiation or inhibition is required. These questions include the identification of the receptors involved in the internalization of bacteria and/or in the activation of DCs, the intracellular signaling routes in DCs, and the strategies whereby microorganisms can evade or can impede DC function, thus escaping immune recognition. Moreover, because deregulation of innate DC functions may be one of the causes inducing inflamma-

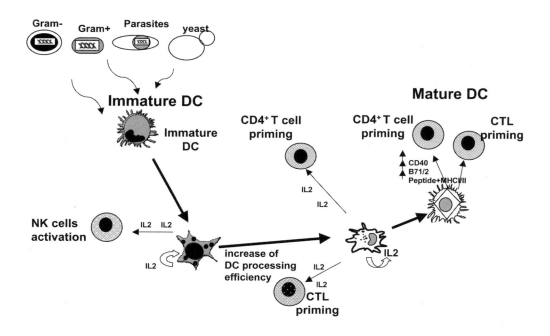

FIGURE 3 DCs link innate and adaptive immune responses. Following microbial encounter, immature DCs increase the efficiency of antigen processing and presentation and express, with a strictly defined kinetic IL-2. At early time points, DC-derived IL-2 helps to activate NK cells (IL-2 pathway; see Fig. 2). At later time points, when DCs have not yet reached the final stage of maturation and still express low levels of costimulatory molecules and peptide-MHC complexes at the cell surface, DC-derived IL-2 cooperates in the activation of T-cell responses (late adaptive response). It cannot be excluded that IL-2 can also act on DCs in an autocrine fashion. CTL, cytotoxic T lymphocyte.

tion as well as autoimmunity, it will be extremely important to define the molecular basis leading to such a DC regulatory role. The adjuvant property of bacteria is explicated by inducing, in DCs, not only the upregulation of costimulatory surface proteins and the maximization of the efficiency in presenting antigens as previously suggested, but also by inducing the production of costimulatory molecules such as IL-2. This seems to be a unique feature of DCs, as it has been found that macrophages are unable to produce IL-2 upon bacterial activation. Two waves of IL-2 production by DCs following bacterial encounter have been observed. The first early wave is between 4 and 8 h after bacterial uptake, and the second wave is between 14 and

18 h following activation. This timing is compatible with the appearance of MHC class II peptide and MHC class I peptide complexes at the cell surface (Rescigno et al., 1998b). Interestingly, DCs are able to present exogenous captured antigens to CD4$^+$ T cells in a few hours, whereas at least 8 h is required to process and present bacterial antigens in association with MHC class I molecules (Rescigno et al., 1998b). Thus, early-activated DCs are perfectly equipped to prime CD4$^+$ cells, despite their relatively low levels of MHC and membrane-associated costimulatory molecules and expression of T-cell inhibitory cytokines, such as IL-10 (Langenkamp et al., 2000). At later time points, IL-2 could represent a key costimulatory protein in activating CD8$^+$ T cells,

even though DCs have not yet reached their terminal maturation stage. These data could explain the ability of activated DCs to prime CD8$^+$ T cells in a CD4-independent manner (Ridge et al., 1998). This ability of DCs to rapidly respond to microbial interaction with IL-2 production is also shown with parasites such as *Leishmania mexicana* or with helminths such as *Schistosoma* (manuscripts in preparation). Interestingly, only inflammatory stages of these two parasites, the *Schistosoma* egg or the *Leishmania* promastigote, are able to induce IL-2 transcription in DCs (manuscripts in preparation).

Pathogen-matured DCs are likely to have an important role not only in stimulating but also in controlling the inflammatory response. As a matter of fact, physiological immune responses originate from a well-controlled inflammatory process.

REFERENCES

Aderem, A., and R. J. Ulevitch. 2000. Toll-like receptors in the induction of the innate immune response. *Nature* **406:**782–787.

Akashi, K., D. Traver, T. Miyamoto, and I. Weissman. 2000. A clonogenic common myeloid progenitor that gives rise to all myeloid lineages. *Nature* **404:** 193–197.

Akbari, O., R. H. DeKruyff, and D. T. Umetsu. 2001. Pulmonary Dc producing IL10 mediate tolerance induced by respiratory exposure to antigen. *Nat. Immunol.* **2:**725–731.

Akira, S., K. Takeda, and T. Kaisho. 2001. Toll-like receptors: critical proteins linking innate and acquired immunity. *Nat. Immunol.* **2:**675–680.

Anderson, D. C., L. J. Miller, F. C. Schmalstieg, R. Rothlein, and T. A. Springer. 1986. Contributions of the Mac-1 glycoprotein family to adherence-dependent granulocyte functions: structure-function assessments employing subunit-specific monoclonal antibodies. *J. Immunol.* **137:**15–27.

Anderson, K. L., H. Perkin, C. D. Surh, S. Venturini, R. A. Maki, and B. E. Torbett. 2000. Transcription factor PU.1 is necessary for development of thymic and myeloid progenitor-derived dendritic cells. *J. Immunol.* **164:**1855–1861.

Austyn, J. M. 1996. New insights into the mobilization and phagocytic activity of dendritic cells. *J. Exp. Med.* **183:**1287–1292.

Austyn, J. M., D. F. Hankins, C. P. Larsen, P. J. Morris, A. S. Rao, and J. A. Roake. 1994. Isolation and characterization of dendritic cells from mouse heart and kidney. *J. Immunol.* **152:**2401–2410.

Banchereau, J., and R. M. Steinman. 1998. Dendritic cells and the control of immunity. *Nature* **392:**245–252.

Banchereau, J., F. Briere, C. Caux, J. Davoust, S. Lebecque, Y. J. Liu, B. Pulendran, and K. Palucka. 2000. Immunobiology of dendritic cells. *Annu. Rev. Immunol.* **18:**767–811.

Bendelac, A., and R. Medzhitov. 2002. Adjuvants of immunity: harnessing innate immunity to promote adaptive immunity. *J. Exp. Med.* **195:**F19–F23.

Biron, C. A., K. B. Nguyen, G. C. Pien, L. P. Cousens, and T. P. Salazar-Mather. 1999. Natural killer cells in antiviral defense: function and regulation by innate cytokines. *Annu. Rev. Immunol.* **17:**189–220.

Blank, C., H. Fuchs, K. Rappersberger, M. Rollinghoff, and H. Moll. 1993. Parasitism of epidermal Langerhans cells in experimental cutaneous leishmaniasis with Leishmania major. *J. Infect. Dis.* **167:**418–425.

Cella, M., M. Salio, Y. Sakakibara, H. Langen, I. Julkunen, and A. Lanzavecchia. 1999. Maturation, activation, and protection of dendritic cells induced by double-stranded RNA. *J. Exp. Med.* **189:**821–829.

Corinti, S., D. Medaglini, A. Cavani, M. Rescigno, G. Pozzi, P. Ricciardi-Castagnoli, and G. Girolomoni. 1999. Human dendritic cells very efficiently present a heterologous antigen expressed on the surface of recombinant gram-positive bacteria to CD4+ T lymphocytes. *J. Immunol.* **163:**3029–3036.

Demangel, C., A. G. Bean, E. Martin, C. G. Feng, A. T. Kamath, and W. J. Britton. 1999. Protection against aerosol Mycobacterium tuberculosis infection using Mycobacterium bovis Bacillus Calmette Guerin-infected dendritic cells. *Eur. J. Immunol.* **29:** 1972–1979.

De Smedt, T., B. Pajak, E. Muraille, L. Lespagnard, E. Heinen, P. De Baetselier, J. Urbain, O. Leo, and M. Moser. 1996. Regulation of dendritic cell numbers and maturation by lipopolysaccharide in vivo. *J. Exp. Med.* **184:**1413–1424.

d'Ostiani, C. F., G. Del Sero, A. Bacci, C. Montagnoli, A. Spreca, A. Mencacci, P. Ricciardi-Castagnoli, and L. Romani. 2000. Dendritic cells discriminate between yeasts and hyphae of the fungus Candida albicans. Implications for initiation of T helper cell immunity in vitro and in vivo. *J. Exp. Med.* **191:**1661–1674.

Ferlazzo, G., M. L. Tsang, L. Moretta, G. Melioli, R. M. Steinman, and C. Munz. 2002. Human dendritic cells activate resting natural killer (NK) cells and are recognized via the NKp30 receptor by activated NK cells. *J. Exp. Med.* **195:**343–351.

Fernandez, N. C., A. Lozier, C. Flament, P. Ricciardi-Castagnoli, D. Bellet, M. Suter, M. Perricaudet, T. Tursz, E. Maraskovsky, and L.

Zitvogel. 1999. Dendritic cells directly trigger NK cell functions: cross-talk relevant in innate antitumor immune responses in vivo. *Nat. Med.* **5:**405–411.

Filgueira, L., F. O. Nestle, M. Rittig, H. I. Joller, and P. Groscurth. 1996. Human dendritic cells phagocytose and process Borrelia burgdorferi. *J. Immunol.* **157:**2998–3005.

Galli, S. J., M. Maurer, and C. S. Lantz. 1999. Mast cells as sentinels of innate immunity. *Curr. Opin. Immunol.* **11:**53–59.

Gerosa, F., B. Baldani-Guerra, C. Nisii, V. Marchesini, G. Carra, and G. Trinchieri. 2002. Reciprocal activating interaction between natural killer cells and dendritic cells. *J. Exp. Med.* **195:**327–333.

Girolomoni, G., C. Caux, C. Dezutter-Dambuyant, S. Lebecque, and P. Ricciardi-Castagnoli. 2001. Langerhans cells: still a fundamental paradigm for studying the immunobiology of dendritic cells. *Trends Immunol.* **23:**6–8.

Grakoui, A., S. K. Bromley, C. Sumen, M. M. Davis, A. S. Shaw, P. M. Allen, and M. L. Dustin. 1999. The immunological synapse: a molecular machine controlling T cell activation. *Science* **28:**221–227.

Granucci, F., C. Vizzardelli, E. Virzi, M. Rescigno, and P. Ricciardi-Castagnoli. 2001a. Transcriptional reprogramming of dendritic cells by differentiation stimuli. *Eur. J. Immunol.* **31:**2539–2546.

Granucci, F., C. Vizzardelli, N. Pavelka, S. Feau, M. Persico, E. Virzi, M. Rescigno, G. Moro, and P. Ricciardi-Castagnoli. 2001b. Inducible IL2 production by dendritic cells revealed by global gene expression analysis. *Nat. Immunol.* **2:**883–888.

Granucci, F., S. Feau, V. Angeli, F. Trottein, and P. Ricciardi-Castagnoli. 2003. Early IL-2 production by mouse dendritic cells is the result of microbial induced priming. *J. Immunol.* **170:**5075–5081.

Groux, H., A. O'Garra, M. Bigler, M. Rouleau, S. Antonenko, J. E. de Vries, and M. G. Roncarolo. 1997. A CD4+ T cell subset inhibits antigen-specific T cell responses and prevents colitis. *Nature* **389:**737–742.

Guerriero, A., P. B. Langmuir, L. M. Spain, and E. W. Scott. 2000. PU.1 is required for myeloid-derived but not lymphoid-derived dendritic cells. *Blood* **95:**879–885.

Henderson, R. A., S. C. Watkins, and J. L. Flynn. 1997. Activation of human dendritic cells following infection with Mycobacterium tuberculosis. *J. Immunol.* **159:**635–643.

Henz, B. M., M. Maurer, U. Lippert, M. Worm, and M. Babina. 2001. Mast cells as initiators of immunity and host defense. *Exp. Dermatol.* **10:**1–10.

Hirschfeld, M., C. J. Kirschning, R. Schwandner, H. Wesche, J. H. Weis, R. M. Wooten, and J. J. Weis. 1999. Cutting edge: inflammatory signaling by

Borrelia burgdorferi lipoproteins is mediated by toll-like receptor 2. *J. Immunol.* **163:**2382–2386.

Hofer, S., M. Rescigno, F. Granucci, S. Citterio, M. Francolini, and P. Ricciardi-Castagnoli. 2001. Differential activation of NF-kB subunits in dendritic cells in response to Gram negative bacteria and to Lipopolysaccharide. *Microb. Infect.* **3:**259–265.

Hugot, J. P., M. Chamaillard, H. Zouali, S. Lesage, J. P. Cezard, J. Belaiche, S. Almer, C. Tysk, C. A. O'Morain, M. Gassull, V. Binder, Y. Finkel, A. Cortot, R. Modigliani, P. Laurent-Puig, C. Gower-Rousseau, J. Macry, J. F. Colombel, M. Sahbatou, and G. Thomas. 2001. Association of NOD2 leucine-rich repeat variants with susceptibility to Crohn's disease. *Nature* **411:**599–603.

Inaba, K., M. Inaba, M. Naito, and R. M. Steinman. 1993. Dendritic cell progenitors phagocytose particulates, including bacillus Calmette-Guerin organisms, and sensitize mice to mycobacterial antigens in vivo. *J. Exp. Med.* **178:**479–488.

Ingulli, E., A. Mondino, A. Khoruts, and M. K. Jenkins. 1997. In vivo detection of dendritic cell antigen presentation to CD4 (+) T cells. *J. Exp. Med.* **185:**2133–2141.

Inohara, N., and G. Nunez. 2002. NODs: a family of cytosolic proteins that regulate the response to pathogens. *Curr. Opin. Microbiol.* **5:**76–80.

Iwasaki, A., and B. L. Kelsall. 1999. Freshly isolated Peyer's patch, but not spleen DC produce IL10 and induce the differentiation of Th2 cells. *J. Exp. Med.* **190:**229–239.

Iwasaki, A., and B. L. Kelsall. 2000. Localization of distinct Peyer's patch dendritic cell subsets and their recruitment by chemokines macrophage inflammatory protein (MIP)-3alpha, MIP-3beta, and secondary lymphoid organ chemokine. *J. Exp. Med.* **191:**1381–1394.

Kelsall, B. L., and W. Strober. 1996. Distinct populations of dendritic cells are present in subepithelial dome and T cell regions of the murine Peyer's patch. *J. Exp. Med.* **183:**237–247.

Kim, J., S. Sif, B. Jones, A. Jackson, J. Koipally, E. Heller, S. Winandy, A. Viel, A. Sawyer, T. Ikeda, R. Kingston, and K. Georgopoulos. 1999. DNA-binding proteins direct formation of chromatin remodeling complexes in lymphocytes. *Immunity* **10:**345–355.

Kohbata, S., H. Yokoyama, and E. Yabuuchi. 1986. Cytopathogenic effect of Salmonella typhi GIFU 10007 on M cells of murine ileal Peyer's patches in ligated ileal loops: an ultrastructural study. *Microbiol. Immunol.* **30:**1225–1232.

Langenkamp, A., M. Messi, A. Lanzavecchia, and F. Sallusto. 2000. Kinetics of dendritic cell activation: impact on priming of TH1, TH2 and nonpolarized T cells. *Nat. Immunol.* **1:**311–316.

Lemaitre, B., E. Nicolas, L. Michaut, J. M. Reichhart, and J. A. Hoffmann. 1996. The dorsoventral regulatory gene cassette spatzle/Toll/cactus controls the potent antifungal response in Drosophila adults. *Cell* **86**:973–983.

Maric, I., P. G. Holt, M. H. Perdue, and J. Bienstock. 1996. Class II MHC antigen (Ia)-bearing dendritic cells in the epithelium of the rat intestine. *J. Immunol.* **156**:1408–1414.

Matsuno, K., T. Ezaki, S. Kudo, and Y. Uehara. 1996. A life stage of particle-laden rat dendritic cells in vivo: their terminal division, active phagocytosis, and translocation from the liver to the draining lymph. *J. Exp. Med.* **183**:1865–1878.

Mbow, M. L., N. Zeidner, N. Panella, R. G. Titus, and J. Piesman. 1997. Borrelia burgdorferi-pulsed dendritic cells induce a protective immune response against tick-transmitted spirochetes. *Infect. Immun.* **65**:3386–3390.

McWilliam, A. S., D. Nelson, J. A. Thomas, and P. G. Holt. 1994. Rapid DC recruitment is a hallmark of acute inflammatory responses at mucosal surfaces. *J. Exp. Med.* **179**:1331–1336.

McWilliam, A. S., S. Napoli, A. M. Marsh, D. J. Pemper, D. Nelson, C. L. Primm, P. A. Stumbles, T. N. Wells, and P. G. Holt. 1996. DC are recruited into the airway epithelium during the inflammatory response to a broad spectrum of stimuli. *J. Exp. Med.* **184**:2429–2432.

Medzhitov, R., and C. A. J. Janeway. 1997. Innate immunity: the virtues of a nonclonal system of recognition. *Cell* **91**:295–298.

Merad, M., M. Manz, H. Karunsky, A. Wagers, W. Peters, I. Charo, I. L. Weissman, J. G. Cyster, and E. G. Engleman. 2002. Langerhans cells renew in the skin throughout life under steady-state conditions. *Nat. Immunol.* **3**:1135–1141.

Miller, L. J., D. F. Bainton, N. Borregaard, and T. A. Springer. 1987. Stimulated mobilization of monocyte Mac-1 and p150,95 adhesion proteins from an intracellular vesicular compartment to the cell surface. *J. Clin. Investig.* **80**:535–544.

Moretta, A. 2002. Natural killer cells and dendritic cells: rendezvous in abused tissues. *Nat. Rev. Immunol.* **2**:957–965.

Ogura, Y., D. K. Bonen, N. Inohara, D. L. Nicolae, F. F. Chen, R. Ramos, H. Britton, T. Moran, R. Karaliuskas, R. H. Duerr, J. P. Achkar, S. R. Brant, T. M. Bayless, B. S. Kirschner, S. B. Hanauer, G. Nunezm, and J. H. Cho. 2001. A frameshift mutation in NOD2 associated with susceptibility to Crohn's disease. *Nature* **411**:603–606.

Parr, M. B., L. Kepple, and E. L. Parr. 1991. Langerhans cells phagocytose vaginal epithelial cells undergoing apoptosis during the murine estrous cycle. *Biol. Reprod.* **45**:252–260.

Piccioli, D., S. Sbrana, E. Melandri, and N. M. Valiante. 2002. Contact-dependent stimulation and inhibition of dendritic cells by natural killer cells. *J. Exp. Med.* **195**:335–341.

Poltorak, A., X. He, I. Smirnova, M. Y. Liu, C. V. Huffel, X. Du, D. Birdwell, E. Alejos, M. Silva, C. Galanos, M. Freudenberg, P. Ricciardi-Castagnoli, B. Layton, and B. Beutler. 1998. Defective LPS signaling in C3H/HeJ and C57BL/10ScCr mice: mutations in Tlr4 gene. *Science* **282**:2085–2088.

Qureshi, S. T., L. Lariviere, G. Leveque, S. Clermont, K. J. Moore, P. Gros, and D. Malo. 1999. Endotoxin-tolerant mice have mutations in Toll-like receptor 4 (Tlr4). *J. Exp. Med.* **189**:615–625.

Reis e Sousa, C., P. D. Stahl, and J. M. Austyn. 1993. Phagocytosis of antigens by Langerhans cells in vitro. *J. Exp. Med.* **178**:509–519.

Rescigno, M., M. Martino, C. L. Sutherland, M. R. Gold, and P. Ricciardi-Castagnoli. 1998a. Dendritic cell survival and maturation are regulated by different signaling pathways. *J. Exp. Med.* **188**:2175–2180.

Rescigno, M., S. Citterio, C. Théry, M. Rittig, D. Medaglini, G. Pozzi, S. Amigorena, and P. Ricciardi-Castagnoli. 1998b. Bacteria-induced neo-biosynthesis, stabilization, and surface expression of functional class I molecules in mouse dendritic cells. *Proc. Natl. Acad. Sci. USA* **95**:5229–5234.

Rescigno, M., F. Granucci, S. Citterio, M. Foti, and P. Ricciardi-Castagnoli. 1999. Coordinated events during bacteria-induced DC maturation. *Immunol. Today* **20**:200–203.

Rescigno, M., M. Urbano, B. Valzasina, M. Francolini, G. Rotta, R. Bonasio, F. Granucci, J. P. Kraehenbuhl, and P. Ricciardi-Castagnoli. 2001. Dendritic cells express tight junction proteins and penetrate gut epithelial monolayers to sample bacteria. *Nat. Immunol.* **2**:361–368.

Rescigno, M., M. Urbano, M. Rimoldi, B. Valzasina, G. Rotta, F. Granucci, and P. Ricciardi-Castagnoli. 2002. Toll-like receptor 4 is not required for the full maturation of dendritic cells nor for the degradation of gram-negative bacteria. *Eur. J. Immunol.* **32**:2800–2806.

Ricciardi-Castagnoli, P., and F. Granucci. 2002. Interpretation of innate immune response complexity by functional genomics. *Nat. Rev. Immunol.* **21**:881–889.

Ridge, J. P., F. Di Rosa, and P. Matzinger. 1998. A conditioned dendritic cell can be a temporal bridge between a CD4+ T-helper and a T-killer cell. *Nature* **393**:474–478.

Rittig, M., T. Haupl, and G. R. Burmester. 1994. Coiling phagocytosis—a way for MHC class I presentation of bacterial antigens? *Int. Arch. Allergy Immunol.* **103**:4–10.

Rittig, M. G., K. Kuhn, C. Dechant, A. Gauckler, M. Modolell, P. Ricciardi-Castagnoli, A. Krause, and G. R. Burmester. 1996. Phagocytes from both vertebrate and invertebrate species use coiling phagocytosis. *Dev. Comp. Immunol.* **20**:393–406.

Rodriguez, A., A. Regnault, M. Kleijmeer, P. Ricciardi-Castagnoli, and S. Amigorena.

1999. Selective transport of internalized antigens to the cytosol for MHC class I presentation in dendritic cells. *Nat. Cell Biol.* **6:**362–368.

Ruedl, C., and S. Hubele. 1997. Maturation of Peyer's patch dendritic cells in vitro upon stimulation via cytokines or CD40 triggering. *Eur. J. Immunol.* **27:**1325–1330.

Sallusto, F., P. Schaerli, P. Loetscher, C. Schaniel, D. Lenig, C. R. Mackay, S. Qin, and A. Lanzavecchia. 1998. Rapid and coordinated switch in chemokine receptor expression during dendritic cell maturation. *Eur. J. Immunol.* **28:**2760–2769.

Sato, N., S. K. Ahuja, M. Quinones, V. Kostecki, R. L. Reddick, P. C. Melby, W. A. Kuziel, and S. S. Ahuja. 2000. CC chemokine receptor (CCR)2 is required for LC migration and localization of T helper cell type 1 (Th1)-inducing dendritic cells. *J. Exp. Med.* **192:**205–218.

Schimpl, A., I. Berberich, B. Kneitz, S. Kramer, B. Santner-Nanan, S. Wagner, M. Wolf, and T. Hunig. 2002. IL2 and autoimmune disease. *Cytokine Growth Factor Rev.* **13:**369–378.

Steinman, R. M. 1991. The dendritic cell system and its role in immunogenicity. *Annu. Rev. Immunol.* **9:**271–279.

Steinman, R. M. 2000. DC-SIGN: a guide to some mysteries of dendritic cells. *Cell* **100:**491–494.

Steinman, R. M., and M. C. Nussenzweig. 2002. Avoiding horror autotoxicus: the importance of dendritic cells in peripheral T cell tolerance. *Proc. Natl. Acad. Sci. USA* **99:**351–358.

Su, H., R. Messer, W. Whitmire, E. Fischer, J. C. Portis, and H. D. Caldwell. 1998. Vaccination against chlamydial genital tract infection after immunization with dendritic cells pulsed ex vivo with nonviable Chlamydiae. *J. Exp. Med.* **188:**809–818.

Svensson, M., B. Stockinger, and M. J. Wick. 1997. Bone marrow-derived dendritic cells can process bacteria for MHC-I and MHC-II presentation to T cells. *J. Immunol.* **158:**4229–4236.

Takeuchi, O., K. Hoshino, T. Kawai, H. Sanjo, H. Takada, T. Ogawa, K. Takeda, and S. Akira. 1999. Differential roles of TLR2 and TLR4 in recognition of gram-negative and gram-positive bacterial cell wall components. *Immunity* **11:**443–451.

Tan, M. C., A. M. Mommaas, J. W. Drijfhout, R. Jordens, J. J. Onderwater, D. Verwoerd, A. A. Mulder, A. N. van der Heiden, D. Scheidegger, L. C. Oomen, T. H. Ottenhoff, A. Tulp, J. J. Neefjes, and F. Koning. 1997. Mannose receptor-mediated uptake of antigens strongly enhances HLA class II-restricted antigen presentation by cultured dendritic cells. *Eur. J. Immunol.* **27:**2426–2435.

Tanaka, Y., T. Imai, M. Baba, I. Ishikawa, M. Uehira, H. Nomiyama, and O. Yoshie. 1999. Selective expression of activation-regulated chemokine in intestinal epithelium in mice and human. *Eur. J. Immunol.* **29:**633–642.

Thurnher, M., R. Ramoner, G. Gastl, C. Radmayr, G. Böck, M. Herold, H. Klocker, and G. Bartsch. 1997. Bacillus calmette-guérin mycobacteria stimulate human blood dendritic cells. *Int. J. Cancer* **70:**128–134.

Traver, D., K. Akashi, M. Manz, M. Merad, T. Miyamoto, E. G. Engleman, and I. L. Weissman. 2000. Development of CD8alpha-positive dendritic cells from a common myeloid progenitor. *Science* **290:**2152–2154.

Underhill, D. M., A. Ozinsky, A. M. Hajjar, A. Stevens, C. B. Wilson, M. Bassetti, and A. Aderem. 1999. The Toll-like receptor 2 is recruited to macrophage phagosomes and discriminates between pathogens. *Nature* **401:**811–815.

Valladeau, J., O. Ravel, C. Dezutter-Dambuyant, K. Moore, M. Kleijmeer, Y. Liu, V. Duvert-Frances, C. Vincent, D. Schmitt, J. Davoust, C. Caux, S. Lebecque, and S. Saeland. 2000. Langerin, a novel C-type lectin specific to Langerhans cells, is an endocytic receptor that induces the formation of Birbeck granules. *Immunity* **12:**71–81.

Vanbervliet, B., B. Homey, I. Durand, C. Massacrier, S. Ait-Yahia, O. de Bouteiller, A. Vicari, and C. Caux. 2002. Sequential involvement of CCR2 and CCR6 ligands for immature dendritic cell recruitment: possible role at inflamed epithelial surfaces. *Eur. J. Immunol.* **32:**231–242.

Wedemeyer, J., M. Tsai, and S. J. Galli. 2000. Roles of mast cells and basophils in innate and acquired immunity. *Curr. Opin. Immunol.* **12:**624–631.

Weih, F., D. Carrasco, S. K. Durham, D. S. Barton, C. A. Rizzo, R. P. Ryseck, S. A. Lira, and R. Bravo. 1995. Multiorgan inflammation and hematopoietic abnormalities in mice with a targeted disruption of RelB, a member of the NF-kappa B/Rel family. *Cell* **80:**331–340.

Wills-Karp, M. 1999. Immunological basis of antigen-induced airway hyperresponsiveness. *Annu. Rev. Immunol.* **17:**225–281.

Winzler, C., P. Rovere, M. Rescigno, F. Granucci, G. Penna, L. Adorini, V. S. Zimmermann, J. Davoust, and P. Ricciardi-Castagnoli. 1997. Maturation stages of mouse dendritic cells in growth factor-dependent long-term cultures. *J. Exp. Med.* **185:**317–328.

Wu, L., A. Nichogiannopoulou, K. Shortman, and K. Geogopoulos. 1997. Cell-autonomous defects in dendritic cell populations of Ikaros mutant mice point to a developmental relationship with the lymphoid lineage. *Immunity* **7:**483–492.

Yoshimura, A., E. Lien, R. R. Ingalls, E. Tuomanen, R. Dziarski, and D. Golenbock. 1999. Cutting edge: recognition of Gram-positive bacterial cell wall components by the innate immune system occurs via Toll-like receptor 2. *J. Immunol.* **163:**1–5.

ROLES OF MAST CELLS AND BASOPHILS IN INNATE IMMUNITY

Stephen J. Galli, Devavani Chatterjea, and Mindy Tsai

6

Mast cells and basophils have long been regarded as representing critical effector cells in Th2 cell- and immunoglobulin E (IgE)-associated immune responses (Metcalfe et al., 1997; Galli and Lantz, 1999; Williams and Galli, 2000; Galli et al., 2001; Kawakami and Galli, 2002). In addition to contributing to the pathogenesis of asthma, anaphylaxis, and other allergic disorders, such IgE-associated immune responses are thought to promote host resistance to certain parasites (Woodbury et al., 1984; Miller, 1996; Metcalfe et al., 1997; Galli and Lantz, 1999; Williams and Galli, 2000; Galli et al., 2001; Kawakami and Galli, 2002). More recently, it has become clear that mast cells can also function as important effector cells in certain innate immune responses to bacteria, at least in mice (Galli et al., 1999, 2002; Mekori and Metcalfe, 2000; Patella et al., 2000a; Feger et al., 2002). In this chapter we review basic aspects of mast cell and basophil development and function, describe a mouse model for analyzing mast cell function in vivo,

and then outline the evidence that mast cells and/or basophils can contribute to innate immune responses. We especially emphasize findings derived from in vivo studies conducted with genetically mast cell-deficient and congenic normal mice and with genetically mast cell-deficient mice that have been selectively repaired of their mast cell deficiency, so-called "mast cell knock-in mice."

MAST CELL AND BASOPHIL BIOLOGY

Both mast cells and basophils are derived from $CD34^+$ hematopoietic progenitor cells present in adult blood and bone marrow, and these two cell types share many similarities in mediator content, surface receptor expression, and function (Valent et al., 1989; Metcalfe et al., 1997; Galli and Lantz, 1999; Galli, 2000; Galli et al., 2001; Wedemeyer and Galli, 2001) (Table 1). However, basophils (like other granulocytes) typically mature in the bone marrow and then circulate in the peripheral blood in low numbers, from where they are recruited into the tissues at sites of inflammation or immune responses; by contrast, mature mast cells typically do not circulate in the blood but complete their differentiation in vascularized tissues (Galli and Lantz, 1999; Galli et al.,

Stephen J. Galli, Departments of Pathology and Microbiology and Immunology, Stanford University School of Medicine, 300 Pasteur Drive, L-235, Stanford, CA 94305-5324. *Devavani Chatterjea and Mindy Tsai*, Department of Pathology, Stanford University School of Medicine, 300 Pasteur Drive, L-235, Stanford, CA 94305-5324.

The Innate Immune Response to Infection
Ed. by S. H. E. Kaufmann, R. Medzhitov, and S. Gordon
©2004 ASM Press, Washington, D.C.

TABLE 1 Natural history, major mediators, and surface membrane structures of human mast cells and basophils[a]

Characteristics	Basophils	Mast cells
Natural history		
Origin of precursor cells	Marrow	Marrow
Site of maturation	Marrow	Connective tissue (a few in marrow)
Mature cells in circulation	Yes (usually <1% of blood leukocytes)	No
Mature cells recruited into tissues from circulation	Yes (during immunologic, inflammatory responses)	No
Mature cells normally residing in connective tissues	No (not detectable by microscopy)	Yes
Proliferative ability of morphologically mature cells	None reported	Yes (limited; under certain circumstances)
Life span	Days (like other granulocytes)	Weeks to months (according to studies in rodents)
Major growth factor	IL-3	SCF
Mediators		
Major mediators stored preformed in cytoplasmic granules	Histamine, chondroitin sulfates, neutral protease with bradykinin-generating activity, β-glucuronidase, elastase, cathepsin G-like enzyme, major basic protein, Charcot-Leyden crystal protein, peroxidase,[b] carboxypeptidase A[c]	Histamine, heparin, and/or chondroitin sulfates, neutral proteases (chymase and/or tryptase[c]), major basic protein, many acid hydrolases, cathepsin, carboxypeptidases, peroxidase
Major lipid mediators produced on appropriate activation	Leukotriene C_4	Prostaglandin D_2, leukotriene C_4, platelet-activating factor
Cytokines released on appropriate activation[d]	IL-4, IL-13	TNF-α, MIP-1α, VPF/VEGF, IL-3, IL-4, IL-5, IL-6, IL-8, IL-10, IL-11, IL-13, IL-16, GM-CSF, MCP-1 (mouse and human mast cells produce many more)[e]
Immunoglobulin receptors	FcεRI, FcγRII (CDw32)	FcεRI, FcγRI, FcγRII, FcγRIII (only mRNA)[e]
Cytokine and growth factor receptors	IL-1RII (CD121b), IL-2Rα (CD25), IL-3R, IL-4R (CD124), IL-5R (CD125), and IL-8R (CD128) and GM-CSFR (CD116), IFN-α/βR (CD118), IFN-γR (CD119); c-kit (CD117) (some basophils express low numbers of c-kit receptors[f])	c-kit (CD117) (only mRNA: IL-3R, IL-4R, IL-5R, cIL-6R)
Complement receptors and proteins	CR1 (CD35), CR3/C3biR (CD11b/18), CR4 (CD11c/18), C5aR (CD88), C3aR, MCP (CD46), DAF (CD55), MACIF (CD59)	C5aR (CD88), CMCP (CD46), DAF (CD55), MACIF (CD59)
Chemokine receptors	CCR1, CCR2, CCR3, CCR5, CXCR1, CXCR2, CXCR4[g]	CXCR-1, CXCR-2, CCR3[h]
Other immune receptors and ligands	CD40L (CD154), CD40, CD4[i]	CD40L (CD154), HLA-DR, HLA-DQ
Other receptors	fMLPR, PAFR, histamine H_2 receptor, PGD_2 receptor, TLR2, TLR4[j]	histamine H_2 receptor, PGD_2 receptor, urokinase receptor (CD87), TLR1, TLR2, TLR6[k]

Transmembrane 4 superfamily	CD37, CD53, CD63, CD81	CD53, CD63, CD81
Cell adhesion structures	P24 (CD09), LFA-1β chain, PECAM (CD31), β$_1$ integrins (CD29, CD49d, CD49e), ICAM-1 (CD54) (low level), ICAM-2 (CD102), ICAM-3 (CD50), β$_2$ integrins (CD18, CD11a, CD11b, CD11c), VCAM-1, LFA-1 (CD11a/18), LFA-3(CD58), leukosialin (CD43), Pgp-1(CD44)	P24 (CD09), LFA-1β chain, β$_1$ integrins (CD29, CD49d, CD49e), ICAM-1 (CD54) (low level), ICAM-2 (CD102), ICAM-3 (CD50)(+), β$_3$ integrins (CD61, CD51), LFA-3(CD58), leukosialin (CD43), Pgp-1(CD44)
Others	LCA (CD45), ME491 (CD63), bsp-1, CD46, CD54, CD13, CD26	LCA (CD45), ME491 (CD63), CD46, CD54

[a]Abbreviations: LFA, lymphocyte function-associated antigen; VLA, very late antigen; ICAM, intercellular adhesion molecule; VNR, vitronectin receptor; fMLPR, f-Met-Leu-Phe receptor; PAFR, platelet-activating factor receptor; PECAM, platelet endothelial cell adhesion molecule; VCAM, vascular cell adhesion molecule; LCA, leukocyte common antigen; MACIF, membrane attack complex inhibitory factor; GM-CSF, granulocyte–macrophage colony-stimulating factor. Data regarding CD antigens are from analysis of blood basophils (Valent, 1994, 1995; Agis et al., 1996; Toba et al., 1999) and lung or uterine mast cells (Valent, 1994, 1995; Agis et al., 1996).

[b]Under certain conditions, tryptase$^+$, chymase$^+$, carboxypeptidase A$^+$, and c-kit$^+$ granulated cells, which appear to be basophils by morphology and are reactive with an antibody against BSP-1 (which stains basophils but not mast cells), can be observed in the peripheral blood (Li et al., 1998).

[c]The peroxidase of basophil granules may be similar or identical to eosinophil peroxidase (Toba et al., 1999).

[d]Several lines of evidence indicate that certain cytokines produced by mast cells, such as TNF-α and VPF/VEGF, are released in part from preformed stores, some of which may be physically associated with the cells' cytoplasmic granules (Young et al., 1987; Gordon and Galli, 1990, 1991; Boesiger et al., 1998).

[e]See Okayama et al. (2001a, 2001b).

[f]See Columbo et al. (1992) and Li et al. (1998).

[g]See Iikura et al. (2001).

[h]See de Paulis et al. (2001).

[i]It appears that at least some peripheral blood basophils can express CD4 (Thonnard-Neuman, 1963).

[j]See Sabroe et al. (2002).

[k]See McCurdy et al. (2003).

2001). Under physiological conditions, basophils have a life span of only several days (Galli et al., 2001). Interleukin-3 (IL-3) can promote the production and survival of human basophils in vitro and can induce basophilia in vivo (Valent et al., 1989; Lantz et al., 1998; Galli, 2000). Unlike basophils, mast cells can be very long-lived, and mast cells that are apparently mature can proliferate under certain conditions (Galli and Lantz, 1999). Many aspects of mast cell development and survival are critically regulated by the stem cell factor (SCF)—the ligand for the c-*kit* receptor (a member of the receptor tyrosine kinase III family of growth factor receptors) that is highly expressed on the mast cell surface (Galli et al., 1994, 1999; Metcalfe et al., 1997; Galli and Lantz, 1999; Tsai et al., 2000b).

The lineage relationship between mast cells and basophils remains to be fully defined. The evidence that tissue mast cells are derived from circulating bone marrow-derived precursors has suggested to some that basophils might represent the circulating precursors of mast cells (reviewed by Galli et al., 2001). However, no evidence has been presented indicating that mature circulating basophils actually can divide or differentiate into mast cells (Galli et al., 2001). An alternative hypothesis, based on studies in mice, is that basophils may actually represent senescent mast cells destined for apoptosis (Friend et al., 2000). This notion does not readily explain why genetically mast cell-deficient Kit^W/Kit^{W-v} mice, which virtually lack mature mast cells, express nearly normal levels of basophils (Lantz et al., 1998). As reviewed elsewhere (Galli et al., 2001), the weight of current evidence indicates that mast cells and basophils are distinct lineages of hematopoietic cells, with basophils being more closely related to the other granulocytes (especially eosinophils) than to mast cells.

Both mast cells and basophils express the $\alpha\beta\gamma_2$ form of the high-affinity receptor for IgE (FcεRI) on their surface, and both cell types can be activated to release diverse preformed mediators and lipid mediators (synthesized de novo), as well as cytokines, after the cross-linking of FcεRI-bound IgE with bivalent or multivalent antigen (Metzger, 1992; Metcalfe et al., 1997; Turner and Kinet, 1999; Williams and Galli, 2000; Kawakami and Galli, 2002). The preformed, cytoplasmic granule-associated mediators of mast cells and basophils include histamine, serotonin (in rodents, not humans) proteoglycans, and neutral proteases, whereas the lipid mediators include leukotriene C_4, platelet-activating factor, and prostaglandin D_2 (in mast cells only) (Table 1). Furthermore, mouse or human mast cells represent potential sources of many cytokines, chemokines, and growth factors with diverse effects in inflammation, immunity, hematopoiesis, tissue remodeling, and other biological processes (e.g., IL-1, IL-3, IL-4, IL-5, IL-6, IL-8, IL-10, IL-11, IL-13, IL-16, tumor necrosis factor alpha [TNF-α], basic fibroblast growth factor [bFGF], vascular endothelial growth factor [VPF/VEGF], transforming growth factor β [TGF-β], and many C-C chemokines, including macrophage inflammatory protein-1α [MIP-1α] and monocyte chemoattractant protein-1 [MCP-1] [Metcalfe et al., 1997; Williams and Galli, 2000; Galli et al., 2001; Sayama et al., 2002]). The spectrum of basophil-derived cytokines appears to be more limited and includes IL-4 and IL-13 (Brunner et al., 1993; MacGlashan et al., 1994; Li et al., 1996). At least certain mast cell populations, both in fish (Silphaduang and Noga, 2001) and in mammals (Di Nardo et al., 2003), represent a potential source of antimicrobial peptides, including the cathelin-related antimicrobial peptides in mice and the cathelicidin LL-37 in humans (Di Nardo et al., 2003).

The prominent cytoplasmic granules of both mast cells and basophils stain metachromatically with certain basic dyes, primarily reflecting their content of proteoglycans such as chondroitin sulfates (in basophils and mast cells) and heparin (thought to be produced exclusively by mast cells). The biological functions of basophil and mast cell proteoglycans are not fully understood; however, in mice, heparin is required for the normal packaging of certain neutral proteases in mast cell cytoplasmic granules (Forsberg et al., 1999; Humphries et al., 1999). Mast cells in different tissues or species, or at different stages of development, can vary in proteoglycan and/or protease content and in many other aspects of phenotype and function, a phenomenon called "mast cell heterogeneity" (Metcalfe et al., 1997; Galli and Lantz, 1999; Galli et al., 1999, 2001; Galli, 2000; Williams and Galli, 2000). Recent evidence suggests that basophils can also exhibit heterogeneity in mediator content (Li et al., 1998; Galli et al., 2001).

In addition to IgE and antigen, a large variety of other agents can induce activation and mediator and/or cytokine release from mast cells and/or basophils. These include products of pathogens (bacteria, viruses, and parasites), products of leukocytes or of complement activation, neuropeptides and neurotrophins, certain hormones, endothelins, components of venoms and other toxins, several cytokines and chemokines, some defensins, the cathelicidin LL-37 (that also can be produced by certain mast cell populations [Di Nardo et al., 2003]), and many other agents (reviewed by Metcalfe et al., 1997; Befus et al., 1999; Mekori and Metcalfe, 2000; Patella et al., 2000a; Marone et al., 2001; Niyonsaba et al., 2001; Feger et al., 2002; and Galli et al., 2002).

Many of these agents can induce a pattern of mediator and/or cytokine release that differs in composition, magnitude, or kinetics from that induced by IgE and antigen in the same cell populations (e.g., some bacterial products induce mast cells to release certain cytokines, but not stored mediators, whereas certain neuropeptides induce the release of stored products preferentially over products that must be synthesized de novo) (Galli et al., 1994, 1999; Leal-Berumen et al., 1994; Metcalfe et al., 1997; Galli and Lantz, 1999; Galli, 2000; Mekori and Metcalfe, 2000; Patella et al., 2000a; Williams and Galli, 2000; Marone et al., 2001; Wedemeyer and Galli, 2001). Moreover, some of the agents that can induce mast cell activation under some circumstances, including some neurotrophins, endothelins, cytokines, chemokines, SCF, and even the cathelicidin LL-37, also can be produced by certain mast cell populations (reviewed by Metcalfe et al., 1997; Galli and Lantz, 1999; Mekori and Metcalfe, 2000; Williams and Galli, 2000; Di Nardo et al., 2003). Many of the bacterial products that have been reported to elicit mast cell mediator release are reviewed by Galli et al. (1999), Mekori and Metcalfe (2000), Patella et al. (2000a), Marone et al. (2001), and Feger et al. (2002). Many of the surface receptors through which such stimuli activate mast cells or basophils have been identified, including Toll-like receptors (TLRs) for bacterial products (Supajatura et al., 2001, 2002b; Sabroe et al., 2002; McCurdy et al., 2003) and several chemokine receptors (de Paulis et al., 2001; Iikura et al., 2001; Li et al., 2001).

ANALYZING MAST CELL AND BASOPHIL FUNCTION IN VIVO

Mice that genetically lack only mast cells or basophils would represent ideal model animals for investigating the contributions of these two cell types to specific pathological or physiological processes. Although mice that *selectively* lack either mast cells or basophils as their only abnormality have not been reported, genetically mast cell-deficient WBB6F$_1$-Kit^W/Kit^{W-v} mice (Kit^W/Kit^{W-v} mice) can be used to investigate the expression of biological responses in mice that differ solely in virtually lacking, or possessing, mast cell populations (Kitamura et al., 1978; Nakano et al., 1985; Tsai et al., 2000a, 2002).

Kit^W/Kit^{W-v} mice lack expression of a functional c-kit receptor due to spontaneous mutations in both copies of c-kit (Nocka et al., 1990; Galli et al., 1994). Adult Kit^W/Kit^{W-v} mice ordinarily have less than 1% of the wild-type (WT) levels of cutaneous mast cells and no detectable mature mast cells in the peritoneal cavity, respiratory system, or gastrointestinal tract (Kitamura et al., 1978). However, these mice also have other abnormalities due to the lack of adequate c-kit function, including a virtually complete lack of germ cells, interstitial cells of Cajal and cutaneous melanocytes, a moderate anemia, and additional more subtle abnormalities (Kitamura et al., 1978; Galli et al., 1994, 2002; Galli, 2000).

Although Kit^W/Kit^{W-v} mice express multiple phenotypic abnormalities related to their c-*kit* deficiency, mast cells can be selectively reconstituted in Kit^W/Kit^{W-v} mice by the adoptive transfer of genetically compatible in vitro-derived mast cells (Nakano et al., 1985; Tsai et al., 2000a). Such mast cells can be generated from the bone marrow or other hematopoietic cells of either WBB6F$_1$-+/+ mice (WT mice that are congenic to WBB6F$_1$-Kit^W/Kit^{W-v} mice) or other genetically compatible normal, transgenic, or knockout mice (Nakano et al., 1985; Tsai et al., 2000a). Alternatively, mast cells can be generated in vitro directly from embryonic stem cells, including those carrying mutations that influence mast cell phenotype or function (Tsai et al., 2000a, 2002). Such in vitro-derived mast cells can be administered by intravenous, intraperitoneal (i.p.), or intradermal injection or by direct injection into the anterior wall of the stomach of mast cell-deficient Kit^W/Kit^{W-v} mice, thus producing the so-called mast cell knock-in mice (Nakano et al., 1985; Galli and Lantz, 1999; Tsai et al., 2000a). These mice can be used to assess the extent to which differences in the expression of biological responses observed in Kit^W/Kit^{W-v} mice and the congenic WT mice reflect the absence of mast cells in the Kit^W/Kit^{W-v} mice. Moreover, by adoptively transferring to Kit^W/Kit^{W-v} mice in vitro-derived mast cells that express genetic alterations in specific receptors, mediators, or signaling pathways, one can assess the roles of these individual mast cell products in the expression of biological responses in vivo (Nakano et al., 1985; Tsai et al., 2000a, 2002; Williams and Galli, 2000).

An analogous "basophil knock-in" system is not currently available.

Although IL-3$^{-/-}$ mice fail to develop the striking basophilia that occurs in response to infections with *Strongyloides venezuelensis* or *Nippostrongylus brasiliensis*, IL-3$^{-/-}$ mice typically express normal baseline levels of bone marrow basophils and circulating basophils (Lantz et al.,

1998, 1999). As a result, if one observed normal expression in IL-3$^{-/-}$ mice of biological responses that are thought to be basophil dependent, this could reflect the residual function of the small numbers of basophils present in these animals in the absence of IL-3.

ROLES OF MAST CELLS AND BASOPHILS IN ANTIBACTERIAL IMMUNE RESPONSES

Several lines of evidence, including data derived from mast cell knock-in mice, indicate that mast cells are exceedingly good at initiating and/or amplifying inflammatory responses (Galli et al., 1999, 2002; Williams and Galli, 2000). This role is expressed in the context of both IgE-associated and IgE-independent inflammatory processes (Galli et al., 1999, 2002; Williams and Galli, 2000). For example, studies in mast cell knock-in mice show that mast cells are essential for optimal expression of certain immunologically nonspecific acute inflammatory responses, such as those induced by the application of the phorbol ester, phorbol myristate acetate, to the skin surface (Wershil et al., 1988) or by the intradermal (Yano et al., 1989) or subcutaneous (Matsuda et al., 1989) injection of the neuropeptide, substance P.

Although the mast cell-associated inflammation observed in immunological or nonimmunological inflammatory responses reflects the direct and indirect actions of diverse mast cell products, TNF-α represents one mast cell-derived cytokine that has been implicated in mast cell-dependent leukocyte recruitment. For example, the mast cell-dependent leukocyte recruitment that occurs upon IgE-dependent mast cell activation in the skin (Wershil et al., 1991, 1995) or stomach wall (Wershil et al., 1996) is, in part, mediated by TNF-α, and TNF-α also contributes to the mast cell-dependent neutrophil recruitment that has been reported in certain models of immune complex-induced i.p. inflammation (Zhang et al., 1992) or cutaneous contact sensitivity (Biedermann et al., 2000).

The mast cell knock-in mouse model has been used by several groups to show that mast cells can represent an important component of host defense against bacterial infection. The majority of these studies have been performed with experimental models of i.p. infection, especially cecal ligation and puncture (CLP). These studies indicate that an intact complement system, mast cell expression of TLR4, a functional Janus kinase 3 (JAK3), and TNF-α production by mast cells can play important roles in these responses.

In papers published back to back, two groups used mast cell knock-in mice to demonstrate that mast cells and TNF-α can be required for optimal expression of innate immunity to bacterial infection (Echtenacher et al., 1996; Malaviya et al., 1996a). Malaviya et al. (1996a) showed that mast cells can promote the clearance of large numbers (10^7 to 10^8) of *Klebsiella pneumoniae* (10^6 to 10^8) that had been injected into the peritoneal cavity (or lungs) of mice, as assessed 2 to 6 h postinoculation. In other experiments, 80% of mast cell-deficient Kit^W/Kit^{W-v} mice died within 24 h of being injected with 6.0 x 10^7 *K. pneumoniae* bacteria, in contrast to 0% mortality at 24 h in WT mice or in Kit^W/Kit^{W-v} mice that contained adoptively transferred WT mast cells (Malaviya et al., 1996a). Studies employing a neutralizing antibody to TNF-α, and i.p. injection of *Escherichia coli* bearing either the WT or a mutant form of the *K. pneumoniae* FimH protein, indicated that mast cell-dependent production of TNF-α (that at least in part reflected mast cell activation by type I fimbriae) was required for optimal neutrophil influx into the peritoneal cavity (Malaviya et al., 1996a).

More recently, using an in vivo model in which *E. coli* bearing the WT FimH were injected i.p., Malaviya et al. (2001) showed that JAK3 plays a role in the early stages (~2 h) of mast cell-mediated TNF-α release, neutrophil recruitment, and bacterial clearance. Employing a different strain of *E. coli*, this group showed that survival after i.p. injection of 4.0 × 10^7 bacteria in Kit^W/Kit^{W-v} mice that had been reconstituted with JAK3$^{+/+}$ mast cells was significantly enhanced compared with that in Kit^W/Kit^{W-v} mice that had been reconstitut-

ed with JAK3$^{-/-}$ mast cells (Malaviya et al., 2001). In a similar model system, it has also been shown that a leukotriene synthesis inhibitor can reduce neutrophil influx and bacterial clearance in mice with normal mast cells (Malaviya and Abraham, 2000).

Taken together, studies in which gram-negative bacteria have been directly injected into the peritoneal cavity of mice indicate that mast cells and TNF-α can be required for optimal neutrophil recruitment and bacterial clearance 1 to 6 h after injection of bacteria and that mast cell-dependent neutrophil recruitment and/or activation may involve leukotrienes as well as TNF-α. Mast cell functions in this model of infection also may be required for optimal survival, at least in the early period after injection of bacteria. Studies in another model of bacterial infection (in mice) have implicated the human mast cell-derived serine protease, tryptase beta 1, in the leukocyte recruitment associated with innate immunity to bacteria (Huang et al., 2001).

The direct i.p. injection of large numbers of bacteria represents one experimental model of infection or septic shock. An alternate model, CLP, produces a polymicrobial acute peritonitis that mimics the acute septic peritonitis that can occur in several clinically important settings such as intestinal perforation due to trauma, ischemia, or complications of inflammatory bowel disease (reviewed by Wichterman et al., 1980). In CLP, the severity of the i.p. infection, and the survival rate in normal mice, can be regulated by varying the amount of the cecum that is ligated, the number and/or size of the perforation(s) made in the cecal wall, or the extent to which the cecum is manipulated to promote entry of cecal contents into the peritoneal cavity (Wichterman et al., 1980; Echtenacher et al., 1990, 1996; Maurer et al., 1998).

Echtenacher et al. (1996) found that i.p. reconstitution of mast cell-deficient $Kit^W/$ Kit^{W-v} mice with WT BMCMC markedly reduced death from CLP and that this effect was abolished by the administration of neutralizing antibodies to TNF-α. Injection of mast cell-deficient $Kit^W/Kit^{W-\nu}$ mice with TNF-α alone could also confer protection, but only when the cytokine was provided at a certain dose; administration of either smaller or larger amounts of TNF-α did not improve survival (Echtenacher et al., 1996). It has been shown subsequently that TLR4, but not TLR2, is required for optimal mast cell-dependent enhancement of TNF-α production, neutrophil recruitment, and survival in this model (Supajatura et al., 2001, 2002b). For example, mast cell-deficient $Kit^W/Kit^{W-\nu}$ mice reconstituted with BMCMC that lacked TLR4 (either BMCMC of C3H/HeJ origin or derived from $TLR4^{-/-}$ mice) had significantly higher mortality from CLP than did $Kit^W/Kit^{W-\nu}$ mice reconstituted with BMCMC that expressed WT TLR4; in vitro, intact TLR4 was required for BMCMC to respond fully to lipopolysaccharide stimulation, as assessed by activation of the NF-κB signaling pathway and production of TNF-α and other cytokines, including IL-1β, IL-6, and IL-13 (Supajatura et al., 2001, 2002b).

Although lipopolysaccharide and fimbrial adhesin (and many other bacterial products) can directly activate mast cells to release mediators (reviewed by Galli et al., 1999; Mekori and Metcalfe, 2000; Patella et al., 2000a; Feger et al., 2002; Supajatura et al., 2002a), pathogens can also activate mast cells indirectly, e.g., via the complement system. For example, products of complement activation, as well as prod-

ucts of other cells activated by complement-dependent mechanisms, can activate mast cells (reviewed by Metcalfe et al., 1997; Galli and Lantz, 1999; Galli et al., 1999; Gommerman et al., 2000; Mekori and Metcalfe, 2000; Patella et al., 2000a).

Prodeus et al. (1997) showed that mice that genetically lacked C3 were much more sensitive to the lethal effects of CLP than were WT mice (100% versus 20% mortality at 24 h, respectively; Table 2). After CLP, $C3^{-/-}$ mice also exhibited diminished (i) degranulation of peritoneal mast cells, (ii) i.p. TNF-α production, (iii) neutrophil recruitment and phagocytosis of opsonized bacteria, and (iv) bacterial clearance from the peritoneal cavity. All of these defects, as well as the associated lethality, were ameliorated by i.p. treatment of the mice with purified human C3 protein (Table 2). It has also been shown that complement receptor CD21/CD35-deficient mice (Cr2[null]) and CD19[null] mice also have decreased survival following CLP and that survival in these mice is only partially improved by injection of IgM (Gommerman et al., 2000). Such studies implicate CD21/CD35 and CD19 in the activation of mast cells for optimal expression of mast cell-dependent innate immunity during CLP (Gommerman et al., 2000).

Mice that lack Mac-1, a β2 integrin important in leukocyte migration, have significantly reduced mast cell numbers in the peritoneal cavity (~70% reduction versus WT levels),

TABLE 2 Features of CLP in WT (+/+), $C3^{-/-}$, or human C3 (HuC3)-treated $C3^{-/-}$ mice[a]

Feature	+/+	$C3^{-/-}$	$C3^{-/-}$ + HuC3
CLP mortality (24 h)	20%	100%	40%
Peritoneal mast cell degranulation (3 h)	++++	+/++	++++
Peritoneal TNF-α (3 h, % of +/+ value)	100	33	79
Neutrophil influx (3 h, % of +/+ value)	100	52	102
Bacterial clearance (*E. coli*, 10⁴ CFU in peritoneal fluid)			
1 h	1.6	35	2.1
3 h	5.7	116	34

[a]From Prodeus et al. (1997) with permission of the publisher.

peritoneal wall (~44% reduction), and back skin (~33% reduction), and these mice were significantly more susceptible to CLP-induced mortality (Rosenkranz et al., 1998). Whether this reflected simply the consequence of the reduced numbers of mast cells in these mice, and/or other effects of the Mac-1 deficiency, is not yet clear. Mice that lack the p85α regulatory subunit of phosphatidylinositol-3 kinase (PI3K) essentially lack gastrointestinal mast cells and exhibit an approximately 10-fold reduction in levels of peritoneal mast cells (Fukao et al., 2002). When PI3K$^{-/-}$ mice were tested in an approximation of the CLP model, in which a bacterial inoculum prepared from the ceca of BALB/c mice was injected i.p. to induce peritonitis, these mice had markedly reduced levels of bacterial clearance in the peritoneal cavity 3 h postinoculation (Fukao et al., 2002). Normal (i.e., WT) levels of bacterial clearance (as well as TNF-α levels at 1 h after injection of bacteria) were restored by reconstitution of PI3K$^{-/-}$ mice with PI3K$^{+/+}$ BMCMC. This study confirms a protective role for peritoneal mast cells in septic peritonitis and highlights the involvement of PI3K in this process.

Beyond the now well-established roles of initiating and amplifying inflammatory responses to bacterial pathogens, many additional potential roles for mast cells in defense against bacterial infection have been proposed. In many cases, such additional roles have been based on findings obtained with populations of mouse or, occasionally, human mast cells generated in vitro. In interpreting findings such as these, it is important to keep in mind that the phenotypic characteristics, and functions, of in vitro-derived mast cells may differ from those of native mast cell populations in vivo. Moreover, to date, we are not aware of data demonstrating that any roles for mast cells in innate immunity, other than their roles in initiating and amplifying the inflammatory response elicited by pathogens, are significant in vivo, even in mouse models.

At least certain populations of in vitro-derived mast cells have been shown to exhibit the ability to phagocytose bacteria (Malaviya et al., 1994, 1996b), in some cases with the concomitant release of TNF-α (Arock et al., 1998), to kill bacteria via the production of cathelin-related AMP (Di Nardo et al., 2003) or to function as antigen-processing or -presenting cells via major histocompatibility complex class I molecules (Malaviya et al., 1994, 1996b; Mecheri and David, 1997). In addition, in opsonin-deficient environments, certain bacteria can express adhesins that can subvert the phagocytosis machinery of mouse mast cells such that the cells become reservoirs of viable bacteria (Shin et al., 2000). Shin et al. (2000) demonstrated that, under serum-deficient conditions, type I fimbriated E. coli can enter in vitro-derived mouse mast cells, evading the classical endosome-lysosome pathway, and localizing to the plasmalemmal caveolae in vitro; the internalized bacteria remain viable inside the cells and may even leave the mast cells subsequently without loss of viability. These very interesting observations suggest that the mast cell might represent a refuge for bacteria within the host and thereby could contribute to either the delayed clearance or recurrence of bacterial infections. However, the in vivo occurrence, and importance, of these observations remain to be established.

THERAPEUTIC ENHANCEMENT OF MAST CELL-DEPENDENT CONTRIBUTIONS TO INNATE IMMUNITY

Can the ability of mast cells to promote innate immunity be manipulated therapeutically? Although this has not yet been demonstrated in humans, in mice the answer appears to be yes. Maurer et al. (1998) assessed whether the repetitive administration of the c-kit ligand, SCF, could enhance survival in mice subjected to CLP and, if so, whether this reflected an effect of the cytokine on mast cells.

It already had been shown that SCF treatment could increase the numbers of mast cells in the tissues of mice (Tsai et al., 1991; Ando et al., 1993; Iemura et al., 1994) and that SCF also can promote mast cell mediator and cytokine secretion, both in vitro and in vivo (reviewed by Wershil et al., 1992; Galli et al., 1994; Costa et al., 1996; Galli and Lantz, 1999; and Tsai et al., 2000b). Maurer et al. (1998) showed that repetitive administration of SCF not only increased the numbers of cutaneous and peritoneal mast cells in C57BL/6 mice (Fig. 1A and B, respectively), but also significantly improved the ability of the mice to survive CLP (Fig. 1C). Experiments conducted with mast cell knock-in mice, in which the

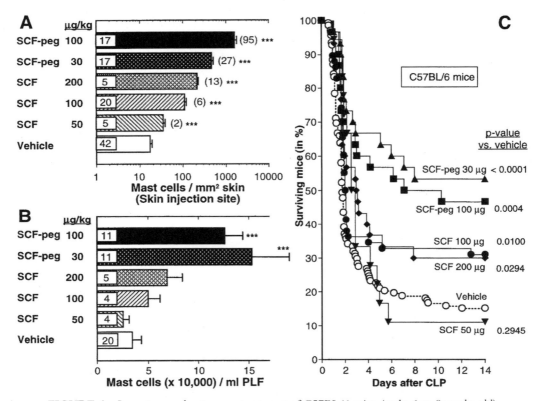

FIGURE 1 Long-term subcutaneous treatment of C57BL/6 mice (male, 6 to 9 weeks old) with SCF results in increased numbers of dermal and peritoneal mast cells and enhanced survival after CLP. (A and B) Some mice were killed after the last of 21 daily subcutaneous injections with vehicle, rat recombinant SCF (Maurer et al., 1998) (rrSCF, 50, 100, or 200 μg/kg per day), or polyethylene glycol–derivatized rrSCF (Maurer et al., 1998) (rrSCF-peg, 30 or 100 μg/kg per day), for assessment of (A) the numbers of mast cells per mm² of dermis at the site of injections and (B) the numbers of mast cells in peritoneal lavage fluid; data in panel A also include values for some mice in panel C that died within 2 days of CLP. Numbers of mice per group are indicated inside the bars; in A, fold change (i.e., value for SCF-treated group and value for vehicle-treated group) is given in parentheses. ★★★ $P < 0.005$ versus values for mice treated with vehicle alone. (C) Some mice (male, 6 to 9 weeks old) were treated daily for 21 days before CLP and for 14 days or until death after CLP (~50% ligation, single puncture with a 0.7-mm needle); mice received subcutaneous injections of vehicle, 50-, 100-, or 200-μg/kg per day rrSCF, or 30- or 100-μg/kg per day rrSCF-peg ($n = 138, 18, 58, 30, 30,$ and 30, respectively). Data were pooled from at least three independent experiments per treatment group. PLF, peritoneal lavage fluid. Reproduced from Fig. 1 of Maurer et al. (1998) with permission of the publisher.

only cells present in these mice that expressed a WT c-kit were the adoptively transferred WT BMCMC, demonstrated that the therapeutic benefit of SCF in this setting reflected, at least in part, actions of SCF on mast cells (Fig. 2).

The same study also demonstrated that TNF-$\alpha^{-/-}$ mice (that had numbers of peritoneal mast cells that were not significantly different from those in the corresponding WT mice) exhibited significantly reduced survival after CLP compared with the WT mice (Maurer et al., 1998). In light of the work of Malaviya et al. (1996a) and Echtenacher et al. (1996), this result was expected. However, the beneficial effect of SCF treatment on survival after CLP not only occurred in TNF-$\alpha^{-/-}$ mice, but was even greater than that observed in the identically treated WT mice (Maurer et al., 1998). Thus, SCF can enhance survival in CLP by mechanisms that are, at least in part, independent of TNF-α. Moreover, the therapeutic benefit of SCF treatment on survival after CLP was observed in both TNF-$\alpha^{-/-}$ mice and the corresponding WT mice, even though the treatment protocol did not result in significantly increased numbers of peritoneal mast cells in these animals (Maurer et al., 1998). This result suggests that the ability of SCF to enhance mast cell-dependent host defense in this model may reflect actions of SCF other than its ability simply to expand numbers of peritoneal mast cells. Finally, in confirmation of the results of our earlier experiments with WBB6F$_1$-+/+ mice (Ando et al., 1993), we found that mice treated repetitively with SCF did not appear to be at substantially increased risk (versus vehicle-treated mice) for death when IgE-dependent systemic anaphylaxis was induced by intravenous (Ando et al., 1993) or i.p. (Maurer et al., 1998) challenge with specific antigen.

The findings of Maurer et al. (1998) showed that survival in a model of innate immunity can be enhanced by treatment with SCF, a cytokine with diverse effects on mast cells as well as on other cell types. These observations also showed that normal animals that have been treated to develop higher-than-baseline levels of mast cells can exhibit enhanced resistance to bacterial infection. Although great caution must be exercised when extrapolating from mouse studies to human medicine, these findings suggest a new approach for attempting to manage patients at risk for bacterial infection. It may be of particular interest to evaluate approaches that attempt to enhance the contributions of mast cells to innate immunity in patients with congenital or acquired immunodeficiency disorders, since a study of a small group of such individuals found that they had greatly decreased numbers of mast cells in the gastrointestinal mucosa (Irani et al., 1987).

MAST CELLS AND BASOPHILS IN HOST DEFENSE AGAINST PARASITES

Studies of mast cells and basophils in host defense against parasites have focused predominantly on the potential roles of these cells in acquired, rather than innate, immune responses. Infections with many species of parasites, particularly helminths, can be associated with increased levels of basophils and eosinophils in the circulation, enhanced serum IgE levels, and increased numbers of mast cells and basophils in the tissues (Askenase, 1977; Woodbury et al., 1984; Miller, 1996; Lantz et al., 1998). Most studies in mice of the roles of mast cells, or their products, in acquired immunity to parasites have investigated primary infections with nematodes. For example, several lines of evidence indicate that mast cells are required for optimal expulsion of *Trichinella spiralis* during primary infection (Knight et al., 2000; Urban et al., 2000), but not for *Nippostrongylus brasiliensis* expulsion in mice (reviewed by Reed, 1989; Arizono et al., 1993; Nawa et al., 1994; Newlands et al., 1995; and Lantz et al., 1998); the response to *T. spiralis* appears to be dependent on Stat6 activation (Urban et al., 2000) and expression of mast cell protease 1 (Knight et al., 2000). Moreover, Kit^W/Kit^{W-v} mice exhibited a delay in *T. spiralis* expulsion compared with Kit^W/Kit^{W-v} mice that had been nonselectively reconstituted with mast cells by

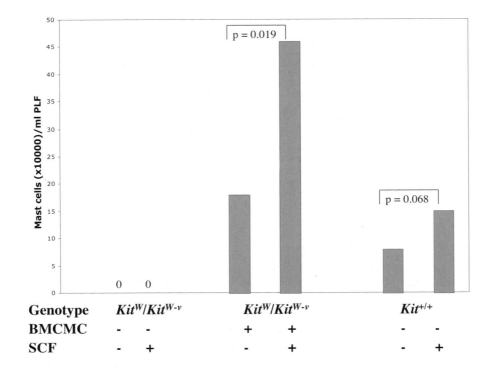

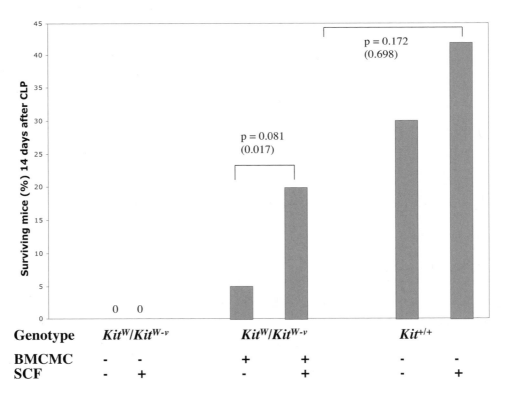

adoptive transfer of WT bone marrow cells (Vallance et al., 2001).

Studies of the primary immune response to the nematodes *S. venezuelensis* and *N. brasiliensis* reveal the complexity of analyzing the roles of individual potential components of host resistance to parasites. Although both parasites induced substantial increases in local populations of intestinal mast cells and basophils, mast cells (and perhaps basophils) appeared to contribute to the primary immune expulsion of *S. venezuelensis* but not *N. brasiliensis* (reviewed by Lantz et al., 1998). Thus, Kit^W/Kit^{W-v} mice that were also IL-3 deficient did not develop basophilia, remained profoundly mast cell-deficient during nematode infection, and exhibited a striking impairment in their ability to expel the nematode *S. venezuelensis* during the primary infection, but no defect in their ability to expel *N. brasiliensis* (Lantz et al., 1998). The defect in the primary immune responses to *S. venezuelensis* in Kit^W/Kit^{W-v} IL-3$^{-/-}$ mice was significantly greater than that observed in either Kit^W/Kit^{W-v} IL-3$^{+/+}$ or $Kit^{+/+}$ IL-3 $^{-/-}$ mice (Lantz et al., 1998). This finding may be representative of a general principle that mast cells often may be part of a complex host defense strategy, in which more than one element (e.g., mast cells plus IL-3) must be impaired before significant effects on the host defense response can be appreciated.

Similarly, mice lacking functional PI3K were found to be highly susceptible to infection with *S. venezuelensis* (Fukao et al., 2002). However, reconstitution with PI3K$^{+/+}$ BMCMC (the PI3K$^{-/-}$ mice lack peritoneal and gastrointestinal mast cells, as noted above) did not restore antinematode immunity; transfer of Th2-conditioned BMCMC grown in the presence of IL-4 and IL-10 was required, suggesting the importance of distinct local populations of mast cells at different anatomical sites for appropriate immune response (Fukao et al., 2002).

Mast cells and basophils may provide similar or overlapping effector functions in acquired immunity to parasites, with the relative contributions of these cell types varying according to species of parasite, species of host, and site of infection. Evidence for this notion comes from studies of *S. venezuelensis* infection in Kit^W/Kit^{W-v} and IL-3$^{-/-}$ mice (Lantz et al., 1998), as well as from studies with ixodid ticks. Thus, experiments in Kit^W/Kit^{W-v} mice showed that the expression of an IgE-dependent immune response to cutaneous feeding by larval *Haemaphysalis longicornis* ticks required mast cells (Matsuda et al., 1990). By contrast, immune resistance to the feeding of larval *Dermacentor variabilis* ticks was not significantly impaired in Kit^W/Kit^{W-v} mice, perhaps because basophils had a dominant role in that response (Steeves and Allen, 1990). Studies with antibodies against basophils or eosinophils showed that basophils were required for optimal expression of an immune response that impaired the skin feeding and survival of larval

---

FIGURE 2 Long-term subcutaneous treatment with SCF increases (A) the numbers of mast cells in the peritoneal lavage fluid (PLF) and (B) survival (%) at day 14 after CLP in WT $Kit^{+/+}$ mice and in mast cell-reconstituted Kit^W/Kit^{W-v} mice, but not in mast cell-deficient Kit^W/Kit^{W-v} mice. (A) Number of mast cells in the PLF: three to five mice per group (male, 11 to 13 weeks old at time of death or CLP) were killed after the last of 21 daily subcutaneous injections with vehicle or rrSCF-peg (30 μg/kg per day) for assessment of the numbers of mast cells in PLF. (B) Survival (%) of mice at 14 days after CLP: 24 to 27 mice per group were treated daily for 21 days before CLP and for 14 days or until death after CLP (~50% ligation, single puncture with a 0.7-mm needle). *P* values in parentheses are for survival after day 3. Data were pooled from two independent experiments per treatment group. Significance of differences in overall (0 to 14 days) or late-phase (>3 days after CLP) survival in the mice was calculated by the Mantel-Cox log rank test. Modified, with permission, from Fig. 2 of Maurer et al. (1998) with permission of the publisher.

ixodid ticks of the species *Amblyomma americanum* in guinea pigs (Brown et al., 1982). Finally, elevated numbers of IL-4-producing MMCP-8[+] cells that were identified as basophil-like were observed in the spleens of mice infected with the malarial parasite *Plasmodium chabaudi chabaudi*; by contrast, none of the classical mouse mast cell serine proteases were upregulated in this setting (Poorafshar et al., 2000). Whether these putative basophils contribute to resistance to this parasite in mice remains to be determined.

It will be of interest to assess whether mast cells (or basophils) might represent important elements of innate immunity to parasites. Another promising area of investigation is whether the pathogen-stimulated production of cytokines such as IL-4 or IL-13 by mast cells or basophils can serve as a link between the innate and the acquired immune responses to these organisms.

MAST CELLS AND BASOPHILS IN IMMUNE RESPONSES TO VIRUSES

So far there is no proof that mast cells or basophils represent a critical component of innate or acquired immunity to viral infection. On the other hand, some tantalizing evidence suggests such roles. For example, Patella et al. (1998, 2000b) recently demonstrated that mast cells and basophils can be activated by certain viral proteins in an IgE-dependent manner. The human immunodeficiency virus (HIV) glycoprotein 120 (gp120), as well as protein Fv—which is released into the intestinal tract in patients with viral hepatitis—can interact with the V_H3 domain of IgE and thereby induce histamine, IL-4, and IL-13 release from human basophils and mast cells (Patella et al., 1998, 2000b). Accordingly, it has been proposed that basophils and/or mast cells activated by an interaction between gp120 and whatever IgE antibodies are present on the cells' surface may represent a source of IL-4 and IL-13 during the early stages of HIV-1 infections—which are characterized by a switch from a Th1-type toward a Th2-type pattern of cytokine production—as well as during later phases of

HIV infection, when Th2 cells are reduced in number (Patella et al., 2000b; Marone et al., 2001).

Interestingly, it has also been shown that metachromatic cells with many features of basophils, such as those previously identified in the blood of severely allergic patients (Li et al., 1998), can be detected in the blood of patients with AIDS (Li et al., 2001). These cells, which express the chemokine receptors CCR3, CCR5, and CXCR4, had become infected with HIV-1 in vivo, and populations of these cells that were maintained ex vivo and populations of cells with similar phenotypic characteristics that were generated in vitro were susceptible to infection by a so-called "M-tropic" strain of HIV-1 (Li et al., 2001). Such findings suggest that basophils (and perhaps mast cells) may represent yet another potential cellular reservoir for HIV in patients with AIDS.

MAST CELL-ASSOCIATED PATHOLOGY DURING HOST RESPONSES TO PATHOGENS

Clearly, one of the potential consequences of the mast cell or basophil activation that occurs during host responses to pathogens (whether in the context of innate or acquired immunity) is the promotion of local, or systemic, pathology. Indeed, the possibility that mast cell activation in the course of innate immune responses may have negative consequences for the host, at least in certain circumstances, is reminiscent of the mast cell's role in acquired immune responses. Although mast cells and basophils can contribute to host defense in the context of acquired immunity to certain parasites (see above), mast cell and basophil activation during acquired immune responses also can promote disease. This outcome occurs when the IgE (or, in the mouse, IgG1) antibodies that confer on the cells the ability to undergo antigen-specific activation are themselves directed against otherwise innocuous exogenous antigens, e.g., in the setting of allergic diseases (Metcalfe et al., 1997; Galli and Lantz, 1999; Williams and Galli, 2000; Kawakami and Galli, 2002).

Moreover, it has recently been shown in mouse model systems that Th2-associated antibodies can also produce pathology, even including fatal anaphylaxis, if they are directed against certain self-antigens. In these experiments, which tested whether certain self-peptide preparations could ameliorate the course of experimentally induced or spontaneous autoimmune disorders, IgG1 antibodies may have played a more significant role than IgE (Pedotti et al., 2001, 2003; Liu et al., 2002). In addition, it is not yet clear to what extent, if any, the products of mast cells, as opposed to mediators derived from other potential effector cells, contributed to the anaphylaxis observed in these settings. By contrast, studies employing mast cell knock-in mice have shown that mast cell activation, presumably via antibody-dependent mechanisms, can significantly contribute to the pathology associated with mouse models of autoimmune disorders, such as experimental autoimmune encephalomyelitis (Secor et al., 2000; Robbie-Ryan et al., 2003) or an antibody-dependent form of arthritis (Lee et al., 2002).

Yet even in the context of Th2-associated acquired immunity to parasites (in which mast cells are generally thought to contribute to host defense), the net effect of mast cell activation during the responses to certain organisms may be to promote pathology. As discussed above, several lines of evidence indicate that mast cells do not contribute significantly to the expression of immune resistance to *N. brasiliensis*. Remarkably, Arizono et al. (1993) demonstrated that egg production by *N. brasiliensis* during primary infections in rats was significantly increased in WT as opposed to mast cell-deficient *Ws/Ws* rats. In accord with these findings, Newlands et al. (1995) showed that *N. brasiliensis* egg production also was increased in control rats as opposed to those experiencing depletion of intestinal mast cells as a result of treatment with a neutralizing antibody to SCF. Although these studies suggest that mast cells may contribute to the fecundity of this parasite, it has not yet been formally proven that mast cell depletion, as opposed to other effects of either the *c-kit* mutations in the *Ws/Ws* rats or the administration of the anti-SCF antibodies in the WT rats, was responsible for the increased egg production in these experiments. By contrast, studies in mast cell knock-in mice clearly showed that mast cells can contribute to both the magnitude and the duration of the cutaneous pathology induced by the intradermal injection of *Leishmania major* promastigotes, unfortunately without a detectable corresponding benefit in terms of host resistance to this pathogen (Wershil et al., 1994).

As discussed above, many direct and/or indirect mechanisms of mast cell or basophil activation may occur during host responses to pathogens. One of these potential mechanisms, that is of particular interest because of its possible consequences for immunoregulation, involves the Ig-dependent, but antigen-independent, activation of the cells by products of pathogens. For example, protein L of *Pneumococcus magnus* and protein A of *Staphylococcus aureus* are bacterial superantigens that can interact with distinct regions of IgE and therefore can induce mediator release from basophils and mast cells in vitro (Patella et al., 2000a). However, it remains to be determined whether such mechanisms of mast cell or basophil activation occur in vivo and, if so, whether they contribute significantly to the pathology associated with the underlying disorders.

The mechanisms by which mast cell activation during host responses to pathogens can result in tissue injury are diverse, and this represents a very broad area of research. For example, an in vitro study with bone marrow-derived cultured mast cells has shown that VacA—the vacuolating cytotoxin of *Helicobacter pylori*—can directly activate mast cells for migration and production of proinflammatory cytokines, including TNF-α and IL-6 (Supajatura et al., 2002a). These findings suggest that mast cell activation by VacA may represent an important part of the host's early response to this pathogen, perhaps contributing to both bacterial clearance and *H. pylori*-induced gastritis.

However, to our knowledge, these hypotheses have not yet been evaluated using mast cell knock-in mice.

By contrast, other potential mechanisms by which mast cells can influence the pathology associated with innate or acquired immune responses already have been investigated in studies employing mast cell-reconstituted mice. For example, studies in Kit^W/Kit^{W-v} mice that contained mast cells derived from adoptively transferred WT bone marrow cells support the hypotheses that mast cells can (i) promote epithelial chloride secretion in a model of intestinal anaphylaxis, probably in part via effects on enteric nerves (Perdue et al., 1991); (ii) promote colonic mucin release in a mouse model of immobilization stress (Castagliuolo et al., 1998); and (iii) contribute to both neutrophil recruitment and intestinal fluid secretion in a model of enteritis that is induced by *Clostridium difficile* toxin A (Wershil et al., 1998). In settings such as these, whether the net effect of mast cell activation is positive or negative for the host may vary considerably, depending on the circumstances.

CONCLUSIONS

Multiple lines of evidence suggest that mast cells, and perhaps basophils, can have important effector functions and other beneficial roles in natural immune responses; however, very few studies provide convincing in vivo evidence for such roles. Studies in genetically mast cell-deficient Kit^W/Kit^{W-v} mice, the congenic WT ($Kit^{+/+}$) mice, and mast cell knock-in mice provide direct evidence that mast cells can contribute to optimal expression of innate immunity and can enhance survival in mice subjected to CLP (Echtenacher et al., 1996; Maurer et al., 1998; Supajatura et al., 2001, 2002b), as well as in some other models of i.p. infection (Malaviya et al., 1996a). Moreover, the mast cell-dependent protective function(s) in CLP can be enhanced in mice that receive repetitive injections of the c-*kit* ligand SCF (Maurer et al., 1998). Although the studies of the role of mast cells in responses to CLP obviously have

been performed in only one species (the mouse) and only in one model of innate immunity (CLP), this work establishes proof of principle that the beneficial role(s) of mast cells in innate immune responses to bacterial infection can be enhanced therapeutically.

The studies in the CLP model in mice, and other lines of evidence, thus support the view that mast cells can have sentinel and effector functions in innate immunity to bacteria. Poised at the ready in serosal cavities and immediately beneath epithelial surfaces, as well as near blood vessels, nerves, and glands, mast cells are strategically positioned to sense the presence of pathogens both directly and indirectly (e.g., via complement activation); these cells then can respond by releasing proinflammatory and immunoregulatory cytokines and many other mediators, including some that may have direct antimicrobial activities. In this way, the mast cell can help to initiate, orchestrate, and amplify the inflammatory response at sites of pathogen invasion.

However, many questions remain about the specific roles of mast cells in response to individual pathogens and in different types or stages of infection. Even if we focus on the role of mast cells as initiators, amplifiers, and regulators of inflammatory reactions to pathogens, it is not yet clear how important these roles are across the full spectrum of infectious disorders. For example, most of the studies in antibacterial immunity have been performed either by using the CLP model or by injecting i.p. large numbers of gram-negative bacteria.

Similarly, although the roles of mast cells in innate immunity probably extend beyond those of representing sentinels and effectors of the response (including positive roles in maintaining epithelial barrier function, the phagocytosis and killing of organisms, antigen processing and presentation, the initiation and regulation of acquired immune responses to the pathogen, and the resolution of inflammation and other pathologies associated with the response), the biological importance of these additional functions in vivo remains to be established. The same is true of the potential roles of mast cells or basophils as reservoirs of bacteria or viruses.

Mast cell knock-in mice, especially those that have been reconstituted with mast cells expressing genetic alterations in receptors, signaling pathways or cytokines, and other mediators, should continue to be very helpful in efforts to characterize the importance and nature of the mast cells' potential contributions to innate immunity. However, if the mast cell is only one of multiple elements providing overlapping functions in these settings, as will typically be the case, then the contribution of the mast cell may be difficult to identify without manipulating precisely and systematically the other components involved in such responses. These efforts will be particularly challenging in light of the fact that mast cells can live a long time, can undergo alterations in phenotype and functional properties, and may have different roles in immune reactions and other biological responses at different points in their natural history.

Finally, it should be kept in mind that, in some circumstances, the mast cell and/or basophil activation that occurs during immune responses to infection (as a result of either direct or indirect interactions between these cells and the pathogens) may not be associated with a corresponding direct contribution of the mast cells or basophils to host resistance. Even worse (from the standpoint of host defense), it is possible that certain consequences of mast cell activation during bacterial, viral, or parasite infections may benefit the pathogen more than the host.

The mast cell, so rightly considered a key "part of the problem" in the expression of anaphylaxis, atopic asthma, and other IgE-associated disorders, clearly can provide significant benefit in host defense during certain examples of bacterial infection, at least in mice. However, it seems likely that, in different circumstances, mast cells may also promote tissue injury associated with innate immunity and/or may express functions that can benefit the pathogen more than the host. This mercurial nature of the mast cell—the potential of its

activation, depending on the circumstances, either to cause harm or to promote health— suggests that much caution should be exercised during any attempts to augment certain mast cell functions (such as those in innate immunity) for therapeutic ends.

REFERENCES

Agis, H., W. Fureder, H. C. Bankl, M. Kundi, W. R. Sperr, M. Willheim, G. Boltz-Nitulescu, J. H. Butterfield, K. Kishi, K. Lechner, and P. Valent. 1996. Comparative immunophenotypic analysis of human mast cells, blood basophils and monocytes. *Immunology* **87:**535–543.

Ando, A., T. R. Martin, and S. J. Galli. 1993. Effects of chronic treatment with the c-kit ligand, stem cell factor, on immunoglobulin E-dependent anaphylaxis in mice. Genetically mast cell-deficient *Sl/Sl^d* mice acquire anaphylactic responsiveness, but the congenic normal mice do not exhibit augmented responses. *J. Clin. Invest.* **92:**1639–1649.

Arizono, N., T. Kasugai, M. Yamada, M. Okada, M. Morimoto, H. Tei, G. F. J. Newlands, H. R. P. Miller, and Y. Kitamura. 1993. Infection of *Nippostrongylus brasiliensis* induces development of mucosal-type but not connective tissue-type mast cells in genetically mast cell-deficient *Ws/Ws* rats. *Blood* **81:**2572–2578.

Arock, M., E. Ross, R. Lai-Kuen, G. Averlant, Z. Gao, and S. N. Abraham. 1998. Phagocytic and tumor necrosis factor alpha response of human mast cells following exposure to gram-negative and gram-positive bacteria. *Infect. Immun.* **66:**6030–6034.

Askenase, P. W. 1977. Immune inflammatory responses to parasites: the role of basophils, mast cells and vasoactive amines. *Am. J. Trop. Med. Hyg.* **26:**96–103.

Befus, A. D., C. Mowat, M. Gilchrist, J. Hu, S. Solomon, and A. Bateman. 1999. Neutrophil defensins induce histamine secretion from mast cells: mechanisms of action. *J. Immunol.* **163:**947–953.

Biedermann, T., M. Kneilling, R. Mailhammer, K. Maier, C. A. Sander, G. Kollias, S. L. Kunkel, L. Hultner, and M. Rocken. 2000. Mast cells control neutrophil recruitment during T cell-mediated delayed-type hypersensitivity reactions through tumor necrosis factor and macrophage inflammatory protein 2. *J. Exp. Med.* **192:**1441–1452.

Boesiger, J., M. Tsai, M. Maurer, M. Yamaguchi, L. F. Brown, K. P. Claffey, H. F. Dvorak, and S. J. Galli. 1998. Mast cells can secrete vascular permeability factor/vascular endothelial cell growth factor and exhibit enhanced release after immunoglobulin E-dependent upregulation of Fc epsilon RI expression. *J. Exp. Med.* **188:**1135–1145.

Brown, S. J., S. J. Galli, G. J. Gleich, and P. W. Askenase. 1982. Ablation of immunity to Amblyomma americanum by anti-basophil serum: cooperation between basophils and eosinophils in expression of immunity to ectoparasites (ticks) in guinea pigs. *J. Immunol.* **129:**790–796.

Brunner, T., C. H. Heusser, and C. A. Dahinden. 1993. Human peripheral blood basophils primed by interleukin 3 (IL-3) produce IL-4 in response to immunoglobulin E receptor stimulation. *J. Exp. Med.* **177:**605–611.

Castagliuolo, I., B. K. Wershil, K. Karalis, A. Pasha, S. T. Nikulasson, and C. Pothoulakis. 1998. Colonic mucin release in response to immobilization stress is mast cell dependent. *Am. J. Physiol.* **274:**G1094–G1100.

Columbo, M., E. M. Horowitz, L. M. Botana, D. W. MacGlashan, Jr., B. S. Bochner, S. Gillis, K. M. Zsebo, S. J. Galli, and L. M. Lichtenstein. 1992. The human recombinant c-kit receptor ligand, rhSCF, induces mediator release from human cutaneous mast cells and enhances IgE-dependent mediator release from both skin mast cells and peripheral blood basophils. *J. Immunol.* **14:**599–608.

Costa, J. J., G. D. Demetri, T. J. Harrist, A. M. Dvorak, D. F. Hayes, E. A. Merica, D. M. Menchaca, A. J. Gringeri, L. B. Schwartz, and S. J. Galli. 1996. Recombinant human stem cell factor (kit ligand) promotes human mast cell and melanocyte hyperplasia and functional activation *in vivo. J. Exp. Med.* **183:**2681–2686.

de Paulis, A., F. Annunziato, L. Di Gioia, S. Romagnani, M. Carfora, C. Beltrame, G. Marone, and P. Romagnani. 2001. Expression of the chemokine receptor CCR3 on human mast cells. *Int. Arch. Allergy Immunol.* **124:**146–150.

Di Nardo, A., A. Vitiello, and R. L. Gallo. 2003. Cutting edge: mast cell antimicrobial activity is mediated by expression of cathelicidin antimicrobial peptide. *J. Immunol.* **170:**2274–2278.

Echtenacher, B., W. Falk, D. N. Mannel, and P. H. Krammer. 1990. Requirement of endogenous tumor necrosis factor/cachectin for recovery from experimental peritonitis. *J. Immunol.* **145:**3762–3766.

Echtenacher, B., D. N. Mannel, and L. Hultner. 1996. Critical protective role of mast cells in a model of acute septic peritonitis. *Nature* **381:**75–77.

Feger, F., S. Varadaradjalou, Z. Gao, S. N. Abraham, and M. Arock. 2002. The role of mast cells in host defense and their subversion by bacterial pathogens. *Trends Immunol.* **23:**151–158.

Forsberg, E., G. Pejler, M. Ringvall, C. Lunderius, B. Tomasini-Johansson, M. Kusche-Gullberg, I. Eriksson, J. Ledin, L. Hellman, and L. Kjellen. 1999. Abnormal mast cells in mice deficient in a heparin-synthesizing enzyme. *Nature* **400:**773–776.

Friend, D. S., M. F. Gurish, K. F. Austen, J. Hunt, and R. L. Stevens. 2000. Senescent jejunal mast cells and eosinophils in the mouse preferentially translocate to the spleen and draining lymph node, respectively, during the recovery phase of helminth infection. *J. Immunol.* **165:**344–352.

Fukao, T., T. Yamada, M. Tanabe, Y. Terauchi, T. Ota, T. Takayama, T. Asano, T. Takeuchi, T. Kadowaki, J. Hata Ji, and S. Koyasu. 2002. Selective loss of gastrointestinal mast cells and impaired immunity in PI3K-deficient mice. *Nat. Immunol.* **3:**295–304.

Galli, S. J. 2000. Mast cells and basophils. *Curr. Opin. Hematol.* **7:**32–39.

Galli, S. J., and C. S. Lantz. 1999. Allergy, p. 1137–1184. *In* W. E. Paul (ed.), *Fundamental Immunology,* 4th ed. Lippincott Raven Press, Philadelphia, Pa.

Galli, S. J., K. M. Zsebo, and E. N. Geissler. 1994. The kit ligand, stem cell factor. *Adv. Immunol.* **55:**1–96.

Galli, S. J., M. Maurer, and C. S. Lantz. 1999. Mast cells as sentinels of innate immunity. *Curr. Opin. Immunol.* **11:**53–59.

Galli, S. J., D. Metcalfe, and A. M. Dvorak. 2001. Basophils and mast cells and their disorders, p. 801–815. *In* E. Beutler, M. A. Lichtman, B. S. Coller, T. J. Kipps, and U. Seligsohn (ed.), *Williams Hematology,* 6th ed. McGraw-Hill, New York, N.Y.

Galli, S. J., J. Wedemeyer, and M. Tsai. 2002. Analyzing the roles of mast cells and basophils in host defense and other biological responses. *Int. J. Hematol.* **75:**363–369.

Gommerman, J. L., D. Y. Oh, X. Zhou, T. F. Tedder, M. Maurer, S. J. Galli, and M. C. Carroll. 2000. A role for CD21/CD35 and CD19 in responses to acute septic peritonitis: a potential mechanism for mast cell activation. *J. Immunol.* **165:**6915–6921.

Gordon, J. R., and S. J. Galli. 1990. Mast cells as a source of both preformed and immunologically inducible TNF-alpha/cachectin. *Nature* **346:**274–276.

Gordon, J. R., and S. J. Galli. 1991. Release of both preformed and newly synthesized tumor necrosis factor alpha (TNF-alpha)/cachectin by mouse mast cells stimulated via the Fc epsilon RI. A mechanism for the sustained action of mast cell-derived TNF-alpha during IgE-dependent biological responses. *J. Exp. Med.* **174:**103–107.

Huang, C., G. T. De Sanctis, P. J. O'Brien, J. P. Mizgerd, D. S. Friend, J. M. Drazen, L. F. Brass, and R. L. Stevens. 2001. Evaluation of the substrate specificity of human mast cell tryptase beta I and demonstration of its importance in bacterial infections of the lung. *J. Biol. Chem.* **276:**26276–26284.

Humphries, D. E., G. W. Wong, D. S. Friend, M. F. Gurish, W. T. Qiu, C. Huang, A. H. Sharpe, and R. L. Stevens. 1999. Heparin is essential for the storage of specific granule proteases in mast cells. *Nature* **400:**769–772.

Iemura, A., M. Tsai, A. Ando, B. K. Wershil, and S. J. Galli. 1994. The c-kit ligand, stem cell factor, promotes mast cell survival by suppressing apoptosis. *Am. J. Pathol.* **144:**321–328.

Iikura, M., M. Miyamasu, M. Yamaguchi, H. Kawasaki, K. Matsushima, M. Kitaura, Y. Morita, O. Yoshie, K. Yamamoto, and K. Hirai. 2001. Chemokine receptors in human basophils: inducible expression of functional CXCR4. *J. Leukoc. Biol.* **70:** 113–120.

Irani, A. M., S. S. Craig, G. DeBlois, C. O. Elson, N. M. Schechter, and L. B. Schwartz. 1987. Deficiency of the tryptase-positive, chymase-negative mast cell type in gastrointestinal mucosa of patients with defective T lymphocyte function. *J. Immunol.* **138:**4381–4386.

Kawakami, T., and S. J. Galli. 2002. Regulation of mast-cell and basophil function and survival by IgE. *Nat. Rev. Immunol.* **2:**773–786.

Kitamura, Y., S. Go, and K. Hatanaka. 1978. Decrease of mast cells in *W/W*ᵛ mice and their increase by bone marrow transplantation. *Blood* **52:**447–452.

Knight, P. A., S. H. Wright, C. E. Lawrence, Y. Y. Paterson, and H. R. P. Miller. 2000. Delayed expulsion of the nematode *Trichinella spiralis* in mice lacking the mucosal mast cell-specific granule chymase, mouse mast cell protease-1. *J. Exp. Med.* **192:** 1849–1856.

Lantz, C. S., J. Boesiger, C. H. Song, N. Mach, T. Kobayashi, R. C. Mulligan, Y. Nawa, G. Dranoff, and S. J. Galli. 1998. Role for interleukin-3 in mast-cell and basophil development and in immunity to parasites. *Nature* **392:**90–93.

Lantz, C. S., C. H. Song, G. Dranoff, and S. J. Galli. 1999. Interleukin-3 (IL-3) is required for blood basophilia, but not for increased basophil IL-4 production, in response to parasite infection in mice. *FASEB J.* **13:**A235.

Leal-Berumen, I., P. Conlon, and J. S. Marshall. 1994. IL-6 production by rat peritoneal mast cells is not necessarily preceded by histamine release and can be induced by bacterial lipopolysaccharide. *J. Immunol.* **152:**5468–5476.

Lee, D. M., D. S. Friend, M. F. Gurish, C. Benoist, D. Mathis, and M. B. Brenner. 2002. Mast cells: a cellular link between autoantibodies and inflammatory arthritis. *Science* **297:**1689–1692.

Li, H., T. C. Sim, and R. Alam. 1996. IL-13 released by and localized in human basophils. *J. Immunol.* **156:**4833–4838.

Li, L., Y. Li, S. W. Reddel, M. Cherrian, D. S. Friend, R. L. Stevens, and S. A. Krilis. 1998. Identification of basophilic cells that express mast cell granule proteases in the peripheral blood of asthma, allergy, and drug-reactive patients. *J. Immunol.* **161:**5079–5086.

Li, Y., L. Li, R. Wadley, S. W. Reddel, J. C. Qi, C. Archis, A. Collins, E. Clark, M. Cooley, S. Kouts, H. M. Naif, M. Alali, A. Cunningham, G. W. Wong, R. L. Stevens, and S. A. Krilis. 2001. Mast cells/basophils in the peripheral blood of allergic individuals who are HIV-1 susceptible due to their surface expression of CD4 and the chemokine receptors CCR3, CCR5, and CXCR4. *Blood* **97:**3484–3490.

Liu, E., H. Moriyama, N. Abiru, D. Miao, L. Yu, R. M. Taylor, F. D. Finkelman, and G. S. Eisenbarth. 2002. Anti-peptide autoantibodies and fatal anaphylaxis in NOD mice in response to insulin self-peptides B:9-23 and B:13-23. *J. Clin. Invest.* **110:**1021–1027.

MacGlashan, D., Jr., J. M. White, S. K. Huang, S. J. Ono, J. T. Schroeder, and L. M. Lichtenstein. 1994. Secretion of IL-4 from human basophils. The relationship between IL-4 mRNA and protein in resting and stimulated basophils. *J. Immunol.* **152:**3006–3016.

Malaviya, R., and S. N. Abraham. 2000. Role of mast cell leukotrienes in neutrophil recruitment and bacterial clearance in infectious peritonitis. *J. Leukoc. Biol.* **67:**841–846.

Malaviya, R., E. A. Ross, J. I. MacGregor, T. Ikeda, J. R. Little, B. A. Jakschik, and S. N. Abraham. 1994. Mast cell phagocytosis of FimH-expressing enterobacteria. *J. Immunol.* **152:**1907–1914.

Malaviya, R., T. Ikeda, E. Ross, and S. N. Abraham. 1996a. Mast cell modulation of neutrophil influx and bacterial clearance at sites of infection through TNF-alpha. *Nature* **381:**77–80.

Malaviya, R., N. J. Twesten, E. A. Ross, S. N. Abraham, and J. D. Pfeifer. 1996b. Mast cells process bacterial Ags through a phagocytic route for class I MHC presentation to T cells. *J. Immunol.* **156:**1490–1496.

Malaviya, R., C. Navara, and F. M. Uckun. 2001. Role of Janus kinase 3 in mast cell-mediated innate immunity against gram-negative bacteria. *Immunity* **15:**313–321.

Marone, G., G. Florio, A. Petraroli, M. Triggiani, and A. de Paulis. 2001. Role of human Fc epsilon RI+ cells in HIV-1 infection. *Immunol. Rev.* **179:**128–138.

Matsuda, H., K. Kawakita, Y. Kiso, T. Nakano, and Y. Kitamura. 1989. Substance P induces granulocyte infiltration through degranulation of mast cells. *J. Immunol.* **142:**927–931.

Matsuda, H., N. Watanabe, Y. Kiso, S. Hirota, H. Ushio, Y. Kannan, M. Azuma, H. Koyama, and Y. Kitamura. 1990. Necessity of IgE antibodies and mast cells for manifestation of resistance against larval Haemaphysalis longicornis ticks in mice. *J. Immunol.* **144:**259–262.

Maurer, M., B. Echtenacher, L. Hultner, G. Kollias, D. N. Mannel, K. E. Langley, and S. J.

Galli. 1998. The c-kit ligand, stem cell factor, can enhance innate immunity through effects on mast cells. *J. Exp. Med.* **188:**2343–2348.

McCurdy, J. D., T. J. Olynych, L. H. Maher, and J. S. Marshall. 2003. Cutting edge: distinct toll-like receptor 2 activators selectively induce different classes of mediator production from human mast cells. *J. Immunol.* **170:**1625–1629.

Mecheri, S., and B. David. 1997. Unravelling the mast cell dilemma: culprit or victim of its generosity? *Immunol. Today* **18:**212–215.

Mekori, Y. A., and D. D. Metcalfe. 2000. Mast cells in innate immunity. *Immunol. Rev.* **173:**131–140.

Metcalfe, D. D., D. Baram, and Y. A. Mekori. 1997. Mast cells. *Physiol. Rev.* **77:**1033–1079.

Metzger, H. 1992. The receptor with high affinity for IgE. *Immunol. Rev.* **125:**37–48.

Miller, H. R. P. 1996. Mucosal mast cells and the allergic response against nematode parasites. *Vet. Immunol. Immunopathol.* **54:**331–336.

Nakano, T., T. Sonoda, C. Hayashi, A. Yamatodani, Y. Kanayama, T. Yamamura, H. Asai, T. Yonezawa, Y. Kitamura, and S. J. Galli. 1985. Fate of bone marrow-derived cultured mast cells after intracutaneous, intraperitoneal, and intravenous transfer into genetically mast cell-deficient *W/W^v* mice. Evidence that cultured mast cells can give rise to both connective tissue type and mucosal mast cells. *J. Exp. Med.* **162:**1025–1043.

Nawa, Y., N. Ishikawa, K. Tsuchiya, Y. Horii, T. Abe, A. I. Khan, S. Bing, H. Itoh, H. Ide, and F. Uchiyama. 1994. Selective effector mechanisms for the expulsion of intestinal helminths. *Parasite Immunol.* **16:**333–338.

Newlands, G. F. J., H. R. P. Miller, A. MacKellar, and S. J. Galli. 1995. Stem cell factor contributes to intestinal mucosal mast cell hyperplasia in rats infected with *Nippostrongylus brasiliensis* or *Trichinella spiralis*, but anti-stem cell factor treatment decreases parasite egg production during *N. brasiliensis* infection. *Blood* **86:**1968–1976.

Niyonsaba, F., A. Someya, M. Hirata, H. Ogawa, and I. Nagaoka. 2001. Evaluation of the effects of peptide antibiotics human beta-defensins-1/-2 and LL-37 on histamine release and prostaglandin D(2) production from mast cells. *Eur. J. Immunol.* **31:**1066–1075.

Nocka, K., J. C. Tan, E. Chiu, T. Y. Chu, P. Ray, P. Traktman, and P. Besmer. 1990. Molecular bases of dominant negative and loss of function mutations at the murine c-kit/white spotting locus: *W^{37}*, *W^v*, *W^{41}* and *W. EMBO J.* **9:**1805–1813.

Okayama, Y., D. D. Hagaman, and D. D. Metcalfe. 2001a. A comparison of mediators released or generated by IFN-gamma-treated human mast cells following aggregation of Fc gamma RI or Fc epsilon RI. *J. Immunol.* **166:**4705–4712.

Okayama, Y., D. D. Hagaman, M. Woolhiser, and D. D. Metcalfe. 2001b. Further characterization of Fc gamma RII and Fc gamma RIII expression by cultured human mast cells. *Int. Arch. Allergy Immunol.* **124:**155–157.

Patella, V., A. Giuliano, J. P. Bouvet, and G. Marone. 1998. Endogenous superallergen protein Fv induces IL-4 secretion from human Fc epsilon RI+ cells through interaction with the VH3 region of IgE. *J. Immunol.* **161:**5647–5655.

Patella, V., G. Florio, A. Oriente, G. Spadaro, V. Forte, A. Genovese, and G. Marone. 2000a. Human mast cells and basophils in immune responses to infectious agents, p. 397–418. *In* G. Marone, L. M. Lichtenstein, and S. J. Galli (ed.), *Mast Cells and Basophils.* Academic Press, San Diego, Calif.

Patella, V., G. Florio, A. Petraroli, and G. Marone. 2000b. HIV-1 gp120 induces IL-4 and IL-13 release from human Fc epsilon RI+ cells through interaction with the VH3 region of IgE. *J. Immunol.* **164:**589–595.

Pedotti, R., D. Mitchell, J. Wedemeyer, M. Karpuj, D. Chabas, E. M. Hattab, M. Tsai, S. J. Galli, and L. Steinman. 2001. An unexpected version of horror autotoxicus: anaphylactic shock to a self-peptide. *Nat. Immunol.* **2:**216–222.

Pedotti, R., M. Sanna, M. Tsai, J. J. DeVoss, L. Steinman, H. McDevitt, and S. J. Galli. 2003. Severe anaphylactic reactions to glutamic acid decarboxylase (GAD) self peptides in NOD mice that spontaneously develop autoimmune type 1 diabetes mellitus. *BMC Immunol.* **4:**2, http://www.biomedcentral.com/1471-2172/4/2.

Perdue, M. H., S. Masson, B. K. Wershil, and S. J. Galli. 1991. Role of mast cells in ion transport abnormalities associated with intestinal anaphylaxis. Correction of the diminished secretory response in genetically mast cell-deficient *W/W^v* mice by bone marrow transplantation. *J. Clin. Invest.* **87:**687–693.

Poorafshar, M., H. Helmby, M. Troye-Blomberg, and L. Hellman. 2000. MMCP-8, the first lineage-specific differentiation marker for mouse basophils. Elevated numbers of potent IL-4-producing and MMCP-8-positive cells in spleens of malaria-infected mice. *Eur. J. Immunol.* **30:**2660–2668.

Prodeus, A. P., X. Zhou, M. Maurer, S. J. Galli, and M. C. Carroll. 1997. Impaired mast cell-dependent natural immunity in complement C3-deficient mice. *Nature* **390:**172–175.

Reed, N. 1989. Function and regulation of mast cells in parasite infections, p. 205–215. *In* S. Galli and K. F. Austen (ed.), *Mast Cell and Basophil Differentiation and Function in Health and Disease.* Raven Press, New York, N.Y.

Robbie-Ryan, M., M. B. Tanzola, V. H. Secor, and M. A. Brown. 2003. Cutting edge: both activating and inhibitory Fc receptors expressed on mast cells regulate experimental allergic encephalomyelitis disease severity. *J. Immunol.* **170:**1630–1634.

Rosenkranz, A. R., A. Coxon, M. Maurer, M. F. Gurish, K. F. Austen, D. S. Friend, S. J. Galli, and T. N. Mayadas. 1998. Impaired mast cell development and innate immunity in Mac-1 (CD11b/CD18, CR3)-deficient mice. *J. Immunol.* **161:**6463–6467.

Sabroe, I., E. C. Jones, L. R. Usher, M. K. Whyte, and S. K. Dower. 2002. Toll-like receptor (TLR)2 and TLR4 in human peripheral blood granulocytes: a critical role for monocytes in leukocyte lipopolysaccharide responses. *J. Immunol.* **168:**4701–4710.

Sayama, K., M. Diehn, K. Matsuda, C. Lunderius, M. Tsai, S. Y. Tam, D. Botstein, P. O. Brown, and S. J. Galli. 2002. Transcriptional response of human mast cells stimulated via the FceRI and identification of mast cells as a source of IL-11. *BMC Immunol.* **3:**5, http://www.biomedcentral.com/1471-2172/3/5.

Secor, V. H., W. E. Secor, C. A. Gutekunst, and M. A. Brown. 2000. Mast cells are essential for early onset and severe disease in a murine model of multiple sclerosis. *J. Exp. Med.* **191:**813–822.

Shin, J. S., Z. Gao, and S. N. Abraham. 2000. Involvement of cellular caveolae in bacterial entry into mast cells. *Science* **289:**785–788.

Silphaduang, U., and E. J. Noga. 2001. Antimicrobials: peptide antibiotics in mast cells of fish. *Nature* **414:**268–269.

Steeves, E. B., and J. R. Allen. 1990. Basophils in skin reactions of mast cell–deficient mice infested with *Dermacentor variabilis. Int. J. Parasitol.* **20:**655–667.

Supajatura, V., H. Ushio, A. Nakao, K. Okumura, C. Ra, and H. Ogawa. 2001. Protective roles of mast cells against enterobacterial infection are mediated by Toll-like receptor 4. *J. Immunol.* **167:**2250–2256.

Supajatura, V., H. Ushio, A. Wada, K. Yahiro, K. Okumura, H. Ogawa, T. Hirayama, and C. Ra. 2002a. Cutting edge:VacA, a vacuolating cytotoxin of *Helicobacter pylori,* directly activates mast cells for migration and production of proinflammatory cytokines. *J. Immunol.* **168:**2603–2607.

Supajatura, V., H. Ushio, A. Nakao, S. Akira, K. Okumura, C. Ra, and H. Ogawa. 2002b. Differential responses of mast cell Toll-like receptors 2 and 4 in allergy and innate immunity. *J. Clin. Invest.* **109:**1351–1359.

Thonnard-Neuman, E. 1963. Studies of basophils: variations with age and sex. *Acta Haematol.* **30:**221.

Toba, K., T. Koike, A. Shibata, S. Hashimoto, M. Takahashi, M. Masuko, T. Azegami, H. Takahashi, and Y. Aizawa. 1999. Novel technique for the direct flow cytofluorometric analysis of human basophils in unseparated blood and bone marrow, and the characterization of phenotype and peroxidase of human basophils. *Cytometry* **35:**249–259.

Tsai, M., L. S. Shih, G. F. J. Newlands, T. Takeishi, K. E. Langley, K. M. Zsebo, H. R. P. Miller, E. N. Geissler, and S. J. Galli. 1991. The rat c-kit ligand, stem cell factor, induces the development of connective tissue-type and mucosal mast cells *in vivo.* Analysis by anatomical distribution, histochemistry, and protease phenotype. *J. Exp. Med.* **174:**125–131.

Tsai, M., J. Wedemeyer, S. Ganiatsas, S. Y. Tam, L. I. Zon, and S. J. Galli. 2000a. *In vivo* immunological function of mast cells derived from embryonic stem cells: an approach for the rapid analysis of even embryonic lethal mutations in adult mice *in vivo. Proc. Natl. Acad. Sci. USA* **97:**9186–9190.

Tsai, M., C. S. Lantz, and S. J. Galli. 2000b. Regulation of mast cell and basophil development by stem cell factor and interleukin-3, p. 3–20. *In* G. Marone and S. J. Galli (ed.), *Mast Cells and Basophils.* Academic Press, London, United Kingdom.

Tsai, M., S. Y. Tam, J. Wedemeyer, and S. J. Galli. 2002. Mast cells derived from embryonic stem cells: a model system for studying the effects of genetic manipulations on mast cell development, phenotype, and function *in vitro* and *in vivo. Int. J. Hematol.* **75:**345–349.

Turner, H., and J. P. Kinet. 1999. Signalling through the high-affinity IgE receptor Fc epsilon RI. *Nature* **402**(Suppl.)**:**B24–B30.

Urban, J. F., Jr., L. Schopf, S. C. Morris, T. Orekhova, K. B. Madden, C. J. Betts, H. R. Gamble, C. Byrd, D. Donaldson, K. Else, and F. D. Finkelman. 2000. Stat6 signaling promotes protective immunity against *Trichinella spiralis* through a mast cell- and T cell-dependent mechanism. *J. Immunol.* **164:**2046–2052.

Valent, P. 1994. The phenotype of human eosinophils, basophils, and mast cells. *J. Allergy Clin. Immunol.* **94:**1177–1183.

Valent, P. 1995. Immunophenotypic characterization of human basophils and mast cells. *Chem. Immunol.* **61:**34–48.

Valent, P., G. Schmidt, J. Besemer, P. Mayer, G. Zenke, E. Liehl, W. Hinterberger, K. Lechner, D. Maurer, and P. Bettelheim. 1989. Interleukin-3 is a differentiation factor for human basophils. *Blood* **73:**1763–1769.

Vallance, B. A., P. A. Blennerhassett, J. D. Huizinga, and S. M. Collins. 2001. Mast cell-independent impairment of host defense and muscle contraction in *T. spiralis*-infected *W/W^v* mice. *Am. J. Physiol. Gastrointest. Liver Physiol.* **280:**G640–G648.

Wedemeyer, J., and S. J. Galli. 2001. Mast cells and basophils, p. 23.1–23.13. *In* R. R. Rich, T. A. Fleisher, W. T. Shearer, B. L. Kotzin, and H. W. Schroeder, Jr. (ed.), *Clinical Immunology: Principles and Practice.* Mosby, London, United Kingdom.

Wershil, B. K., T. Murakami, and S. J. Galli. 1988. Mast cell-dependent amplification of an immunologically nonspecific inflammatory response. Mast cells are required for the full expression of cutaneous acute inflammation induced by phorbol 12-myristate 13-acetate. *J. Immunol.* **140:**2356–2360.

Wershil, B. K., Z. S. Wang, J. R. Gordon, and S. J. Galli. 1991. Recruitment of neutrophils during IgE-dependent cutaneous late phase reactions in the mouse is mast cell-dependent. Partial inhibition of the reaction with antiserum against tumor necrosis factor-alpha. *J. Clin. Invest.* **87:**446–453.

Wershil, B. K., M. Tsai, E. N. Geissler, K. M. Zsebo, and S. J. Galli. 1992. The rat c-kit ligand, stem cell factor, induces c-kit receptor-dependent mouse mast cell activation *in vivo*. Evidence that signaling through the c-kit receptor can induce expression of cellular function. *J. Exp. Med.* **175:**245–255.

Wershil, B. K., C. M. Theodos, S. J. Galli, and R. G. Titus. 1994. Mast cells augment lesion size and persistence during experimental *Leishmania major* infection in the mouse. *J. Immunol.* **152:**4563–4571.

Wershil, B. K., G. T. Furuta, J. A. Lavigne, A. R. Choudhury, Z. S. Wang, and S. J. Galli. 1995. Dexamethasone or cyclosporin A suppress mast cell-leukocyte cytokine cascades. Multiple mechanisms of inhibition of IgE- and mast cell-dependent cutaneous inflammation in the mouse. *J. Immunol.* **154:**1391–1398.

Wershil, B. K., G. T. Furuta, Z. S. Wang, and S. J. Galli. 1996. Mast cell-dependent neutrophil and mononuclear cell recruitment in immunoglobulin E-induced gastric reactions in mice. *Gastroenterology* **110:**1482–1490.

Wershil, B. K., I. Castagliuolo, and C. Pothoulakis. 1998. Direct evidence of mast cell involvement in Clostridium difficile toxin A-induced enteritis in mice. *Gastroenterology* **114:**956–964.

Wichterman, K. A., A. E. Baue, and I. H. Chaudry. 1980. Sepsis and septic shock—a review of laboratory models and a proposal. *J. Surg. Res.* **29:**189–201.

Williams, C. M., and S. J. Galli. 2000. The diverse potential effector and immunoregulatory roles of mast cells in allergic disease. *J. Allergy Clin. Immunol.* **105:**847–859.

Woodbury, R. G., H. R. P. Miller, J. F. Huntley, G. F. J. Newlands, A. C. Palliser, and D. Wakelin. 1984. Mucosal mast cells are functionally active during spontaneous expulsion of intestinal nematode infections in rat. *Nature* **312:**450–452.

Yano, H., B. K. Wershil, N. Arizono, and S. J. Galli. 1989. Substance P-induced augmentation of cutaneous vascular permeability and granulocyte infiltration in mice is mast cell dependent. *J. Clin. Invest.* **84:**1276–1286.

Young, J. D.-E., C. C. Liu, G. Butler, Z. A. Cohn, and S. J. Galli. 1987. Identification, purification, and characterization of a mast cell-associated cytolytic factor related to tumor necrosis factor. *Proc. Natl. Acad. Sci. USA* **84:**9175–9179.

Zhang, Y., B. F. Ramos, and B. A. Jakschik. 1992. Neutrophil recruitment by tumor necrosis factor from mast cells in immune complex peritonitis. *Science* **258:**1957–1959.

INNATE NATURAL KILLER CELL RESPONSES TO INFECTION

Wayne M. Yokoyama

7

Initial studies on natural killer (NK) cells focused on their tumor-killing properties and their role in tumor surveillance (Herberman, 1982). However, NK cells also provide clinically significant host responses against microbial pathogens. In this chapter I describe and review the functions of NK cells, primarily from studies of their antitumor properties, and then discuss recent advances in the understanding of NK cell responses in host defense against pathogens.

GENERAL DESCRIPTION OF NK CELLS

"Natural killing" was originally described in studies demonstrating the capacity of unfractionated lymphocytes to spontaneously kill tumor cells in vitro (Herberman et al., 1975; Kiessling et al., 1975). This property appeared to be innate because it did not require prior host exposure to the tumor (Trinchieri, 1989; Yokoyama, 1999). Subsequent studies indi-

cated that a unique cell population, NK cells, possessed this property; was found in peripheral lymphoid tissues and blood; and could be distinguished from other lymphocytes (Lanier et al., 1986).

NK cells are now differentiated from B and T lymphocytes by the absence of antigen receptors, i.e., surface immunoglobulin (Ig) (B-cell receptor) and T-cell receptor (TCR), respectively. Yet, NK cells more closely resemble T cells in terms of effector mechanisms (see below). Freshly isolated NK cells express molecules also found on T cells such as the ζ chain of the TCR/CD3 complex (Anderson et al., 1989; Lanier et al., 1989). However, they do not display other TCR/CD3 components, do not express mRNA for mature TCR chains, and do not rearrange TCR genes (Lanier et al., 1986). Whereas mice with defects in the antigen receptor recombination pathway, such as *scid* and RAG-1 or -2 deficiency, lack mature T cells, NK cells are present (Hackett et al., 1986a). Morphologically, NK cells typically display a large, granular appearance, but this is not absolutely specific because activated T cells may demonstrate this morphology and small granular NK cells have been described (Inverardi et al., 1991).

Wayne M. Yokoyama, Howard Hughes Medical Institute, Rheumatology Division, Box 8045, Washington University Medical Center, 660 South Euclid Avenue, St. Louis, MO 63110.

The Innate Immune Response to Infection
Ed. by S. H. E. Kaufmann, R. Medzhitov, and S. Gordon
©2004 ASM Press, Washington, D.C.

Currently, most investigators in the NK cell field generally agree on the following to be characteristic marker phenotypes for NK cells (Lanier et al., 1986; Yokoyama, 1999). Human NK cells are typically $CD56^+ CD3^-$, and in C57BL/6 mice they are $NK1.1^+ CD3^-$. In mouse strains other than C57BL/6, NK cells often do not express the allele of NK1.1 (NKR-P1C) recognized by the anti-NK1.1-specific monoclonal antibody (MAb) PK136. In these strains, NK cells can be detected with the DX5 MAb (Pharmingen, La Jolla, Calif.). The DX5 epitope was recently determined to be the integrin $\alpha 2$ (CD49b) chain (Arase et al., 2001) and is expressed on some non-NK cells. In the older literature, antisera against asialo-GM1 were also used frequently, although this marker is also more widely expressed than NK1.1.

Both human and mouse NK cells express the low-affinity Fc receptor for IgG, FcγRIII (CD16) (Ravetch and Kinet, 1991). Human NK cells specifically express the FcγRIIIA transmembrane isoform. In mice, there is only one FcγRIII isoform that is recognized by the anti-mouse FcγRIII MAb 2.4G2 that also recognizes FcγRII. (Although NK cells use their Fc receptors to mediate antibody-dependent cellular cytotoxicity against antibody-coated targets, the role of these receptors in innate immunity in a naive host is unclear because specific antibody production implies a previous specific immune encounter.) Thus, the NK cell phenotype in humans ($CD56^+$ $FcγRIII^+ CD3^-$) and mice ($NK1.1^+$ [or $DX5^+$ or asialo-$GM1^+$] $FcγRII/III^+ CD3^-$) can be used to isolate NK cells for in vitro analysis.

Note that the relationship between these markers and NK cells is primarily correlative, i.e., the markers are associated with natural killing activity by $CD3^-$ lymphocytes. There is no consensus on how to define NK cells in molecular terms, such as by expression of a specific function-defining receptor akin to the TCR on T cells. Until such an advance is made or a consensus is reached, the definition of NK cells is by exclusion of other lymphocytes and by correlation to markers associated with NK cell killing capacity.

EXPERIMENTAL ANALYSIS OF NK CELLS

Regardless of difficulties in defining NK cells in molecular terms, experimental approaches to determine NK cell-dependent effects in mice have made use of the markers associated with NK cell activity. For example, in vivo administration of polyclonal rabbit anti-asialo-GM1 antiserum or the anti-NK1.1 MAb (PK136) is effective for NK cell depletion. Such studies may be compromised by the reactivity of the antibodies with other cell populations. For example, anti-asialo-GM1 also reacts with activated T cells and perhaps other cells whereas anti-NK1.1 reacts with NK T cells (innate $CD3^+$ T cells with NK markers). To date, there is less experience with the DX5 MAb in vivo. Nonetheless, the NK cell-specific effect of these antibodies can be confirmed when they are used in combination with studies on *scid* or $RAG^{-/-}$ mice that do not have mature T cells or $CD1^{-/-}$ mice that lack NK T cells. With these caveats, the anti-NK1.1 MAb has become the standard for NK cell depletion in C57BL/6 and related mouse strains because the anti-NK1.1 MAb is very effective (Seaman et al., 1987) and reacts with the best serological determinant on mouse NK cells (Hackett et al., 1986b).

A number of targeted mutant mice defective in development of $CD3^-$ NK cells have been helpful in studies of NK cells in innate immunity. These mice have mutations in the genes for Ikaros, interleukin-2 receptor-γ (IL-2Rγ), IL-2Rβ, interferon regulatory factor-1, IL-15, and IL-15Rα (DiSanto et al., 1995; Duncan et al., 1996; Georgopoulos et al., 1994; Kennedy et al., 2000; Lodolce et al., 1998; Ogasawara et al., 1998; Ohteki et al., 1998; Suzuki et al., 1997). Although results from experimental infections in these mice may be revealing, the mice also have defects in other lymphoid compartments and the deficient factor, potentially compromising attributions of these effects to NK cell deficiency.

Mutant mice with defects in NK cell effector mechanisms also are helpful in dissection of innate immunity. Natural killing of targets is severely impaired in mice with mutations in molecules involved in this effector function, i.e., perforin or granzyme B (Ebnet et al., 1995; Heusel et al., 1994; Kagi et al., 1994; Lowin et al., 1994; Walsh et al., 1994) (see more detailed discussion of granule exocytosis below). Beige (*bg*) mice, deficient in Lyst (see below), also fit in this category and were frequently used in the older literature. However, all of these mice have other non-NK cell abnormalities, such as defective cytotoxic T cells, making some results difficult to interpret with respect to NK cell defects.

Among transgenic mice with NK cell defects, the transgenic Tgε26 mouse overexpresses a human CD3ε transgenic construct and has been useful due to an absolute deficiency in NK cells. However, it also has a prominent defect in T-cell development (Wang et al., 1994, 1996). Recent studies also indicate that a mouse transgenic for a granzyme A-Ly49A construct appears to have a selective NK cell deficiency (Kim et al., 2000). However, these mice are less well characterized.

It has thus been particularly challenging to study NK cells in vivo because there is no clear-cut animal model in which CD3⁻ NK cell activity is genetically and selectively deficient. Nevertheless, in vivo studies using antibody-mediated NK cell depletion, gene-targeted or spontaneously mutant mice may be consistent with NK cell-dependent resistance to infection. A role for NK cell involvement in infection control may be supported by experiments utilizing complementary in vitro approaches.

Standard ^{51}Cr-release assays of natural killing and other in vitro assays for NK cell function may support a role for NK cells in pathogen resistance. Most in vitro studies of mouse NK cells utilize NK cells that are generally propagated in high concentrations of IL-2. Several general effects result from IL-2 stimulation, including induction of more potent killing capacity and the killing of a broader panel of targets than freshly isolated NK cells for reasons that are not fully understood. This activity is related to the phenotype of lymphokine-activated killer (LAK) cells, originally found when human peripheral blood leukocytes were cultured in 1,000 U of IL-2 per ml (Grimm et al., 1982). In high-dose IL-2 cultures, there may be contaminating T cells that are also "promiscuous killers" (Brooks et al., 1985). CD3⁻ NK cells adhere better to plastic, so adherent LAK cells are enriched for NK cells (Gunji et al., 1989). Unfortunately, in vitro expansion of mature mouse NK cells is self-limited, requiring regeneration of primary cultures.

The in vitro NK cell proliferative response to high concentrations of IL-2 is unlikely to be mimicked in vivo. Because NK cells are apparently normal in mice with a targeted mutation in the IL-2 gene or the IL-2Rα chain (Schorle et al., 1991; Suzuki et al., 1997; Willerford et al., 1995), IL-2 itself does not seem to be required for normal NK cell development. However, the IL-2R complex shares two subunits, IL-2Rβ and IL-2Rγ, with the IL-15R complex that also contains the IL-15 binding subunit IL-15Rα. IL-15 plays a more important physiological role in NK cell responses in vivo because mice deficient in IL-15 or IL-15Rα fail to develop NK cells (Kennedy et al., 2000; Lodolce et al., 1998). Recent studies indicate that IL-15 can stimulate in *trans*. Cells expressing IL-15Rα can present IL-15 to cells having only IL-15Rβγ (Dubois et al., 2002), although it is not known if this is physiologically important for NK cells in vivo. Recent studies also suggest that IL-15 may promote the in vivo survival of mature peripheral NK cells (Cooper et al., 2002). Thus, IL-15 is important to the development, survival, and stimulation of NK cells.

Finally, NK cells are frequently isolated from human peripheral blood or mouse spleen. These populations are not homogeneous and are best considered to be "polyclonal" in terms of receptors and function (see below). In humans, NK cell clones can be generated from peripheral blood lymphocytes and have been helpful in dissecting the molecular basis for NK cell tumor target recognition (Colonna, 1997; Lanier et al., 1997; Moretta et al., 1997).

Mouse NK cell clones have been difficult to produce unless they are made in relatively unusual circumstances, such as from p53-deficient mice or from fetal organs (Karlhofer et al., 1995; Manoussaka et al., 1998), limiting this approach in mice.

ROLE OF NK CELLS IN INFECTIONS

The role of NK cells in infection is highlighted by the case of an adolescent woman with a selective NK cell deficiency in whom there were frequent, recurrent septicemic episodes due to uncontrolled viral infections, including cytomegalovirus (CMV), varicella–zoster virus, and herpes simplex virus (Biron et al., 1989). Other case reports also support the notion that NK cell-deficient patients appear to have a common propensity for severe and/or recurrent virus infections (Jawahar et al., 1996).

NK cell activity has long been noted to be significantly diminished in AIDS patients (Bonavida et al., 1986; Rook et al., 1983). This appears to be related to diminished NK cell number. NK cell infection with herpesvirus 6 induces cytopathic changes and de novo expression of CD4, a cellular receptor for human immunodeficiency virus type 1 (HIV-1) not normally expressed by NK cells (Lusso et al., 1993). This renders NK cells susceptible to infection by HIV-1, perhaps accounting, in part, for increased susceptibility of patients to other infections, such as CMV. These coinfections may be particularly severe and may be characterized by relatively unusual manifestations, such as CMV retinitis.

The NK cell compartment is not fully developed at birth, as indicated by lower natural killing by human cord blood lymphocytes and corroborated by studies on the ontogeny of NK cells in rodents (Cook et al., 1995; Seki et al., 1985). Immature NK cell number and function in the developing fetus may be clinically relevant to the classic "TORCH" syndrome, birth defects, and severe fetal anomalies that are associated with maternal *Toxoplasma*, rubella virus, CMV, and herpesvirus infections (Greenough, 1994).

NK cell responses against a variety of gram-positive, gram-negative, and intracellular bacteria and protozoan parasites have been studied (summarized by Bancroft [1993]), but analysis of the NK cell responses against many of these organisms has been limited. On the other hand, detailed and ongoing evaluations of mouse NK cell responses, especially against *Listeria* and viral infections, have been revealing (summarized by Biron et al. [1999] and Unanue [1997]).

In mouse models, there is abundant experimental in vivo evidence supporting a role for NK cells in resisting certain infections. Shellam and colleagues found that beige mice are susceptible to murine CMV (MCMV) infections (Shellam et al., 1981). Furthermore, Welsh and coworkers eliminated NK cells in vivo by administration of the anti-NK1.1 MAb or other anti-NK cell antibodies (Bukowski et al., 1983, 1984; Welsh et al., 1990). When mice were then infected with murine CMV (MCMV), vaccinia virus, or mouse hepatitis virus, there was marked viral replication in internal organs (spleen, liver) and lethality. A similar phenotype was observed in the Tgε26 mouse, which lacks NK and T cells (Orange and Biron, 1996a), indicating the importance of NK cells in resisting infection. Interestingly, the antibody depletion studies further showed that if anti-NK cell antibody was given to wild-type mice later in the infection, there was no untoward effect (Bukowski et al., 1984). Finally, in listeriosis, NK cells provide acute protective effects in *scid* mice, but mice do succumb to a late death (Bancroft et al., 1991; Dunn and North, 1991; Tripp et al., 1993). Thus, NK cells are significant in early, innate immunity to infections.

NK CELL EFFECTOR RESPONSES IN INFECTIONS

How do NK cells help control infections? In this section, I consider their two major effector mechanisms, target killing triggered by activation receptors and cytokine production.

Target Killing

Classically, NK cells kill their targets by the triggered and directional release of preformed cytoplasmic granules containing perforin and granzymes, a process termed granule exocytosis (Henkart, 1994). Conventionally, it has been thought that perforin polymerizes in the target cell plasma membrane, producing a pore through which the granzymes enter and then are activated to trigger target cell apoptosis. Although recent studies suggest that granzymes may enter the cell via the mannose-6-phosphate receptor, rather than through the perforin-formed pore (Motyka et al., 2000), both perforin and granzymes are required for the full apoptotic "hit" from granule exocytosis.

Successful granule exocytosis also requires events involving Lyst, a molecule contained in lysosomes (Introne et al., 1999). This is illustrated by the phenotype of *bg* mice and the corresponding human disease, Chediak-Higashi syndrome, which is due to mutations in Lyst and associated with abnormal granules. Although the function of Lyst has yet to be understood, it appears to be involved in vesicle formation, fusion, or trafficking.

Recent studies also suggest that NK cells can kill certain targets through other means, including Fas and TRAIL (TNF [tumor necrosis factor]-related apoptosis-inducing ligand), but the functional significance of these pathways to in vivo infections is not yet clear (Zamai et al., 1998). In addition, resting NK cells apparently do not express Fas ligand on their cell surface and therefore must be triggered to mediate Fas-induced death (Bradley et al., 1998). Thus, activation of NK cells by their targets is a critical element in the function of NK cells.

Two-Receptor Model for NK Cell Recognition of Cellular Targets.

The role of NK cells in infection control is related to their receptors that regulate the natural killing function. Early studies described an inverse correlation between target cell expression of major histocompatibility complex (MHC) class I and susceptibility to NK cells (Kärre et al., 1986). Targets that do not express MHC class I are killed by NK cells, whereas MHC class I-bearing targets are generally resistant (Ljunggren and Kärre, 1990). These studies provided major insight into NK cell recognition, particularly with a teleological explanation termed the "missing-self hypothesis." Kärre postulated that NK cells survey tissues for normal ubiquitous expression of MHC class I (Kärre, 1985). A cell may downregulate expression of MHC class I, such as occurs in tumorigenesis or viral infection to evade MHC class I-restricted T cells. However, the MHC class I-deficient cell would then lose the chronic inhibitory influence of MHC class I, permitting lysis by NK cells. This hypothesis suggested a potential rationale for why the inhibitory influence of MHC class I should be a physiologically relevant phenomenon for NK cell function.

It is now clear that NK cell recognition of tumor targets involves inhibitory receptors specific for target cell MHC class I and target cell ligand-specific NK cell activation receptors, compatible with a two-receptor model (Yokoyama, 1995). This model predicts that the fate of a target cell is determined by the engagement (or not) of both activation and inhibitory receptors on the NK cell by their target cell ligands and integration of signals transduced by such receptors. In other words, inhibitory receptors appear to regulate activation receptors (or vice versa) that may have their own specificity for ligands on targets. Although the nature and specificity of putative activation receptors are less well understood, there has been significant progress in understanding the inhibitory receptors.

Inhibitory Receptors. It is now appreciated that NK cells express MHC class I-specific inhibitory receptors, as first shown by studies on the mouse receptor Ly49A (Karlhofer et al., 1992b). The inhibitory NK cell receptors fall into two general structural types (reviewed by Yokoyama, 1997). Human killer Ig-like receptors (KIRs) are type I integral membrane proteins with Ig-like domains encoded in the leukocyte receptor complex (Long, 1999). By contrast, human and rodent CD94/NKG2A and rodent Ly49 receptors have type II orientation and are disulfide-linked dimers with domains that are distantly related to the C-type lectins and encoded in the NK gene complex (NKC) (Yokoyama and Plougastel, 2003). Despite their structural differences, the inhibitory receptors have several shared features. In addition to relatively restricted expression on NK cells (and NK T cells for the lectinlike molecules), the receptors generally belong to families of highly related molecules. Importantly, all inhibitory receptors to date contain immunoreceptor tyrosine-based inhibitory motifs (ITIMs) in their cytoplasmic domains (reviewed by Long, 1999). Upon receptor cross-linking and subsequent ITIM phosphorylation, the ITIMs recruit and activate the cytoplasmic tyrosine phosphatase SHP-1. This recruitment then presumably leads to dephosphorylation of molecules involved in cellular activation, particularly pathways involving immunoreceptor tyrosine-based activation motif (ITAM)-containing signaling chains. These general mechanisms are now appreciated as being applicable to a large number of other inhibitory receptors that are expressed on a wide variety of hematopoietic cells (Long, 1999).

Initial studies noted the discrepancy between the types of NK cell inhibitory receptors that were found on human (Ig-like, KIR) and mouse (lectinlike, Ly49) NK cells, although it is now apparent that they are functionally related as MHC class I-specific inhibitory receptors. Furthermore, both structural types of inhibitory receptors are expressed on NK cells from both species, and strict structural and functional orthologues also have been identified. For example, both human and mouse NK cells express the CD94/NKG2A heterodimers, a lectinlike receptor (Ho et al., 1998; Lopez-Botet et al., 1997; Philbrick et al., 1990; Phillips et al., 1996; Vance et al., 1997). Human CD94/NKG2A recognizes the nonclassical MHC class I molecule HLA-E that predominantly binds peptides derived from classical HLA molecules (Braud et al., 1998). In mice, CD94/NKG2A recognizes the HLA-E orthologue, Qa-1 (Vance et al., 1998), demonstrating the conservation of NK cell receptors across species.

By contrast to T cells, NK cell receptors for MHC class I have different requirements for MHC-associated peptides. Some receptors appear to have no peptide selectivity. For example, Ly49A binds its MHC class I ligand regardless of bound peptide, although it does not appear to recognize "empty" MHC class I (Correa and Raulet, 1995; Orihuela et al., 1996). On the other hand, other NK cell receptors appear to have peptide selectivity (Mandelboim et al., 1997; Michaelsson et al., 2000). An appreciation for how peptides could alter recognition is now beginning to be recognized with the crystallization of NK cell receptor-ligand complexes (Fan et al., 2001; Tormo et al., 1999). These data indicate that the NK cell receptors engage MHC class I in a manner distinct from TCR binding.

Activation Receptors and Signaling Chains. The inhibitory receptors do not explain all aspects of NK cell specificity. As predicted by the two-receptor model, NK cell recognition also appears to involve activation receptors (Yokoyama, 1995). Insight into the nature of the activation receptors came largely from studies indicating that a number of receptors resembling the inhibitory receptors did not contain cytoplasmic ITIMs (Biassoni et al., 1996; Smith et al., 1994). Other candidate activation receptors were identified because of their ability to stimulate NK cell activities when cross-linked by their specific MAbs. For example, cross-linking of the rat NKR-P1 molecule results in NK cell killing of targets that are not usually killed (Chambers et al., 1989). Although the cytoplasmic domains of these molecules do not contain obvious signaling motifs, such as ITAMs, cross-linking of several of these molecules appeared to stimulate NK cells (Mason et al., 1996). Interestingly, these ITAM- and ITIM-less molecules generally have charged residues in their transmembrane domains, implying membrane coassociation with other molecules. Indeed, coimmunoprecipitation experiments have shown that such receptors are noncovalently associated with proteins that are phosphorylated upon receptor cross-linking or pervanadate stimulation (Mason et al., 1998).

Thus, like the TCR and B-cell receptor, NK cell activation receptors are expressed in signaling complexes.

Major insight into the nature of NK cell activation receptor complexes came from studies of the DAP12 (also known as KARAP) molecule, identified as a signaling chain that is associated with several ITIM-less NK cell receptors with charged transmembrane residues (Lanier et al., 1998a; Tomasello et al., 2000a). Like the contribution of CD3ζ chain to the assembly and signaling of the TCR/CD3 complex, DAP12 is required for efficient expression of putative NK cell activation receptors, such as CD94/NKG2C, Ly49D, and Ly49H (Bakker et al., 2000). Moreover, DAP12 is phosphorylated when the associated receptor is cross-linked (Lanier et al., 1998a, 1998b). Recent studies on DAP12-deficient or DAP12-mutant mice support the role of DAP12 as a signaling molecule associated with certain NK cell activation receptors (Bakker et al., 2000; Tomasello et al., 2000b).

NK cells also express other ITAM-associated signaling chains, including CD3ζ and FcεRIγ. These signaling chains provide functions similar to those of DAP12, but they are associated with other ligand-binding receptors, such as CD16 or NKR-P1C (Anderson et al., 1989; Arase et al., 1997; Lanier et al., 1989). Thus, NK cells express several distinct ITAM-containing signaling chains that are associated with a myriad of activation receptors. Yet the function and ligand specificity of most "activation" receptors have yet to be described; most are orphan receptors.

It is also important to note that an individual NK cell often expresses simultaneously more than one activation receptor, unlike the clonotypic distribution of TCRs on individual T cells. Moreover, each NK cell usually expresses more than one inhibitory receptor. The repertoire of receptors expressed by an individual NK cell is subject to both stochastic and nonstochastic events (Raulet et al., 2001; Smith et al., 2000a), resulting in a complex overlap of NK cell subsets as determined by expression of NK cell receptors.

The downstream signaling events following activation receptor engagement have not yet been fully described (Brumbaugh et al., 1998). Nonetheless, it is likely that the pathway will resemble the tyrosine kinase activation cascade in T and B cells. The proximal Syk family tyrosine kinases, ZAP-70 and Syk itself, are expressed in NK cells and can be phosphorylated upon cross-linking of activation receptors (Lanier et al., 1998b; Viver et al., 1993) or exposure to sensitive targets (Brumbaugh et al., 1997). However, NK cells in ZAP-70 and Syk double-deficient mice can develop unlike T and B cells, and the double-deficient NK cells retain some capacity for target killing (Colucci et al., 2002). Many of the subsequent downstream effector and adapter molecules are also present but their contribution to NK cell activities may differ from that in other lymphocytes (Jevremovic et al., 1999; Peterson et al., 1999).

Recent studies indicate a role for phosphoinositide-3-kinase (PI-3-kinase) and mitogen-activated protein kinase pathways in NK cell cytotoxicity against tumor targets (Jiang et al., 2000). In this regard, the lectinlike NK cell receptor NKG2D deserves special mention because it can couple to DAP10 that has a PI-3-kinase docking site and no ITAMs (Wu et al., 2000, 1999). Indeed, analogous to CD28 and PI-3-kinase and Akt-dependent costimulation of T cells (Kane et al., 2001), NKG2D can costimulate NK and T-cell functions (Groh et al., 2001; Ho et al., 2002). Recent studies also indicate that an alternatively spliced form of mouse NKG2D can be expressed that is coupled to DAP12 and function as a primary NK cell activation receptor (Diefenbach et al., 2002; Gilfillan et al., 2002), demonstrating the polygamous nature of certain NK cell receptors, such as NKG2D.

The function of NK cell activation receptors is regulated by the inhibitory receptors. In general, simultaneous engagement of activation and inhibitory receptors is associated with inhibition, indicating that inhibition dominates over activation (Correa et al., 1994; Karlhofer et al., 1992a). However, earlier studies demonstrated that the degree of NK cell inhibition can be directly correlated to the level of MHC class I expression on the targets (Storkus et al., 1989), indicating that the outcome of activation or inhibition is likely to result from a balance between the kinases and the phosphatases activated by respective receptor–ligand interactions.

The ligand specificity of NK cell activation receptors is an area under intense investigation. Some of the activation receptors are responsible for target specificity (Biassoni et al., 1996; Idris et al., 1999) and appear to be specific for MHC class Ia and Ib molecules (Biassoni et al., 1996; Furukawa et al., 2002; George et al., 1999; Nakamura et al., 1999; Vance et al., 1999). Their relationship to inhibitory receptors binding the same ligand is incompletely understood.

To date, the best-characterized NK cell activation receptor ligands are those for NKG2D. All are related to MHC class I molecules by sequence and crystallographic structure (Li et al., 2002, 2001; Radaev et al., 2001; Yokoyama, 2000). In humans, these ligands include the MIC and ULBP molecules, whereas in mice they include the RAE1, H60, and MULT1 molecules (Bauer et al., 1999; Diefenbach et al., 2000; Carayannopoulos et al., 2002; Cerwenka et al., 2000; Cosman et al., 2001). With respect to innate immunity against viruses, NKG2D and its ligands are particularly notable because some appear to be inducible by virus infection (Groh et al., 2001). Moreover, human CMV (HCMV) and MCMV have evolved molecules that block NKG2D function (see below).

Thus, there is accumulating evidence that NK cells express activation receptors that can trigger through their associated signaling chains, and the action of these receptors is regulated by inhibitory receptors. These activation receptors, originally defined in terms of tumor killing, are also important in NK cell responses in innate immunity.

Viral Evasion Strategies Implicate NK Cell Activation Receptors in Viral Resistance. Although the role of NK cell activation receptors in NK cell-mediated resistance to infections is just beginning to be understood, there are several important observations indicating that such receptors are likely to be important in this context. Probably the most significant findings are from studies of viral evasion tactics targeting NK cells (for a recent review, see Orange et al., 2002). Because viruses have evolved numerous strategies to downregulate MHC class I molecules on infected cells to avoid MHC class I-restricted cytotoxic T lymphocytes (Tortorella et al., 2000), virally infected cells should have enhanced susceptibility to NK cell lysis. However, viruses encode proteins that interfere with natural killing.

In many cases, viral interference of natural killing is due to enhanced function of inhibitory MHC class I-specific NK cell receptors. For example, herpesviruses encode MHC class I mimics that bind inhibitory NK cell receptors. MCMV and rat CMV contain open reading frames (ORFs) *m144* and *r144*, respectively, which encode molecules with sequence homology to MHC class I and enhance in vivo virulence presumably by interacting with an as yet unidentified NK cell inhibitory receptor (Cretney et al., 1999; Farrell et al., 1997; Kloover et al., 2002; Kubota et al., 1999). HCMV encodes an MHC class I-like molecule (UL18) that interacts with LIR-1/ILT-2, an Ig superfamily inhibitory receptor on NK cells (Cosman et al., 1997; Reyburn et al., 1997). HCMV also encodes a peptide that binds HLA-E, an MHC class Ib molecule that predominantly binds leader peptides derived from MHC class Ia molecules (Tomasec et al., 2000; Ulbrecht et al., 2000). The HCMV peptide permits enhanced expression of HLA-E that in turn binds CD94/NKG2A, a lectinlike NK cell inhibitory receptor. Another elegant example of viral evasion of NK cells is the selective downregulation of MHC class I by HIV-1 (Cohen et al., 1999). In this case, the virus downregulates HLA-A and -B but not HLA-C or -E; the former HLA molecules tend to be restricting elements for MHC class I-restricted cytotoxic T cells, whereas the latter are selectively recognized by human KIRs and

CD94/NKG2A. Therefore, viruses have evolved mechanisms that result in inhibition due to selective engagement of inhibitory receptors.

Importantly, the inhibitory receptors should not block NK responses to inflammatory cytokines because the inhibitory receptors generally do not affect cytokine receptor signaling. Rather, as described above for natural killing of tumors, NK cell inhibitory receptors prevent in vitro killing by blocking signals from activation receptors that are coupled to ITAM-containing molecules (Long, 1999; Ravetch and Lanier, 2000). This has been directly demonstrated by the transfected expression of UL18 or UL40 that blocks killing of tumor targets (Cosman et al., 1997; Tomasec et al., 2000; Ulbrecht et al., 2000). These data suggest that these viral strategies have evolved to limit NK cell activation receptors involved in target killing rather than limit NK cell responses to cytokines.

Consistent with this explanation, viruses can also directly block triggering of NK cell activation receptors. In one recent example, the HCMV ORF UL16 binds ULBP molecules that are ligands for human NKG2D (Cosman et al., 2001). As such, UL16 expression on an HCMV-infected cell may somehow prevent recognition of ULBP and prevent killing by an NKG2D-expressing NK cell (Cosman et al., 2001; Yokoyama, 2000). Although the molecular basis for UL16 function is still being investigated, other recent studies indicate the relevance of NKG2D in infection. MCMV encodes m152 that downregulates MHC class I and also NKG2D ligands with functional consequences on NK cell responses in vitro and in vivo (Krmpotic et al., 2002). Thus, NKG2D function is specifically targeted by CMV, indicating its importance in antiviral defense.

More generally, the Kaposi's sarcoma–associated herpesvirus (KSHV) has also been shown to have a mechanism to avoid NK cell activation (Ishido et al., 2000). In this case, the KSHV protein K5 downregulates expression of ICAM-1 and B7-2, which are ligands for NK cell receptors involved in cytotoxicity.

Indeed, the interaction of LFA-1 on the NK cell with ICAM-1 on the target was one of the first recognized receptor–ligand interactions important in NK cell killing of targets (Schmidt et al., 1985). In contrast to the limited distribution of most NK cell activation and inhibitory receptors, LFA-1 in particular is broadly expressed and its function is required for target cytotoxicity.

The in vivo advantage to the virus of enhancing inhibition or blocking activation is obvious. These observations strongly suggest that NK cells mediate in vivo antiviral defense with activation receptors that are functionally related to those that are used in tumor killing.

NK Cell Activation Receptors Critical to Viral Resistance. The NK cell activation receptors involved in antiviral defense are just beginning to be identified. The human NK cell activation receptor NKp46 binds hemagglutinin of influenza virus and hemagglutinin-neuraminidase of parainfluenza virus, suggesting it may be involved in resistance to these viruses (Mandelboim et al., 2001). However, this interaction is dependent on sialic acid residues that are widely expressed, and the in vivo significance of these findings is difficult to assess in humans.

More data are available on the murine NK cell receptor, Ly49H, recently identified as an NK cell activation receptor required for resistance to MCMV infection in vivo. A genome-wide scan had identified the autosomal dominant *Cmv1* resistance gene as being responsible for the genetically determined resistance of certain strains of mice to MCMV (Scalzo et al., 1990). Abundant genetic mapping data indicated that *Cmv1* maps to the NKC (Depatie et al., 1997; Forbes et al., 1997; Scalzo et al., 1995), which contains clusters of genes encoding the lectinlike NK cell receptors (Brown et al., 1997). These studies implicated NK cell involvement in the resistant phenotype (Brown et al., 1997). Indeed, when NK cells were depleted with the anti-NK1.1 MAb, MCMV-resistant C57BL/6 mice became susceptible (Scalzo et al., 1992).

The successful isolation of the resistant *Cmv1* allele depended on genetic evidence that the BXD-8 recombinant inbred mouse strain, derived from MCMV-resistant C57BL/6 and susceptible DBA/2 inbred strains, appeared to have inherited the entire NKC and flanking genomic segments from its resistant C57BL/6 progenitor but displayed the susceptible phenotype (Scalzo et al., 1992). These mice were subsequently found to specifically lack expression of Ly49H due to a specific deletion in *Ly49h*, whereas other NKC-encoded molecules were expressed normally and were genetically intact (Brown et al., 2001; Lee et al., 2001). Furthermore, when resistant C57BL/6 mice were injected with an anti-Ly49H MAb, they became susceptible as measured by viral titers in the spleen and lethality (Brown et al., 2001; Daniels et al., 2001). These studies established that *Ly49h* is responsible for genetic resistance to MCMV and suggested that Ly49H is an activation receptor that recognizes MCMV-infected cells.

The activation receptor hypothesis was confirmed by a study showing that a DAP12 mutant (Tyr in ITAMs mutated to Phe) mouse could not resist MCMV (Sjolin et al., 2002). This is consistent with predictions from previous in vitro signaling studies showing that Ly49H signals through DAP12 (Brown et al., 2001; Smith et al., 1998). The ligand for Ly49H during MCMV infection was independently identified by two groups (Arase et al., 2002; Smith et al., 2002). As a technical advance, both groups utilized reporter cell assays; Ly49H and DAP12 were transfected into heterologous cell lines with stably integrated reporter constructs activated by ITAM signaling if exposed to MCMV-infected targets. Using deletion mutants of MCMV (Arase et al., 2002) or a bioinformatics approach (Smith et al., 2002), both groups obtained evidence indicating that Ly49H specifically recognized the MCMV ORF, m157.

The identification of Ly49H as a resistance factor for MCMV infections also suggested that it may be involved in defense against other pathogens, such as mousepox (ectromelia)

virus and herpes simplex virus, for which resistance loci have also been genetically mapped to the NKC (Delano and Brownstein, 1995; Pereira et al., 2001). These loci are termed *Rmp1* and *Rhs1*, respectively, and C57BL/6 mice are resistant. However, recent studies have reported that *Rhs1* appears to independently segregate from *Cmv1* (Pereira et al., 2001). Nevertheless, the parallel phenotypes with *Cmv1* suggest that other NKC-encoded NK cell activation receptors may be involved in NK cell-mediated resistance to other viruses.

Specific Triggering of NK Cells In Vitro and In Vivo. In addition to target killing, NK cell activation receptors can also trigger cytokine production in vitro. Whereas NK cells produce gamma interferon (IFN-γ) in response to inflammatory cytokines, it has long been known that cross-linking of NK cell activation receptors such as CD16 leads to cytokine production (Cuturi et al., 1989). Furthermore, engagement of NK1.1 with immobilized anti-NK1.1. MAb also results in NK cell production of TNF alpha (TNF-α) and granulocyte-macrophage colony-stimulating factor, as well as IFN-γ (Kim and Yokoyama, 1998). This receptor-triggered cytokine production can be blocked by engagement of an inhibitory receptor. The relative contribution of this pathway of cytokine secretion to NK cell function in infection is currently unknown. However, the identification of Ly49H and its ligand m157 facilitated the investigation of specific NK cell responses to MCMV infection by permitting analysis of intracellular cytokine production. Intracellular staining for IFN-γ and lymphotactin and ATAC revealed that Ly49H⁺ NK cells can be selectively activated within 6 to 8 h when coincubated in vitro with MCMV-infected macrophages or cell lines transfected with m157 (Smith et al., 2002), indicating that competent NK cells respond within hours of recognizing virus-infected cells.

These findings, however, contrast with the relative "nonspecific" stimulation of NK cells found during early MCMV infection in vivo where IFN-γ production was not confined to the Ly49H⁺ NK cell subset (Dokun et al., 2001b). Moreover, direct assessment of NK cell proliferation by fluorescence-activated cell sorter analysis of in vivo bromodeoxyuridine incorporation (Dokun et al., 2001b) confirmed that infection stimulates NK cell proliferation (Biron et al., 1984; Orange and Biron, 1996b) and also demonstrated that early (days 1 to 2 postinfection) in vivo NK cell proliferation was nonselective with respect to Ly49H expression. This proliferation resembled the cytokine-driven "bystander proliferation" observed in T cells in response to viral infections or stimulation with type I interferons (Tough et al., 1996), suggesting that the initial phase of viral-induced NK cell proliferation represents a nonspecific response to proinflammatory cytokines (IL-12, type I interferons) and proliferative cytokines such as IL-15 (also see below).

On the other hand, the nonselective proliferation phase was followed by a period of preferential proliferation of Ly49H⁺ NK cells peaking at days 4 to 6 of MCMV infection (Dokun et al., 2001b). Specific proliferation was abrogated with anti-Ly49H antibody supporting the hypothesis that Ly49H recognition of MCMV-infected cells stimulates selective proliferation of Ly49H⁺ NK cells. In addition, an initial phase of nonspecific NK cell proliferation was seen with vaccinia virus infection, but the later specific proliferation of Ly49H⁺ NK cells was absent. Thus, initial virus-specific NK cell responses may be masked by generic cytokine responses and only later are detectable.

Cytokine-Induced NK Cell Responses
NK cells can respond to several different cytokines, resulting in production of other cytokines. In the context of infection, the best studied have been the induction of NK cell production of IFN-γ by IL-12 and the type I interferons, some of which may be important in the nonspecific early phase of NK cell responses to MCMV. In listeriosis, the classic model for T-cell-dependent resistance, it was

noted that *scid* mice achieved acute control of infection despite the absence of T cells (Bancroft et al., 1991). Neutralization of IFN-γ or elimination of NK cells by anti-NK cell antibodies (against NK1.1 and other NK cell receptors or anti-asialo-GM1) abrogated control of infection (Dunn and North, 1991). Furthermore, IFN-γ production was also markedly reduced with administration of the anti-NK cell antibodies, indicating that NK cells were responsible for early production of IFN-γ. Interestingly, NK cells do not appear to respond directly to *Listeria* sp. Rather, macrophage production of IL-12 is required for NK cell secretion of IFN-γ and infection control (Tripp et al., 1994, 1993). Furthermore, TNF-α can synergize with IL-12 to induce NK cell production of IFN-γ, whereas IL-10 is antagonistic (Tripp et al., 1993). Studies with mutant mice have indicated the increased susceptibility of mice lacking IL-12 receptor, IFN-γ, IFN-γ receptor, or the IFN-γ receptor signaling pathway (Brombacher et al., 1999; Harty and Bevan, 1995; Huang et al., 1993; Meraz et al., 1996), consistent with this model of *Listeria* infection inducing macrophage production of IL-12 that stimulates IFN-γ secretion by NK cells.

The IL-12-stimulated IFN-γ pathway is quite complex. In immunocompetent mice, CD8⁺ T cells can also produce IFN-γ in response to bacterial infection. Whereas NK cells produce IFN-γ shortly (5 h) after infection, T cells produce IFN-γ after 15 h and represent the dominant source. In addition, IL-18 also contributes to stimulation of IFN-γ by both populations. A role for IL-18 may explain the capacity of IL-12-deficient mice to survive low but not high inoculi of *Listeria* sp. (Brombacher et al., 1999). Also, *Listeria* sp. can induce CD8α⁺ dendritic cells (DCs) to produce IFN-γ in an IL-12-dependent manner (Ohteki et al., 1999). Although the intricacies of the IL-12–IFN-γ pathway and its regulation are still under investigation, it is clear that NK cells play a central role in this pathway.

A similar IL-12–IFN-γ pathway is also operational in MCMV infections (Biron et al.,

1999). As in listeriosis, one component of the NK cell response to MCMV is the production of IFN-γ stimulated by IL-12. Antibody elimination of NK cells abrogates IFN-γ production in MCMV infections (Orange and Biron, 1996a; Orange et al., 1995). Furthermore, anti-IFN-γ increases susceptibility, whereas administration of IL-12 has a protective effect. These effects are abrogated by NK cell elimination or IFN-γ neutralization.

As in listeriosis, IL-18 also contributes somewhat to NK cell control of MCMV infections (Pien et al., 2000). However, IL-12 appears to play a more crucial role than IL-18 because uniform lethality was observed in IL-12p35$^{-/-}$ mice challenged with MCMV, whereas all IL-18$^{-/-}$ mice survived (Pien et al., 2000). In ectromelia virus (EV; mousepox) infections, an important role for IL-18 is indicated by an EV ORF for an IL-18 binding protein (IL18BP) that effectively neutralizes the effects of IL-18 (Born et al., 2000). Neutralization of IL-18 is a common feature of orthopoxviruses (Smith et al., 2000b). IL-18 has two IL-12-independent effects on NK cells, the aforementioned stimulation of IFN-γ production and enhancement of perforin-dependent cytotoxicity (Akira, 2000; Hyodo et al., 1999; Takeda et al., 1998). Infections with an IL-18BP-deficient EV mutant gave rise to higher IFN-γ production and enhanced NK cell cytotoxicity against tumor targets (Born et al., 2000). Although infections with the IL-18BP-deficient EV strain are less virulent, there is only a twofold to threefold decrease in viral titers as compared to wild-type EV. One possible explanation for the very modest effect is the presence of additional poxvirus immune evasion genes, probably related to the ongoing coevolution of the virus and its host immune system, which needs consideration when studying in vivo models (Yewdell and Hill, 2002).

Importantly, not all viral infections are controlled by NK cells, as illustrated by studies of lymphocytic choriomeningitis virus (LCMV) infections (Biron et al., 1999; Bukowski et al., 1985, 1983). Elimination of NK cells has little effect on systemic LCMV infections, such as survival or viral replication. Interestingly, Biron and colleagues have shown that LCMV infection does not induce IL-12-dependent IFN-γ production (Orange and Biron, 1996a). Furthermore, neutralization of IL-12 had no effect on LCMV replication. Yet, many NK cell activities are stimulated by LCMV infection.

During infections, even with LCMV, cytotoxicity of NK cells is enhanced, and proliferation ensues. These events constitute some of the systemic effects directly or indirectly mediated by IL-18 (discussed above) and the type I interferons (Guidotti and Chisari, 2001). However, IFN-γ production is not seen in LCMV infections (Nguyen et al., 2000; Orange and Biron, 1996a). Furthermore, administration of IL-12 does not promote NK cell production of IFN-γ. This apparent paradox was recently shown to be due to an inhibitory effect of the type I interferons on IL-12-dependent IFN-γ production (Nguyen et al., 2000). Inhibition by IFN-α/β is mediated through the STAT1 signaling pathway. In the absence of STAT1, IL-12 responsiveness is restored and IFN-α/β induces IFN-γ production. Although it remains to be determined how the type I interferon response to LCMV differs from the response to MCMV, these studies indicate that the NK cell cytokine response to infection varies with the pathogen even though the responses may appear to be similar.

A challenging area of investigation is the role of IL-15 in NK cell responses in vivo (Waldmann and Tagaya, 1999) since mice deficient in IL-15 or IL-15Rα lack NK cells (Kennedy et al., 2000; Lodolce et al., 1998). Nevertheless, a series of studies indicate that NK cells are stimulated during the course of infection by IL-15 (Ahmad et al., 2000; Fawaz et al., 1999; Gosselin et al., 1999; Tsunobuchi et al., 2000; Waldmann and Tagaya, 1999). As expected from studies of IL-2-activated NK cells (LAK cells), IL-15-stimulated NK cells have increased killing potential against tumor targets (Gosselin et al., 1999). However, the IL-

15-stimulated NK cells also have increased activity against virus-infected cells, which may be physiologically more relevant in innate immunity. Interestingly, several viruses can stimulate human peripheral blood mononuclear cells to secrete IL-15 and induce NK cell activity, resulting in in vitro control of viral replication (Ahmad et al., 2000; Fawaz et al., 1999). This appears to be physiologically important in vivo because IL-15 can provide protection to herpes simplex virus infections in mice (Tsunobuchi et al., 2000). Finally, recent studies suggest that the type I interferons stimulate IL-15 production that can drive NK cell proliferation (Nguyen et al., 2002).

NK cell responses to cytokines are also regulated by other innate lymphocytes. In TCRδ$^{-/-}$ mice, *Listeria* growth at day 1 after infection is significantly enhanced compared with TCRβ$^{-/-}$ mice. This is associated with diminished production of IFN-γ by NK cells and TNF-α production in TCRδ$^{-/-}$ mice, whereas comparable amounts of IL-12 were made, suggesting that γ/δ T cells regulate NK cell responses. Similarly, NK T cells contribute to IFN-γ production by NK cells (Carnaud et al., 1999). Administration of α-galactosylceramide, a potent ligand for the TCR on NK T cells, results in nearly concomitant activation of NK cells, possibly due to release of IFN-γ by the NK T cells. Inasmuch as NK T cells can recognize glycolipid antigens in mycobacteria (Moody et al., 1997, 2000), these studies indicate a potential physiologically important mechanism for NK cell activation in innate immunity to these organisms.

NK cells can also produce several other cytokines that have been less well studied in the context of infection. Also, early NK cell responses appear to be relatively nonspecific with polyclonal activation. Analysis of activation markers that are absent on resting NK cells reveals that all NK cells display these activation markers during MCMV infection (Wang et al., 2000). Although this requires further study, presumably this activation reflects stimulation from a variety of cytokines that are induced upon infection.

Hence, the pathways involving NK cell cytokine responses with resultant production of other cytokines, such as IL-12-stimulated NK cell production of IFN-γ, are intricate and perhaps even more complex than currently appreciated. Nevertheless, the studies defining these pathways in the context of in vivo infections have already yielded important principles that will continue to guide our understanding of NK cell cytokine responses to infections.

NK CELL TRAFFICKING AND INFECTION

For NK cells to effect target killing, they obviously must be in physical proximity of their targets. In situ localization studies of NK cells indicate that normally there are few NK cells in the liver parenchyma, and therefore they need to be recruited from the blood vasculature and sinusoidal compartments to the site of MCMV-infected hepatocytes, a process that takes time (Andrews et al., 2001b; Dokun et al., 2001a). Although accumulation of NK cells at sites of viral replication was independent of IL-12, IFN-γ, and TNF-α in MCMV-infected knockout mice (Dokun et al., 2001a), the number of NK cells in the liver during MCMV infection was decreased in macrophage inflammatory protein 1α (MIP-1α)-deficient mice (Salazar-Mather et al., 2000, 2002, 1998), suggesting that this chemokine plays a significant role in the recruitment of NK cells to hepatic sites of viral replication. In MIP-1α-deficient mice, NK cell migration into the liver and NK cell-dependent IFN-γ production were markedly impaired, whereas spleen NK cell responses were less affected.

By contrast to the liver, NK cells are normally found scattered in the red pulp of the spleen. Relatively minor changes in NK cell localization need to occur in the spleen after infection because MCMV-infected cells line the marginal zone, adjacent to the red pulp (Andrews et al., 2001b; Dokun et al., 2001a). The splenic marginal zone is enriched in macrophages and DCs, suggesting that these cells may be the infected cellular targets of NK cells. Indeed, in situ staining demonstrated that

MCMV infection occurred in CD11b$^+$ macrophages (Andrews et al., 2001a). In addition, in vitro studies showed that bone marrow-derived macrophages are permissive for MCMV infection and effectively display m157, the ligand for Ly49H (Smith et al., 2002). These data indicate that cognate interactions between infected macrophages and NK cells could occur in vivo.

The distribution of NK cells and recruitment therefore may be related to organ-specific differences in the NK cell effector mechanism controlling MCMV replication (Tay and Welsh, 1997). IFN-γ receptor-deficient mice displayed high viral titers in the liver but not the spleen. Conversely, in perforin-deficient mice, liver MCMV replication was unaffected whereas viral replication in the spleen was uncontrolled. The latter phenotype is reminiscent of the effect of *Cmv1* (*Ly49h*) (Scalzo et al., 1990). Because it takes time for NK cells to be recruited to the liver, antiviral effector responses that do not require precise physical proximity, such as IFN-γ secretion, may be more effective at an earlier time point.

Recent studies also have demonstrated "cross talk," i.e., bidirectional regulation, between NK cells and DCs (Ferlazzo et al., 2002; Gerosa et al., 2002; Piccioli et al., 2002; Zitvogel, 2002). During in vivo infection with MCMV, type I interferons and IL-12 are produced primarily by the CD8α$^+$Ly6G/ C$^+$CD11b$^-$ DC subset, also described as plasmacytoid DCs (Cella et al., 2000; Colonna et al., 2002). This phenomenon is not seen in LCMV infections, suggesting that this DC subset is involved in stimulating NK cells in MCMV infections (Dalod et al., 2002). Although the role of these interactions in affecting NK cell function in infections continues to be a topic of ongoing work, over 70% of splenic DCs are infected by day 2 of MCMV infection in vivo, resulting in functional impairment (Andrews et al., 2001a).

CONCLUDING REMARKS

A hallmark of innate immunity is the involvement of "pattern recognition receptors" (PRRs) on other innate immune cells to discriminate among patterns shared by microbes (Medzhitov and Janeway, 1998). The Toll-like receptors, for example, recognize "pathogen-associated molecular patterns" on bacteria and by way of their IL-1R-like cytoplasmic domains signal through MyD88 and ultimately NF-κB (Aderem and Ulevitch, 2000). Thus, the PRRs utilize signaling pathways that are distinct from the Syk family tyrosine kinase pathway stimulated by ITAM-coupled T- and B-cell antigen receptors.

Recent studies, however, indicate that NK cells can recognize virus-infected cells and trigger activation via receptors that do not resemble the PRRs. Instead, by virtue of ITAM signaling, these NK cell activation receptors more closely resemble antigen receptors on T and B cells because of coupling to the Syk family tyrosine kinase pathway. In many respects, these NK cell activation receptors have TCR-like properties. Yet, these receptors are involved in innate host pathogen responses and do not require somatic gene rearrangement for receptor expression. In addition, individual NK cells do not express clonally restricted activation receptors. Rather, they express an array of receptors such that overlapping subsets of NK cells express the same receptor (Smith et al., 2000a). This preformed, widely expressed repertoire of receptors appears to confer upon NK cells the capacity for immediate innate response, in contrast to the days required for clonal expansion of antigen receptor-specific T and B cells. In this way, even though the NK cell population is a small fraction of the total T-cell pool, substantial numbers of NK cells can be specifically activated in innate immune responses to control pathogen invasion during the time required for specific immunity to develop.

Despite this close relationship to lymphocyte antigen-receptor responses, NK cells also respond acutely to infection in a manner that more closely resembles other cells of the innate immune system. A number of different infections trigger non-NK cells to produce similar cytokines that ultimately stimulate NK cell production of still other cytokines that contribute to pathogen control.

Therefore, the emerging picture suggests that NK cells counter infection by both specific activation receptors and nonspecific cytokine responses, displaying the features of traditional acquired immune as well as innate immune cells.

ACKNOWLEDGMENTS

I thank Anthony French, Kevin Latinis, and Sandeep Tripathy for critical review of this manuscript. Work in the Yokoyama laboratory is supported by the Barnes-Jewish Research Foundation, the National Institute of Allergy and Infectious Diseases, and the Howard Hughes Medical Institute.

REFERENCES

Aderem, A., and R. J. Ulevitch. 2000. Toll-like receptors in the induction of the innate immune response. *Nature* **406:**782–787.

Ahmad, A., E. Sharif-Askari, L. Fawaz, and J. Menezes. 2000. Innate immune response of the human host to exposure with herpes simplex virus type 1: in vitro control of the virus infection by enhanced natural killer activity via interleukin-15 induction. *J. Virol.* **74:**7196–7203.

Akira, S. 2000. The role of IL-18 in innate immunity. *Curr. Opin. Immunol.* **12:**59–63.

Anderson, P., M. Caligiuri, J. Ritz, and S. F. Schlossman. 1989. CD3-negative natural killer cells express zeta TCR as part of a novel molecular complex. *Nature* **341:**159–162.

Andrews, D. M., C. E. Andoniou, F. Granucci, P. Ricciardi-Castagnoli, and M. A. Degli-Esposti. 2001a. Infection of dendritic cells by murine cytomegalovirus induces functional paralysis. *Nat. Immunol.* **2:**1077–1084.

Andrews, D. M., H. E. Farrell, E. H. Densley, A. A. Scalzo, G. R. Shellam, and M. A. Degli-Esposti. 2001b. NK1.1+ cells and murine cytomegalovirus infection: what happens in situ? *J. Immunol.* **166:**1796–1802.

Arase, H., T. Saito, J. H. Phillips, and L. L. Lanier. 2001. Cutting edge: the mouse NK cell-associated antigen recognized by DX5 monoclonal antibody is CD49b (alpha 2 integrin, very late antigen-2). *J. Immunol.* **167:**1141–1144.

Arase, H., E. S. Mocarski, A. E. Campbell, A. B. Hill, and L. L. Lanier. 2002. Direct recognition of cytomegalovirus by activating and inhibitory NK cell receptors. *Science* **296:**1323–1326.

Arase, N., H. Arase, S. Y. Park, H. Ohno, C. Ra, and T. Saito. 1997. Association with FcR-γ is essential for activation signal through NKR-P1 (CD161) in natural killer (NK) cells and NK1.1+ T cells. *J. Exp. Med.* **186:**1957–1963.

Bakker, A. B., R. M. Hoek, A. Cerwenka, B. Blom, L. Lucian, T. McNeil, R. Murray, L. H. Phillips, J. D. Sedgwick, and L. L. Lanier. 2000. DAP12-deficient mice fail to develop autoimmunity due to impaired antigen priming. *Immunity* **13:**345–353.

Bancroft, G. J. 1993. The role of natural killer cells in innate resistance to infection. *Curr. Opin. Immunol.* **5:**503–510.

Bancroft, G. J., R. D. Schreiber, and E. R. Unanue. 1991. Natural immunity: a T-cell-independent pathway of macrophage activation, defined in the scid mouse. *Immunol. Rev.* **124:**5–24.

Bauer, S., V. Groh, J. Wu, A. Steinle, J. H. Phillips, L. L. Lanier, and T. Spies. 1999. Activation of NK cells and T cells by NKG2D, a receptor for stress-inducible MICA. *Science* **285:**727–729.

Biassoni, R., C. Cantoni, M. Falco, S. Verdiani, C. Bottino, M. Vitale, R. Conte, A. Poggi, A. Moretta, and L. Moretta. 1996. The human leukocyte antigen (HLA)-C-specific "activatory" or "inhibitory" natural killer cell receptors display highly homologous extracellular domains but differ in their transmembrane and intracytoplasmic portions. *J. Exp. Med.* **183:**645–650.

Biron, C. A., G. Sonnenfeld, and R. M. Welsh. 1984. Interferon induces natural killer cell blastogenesis in vivo. *J. Leukoc. Biol.* **35:**31–37.

Biron, C. A., K. S. Byron, and J. L. Sullivan. 1989. Severe herpesvirus infections in an adolescent without natural killer cells. *N. Engl. J. Med.* **320:**1731–1735.

Biron, C. A., K. B. Nguyen, G. C. Pien, L. P. Cousens, and T. P. Salazar-Mather. 1999. Natural killer cells in antiviral defense: function and regulation by innate cytokines. *Annu. Rev. Immunol.* **17:**189–220.

Bonavida, B., J. Katz, and M. Gottlieb. 1986. Mechanism of defective NK cell activity in patients with acquired immunodeficiency syndrome (AIDS) and AIDS-related complex. I. Defective trigger on NK cells for NKCF production by target cells, and partial restoration by IL 2. *J. Immunol.* **137:**1157–1163.

Born, T. L., L. A. Morrison, D. J. Esteban, T. VandenBos, L. G. Thebeau, N. Chen, M. K. Spriggs, J. E. Sims, and R. M. Buller. 2000. A poxvirus protein that binds to and inactivates IL-18, and inhibits NK cell response. *J. Immunol.* **164:**3246–3254.

Bradley, M., A. Zeytun, A. Rafi-Janajreh, P. S. Nagarkatti, and M. Nagarkatti. 1998. Role of spontaneous and interleukin-2-induced natural killer cell activity in the cytotoxicity and rejection of Fas+ and Fas− tumor cells. *Blood* **92:**4248–4255.

Braud, V. M., D. S. J. Allen, C. A. O'Callaghan, K. Söderström, A. D'Andrea, G. S. Ogg, S. Lazetic, N. T. Young, J. I. Bell, J. H. Phillips, and A. J. McMichael. 1998. HLA-E binds to natural-killer-cell receptors CD94/NKG2A, B and C. *Nature* **391:**795–799.

Brombacher, F., A. Dorfmuller, J. Magram, W. J. Dai, G. Kohler, A. Wunderlin, K. Palmer-Lehmann, M. K. Gately, and G. Alber. 1999. IL-12 is dispensable for innate and adaptive immunity against low doses of *Listeria monocytogenes*. *Int. Immunol.* **11:**325–332.

Brooks, C. G., M. Holscher, and D. Urdal. 1985. Natural killer activity in cloned cytoxic T lymphocytes: regulation by interleukin 2, interferon, and specific antigen. *J. Immunol.* **135:**1145–1152.

Brown, M. G., A. A. Scalzo, K. Matsumoto, and W. M. Yokoyama. 1997. The natural killer gene complex—a genetic basis for understanding natural killer cell function and innate immunity. *Immunol. Rev.* **155:**53–65.

Brown, M. G., A. O. Dokun, J. W. Heusel, H. R. Smith, D. L. Beckman, E. A. Blattenberger, C. E. Dubbelde, L. R. Stone, A. A. Scalzo, and W. M. Yokoyama. 2001. Vital involvement of a natural killer cell activation receptor in resistance to viral infection. *Science* **292:**934–937.

Brumbaugh, K. M., B. A. Binstadt, D. D. Billadeau, R. A. Schoon, C. J. Dick, R. M. Ten, and P. J. Leibson. 1997. Functional role for syk tyrosine kinase in natural killer cell-mediated natural cytotoxicity. *J. Exp. Med.* **186:**1965–1974.

Brumbaugh, K. M., B. A. Binstadt, and P. J. Leibson. 1998. Signal transduction during NK cell activation: balancing opposing forces. *Curr. Top. Microbiol. Immunol.* **230:**103–122.

Bukowski, J. F., B. A. Woda, S. Habu, K. Okumura, and R. M. Welsh. 1983. Natural killer cell depletion enhances virus synthesis and virus-induced hepatitis in vivo. *J. Immunol.* **131:**1531–1538.

Bukowski, J. F., B. A. Woda, and R. M. Welsh. 1984. Pathogenesis of murine cytomegalovirus infection in natural killer cell-depleted mice. *J. Virol.* **52:**119–128.

Bukowski, J. F., J. F. Warner, G. Dennert, and R. M. Welsh. 1985. Adoptive transfer studies demonstrating the antiviral effect of natural killer cells in vivo. *J. Exp. Med.* **161:**40–52.

Carayannopoulos, L., O. Naidenko, D. Fremont, and W. M. Yokoyama. 2002. Cutting edge: murine UL16-binding protein-like transcript 1: a newly described transcript encoding a high-affinity ligand for murine NKG2D. *J. Immunol.* **169:**4079–4083.

Carnaud, C., D. Lee, O. Donnars, S. H. Park, A. Beavis, Y. Koezuka, and A. Bendelac. 1999. Cutting edge: cross-talk between cells of the innate immune system: NKT cells rapidly activate NK cells. *J. Immunol.* **163:**4647–4650.

Cella, M., F. Facchetti, A. Lanzavecchia, and M. Colonna. 2000. Plasmacytoid dendritic cells activated by influenza virus and CD40L drive a potent TH1 polarization. *Nat. Immunol.* **1:**305–310.

Cerwenka, A., A. B. H. Bakker, T. McClanahan, J. Wagner, J. Wu, J. H. Phillips, and L. L. Lanier. 2000. Retinoic acid early inducible genes define a ligand family for the activating NKG2D receptor in mice. *Immunity* **12:**721–727.

Chambers, W. H., N. L. Vujanovic, A. B. DeLeo, M. W. Olszowy, R. B. Herberman, and J. C. Hiserodt. 1989. Monoclonal antibody to a triggering structure expressed on rat natural killer cells and adherent lymphokine-activated killer cells. *J. Exp. Med.* **169:**1373–1389.

Cohen, G. B., R. T. Gandhi, D. M. Davis, O. Mandelboim, B. K. Chen, J. L. Strominger, and D. Baltimore. 1999. The selective downregulation of class I major histocompatibility complex proteins by HIV-1 protects HIV-infected cells from NK cells. *Immunity* **10:**661–671.

Colonna, M. 1997. Specificity and function of immunoglobulin superfamily NK cell inhibitory and stimulatory receptors. *Immunol. Rev.* **155:**127–133.

Colonna, M., A. Krug, and M. Cella. 2002. Interferon-producing cells: on the front line in immune responses against pathogens. *Curr. Opin. Immunol.* **14:**373–379.

Colucci, F., E. Schweighoffer, E. Tomasello, M. Turner, J. R. Ortaldo, E. Vivier, V. L. Tybulewicz, and J. P. Di Santo. 2002. Natural cytotoxicity uncoupled from the Syk and ZAP-70 intracellular kinases. *Nat. Immunol.* **3:**288–294.

Cook, J. L., D. N. Ikle, and B. A. Routes. 1995. Natural killer cell ontogeny in the athymic rat. Relationship between functional maturation and acquired resistance to E1A oncogene-expressing sarcoma cells. *J. Immunol.* **155:**5512–5518.

Cooper, M. A., J. E. Bush, T. A. Fehniger, J. B. VanDeusen, R. E. Waite, Y. Liu, H. L. Aguila, and M. A. Caligiuri. 2002. In vivo evidence for a dependence on interleukin 15 for survival of natural killer cells. *Blood* **100:**3633–3638.

Correa, I., and D. H. Raulet. 1995. Binding of diverse peptides to MHC class I molecules inhibits target cell lysis by activated natural killer cells. *Immunity* **2:**61–71.

Correa, I., L. Corral, and D. H. Raulet. 1994. Multiple natural killer cell-activating signals are inhibited by major histocompatibility complex class I expression in target cells. *Eur. J. Immunol.* **24:**1323–1331.

Cosman, D., N. Fanger, L. Borges, M. Kubin, W. Chin, L. Peterson, and M.-L. Hsu. 1997. A novel immunoglobulin superfamily receptor for cellular and viral MHC class I molecules. *Immunity* **7:**273–282.

Cosman, D., J. Mullberg, C. L. Sutherland, W. Chin, R. Armitage, W. Fanslow, M. Kubin, and N. J. Chalupny. 2001. ULBPs, novel MHC class I-related molecules, bind to CMV glycoprotein UL16 and stimulate NK cytotoxicity through the NKG2D receptor. *Immunity* **14:**123–133.

Cretney, E., M. A. Degli-Esposti, E. H. Densley, H. E. Farrell, N. J. Davis-Poynter, and M. J. Smyth.

1999. m144, a murine cytomegalovirus (MCMV)-encoded major histocompatibility complex class I homologue, confers tumor resistance to natural killer cell-mediated rejection. *J. Exp. Med.* **190:**435–444.

Cuturi, M. C., I. Anegon, F. Sherman, R. Loudon, S. C. Clark, B. Perussia, and G. Trinchieri. 1989. Production of hematopoietic colony stimulating factors by human natural killer cells. *J. Exp. Med.* **169:**569.

Dalod, M., T. P. Salazar-Mather, L. Malmgaard, C. Lewis, C. Asselin-Paturel, F. Briere, G. Trinchieri, and C. A. Biron. 2002. Interferon alpha/beta and interleukin 12 responses to viral infections: pathways regulating dendritic cell cytokine expression in vivo. *J. Exp. Med.* **195:**517–528.

Daniels, K. A., G. Devora, W. C. Lai, C. L. O'Donnell, M. Bennett, and R. M. Welsh. 2001. Murine cytomegalovirus is regulated by a discrete subset of natural killer cells reactive with monoclonal antibody to ly49h. *J. Exp. Med.* **194:**29–44.

Delano, M. L., and D. G. Brownstein. 1995. Innate resistance to lethal mousepox is genetically linked to the NK gene complex on chromosome 6 and correlates with early restriction of virus replication by cells with an NK phenotype. *J. Virol.* **69:**5875–5877.

Depatie, C., E. Muise, P. Lepage, P. Gros, and S. M. Vidal. 1997. High-resolution linkage map in the proximity of the host resistance locus CMV1. *Genomics* **39:**154–163.

Diefenbach, A., A. M. Jamieson, S. D. Liu, N. Shastri, and D. H. Raulet. 2000. Ligands for the murine NKG2D receptor: expression by tumor cells and activation of NK cells and macrophages. *Nat. Immunol.* **1:**119–126.

Diefenbach, A., E. Tomasello, M. Lucas, A. M. Jamieson, J. K. Hsia, E. Vivier, and D. H. Raulet. 2002. Selective associations with signaling molecules determine stimulatory versus costimulatory activity of NKG2D. *Nat. Immunol.* **3:**1142–1149.

DiSanto, J. P., W. Muller, D. Guy-Grand, A. Fischer, and K. Rajewsky. 1995. Lymphoid development in mice with a targeted deletion of the interleukin 2 receptor gamma chain. *Proc. Natl. Acad. Sci. USA* **92:**377–381.

Dokun, A. O., D. T. Chu, L. Yang, A. S. Bendelac, and W. M. Yokoyama. 2001a. Analysis of in situ NK cell responses during viral infection. *J. Immunol.* **167:**5286–5293.

Dokun, A. O., S. Kim, H. R. Smith, H. S. Kang, D. T. Chu, and W. M. Yokoyama. 2001b. Specific and nonspecific NK cell activation during virus infection. *Nat. Immunol.* **2:**951–956.

Dubois, S., J. Mariner, T. A. Waldmann, and Y. Tagaya. 2002. IL-15Ralpha recycles and presents IL-15 in trans to neighboring cells. *Immunity* **17:**537–547.

Duncan, G. S., H. W. Mittrucker, D. Kagi, T. Matsuyama, and T. W. Mak. 1996. The transcription factor interferon regulatory factor-1 is essential for natural killer cell function in vivo. *J. Exp. Med.* **184:**2043–2048.

Dunn, P. L., and R. J. North. 1991. Early gamma interferon production by natural killer cells is important in defense against murine listeriosis. *Infect. Immun.* **59:**2892–2900.

Ebnet, K., M. Hausmann, F. Lehmann-Grube, A. Mullbacher, M. Kopf, M. Lamers, and M. M. Simon. 1995. Granzyme A-deficient mice retain potent cell-mediated cytotoxicity. *EMBO J.* **14:**4230–4239.

Fan, Q. R., E. O. Long, and D. C. Wiley. 2001. Crystal structure of the human natural killer cell inhibitory receptor KIR2DL1-HLA-Cw4 complex. *Nat. Immunol.* **2:**452–460.

Farrell, H. E., H. Vally, D. M. Lynch, P. Fleming, G. R. Shellam, A. A. Scalzo, and N. J. Davis-Poynter. 1997. Inhibition of natural killer cells by a cytomegalovirus MHC class I homologue in vivo. *Nature* **386:**510–514.

Fawaz, L. M., E. Sharif-Askari, and J. Menezes. 1999. Up-regulation of NK cytotoxic activity via IL-15 induction by different viruses: a comparative study. *J. Immunol.* **163:**4473–4480.

Ferlazzo, G., M. L. Tsang, L. Moretta, G. Melioli, R. M. Steinman, and C. Munz. 2002. Human dendritic cells activate resting natural killer (NK) cells and are recognized via the NKp30 receptor by activated NK cells. *J. Exp. Med.* **195:**343–351.

Forbes, C. A., M. G. Brown, R. Cho, G. R. Shellam, W. M. Yokoyama, and A. A. Scalzo. 1997. The Cmv1 host resistance locus is closely linked to the Ly49 multigene family within the natural killer cell gene complex on mouse chromosome 6. *Genomics* **41:**406–413.

Furukawa, H., K. Iizuka, J. Poursine-Laurent, N. Shastri, and W. M. Yokoyama. 2002. A ligand for the murine NK activation receptor Ly-49D: activation of tolerized NK cells from beta(2)-microglobulin-deficient mice. *J. Immunol.* **169:**126–136.

George, T. C., L. H. Mason, J. R. Ortaldo, V. Kumar, and M. Bennett. 1999. Positive recognition of MHC class I molecules by the Ly49D receptor of murine NK cells. *J. Immunol.* **162:**2035–2043.

Georgopoulos, K., M. Bigby, J. H. Wang, A. Molnar, P. Wu, S. Winandy, and A. Sharpe. 1994. The Ikaros gene is required for the development of all lymphoid lineages. *Cell* **79:**143–156.

Gerosa, F., B. Baldani-Guerra, C. Nisii, V. Marchesini, G. Carra, and G. Trinchieri. 2002. Reciprocal activating interaction between natural killer cells and dendritic cells. *J. Exp. Med.* **195:**327–333.

Gilfillan, S., E. L. Ho, M. Cella, W. M. Yokoyama, and M. Colonna. 2002. NKG2D recruits two distinct adapters to trigger natural killer cell activation and costimulation. *Nat. Immunol.* **3:**1150–1155.

Gosselin, J., A. Tomoiu, R. C. Gallo, and L. Flamand. 1999. Interleukin-15 as an activator of natural killer cell-mediated antiviral response. *Blood* **94:**4210–4219.

Greenough, A. 1994. The TORCH screen and intrauterine infections. *Arch. Dis. Childhood Fetal Neonatal Ed.* **70:**F163–F165.

Grimm, E. A., A. Mazumder, H. Z. Zhang, and S. A. Rosenberg. 1982. Lymphokine-activated killer cell phenomenon. Lysis of natural killer-resistant fresh solid tumor cells by interleukin 2-activated autologous human peripheral blood lymphocytes. *J. Exp. Med.* **155:**1823–1841.

Groh, V., R. Rhinehart, J. Randolph-Habecker, M. S. Topp, S. R. Riddell, and T. Spies. 2001. Costimulation of CD8αβ T cells by NKG2D via engagement by MIC induced on virus-infected cells. *Nat. Immunol.* **2:**255–260.

Guidotti, L. G., and F. V. Chisari. 2001. Noncytolytic control of viral infections by the innate and adaptive immune response. *Annu. Rev. Immunol.* **19:** 65–91.

Gunji, Y., N. L. Vujanovic, J. C. Hiserodt, R. B. Herberman, and E. Gorelik. 1989. Generation and characterization of lymphokine-activated killer cells in mice. *J. Immunol.* **142:**1748–1754.

Hackett, J., Jr., G. C. Bosma, M. J. Bosma, M. Bennett, and V. Kumar. 1986a. Transplantable progenitors of natural killer cells are distinct from those of T and B lymphocytes. *Proc. Natl. Acad. Sci. USA* **83:** 3427–3431.

Hackett, J., Jr., M. Tutt, M. Lipscomb, M. Bennett, G. Koo, and V. Kumar. 1986b. Origin and differentiation of natural killer cells. II. Functional and morphologic studies of purified NK-1.1+ cells. *J. Immunol.* **136:**3124–3131.

Harty, J. T., and M. J. Bevan. 1995. Specific immunity to Listeria monocytogenes in the absence of IFN gamma. *Immunity* **3:**109–117.

Henkart, P. A. 1994. Lymphocyte-mediated cytotoxicity: two pathways and multiple effector molecules. *Immunity* **1:**343–346.

Herberman, R. 1982. *NK Cells and Other Natural Effector Cells.* Academic Press, New York, N.Y.

Herberman, R. B., M. E. Nunn, and D. H. Lavrin. 1975. Natural cytotoxic reactivity of mouse lymphoid cells against syngeneic and allogeneic tumors. I. Distribution of reactivity and specificity. *Int. J. Cancer* **16:**216.

Heusel, J. W., R. L. Wesselschmidt, S. Shresta, J. H. Russell, and T. J. Ley. 1994. Cytotoxic lymphocytes require granzyme B for the rapid induction of DNA fragmentation and apoptosis in allogeneic target cells. *Cell* **76:**977–987.

Ho, E. L., J. W. Heusel, M. G. Brown, K. Matsumoto, A. A. Scalzo, and W. M. Yokoyama. 1998. Murine nkg2d and Cd94 are clustered within the natural killer complex and are expressed independently in natural killer cells. *Proc. Natl. Acad. Sci. USA* **95:**6320–6325.

Ho, E. L., L. N. Carayannopoulos, J. Poursine-Laurent, J. Kinder, B. Plougastel, H. R. C. Smith, and W. M. Yokoyama. 2002. Co-stimulation of multiple NK cell activation receptors by NKG2D. *J. Immunol.* **169:**3667–3675.

Huang, S., W. Hendriks, A. Althage, S. Hemmi, H. Bluethmann, R. Kamijo, J. Vilcek, R. M. Zinkernagel, and M. Aguet. 1993. Immune response in mice that lack the interferon-gamma receptor. *Science* **259:**1742–1745.

Hyodo, Y., K. Matsui, N. Hayashi, H. Tsutsui, S. Kashiwamura, H. Yamauchi, K. Hiroishi, K. Takeda, Y. Tagawa, Y. Iwakura, N. Kayagaki, M. Kurimoto, H. Okamura, T. Hada, H. Yagita, S. Akira, K. Nakanishi, and K. Higaashino. 1999. IL-18 up-regulates perforin-mediated NK activity without increasing perforin messenger RNA expression by binding to constitutively expressed IL-18 receptor. *J. Immunol.* **162:**1662–1668.

Idris, A. H., H. R. C. Smith, L. H. Mason, J. H. Ortaldo, A. A. Scalzo, and W. M. Yokoyama. 1999. The natural killer cell complex genetic locus, Chok, encodes Ly49D, a target recognition receptor that activates natural killing. *Proc. Natl. Acad. Sci. USA* **96:** 6330–6335.

Introne, W., R. E. Boissy, and W. A. Gahl. 1999. Clinical, molecular, and cell biological aspects of Chediak-Higashi syndrome. *Mol. Genet. Metab.* **68:** 283–303.

Inverardi, L., J. C. Witson, S. A. Fuad, R. T. Winkler-Pickett, J. R. Ortaldo, and F. H. Bach. 1991. CD3 negative "small agranular lymphocytes" are natural killer cells. *J. Immunol.* **146:**4048–4052.

Ishido, S., J. K. Choi, B. S. Lee, C. Wang, M. DeMaria, R. P. Johnson, G. B. Cohen, and J. U. Jung. 2000. Inhibition of natural killer cell-mediated cytotoxicity by Kaposi's sarcoma-associated herpesvirus K5 protein. *Immunity* **13:**365–374.

Jawahar, S., C. Moody, M. Chan, R. Finberg, R. Geha, and T. Chatila. 1996. Natural Killer (NK) cell deficiency associated with an epitope-deficient Fc receptor type IIIA (CD16-II). *Clin. Exp. Immunol.* **103:**408–413.

Jevremovic, D., D. D. Billadeau, R. A. Schoon, C. J. Dick, B. J. Irvin, W. Zhang, L. E. Samelson, R. T. Abraham, and P. J. Leibson. 1999. Cutting edge: a role for the adaptor protein LAT in human NK cell-mediated cytotoxicity. *J. Immunol.* **162:**2453–2456.

Jiang, K., B. Zhong, D. L. Gilvary, B. C. Corliss, E. Hong-Geller, S. Wei, and J. Y. Djeu. 2000. Pivotal role of phosphoinositide-3 kinase in regulation of cytotoxicity in natural killer cells. *Nat. Immunol.* **1:**419–425.

Kagi, D., B. Ledermann, K. Burki, P. Seiler, B. Odermatt, K. J. Olsen, E. R. Podack, R. M. Zinkernagel, and H. Hengartner. 1994. Cytotoxicity mediated by T cells and natural killer cells is greatly impaired in perforin-deficient mice. *Nature* **369**:31–37.

Kane, L. P., P. G. Andres, K. C. Howland, A. K. Abbas, and A. Weiss. 2001. Akt provides the CD28 costimulatory signal for up-regulation of IL-2 and IFN-gamma but not TH2 cytokines. *Nat. Immunol.* **2**:37–44.

Karlhofer, F. M., M. M. Orihuela, and W. M. Yokoyama. 1995. Ly-49-independent natural killer (NK) cell specificity revealed by NK cell clones derived from p53-deficient mice. *J. Exp. Med.* **181**: 1785–1795.

Karlhofer, F. M., R. K. Ribaudo, and W. M. Yokoyama. 1992a. The interaction of Ly-49 with H-2Dd globally inactivates natural killer cell cytolytic activity. *Trans. Assoc. Am. Phys.* **105**:72–85.

Karlhofer, F. M., R. K. Ribaudo, and W. M. Yokoyama. 1992b. MHC class I alloantigen specificity of Ly-49+ IL-2-activated natural killer cells. *Nature* **358**:66–70.

Kärre, K. 1985. Role of target histocompatibility antigens in regulation of natural killer activity: a reevaluation and a hypothesis, p. 81–92. *In* R. B. Herberman and D. M. Callewaert (ed.), *Mechanisms of Cytotoxicity by NK Cells*. Academic Press, Inc., Orlando, Fla.

Kärre, K., H. G. Ljunggren, G. Piontek, and R. Kiessling. 1986. Selective rejection of H-2-deficient lymphoma variants suggests alternative immune defence strategy. *Nature* **319**:675–678.

Kennedy, M. K., M. Glaccum, S. N. Brown, E. A. Butz, J. L. Viney, M. Embers, N. Matsuki, K. Charrier, L. Sedger, C. R. Willis, K. Brasel, P. J. Morrissey, K. Stocking, J. C. L. Schuh, S. Joyce, and J. J. Peschon. 2000. Reversible defects in natural killer and memory CD8 T cell lineages in interleukin 15-deficient mice. *J. Exp. Med.* **191**:771–780.

Kiessling, R., E. Klein, and H. Wigzell. 1975. Natural killer cells in the mouse. I. Cytotoxic cells with specificity for mouse Moloney leukemia cells: specificity and distribution according to genotype. *Eur. J. Immunol.* **5**:112.

Kim, S., and W. M. Yokoyama. 1998. NK cell granule exocytosis and cytokine production inhibited by Ly-49A engagement. *Cell. Immunol.* **183**:106–112.

Kim, S., K. Iizuka, H. L. Aguila, I. L. Weissman, and W. M. Yokoyama. 2000. In vivo natural killer cell activities revealed by natural killer cell-deficient mice. *Proc. Natl. Acad. Sci. USA* **97**:2731–2736.

Kloover, J. S., G. E. Grauls, M. J. Blok, C. Vink, and C. A. Bruggeman. 2002. A rat cytomegalovirus strain with a disruption of the r144 MHC class I-like gene is attenuated in the acute phase of infection in neonatal rats. *Arch. Virol.* **147**:813–824.

Krmpotic, A., D. H. Busch, I. Bubic, F. Gebhardt, H. Hengel, M. Hasan, A. A. Scalzo, U. H. Koszinowski, and S. Jonjic. 2002. MCMV glycoprotein gp40 confers virus resistance to CD8+

T cells and NK cells in vivo. *Nat. Immunol.* **3**:529–535.

Kubota, A., S. Kubota, H. E. Farrell, N. Davis-Poynter, and F. Takei. 1999. Inhibition of NK cells by murine CMV-encoded class I MHC homologue m144. *Cell. Immunol.* **191**:145–151.

Lanier, L. L., J. H. Phillips, J. Hackett, Jr., M. Tutt, and V. Kumar. 1986. Natural killer cells: definition of a cell type rather than a function. *J. Immunol.* **137**:2735–2739.

Lanier, L. L., G. Yu, and J. H. Phillips. 1989. Co-association of CD3 zeta with a receptor (CD16) for IgG Fc on human natural killer cells. *Nature* **342**:803–805.

Lanier, L. L., B. Corliss, and J. H. Phillips. 1997. Arousal and inhibition of human NK cells. *Immunol. Rev.* **155**:145–154.

Lanier, L. L., B. Corliss, J. Wu, and J. H. Phillips. 1998a. Association of DAP12 with activating CD94/NKG2C NK cell receptors. *Immunity* **8**:693–701.

Lanier, L. L., B. C. Cortiss, J. Wu, C. Leong, and J. H. Phillips. 1998b. Immunoreceptor DAP12 bearing a tyrosine-based activation motif is involved in activating NK cells. *Nature* **391**:703–707.

Lee, S. H., S. Girard, D. Macina, M. Busa, A. Zafer, A. Belouchi, P. Gros, and S. M. Vidal. 2001. Susceptibility to mouse cytomegalovirus is associated with deletion of an activating natural killer cell receptor of the C-type lectin superfamily. *Nat. Genet.* **28**:42–45.

Li, P., D. L. Morris, B. E. Willcox, A. Steinle, T. Spies, and R. K. Strong. 2001. Complex structure of the activating immunoreceptor NKG2D and its MHC class I-like ligand MICA. *Nat. Immunol.* **2**:443–451.

Li, P., G. McDermott, and R. K. Strong. 2002. Crystal structures of RAE-1beta and its complex with the activating immunoreceptor NKG2D. *Immunity* **16**:77–86.

Ljunggren, H. G., and K. Kärre. 1990. In search of the "missing self": MHC molecules and NK cell recognition. *Immunol. Today* **11**:237–244.

Lodolce, J. P., D. L. Boone, S. Chai, R. E. Swain, T. Dassopoulos, S. Trettin, and A. Ma. 1998. IL-15 receptor maintains lymphoid homeostasis by supporting lymphocyte homing and proliferation. *Immunity* **9**:669–676.

Long, E. O. 1999. Regulation of immune responses through inhibitory receptors. *Annu. Rev. Immunol.* **17**: 875–904.

Lopez-Botet, M., J. J. Perezvillar, M. Carretero, A. Rodriguez, I. Melero, T. Bellon, M. Llano, and F. Navarro. 1997. Structure and function of the CD94 C-type lectin receptor complex involved in recognition of HLA class I molecules. *Immunol. Rev.* **155**:165–174.

Lowin, B., F. Beermann, A. Schmidt, and J. Tschopp. 1994. A null mutation in the perforin gene impairs cytolytic T lymphocyte- and natural killer cell-mediated cytotoxicity. *Proc. Natl. Acad. Sci. USA* **91**:11571–11575.

Lusso, P., M. S. Malnati, A. Garzino-Demo, R. W. Crowley, E. O. Long, and R. C. Gallo. 1993. Infection of natural killer cells by human herpesvirus 6. *Nature* **362**:458–462.

Mandelboim, O., S. B. Wilson, M. Vales-Gomez, H. T. Reyburn, and J. L. Strominger. 1997. Self and viral peptides can initiate lysis by autologous natural killer cells. *Proc. Natl. Acad. Sci. USA* **94**:4604–4609.

Mandelboim, O., N. Lieberman, M. Lev, L. Paul, T. I. Arnon, Y. Bushkin, D. M. Davis, J. L. Strominger, J. W. Yewdell, and A. Porgador. 2001. Recognition of haemagglutinins on virus-infected cells by NKp46 activates lysis by human NK cells. *Nature* **409**:1055–1060.

Manoussaka, M. S., R. J. Smith, V. Conlin, J. A. Toomey, and C. G. Brooks. 1998. Fetal mouse NK cell clones are deficient in Ly49 expression, share a common broad lytic specificity, and undergo continuous and extensive diversification in vitro. *J. Immunol.* **160**:2197–2206.

Mason, L. H., S. K. Anderson, W. M. Yokoyama, H. R. C. Smith, R. Winklerpickett, and J. R. Ortaldo. 1996. The Ly-49D receptor activates murine natural killer cells. *J. Exp. Med.* **184**:2119–2128.

Mason, L. H., J. Willettebrown, S. K. Anderson, P. Gosselin, E. W. Shores, P. E. Love, J. R. Ortaldo, and D. W. McVicar. 1998. Characterization of an associated 16-KDa tyrosine phosphoprotein required for Ly-49D signal transduction. *J. Immunol.* **160**:4148–4152.

Medzhitov, R., and C. A. Janeway, Jr. 1998. Innate immune recognition and control of adaptive immune responses. *Semin. Immunol.* **10**:351–353.

Meraz, M. A., J. M. White, K. C. Sheehan, E. A. Bach, S. J. Rodig, A. S. Dighe, D. H. Kaplan, J. K. Riley, A. C. Greenlund, D. Campbell, K. Carver-Moore, R. N. DuBois, R. Clark, M. Arguet, and R. D. Schreiber. 1996. Targeted disruption of the Stat1 gene in mice reveals unexpected physiologic specificity in the JAK-STAT signaling pathway. *Cell* **84**:431–442.

Michaelsson, J., A. Achour, M. Salcedo, A. Kase-Sjostrom, J. Sundback, R. A. Harris, and K. Karre. 2000. Visualization of inhibitory Ly49 receptor specificity with soluble major histocompatibility complex class I tetramers. *Eur. J. Immunol.* **30**:300–307.

Moody, D. B., B. B. Reinhold, M. R. Guy, E. M. Beckman, D. E. Frederique, S. T. Furlong, S. Ye, V. N. Reinhold, P. A. Sieling, R. L. Modlin, G. S. Besra, and S. A. Porcelli. 1997. Structural requirements for glycolipid antigen recognition by CD1b-restricted T cells. *Science* **278**:283–286.

Moody, D. B., T. Ulrichs, W. Muhlecker, D. C. Young, S. S. Gurcha, E. Grant, J. P. Rosat, M. B. Brenner, C. E. Costello, G. S. Besra, and S. A. Porcelli. 2000. CD1c-mediated T-cell recognition of isoprenoid glycolipids in Mycobacterium tuberculosis infection. *Nature* **404**:884–888.

Moretta, A., R. Biassoni, C. Bottino, D. Pende, M. Vitale, A. Poggi, M. C. Mingari, and L. Moretta. 1997. Major histocompatibility complex class I-specific receptors on human natural killer and T lymphocytes. *Immunol. Rev.* **155**:105–117.

Motyka, B., G. Korbutt, M. J. Pinkoski, J. A. Heibein, A. Caputo, M. Hobman, M. Barry, I. Shostak, T. Sawchuk, C. F. Holmes, J. Gauldie, and R. C. Bleackley. 2000. Mannose 6-phosphate/insulin-like growth factor II receptor is a death receptor for granzyme B during cytotoxic T cell-induced apoptosis. *Cell* **103**:491–500.

Nakamura, M. C., P. A. Linnemeyer, E. C. Niemi, L. H. Mason, J. R. Ortaldo, J. C. Ryan, and W. E. Seaman. 1999. Mouse Ly-49D recognizes H-2Dd and activates natural killer cell cytotoxicity. *J. Exp. Med.* **189**:493–500.

Nguyen, K. B., L. P. Cousens, L. A. Doughty, G. C. Pien, J. E. Durbin, and C. A. Biron. 2000. Interferon a/b-mediated inhibition and promotion of interferon-g: STAT1 resolves a paradox. *Nat. Immunol.* **1**:70–76.

Nguyen, K. B., T. P. Salazar-Mather, M. Y. Dalod, J. B. Van Deusen, X. Q. Wei, F. Y. Liew, M. A. Caligiuri, J. E. Durbin, and C. A. Biron. 2002. Coordinated and distinct roles for IFN-alphabeta, IL-12, and IL-15 regulation of NK cell responses to viral infection. *J. Immunol.* **169**:4279–4287.

Ogasawara, K., S. Hida, N. Azimi, Y. Tagaya, T. Sato, T. Yokochifukuda, T. A. Waldmann, T. Taniguchi, and S. Taki. 1998. Requirement for IRF-1 in the microenvironment supporting development of natural killer cells. *Nature* **391**:700–703.

Ohteki, T., H. Yoshida, T. Matsuyama, G. S. Duncan, T. W. Mak, and P. S. Ohashi. 1998. The transcription factor interferon regulatory factor 1 (IRF-1) is important during the maturation of NK1.1+ T cell receptor-αβ+ (NK1+ T) cells, natural killer cells, and intestinal intraepithelial T cells. *J. Exp. Med.* **187**:967–972.

Ohteki, T., T. Fukao, K. Suzue, C. Maki, M. Ito, M. Nakamura, and S. Koyasu. 1999. Interleukin 12-dependent interferon gamma production by CD8alpha+ lymphoid dendritic cells. *J. Exp. Med.* **189**:1981–1986.

Orange, J. S., and C. A. Biron. 1996a. An absolute and restricted requirement for IL-12 in natural killer cell IFN-gamma production and antiviral defense. Studies of natural killer and T cell responses in contrasting viral infections. *J. Immunol.* **156**:1138–1142.

Orange, J. S., and C. A. Biron. 1996b. Characterization of early IL-12, IFN-alphabeta, and TNF effects on antiviral state and NK cell responses during murine cytomegalovirus infection. *J. Immunol.* **156:** 4746–4756.

Orange, J. S., B. Wang, C. Terhorst, and C. A. Biron. 1995. Requirement for natural killer cell-produced interferon gamma in defense against murine cytomegalovirus infection and enhancement of this defense pathway by interleukin 12 administration. *J. Exp. Med.* **182:**1045–1056.

Orange, J. S., M. S. Fassett, L. A. Koopman, J. E. Boyson, and J. L. Strominger. 2002. Viral evasion of natural killer cells. *Nat. Immunol.* **3:**1006–1012.

Orihuela, M., D. H. Margulies, and W. M. Yokoyama. 1996. The natural killer cell receptor Ly-49A recognizes a peptide-induced conformational determinant on its major histocompatibility complex class I ligand. *Proc. Natl. Acad. Sci. USA* **93:**11792–11797.

Pereira, R. A., A. Scalzo, and A. Simmons. 2001. Cutting edge: a NK complex-linked locus governs acute versus latent herpes simplex virus infection of neurons. *J. Immunol.* **166:**5869–5873.

Peterson, E. J., J. L. Clements, Z. K. Ballas, and G. A. Koretzky. 1999. NK cytokine secretion and cytotoxicity occur independently of the SLP-76 adaptor protein. *Eur. J. Immunol.* **29:**2223–2232.

Philbrick, W. M., S. E. Maher, M. M. Bridgett, and A. L. Bothwell. 1990. A recombination event in the 5° flanking region of the Ly-6C gene correlates with impaired expression in the NOD, NZB and ST strains of mice. *EMBO J.* **9:**2485–2492.

Phillips, J. H., C. W. Chang, J. Mattson, J. E. Gumperz, P. Parham, and L. L. Lanier. 1996. CD94 and a novel associated protein (94ap) form a NK cell receptor involved in the recognition of HLA-A, HLA-B, and HLA-C allotypes. *Immunity* **5:**163–172.

Piccioli, D., S. Sbrana, E. Melandri, and N. M. Valiante. 2002. Contact-dependent stimulation and inhibition of dendritic cells by natural killer cells. *J. Exp. Med.* **195:**335–341.

Pien, G. C., A. R. Satoskar, K. Takeda, S. Akira, and C. A. Biron. 2000. Cutting edge: selective IL-18 requirements for induction of compartmental IFN-gamma responses during viral infection. *J. Immunol.* **165:**4787–4791.

Radaev, S., B. Rostro, A. G. Brooks, M. Colonna, and P. D. Sun. 2001. Conformational plasticity revealed by the cocrystal structure of NKG2D and its class I MHC-like ligand ULBP3. *Immunity* **15:**1039–1049.

Raulet, D. H., R. E. Vance, and C. W. McMahon. 2001. Regulation of the natural killer cell receptor repertoire. *Annu. Rev. Immunol.* **19:**291–330.

Ravetch, J. V., and J. P. Kinet. 1991. Fc receptors. *Annu. Rev. Immunol.* **9:**457–491.

Ravetch, J. V., and L. L. Lanier. 2000. Immune inhibitory receptors. *Science* **290:**84–89.

Reyburn, H. T., O. Mandelboim, M. Vales-Gomez, D. M. Davis, L. Pazmany, and J. L. Strominger. 1997. The class I MHC homologue of human cytomegalovirus inhibits attack by natural killer cells. *Nature* **386:**514–517.

Rook, A. H., H. Masur, H. C. Lane, W. Frederick, T. Kasahara, A. M. Macher, J. Y. Djeu, J. F. Manischewitz, L. Jackson, A. S. Fauci, and G. V. Quinnan, Jr. 1983. Interleukin-2 enhances the depressed natural killer and cytomegalovirus-specific cytotoxic activities of lymphocytes from patients with the acquired immune deficiency syndrome. *J. Clin. Invest.* **72:**398–403.

Salazar-Mather, T. P., J. S. Orange, and C. A. Biron. 1998. Early murine cytomegalovirus (MCMV) infection induces liver natural killer (NK) cell inflammation and protection through macrophage inflammatory protein 1-alpha (MIP-1-alpha)-dependent pathways. *J. Exp. Med.* **187:**1–14.

Salazar-Mather, T. P., T. A. Hamilton, and C. A. Biron. 2000. A chemokine-to-cytokine-to-chemokine cascade critical in antiviral defense. *J. Clin. Invest.* **105:**985–993.

Salazar-Mather, T. P., C. A. Lewis, and C. A. Biron. 2002. Type I interferons regulate inflammatory cell trafficking and macrophage inflammatory protein 1alpha delivery to the liver. *J. Clin. Invest.* **110:**321–330.

Scalzo, A. A., N. A. Fitzgerald, A. Simmons, A. B. La Vista, and G. R. Shellam. 1990. Cmv-1, a genetic locus that controls murine cytomegalovirus replication in the spleen. *J. Exp. Med.* **171:**1469–1483.

Scalzo, A. A., N. A. Fitzgerald, C. R. Wallace, A. E. Gibbons, Y. C. Smart, R. C. Burton, and G. R. Shellam. 1992. The effect of the Cmv-1 resistance gene, which is linked to the natural killer cell gene complex, is mediated by natural killer cells. *J. Immunol.* **149:**581–589.

Scalzo, A. A., P. A. Lyons, N. A. Fitzgerald, C. A. Forbes, W. M. Yokoyama, and G. R. Shellam. 1995. Genetic mapping of Cmv1 in the region of mouse chromosome 6 encoding the NK gene complex-associated loci Ly49 and musNKR-P1. *Genomics* **27:**435–441.

Schmidt, R. E., G. Bartley, H. Levine, S. F. Schlossman, and J. Ritz. 1985. Functional characterization of LFA-1 antigens in the interaction of human NK clones and target cells. *J. Immunol.* **135:** 1020–1025.

Schorle, H., T. Holtschke, T. Hunig, A. Schimpl, and I. Horak. 1991. Development and function of T cells in mice rendered interleukin-2 deficient by gene targeting. *Nature* **352:**621–624.

Seaman, W. E., M. Sleisenger, E. Eriksson, and G. C. Koo. 1987. Depletion of natural killer cells in mice by monoclonal antibody to NK-1.1. Reduction in host defense against malignancy without loss of cellular or humoral immunity. *J. Immunol.* **138**:4539–4544.

Seki, H., Y. Ueno, K. Taga, A. Matsuda, T. Miyawaki, and N. Taniguchi. 1985. Mode of in vitro augmentation of natural killer cell activity by recombinant human interleukin 2: a comparative study of Leu-11+ and Leu-11− cell populations in cord blood and adult peripheral blood. *J. Immunol.* **135**:2351–2356.

Shellam, G. R., J. E. Allan, J. M. Papadimitriou, and G. J. Bancroft. 1981. Increased susceptibility to cytomegalovirus infection in beige mutant mice. *Proc. Natl. Acad. Sci. USA* **78**:5104–5108.

Sjolin, H., E. Tomasello, M. Mousavi-Jazi, A. Bartolazzi, K. Karre, E. Vivier, and C. Cerboni. 2002. Pivotal role of KARAP/DAP12 adaptor molecule in the natural killer cell-mediated resistance to murine cytomegalovirus infection. *J. Exp. Med.* **195**:825–834.

Smith, H. R. C., F. M. Karlhofer, and W. M. Yokoyama. 1994. Ly-49 multigene family expressed by IL-2-activated NK cells. *J. Immunol.* **153**:1068–1079.

Smith, H. R., H. H. Chuang, L. L. Wang, M. Salcedo, J. W. Heusel, and W. M. Yokoyama. 2000a. Nonstochastic coexpression of activation receptors on murine natural killer cells. *J. Exp. Med.* **191**:1341–1354.

Smith, H. R., J. W. Heusel, I. K. Mehta, S. Kim, B. G. Dorner, O. V. Naidenko, K. Iizuka, H. Furukawa, D. L. Beckman, J. T. Pingel, A. A. Scalzo, D. H. Fremont, and W. M. Yokoyama. 2002. Recognition of a virus-encoded ligand by a natural killer cell activation receptor. *Proc. Natl. Acad. Sci. USA* **99**:8826–8831.

Smith, K. M., J. Wu, A. B. Bakker, J. H. Phillips, and L. L. Lanier. 1998. Cutting edge: Ly-49D and Ly-49H associate with mouse DAP12 and form activating receptors. *J. Immunol.* **161**:7–10.

Smith, V. P., N. A. Bryant, and A. Alcami. 2000b. Ectromelia, vaccinia and cowpox viruses encode secreted interleukin-18-binding proteins. *J. Gen. Virol.* **81**:1223–1230.

Storkus, W. J., J. Alexander, J. A. Payne, J. R. Dawson, and P. Cresswell. 1989. Reversal of natural killing susceptibility in target cells expressing transfected class I HLA genes. *Proc. Natl. Acad. Sci. USA* **86**:2361–2364.

Suzuki, H., G. S. Duncan, H. Takimoto, and T. W. Mak. 1997. Abnormal development of intestinal intraepithelial lymphocytes and peripheral natural killer cells in mice lacking the IL-2 receptor beta chain. *J. Exp. Med.* **185**:499–505.

Takeda, K., H. Tsutsui, T. Yoshimoto, O. Adachi, N. Yoshida, T. Kishimoto, H. Okamura, K.

Nakanishi, and S. Akira. 1998. Defective NK cell activity and Th1 response in IL-18-deficient mice. *Immunity* **8**:383–390.

Tay, C. H., and R. M. Welsh. 1997. Distinct organ-dependent mechanisms for the control of murine cytomegalovirus infection by natural killer cells. *J. Virol.* **71**:267–275.

Tomasec, P., V. M. Braud, C. Rickards, M. B. Powell, B. P. McSharry, S. Gadola, V. Cerundolo, L. K. Borysiewicz, A. J. McMichael, and G. W. Wilkinson. 2000. Surface expression of HLA-E, an inhibitor of natural killer cells, enhanced by human cytomegalovirus gpUL40. *Science* **287**:1031.

Tomasello, E., C. Cant, H. J. Buhring, F. Vely, P. Andre, M. Seiffert, A. Ullrich, and E. Vivier. 2000a. Association of signal-regulatory proteins beta with KARAP/DAP-12. *Eur. J. Immunol.* **30**:2147–2156.

Tomasello, E., P.-O. Desmoulins, K. Chemin, S. Guia, H. Cremer, J. Ortaldo, P. Love, D. Kaiserlian, and E. Vivier. 2000b. Combined natural killer cell and dendritic cell functional deficiency in KARAP/DAP12 loss-of-function mutant mice. *Immunity* **13**:355–364.

Tormo, J., K. Natarajan, D. H. Margulies, and R. A. Mariuzza. 1999. Crystal structure of a lectin-like natural killer cell receptor bound to its MHC class I ligand. *Nature* **402**:623–631.

Tortorella, D., B. E. Gewurz, M. H. Furman, D. J. Schust, and H. L. Ploegh. 2000. Viral subversion of the immune system. *Annu. Rev. Immunol.* **18**:861–926.

Tough, D. F., P. Borrow, and J. Sprent. 1996. Induction of bystander T cell proliferation by viruses and type I interferon in vivo. *Science* **272**:1947–1950.

Trinchieri, G. 1989. Biology of natural killer cells. *Adv. Immunol.* **47**:187–376.

Tripp, C. S., S. F. Wolf, and E. R. Unanue. 1993. Interleukin 12 and tumor necrosis factor alpha are costimulators of interferon gamma production by natural killer cells in severe combined immunodeficiency mice with listeriosis, and interleukin 10 is a physiologic antagonist. *Proc. Natl. Acad. Sci. USA* **90**:3725–3729.

Tripp, C. S., M. K. Gately, J. Hakimi, P. Ling, and E. R. Unanue. 1994. Neutralization of IL-12 decreases resistance to Listeria in SCID and C.B-17 mice. Reversal by IFN-gamma. *J. Immunol.* **152**:1883–1887.

Tsunobuchi, H., H. Nishimura, F. Goshima, T. Daikoku, H. Suzuki, I. Nakashima, Y. Nishiyama, and Y. Yoshikai. 2000. A protective role of interleukin-15 in a mouse model for systemic infection with herpes simplex virus. *Virology* **275**:57–66.

Ulbrecht, M., S. Martinozzi, M. Grzeschik, H. Hengel, J. W. Ellwart, M. Pla, and E. H. Weiss. 2000. Cutting edge: the human cytomegalovirus

UL40 gene product contains a ligand for HLA-E and prevents NK cell-mediated lysis. *J. Immunol.* **164:** 5019–5022.

Unanue, E. R. 1997. Inter-relationship among macrophages, natural killer cells and neutrophils in early stages of Listeria resistance. *Curr. Opin. Immunol.* **9:**35–43.

Vance, R. E., D. M. Tanamachi, T. Hanke, and D. H. Raulet. 1997. Cloning of a mouse homolog of CD94 extends the family of C-type lectins on murine natural killer cells. *Eur. J. Immunol.* **27:**3236–3241.

Vance, R. E., J. R. Kraft, J. D. Altman, P. E. Jensen, and D. H. Raulet. 1998. Mouse CD94/NKG2A is a natural killer cell receptor for the nonclassical major histocompatibility complex (MHC) class I molecule Qa-1(b). *J. Exp. Med.* **188:**1841–1848.

Vance, R. E., A. M. Jamieson, and D. H. Raulet. 1999. Recognition of the class Ib molecule Qa-1(b) by putative activating receptors CD94/NKG2C and CD94/NKG2E on mouse natural killer cells. *J. Exp. Med.* **190:**1801–1812.

Viver, E., A. J. da Silva, M. Ackerly, H. Levine, C. E. Rudd, and P. Anderson. 1993. Association of a 70-kDa tyrosine phosphoprotein with the CD16: zeta:gamma complex expressed in human natural killer cells. *Eur. J. Immunol.* **23:**1872–1876.

Waldmann, T. A., and Y. Tagaya. 1999. The multifaceted regulation of interleukin-15 expression and the role of this cytokine in NK cell differentiation and host response to intracellular pathogens. *Annu. Rev. Immunol.* **17:**19–49.

Walsh, C. M., M. Matloubian, C. C. Liu, R. Ueda, C. G. Kurahara, J. L. Christensen, M. T. Huang, J. D. Young, R. Ahmed, and W. R. Clark. 1994. Immune function in mice lacking the perforin gene. *Proc. Natl. Acad. Sci. USA* **91:**10854–10858.

Wang, B., C. Biron, J. She, K. Higgins, M. J. Sunshine, E. Lacy, N. Lonberg, and C. Terhorst. 1994. A block in both early T lymphocyte and natural killer cell development in transgenic mice with high-copy numbers of the human CD3E gene. *Proc. Natl. Acad. Sci. USA* **91:**9402–9406.

Wang, B. P., G. A. Hollander, A. Nichogiannopoulou, S. J. Simpson, J. S. Orange, J. C. Gutierrezramos, S. J. Burakoff, C. A. Biron, and C. Terhorst. 1996. Natural killer cell development is blocked in the context of aberrant T lymphocyte ontogeny. *Int. Immunol.* **8:**939–949.

Wang, L. L., D. T. Chu, A. O. Dokun, and W. M. Yokoyama. 2000. Inducible expression of the gp49B inhibitory receptor on NK cells. *J. Immunol.* **164:** 5215–5220.

Welsh, R. M., P. L. Dundon, E. E. Eynon, J. O. Brubaker, G. C. Koo, and C. L. O'Donnell. 1990. Demonstration of the antiviral role of natural killer cells in vivo with a natural killer cell-specific monoclonal antibody (NK 1.1). *Nat. Immun. Cell Growth Regul.* **9:**112–120.

Willerford, D. M., J. Chen, J. A. Ferry, L. Davidson, A. Ma, and F. W. Alt. 1995. Interleukin-2 receptor alpha chain regulates the size and content of the peripheral lymphoid compartment. *Immunity* **3:**521–530.

Wu, J., Y. Song, A. B. Bakker, S. Bauer, T. Spies, L. L. Lanier, and J. H. Phillips. 1999. An activating immunoreceptor complex formed by NKG2D and DAP10. *Science* **285:**730–732.

Wu, J., H. Cherwinski, T. Spies, J. H. Phillips, and L. L. Lanier. 2000. DAP10 and DAP12 form distinct, but functionally cooperative, receptor complexes in natural killer cells. *J. Exp. Med.* **192:**1059–1068.

Yewdell, J. W., and A. B. Hill. 2002. Viral interference with antigen presentation. *Nat. Immunol.* **3:**1019–1025.

Yokoyama, W. M. 1995. Natural killer cell receptors. *Curr. Opin. Immunol.* **7:**110–120.

Yokoyama, W. M. 1997. What goes up must come down: the emerging spectrum of inhibitory receptors. *J. Exp. Med.* **186:**1803–1808.

Yokoyama, W. M. 1999. Natural killer cells, p. 575–603. *In* W. E. Paul (ed.), *Fundamental Immunology.* Lippincott-Raven, New York, N.Y.

Yokoyama, W. M. 2000. Now you see it, now you don't! *Nat. Immunol.* **1:**95–97.

Yokoyama, W. M., and B. Plougastel. 2003. Immune functions encoded by the natural killer gene complex. *Nat. Rev. Immunol.* **3:**304–316.

Zamai, L., M. Ahmad, I. M. Bennett, L. Azzoni, E. S. Alnemri, and B. Perussia. 1998. Natural killer (NK) cell-mediated cytotoxicity: differential use of TRAIL and Fas ligand by immature and mature primary human NK cells. *J. Exp. Med.* **188:**2375–2380.

Zitvogel, L. 2002. Dendritic and natural killer cells cooperate in the control/switch of innate immunity. *J. Exp. Med.* **195:**F9–F14.

URINARY TRACT INFECTION AS A MODEL FOR INNATE MUCOSAL IMMUNITY

M. Samuelsson, G. Bergsten, H. Fischer, D. Karpman,
I. Leijonhufvud, A. C. Lundstedt, P. Samuelsson,
M. L. Svensson, B. Wullt, and C. Svanborg

8

BACKGROUND: MUCOSAL SURFACES RELY ON INNATE IMMUNITY FOR RESISTANCE TO INFECTION

Mucosal surfaces continue where the skin leaves off and complete the body's mechanical barrier to the outside world. This apparently simple compartmentalization serves to protect internal organs and helps define and maintain the integrity of higher organisms. Despite the challenges from the diverse environmental microflora and the frequent attacks by sophisticated pathogens, most tissues remain sterile and infections are relatively rare. So how is this achieved and what are the mechanisms that fail to function in infection-prone individuals who develop severe acute disease and chronic sequels?

The mucosal membranes are protected by multiple and highly diverse effectors of the host defense. The mechanical barrier serves mainly to limit the microbial mass that actually reaches the tissues, but more sophisticated defenses become involved as different responsive cell populations in the mucosal barrier interact with specific microbes and their products. For example, more than half of all B lymphocytes in the human body are localized along the intestinal mucosa, and more secretory immunoglobulin A (sIgA) is produced daily than any other immunoglobulin (Ig) class. sIgA acts mainly by preventing tissue contact with lumenal microbes or toxins and by clearing the subepithelial compartment of viral and possibly bacterial particles that have breached the barrier (Freter, 1972; Lamm et al., 1995). Mucosal T-lymphocyte populations include the intraepithelial lymphocytes and the $\gamma\delta$ T cells, but in addition, the normal effector T cells are present, executing cytotoxic killing of infected target cells (Ogra et al., 2003). Specific mucosal immunity is essential, and immunodeficient patients show increased susceptibility to many viral and bacterial pathogens.

Yet immunodeficient hosts often cope quite well with other common infections. Their relative resistance illustrates the efficiency of the innate defense. Innate host response mechanisms are critically needed to maintain mucosal integrity, and effectors of the innate mucosal defense include mucins and carbohydrate receptor analogues that prevent adhesion;

M. Samuelsson, G. Bergsten, H. Fischer, I. Leijonhufvud, A. C. Lundstedt, P. Samuelsson, M. L. Svensson, B. Wullt, and C. Svanborg, Department of Laboratory Medicine, Division of Microbiology, Immunology, and Glycobiology, Lund University, Lund, Sweden. *D. Karpman,* Department of Pediatrics, Lund University Hospital, Lund, Sweden. *B. Wullt,* Department of Urology, Lund University Hospital, Lund, Sweden.

The Innate Immune Response to Infection
Ed. by S. H. E. Kaufmann, R. Medzhitov, and S. Gordon
©2004 ASM Press, Washington, D.C.

bactericidal defensins and NO derivatives; and complement and recruited cells such as neutrophils, mast cells, and macrophages. In the lungs, upper intestinal tract, or kidneys, the host defense is designed to maintain sterility, but the upper respiratory tract, large intestine, and genital tract are populated by a rich indigenous microflora and need mechanisms to differentiate between the threats from pathogens and the benefits derived from the commensals. Clearly, complex and highly specific host defense strategies are needed to achieve these different endpoints.

By the same token, pathogens and commensals use quite different strategies to overcome the defense and remain in their hosts. Pathogens have evolved mechanisms to first establish a population at the site of infection and to survive the defense at this site. They then attack the host cells and exploit the eukaryotic cell machinery to their own advantage. Like other "danger signals," the pathogens trigger a first wave of host response mediators that later get amplified through a variety of cellular interactions, leading to symptoms and possibly tissue damage. Commensals, in contrast, have evolved mechanisms of persisting without causing an overt host response, a potentially more successful strategy.

EPITHELIAL CELLS ORCHESTRATE THE INNATE MUCOSAL RESPONSE TO INFECTION

Most studies on innate immunity have focused on macrophages, as these cells are crucial defenders against infection of the systemic compartments. The mucosal surfaces rely on partly different cell types for the initial defense against infection, however. Epithelial cells form the mechanic barrier necessary to exclude microbes and protect the tissues. In addition, the epithelial cells are equipped to sense and respond to the molecular contents in the lumen (Fig. 1) (Svanborg et al., 1999). By translating this molecular information into signals that can reach local or distant tissue sites, the epithelial cells can direct the response to invading microbes (Godaly et al., 2001). The epithelium may remain "inert" or be activated to secrete mediators of inflammation, immunity, and cell differentiation. It is fascinating that vast numbers of bacteria may populate the mucous membranes and viruses may persist for long periods of time without provoking a response in perfectly healthy individuals.

UTI AS A MODEL OF INNATE IMMUNITY

The normal urinary tract is sterile, due to an efficient antibacterial defense. Yet bacteriuria is extremely common in all age groups, and symptomatic urinary tract infections (UTIs) are a major cause of morbidity and mortality. The symptomatic infections are accompanied by a rapid innate host response that causes symptoms and tissue pathology. In acute pyelonephritis, the infectious focus is in the kidneys, whereas in acute cystitis the bacteria remain in the bladder. In patients with asymptomatic bacteriuria (ABU) there is no overt host response. This is the most frequent end result, occurring in about 1% of girls, 2% of pregnant women, and 20% of elderly individuals. If left untreated, a single bacterial strain may persist for months or years at $>10^5$ CFU/ml of urine without significant host response induction (Kunin, 1987; Wullt et al., 2001).

FIGURE 1 Innate responses at mucosal surfaces. (A) The epithelial barrier is breached by pathogenic bacteria. Following the initial adherence, the bacteria activate the epithelial cells to release of mediators of inflammation, immunity, and cell differentiation. (B) In our model, attachment is mediated through P fimbriae. Cell surface GSLs serve as recognition receptors and signaling is via TLR4. (C) The two-step model of the innate host response in the human urinary tract. Step 1: the adhering bacteria break the inertia of the mucosal barrier by triggering a cellular cytokine response. Step 2: the IL-8 chemokine family and the CXCR1 receptor support neutrophil migration across the epithelium and into the urine and, in the process, infection is cleared.

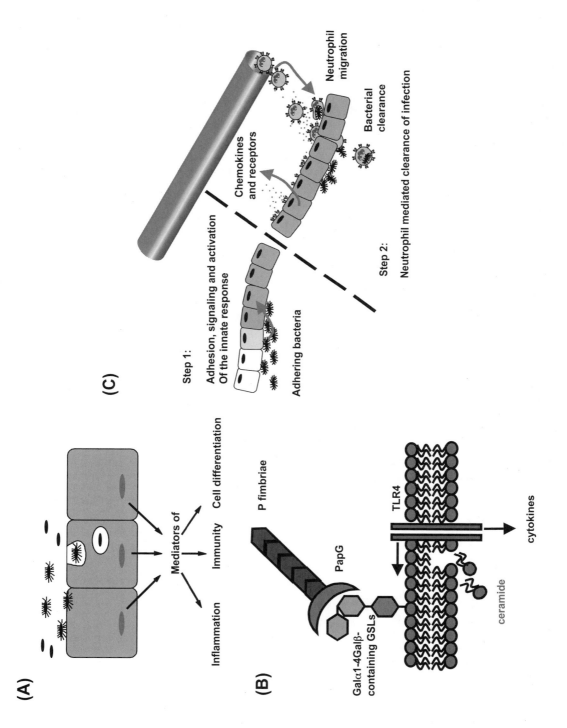

159

The severity of infection reflects the virulence of the infecting strain. Over the past decades, the molecular details of many important virulence factors have been elucidated. The pathogenic *Escherichia coli* clones first adhere to the mucosa and then proceed to interact with the host cells through toxins, capsular polysaccharides, invasins, and other molecules encoded on the chromosomal pathogenicity islands. Indeed, UTIs have served as a very useful model to link specific virulence factors to disease severity (Middendorf et al., 2001; Svanborg-Eden et al., 1976; Svanborg et al., 2002).

The antimicrobial defense of the urinary tract relies on innate immunity (Hagberg et al., 1984; Shahin et al., 1987). There is no preexisting mucosal immune response in the uninfected urinary tract unless the individual has experienced a recent infection. Yet following intravesical inoculation of *E. coli* into the bladder, bacteriuria is cleared within hours or days. Three phases can be distinguished (Fig. 2). A rapid initial reduction in bacterial counts during the first 2 h is followed by a gradual decline until about 24 h, with complete elimination by 2 to 7 days depending on virulence and host background.

The reduction in bacterial numbers during the first 2 h depends largely on the urine flow, but specific host defense molecules like defensins may be involved (Ganz et al., 2001). During this time, the epithelium is activated to produce inflammatory mediators and neutrophils are recruited (step 1, Fig. 1). The subsequent reduction in bacterial numbers depends on these recruited cells, which may

(A)

Kinetics of bacterial clearance

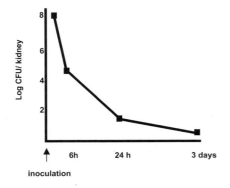

(B)

Impact of specific vs innate immunity defects on UTI

Mouse strain	Genotype	CFU / Ml	p
C 3 H / H eN	Lps^n Lps^n	1.07 ± 1.20	< 0.0001
C 3 H / H eJ	Lps^d Lps^d	3.64 ± 0.31	
BALB/ c	(nu, +)	1.61 ± 1.89	n.s.
BALB/ c	(nu, nu)	0.76 ± 0.97	
N IH Sw iss	(nu, nu)	1.72 ± 0.93	n.s.
N IH Sw iss	(nu, +)	1.07 ± 0.85	
N IH Sw iss	(nu, nu, xid)	2.35 ± 1.02	
C BA / J		1.07 ± 1.29	n.s.
C BA / N	(xid)	1.07 ± 1.56	
A K R		0.20 ± 0.65	n.s.
C BA / J		0.86 ± 1.03	
A / J		1.70 ± 1.46	

FIGURE 2 Bacterial clearance is independent of specific immunity. (A) Kinetics of bacterial clearance. The initial reduction in bacterial numbers and activation of the mucosal response are followed by the neutrophil-dependent phase of bacterial clearance. There is no preexisting specific immune response, and infection is cleared before such a response can be activated. (B) Bacterial clearance is efficient in immunodeficient mice, but deficient in TLR4 mutant mice (Hagberg et al., 1983). These experiments have been repeated in TCR KO and RAG KO mice (Frendeus et al., 2001a). The results show that bacterial clearance from the urinary tract depends on the innate immune system. n.s., not significant.

achieve complete clearance of infection (step 2, Fig. 1) (Haraoka et al., 1999; Shahin et al., 1987). Thus, most infections are cured before a specific immune response is activated, but a specific immune response may occur later in patients who develop severe symptomatic disease or chronic infection.

Further evidence against the involvement of specific immunity in the early defense has been derived from studies in genetically deficient mouse strains. Nude, *xid*, and SCID mice with defective T-lymphocyte, Ig, or B- and T-lymphocyte function were shown to be fully resistant to UTI (Svanborg et al., 1985), as were T-cell receptor α/β (TCR-α/β), TCR-γ/δ, and RAG knockout (KO) mice (Frendeus et al., 2001b), suggesting that specific lymphocyte populations do not contribute to the defense.

In contrast, mouse strains with inherited or induced neutrophil response defects were highly susceptible to pyelonephritis, demonstrating that the innate defense is essential in the urinary tract and that it depends on neutrophils as the main antibacterial effector cells (Haraoka et al., 1999; Shahin et al., 1987). UTIs thus provide one of the clearest examples of innate defense mechanisms maintaining the sterility of the mucosa. In addition, the extensive information about disease pathogenesis makes this a useful model to study the induction of innate responses at mucosal surfaces.

This review concerns (i) the molecular mechanisms used by bacteria to trigger the innate host response, (ii) neutrophils as effectors of the antimicrobial defense of the urinary tract, and (iii) genetic defects in innate host defense pathways that explain the susceptibility to UTI.

BACTERIAL ACTIVATION OF INNATE IMMUNITY: PRIMARY RECOGNITION RECEPTORS AND TLR4-DEPENDENT SIGNALING
Bacterial attachment is the critical event that breaks mucosal inertia (Fig. 3). The urinary tract pathogens achieve tissue-specific attachment through the expression of surface fimbriae with lectinlike domains that bind to

receptor motifs in glycolipids or glycoproteins (Leffler and Svanborg-Eden, 1980). The resulting specific adherence promotes colonization but, in addition, adherence is a virulence factor (Svanborg-Eden et al., 1976). Attachment promotes the delivery of microbial products in a molecular context that allows them to trigger a host response (Hedlund et al., 1996; Linder et al., 1988; Sansonetti, 2001).

P fimbriae, encoded by the *pap* gene clusters, show the most clear-cut association to virulence as defined by acute disease severity (Leffler and Svanborg-Eden, 1981). At least 90% of acute pyelonephritis (but less than 20% of ABU) strains express this phenotype (Leffler and Svanborg-Eden, 1981; Plos et al., 1995) (Fig. 3). P-fimbriated strains remain longer in the intestinal flora, and *pap*-positive strains spread more efficiently to the urinary tract than *pap*-negative strains (Plos et al., 1995; Wold et al., 1988). Once in the urinary tract, P fimbriae enhance the establishment of bacteriuria and may facilitate invasion across the epithelial barrier into the bloodstream (Wullt et al., 2001; Warren et al., 1988). In addition, P fimbriae have a proinflammatory effect, as shown in vitro by stimulation of epithelial cells to secrete interleukin-6 (IL-6) and IL-8 (Godaly et al., 1998; Hedges et al., 1992; Hedlund et al., 1996; Svensson et al., 1994) and by the enhanced cytokine response to *E. coli* in human patients (Wullt et al., 2001).

We have used P-fimbriated *E. coli* to examine the role of recognition receptors and Toll-like receptor-4 (TLR4) coreceptors in epithelial cell activation. We show that cell activation can proceed in two steps, involving a primary ligand-binding receptor and a second receptor responsible for transmembrane signaling, which in this model is TLR4.

GSLs as Ligand Recognition Receptors
E. coli P fimbriae use glycosphingolipids (GSLs) as primary receptors to adhere to the host cells. The receptor specificity is determined by the PapG adhesin, located at the fimbrial tip (Leffler and Svanborg-Eden, 1980;

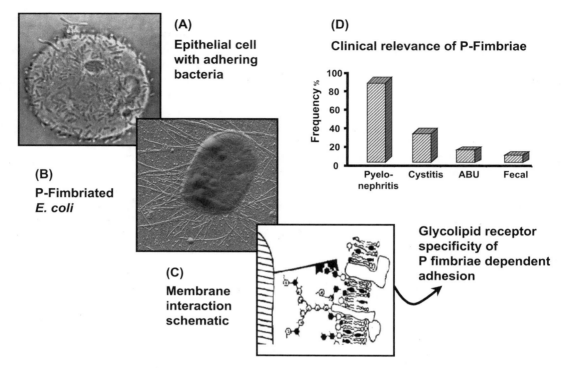

FIGURE 3 Specific adherence as a mechanism of tissue targeting. (A) P-fimbriated *E. coli* adhering to a human urinary tract epithelial cell (bright-field microscopy; enlargement, ×1,000). (B) Fimbriae are adhesive organelles. Fimbrial expression (platinum-shadowed electron microscopy; enlargement, ×15,000). (C) Mechanism of adherence. The PapG adhesin at the fimbrial tip recognizes receptor epitopes defined by the Galα1-4Galβ disaccharide in cell surface GSLs. This interaction initiates the mucosal response. (D) Disease association of P-fimbrial expression. P fimbriae are expressed by >95% of strains causing acute pyelonephritis but <20% of asymptomatic carrier strains and commensal fecal strains.

Lindberg et al., 1987). PapG recognizes oligosaccharide epitopes in the globoseries of GSLs and specifically a Galα1-4Galβ disaccharide motif (Leffler and Svanborg-Eden, 1980; Sung et al., 2001). The GSL-specific binding is critical for cell attachment and cell activation as shown by several experimental approaches. Deletion of the adhesive tip protein PapG abolishes P fimbriae-mediated adherence. The same effect is obtained by the ceramide glycosylation blocker NB-DNJ (*N*-butyldeoxynojirimycin) that selectively removes receptor GSLs from the host cell surface (Svensson et al., 2003). The nonadhesive bacteria fail to trigger the innate host response, even though they carry lipopolysaccharide (LPS) and other surface

molecules that activate a TLR4-specific response in other cell types (Bergstén et al., 2004).

P Fimbriae Release Ceramide from Membrane GSLs

The receptors' GSLs are anchored to ceramide in the outer leaflet of the lipid bilayer and thus lack a transmembrane domain. The binding of P-fimbriated *E. coli* cells to their GSL receptors stimulates an increase in intracellular ceramide levels. Ceramide release and phosphorylation of ceramide are detected within a few minutes after exposure to P-fimbriated *E. coli*, and there is a decrease in surface-expressed receptor-active GSLs, suggesting that ceramide is released by hydrolysis of the receptor itself

(Hedlund et al., 1998, 1996). Signaling involves Ser/Thr protein kinases as shown by the blocking of the chemokine response by Ser/Thr protein kinase inhibitors (Hedlund et al., 1996).

P Fimbriae Recruit TLR4 in Transmembrane Signaling

TLR4 was found to be critical for mucosal responses to P-fimbriated bacteria in early studies using C3H/HeJ mice (Hagberg et al., 1981; Shahin et al., 1987; Svanborg et al., 1985). These "LPS nonresponder" mice carry a point mutation in the Toll-interleukin-resistant domain and express a signaling-deficient form of the TLR4 protein (Poltorak et al., 1998). Subsequent experiments have confirmed that TLR4 mice are unresponsive to UTI with P-fimbriated *E. coli*. In vitro studies in human uroepithelial cells localized TLR4 to the caveoli, adjacent to the GSL receptors, and showed that TLR4 expression is enhanced following challenge with P-fimbriated strains (Frendeus et al., 2001a).

We propose that P fimbriae first bind to the GSL receptors and then recruit TLR4 as coreceptors in signal transduction. This mechanism would allow TLRs to regulate the innate host response without having to be directly involved in the recognition of each specific ligand at the unique sites of infection. The highly specific adherence mechanisms permit each pathogen to first target the appropriate cell and then recruit TLRs for signaling. As ceramide is the membrane-anchoring domain of membrane sphingolipids, this mechanism may allow the TLRs to control responses to a broad range of agonists that perturb membrane lipids. Other microbial ligands with specificity for GSL receptors include cholera toxin, influenza hemagglutinin, or *Pseudomonas* sp. fimbriae.

Role of LPS in the Activation of Epithelial Cells by P-Fimbriated *E. coli*

In CD14-positive cells, LPS binds to the CD14/MD2 complex, which then interacts with TLR4 (Beutler, 2000). Thus, we expected the P fimbriae to activate the cells by delivering LPS to the TLR4 pathway in the uroepithelial cells. The uroepithelial cells lack CD14, however, and thus lack the normal pathway for LPS activation. As a consequence, they respond poorly to LPS challenge in the absence of soluble CD14 (Hedlund et al., 2001, 1999).

The LPS unresponsiveness contradicts the hypothesis of LPS delivery by P-fimbriated *E. coli*. Furthermore, we were surprised to find that the cellular response to whole bacteria is not inhibited by molecules such as polymyxin B or BPI (bactericidal permeability inducer), which inactivate LPS in other systems (Hedlund et al., 1996, 1999). Finally, mutational inactivation of the endotoxic activity of lipid A in whole bacteria did not impair the response to P-fimbriated bacteria. LPS detoxification was achieved by mutating the *msbB* sequences that control myristoylation and toxicity of LPS (Hedlund et al., 1999).

The results suggest that P fimbriae utilize an LPS-like cell activation mechanism in cells that lack CD14 and are refractory to LPS itself (Frendeus et al., 2001b). The prediction would be that the epithelial response is independent of myeloid differentiation marker 88 and IL-1 receptor-associated kinase, which control downstream signaling in LPS-dependent responses. It thus appears that the GSL receptors on epithelial cells serve a function similar to CD14 on macrophages. Whereas LPS targets TLR4 via CD14, the P fimbriae may activate TLR4 via their GSL receptors. In this way they overcome the refractoriness to LPS of the mucosal barrier and succeed in defying the normal control of mucosal inflammation (Fig. 1).

We have speculated that epithelial unresponsiveness to LPS may be essential to maintain mucosal integrity. In the absence of CD14, the indigenous gram-negative microflora is prevented from triggering a continuous and potentially destructive mucosal inflammatory response at colonized mucosal sites.

The urinary tract model also illustrates how the receptor specificity of the fimbriae and the nature of their cell surface receptors may determine the transmembrane signaling pathways that activate innate immunity and direct the cytokine repertoire of infected epithelial cells. By "playing" on the host response keyboard, bacteria may activate different aspects of the host response repertoire.

Clinical Consequences: TLR4-Deficient Mice Develop ABU

The innate response to intravesical infection is abrogated in TLR4-deficient mice. As a consequence, the mice neither clear the infection nor develop symptoms. For example, C3H/HeJ mice became asymptomatic carriers of bacteria in the urinary tract with no evidence of acute inflammation or tissue damage (Fig. 4).

We speculate that similar mechanisms of unresponsiveness may be highly relevant in humans. Asymptomatic bacterial carriage is very common, with frequencies of 1% in schoolgirls, 2% in pregnant women, and about 20% in the elderly (Kunin et al., 1987). We are exploring whether inherited or acquired defects in TLR4 signaling may explain the unresponsiveness in humans as well.

NEUTROPHILS AS EFFECTORS OF THE INNATE DEFENSE

Neutrophils dominate the inflammatory infiltrate during acute UTI and are essential effector cells of the innate host defense (Shahin et al., 1987). Normal mice have a transient neutrophil response, during which bacteria are eliminated from the tissues, but neutrophil-deficient mice fail to clear the infection. The importance of neutrophils has been demonstrated by depletion experiments (Hang et al., 2000; Haraoka et al., 1999) and by infection of mice with genetically determined aberrations in neutrophil migration or activation (Frendeus et al., 2000; Hang et al., 2000).

Molecular Mechanisms of Neutrophil Recruitment

The urinary tract epithelium directs the neutrophil response by secreting IL-8 and other CXC chemokines (Agace et al., 1993a, 1993b). In the Transwell model, recombinant IL-8 was able to replace the bacterial stimulus as the force driving transepithelial neutrophil migration, and anti-IL-8 antibodies blocked the migration in response to the bacteria (Godaly et al., 1997). These in vitro observations have been corroborated in vivo. Epithelial cells in the human urinary tract mucosa synthesize IL-8 (Hang et al., 1998), and intravesical infection causes a rapid IL-8 response (Agace et al., 1993a). Macrophage inflammatory protein 2 (MIP-2) is an important IL-8 equivalent in the murine urinary tract (Hang et al., 1998; Haraoka et al., 1999), and MIP-2 depletion was shown to block neutrophil exit across the epithelial barrier in vivo. Indeed, antibody treatment caused the neutrophils to accumulate under the epithelium, demonstrating that chemokines like IL-8 direct the exodus of neutrophils from the tissues and into the urine.

Fimbria-mediated attachment influences the chemokine response repertoire in that type 1 fimbriated strains elicit mainly neutrophil-activating chemokines (e.g., IL-8 and growth-related oncogene alpha [GRO-α]), whereas the P fimbriae trigger a chemokine repertoire favoring the recruitment of many different cell types, including lymphocytes and monocytes, in addition to neutrophils (e.g., membrane cofactor protein-1 [MCP-1], MIP-1α) (Godaly et al., 2001). For example, the early MCP-1 response may activate mast cells, macrophages, monocytes, and even neutrophils, as receptors for MCP-1 are found on these different cell types.

Infection also enhances the expression of the CXC chemokine receptors on both epithelial cells and neutrophils. IL-8 mediates its biological activity through the G-protein-coupled receptors CXCR1 and CXCR2. Several cell types have been shown to express CXCR1 and CXCR2, including endothelial cells (Middleton et al., 1997), basophils (Ochensberger et al., 1999), dendritic cells (Sallusto et al., 1998), mast cells (Lippert et al., 1998), type 1 helper cells (Bonecchi et al., 1998), and eosinophils (Petering et al., 1999),

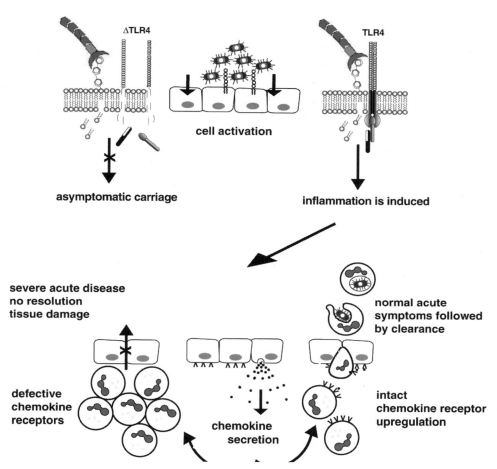

FIGURE 4 Consequences of TLR4 and CXCR1 deficiencies. Step 1: the bacteria bind to the primary targeting receptors and trigger inflammation. The specificity is determined by the PapG protein on the fimbrial tip and the Galα1-4Galβ receptor motif. Activation is through TLR4. Inactivation of the TLR4 signal aborts the inflammatory cascade. This results in asymptomatic bacterial carriage of the bacteria. Step 2: if TLR4 is functional and the response is activated, the epithelium will secrete inflammatory mediators. Neutrophils will be recruited to the site to deal with the infection. In the presence of the human IL-8 receptor, CXCR1, the neutrophils can squeeze through the tight junctions and enter the lumen with their cargo of phagocytosed bacteria. This will eventually result in a clearance of the infection and pyuria, one of the classic signs of an ongoing UTI. In the absence of CXCR1, the neutrophils are trapped under the epithelial barrier. This will inevitably result in tissue damage as the neutrophils release their contents in the tissues.

but these receptors have been most extensively studied on neutrophils. IL-8 mediates its effect on neutrophil chemotaxis predominantly through CXCR1 (Godaly et al., 2000; Green et al., 1996; Hammond et al., 1995; Quan et al., 1996). UTI stimulates CXCR1 and CXCR2 expression in human urinary tract epithelium, and in vitro studies have identified CXCR1 as the crucial receptor required to support neutrophil exit across infected human uroepithelial cell layers (Godaly et al., 2000).

mIL-8Rh$^{-/-}$ Mice Develop Severe Acute Disease and Chronic Tissue Damage

We have used the murine IL-8 receptor homologue (mIL-8Rh$^{-/-}$) mouse to study chemokines and chemokine receptors in the defense against UTI. Mice have a single functional receptor for the IL-8 CXC chemokine family. The neutrophils of the mIL-8Rh$^{-/-}$ mice maintain their sensitivity to other chemoattractants, but fail to respond to the CXC chemokines (Lee et al., 1995).

The mIL-8Rh$^{-/-}$ mice were found to develop severe acute pyelonephritis with bacteremia and symptoms during the first week following intravesical infection. In addition, mice that survived the acute phase of infection developed chronic inflammation and kidney damage. The mIL-8RH$^{-/-}$ mice showed a dysfunctional neutrophil response, in that neutrophils were recruited into the tissues but were unable to cross the epithelial barrier or to kill the bacteria (Color Plate 2). The accumulation of neutrophils resulted in tissue destruction, resembling renal scarring in humans (Hang et al., 2000). After 7 days, mIL-8Rh KO mice had swollen kidneys with neutrophil abscesses. After 35 days, they had developed kidney pathology and renal scarring. Fibrosis was observed under the epithelium and in the perivascular space.

In control mice the neutrophil influx was transient, and the successful exit of neutrophils across the epithelial barrier into the lumen was detected as "pyuria." Infection was cleared in a few days, and there was no evidence of tissue damage.

We conclude that inactivation of a single gene encoding mIL-8Rh is sufficient to convert the mice from a resistant to a susceptible phenotype, as defined both by acute disease susceptibility and by chronic disease development. The chemokine receptors must be functional to avoid the trapping of neutrophils that results in tissue destruction.

These experiments illustrate the compartmentalization of neutrophil migration, with the epithelial barrier shepherding neutrophils out of the tissues. In the mIL-8Rh$^{-/-}$ mice, the neutrophils were unable to cross the epithelium, and thus they accumulated in large numbers under the epithelium and eventually filled the tissues. In the absence of IL-8 receptors, the epithelium appeared to form a virtually impermeable barrier to the neutrophils.

Low-Level Expression of the Human IL-8 Receptor CXCR1 in Patients Prone to Acute Pyelonephritis

There is considerable intraindividual variation in the susceptibility to UTI and in the tendency to develop renal scarring following acute pyelonephritis. The recurrence rate following a first episode of acute pyelonephritis in children is about 30%, and for about 60% of these patients the disease keeps recurring. Failure to resolve the local phase of acute infection may cause renal scarring in children and lead to permanent renal damage. Until recently, no molecular explanations for the differences in disease susceptibility have been offered.

mIL-8Rh shares 69% amino acid identity with the human IL-8 receptor CXCR1 (Cacalano et al., 1994). Based on the results in mIL-8Rh KO mice, we hypothesized that variant receptor expression might also underlie disease susceptibility in the patients who develop acute pyelonephritis and renal scarring. CXCR1 expression was examined in children with documented episodes of acute pyelonephritis and was found to be much lower than in age-matched controls. Furthermore, the CXCR1 mRNA levels were reduced in the patients as compared with the controls. In contrast, we detected no decrease in CXCR2 expression (Frendeus et al., 2000).

SNPs in the *CXCR1* Gene of Pyelonephritis–Prone Individuals

Both IL-8 receptor genes and a homologous pseudogene have been mapped to position 2q34-35 in the human genome (Ahuja et al., 1992; Lloyd et al., 1993). We have obtained DNA from pyelonephritis-prone and age-matched control children. Sequencing of the

CXCR1 gene revealed the presence of single nucleotide polymorphisms (SNPs) in patient DNA but not in the controls. Five heterozygous mutations were identified across the *CXCR1* gene in pyelonephritis-prone children; much less of the CXCR1 receptor protein was expressed in these children than in the age-matched children without UTI, and the CXCR1 sequences in the control population all matched the published consensus sequence. The results demonstrate that pyelonephritis-prone individuals carry new mutations in *CXCR1*.

Ongoing family studies have confirmed the inheritance of the SNPs both from the maternal and from the paternal sides of the family. Through structured interviews, the UTI morbidity in the families is being matched with the presence or absence of the specific SNPs or with the low-level CXCR1 expression phenotype. There is a belief among many clinicians that pyelonephritis runs in families, but no genetic parameter has been found to substantiate this inheritance. Low-level CXCR1 expression and the SNPs thus offer a first molecular handle on the genetic basis of disease susceptibility in the pyelonephritis-prone patient group.

THE TWO-STEP MODEL OF INNATE IMMUNITY IN THE HUMAN URINARY TRACT

Based on the experiments described above, we have proposed a model of innate immunity in the urinary tract, which is illustrated in Fig. 1. Step 1 determines the activation of the innate response. In the case of P-fimbriated *E. coli*, step 1 requires specific GSL receptors for tissue targeting and TLR4 for transmembrane signaling and cell activation. Step 2 is the effector phase involved in bacterial clearance and relies on neutrophils and their IL-8/CXCR1-directed migration and their ability to remove lingering inflammatory cells and bacteria.

Without step 1, the host is not alerted to the presence of bacteria, and the mucosal surfaces maintain their inertia. This can be achieved

either by lack of bacterial virulence or by the inactivation TLR4-dependent signaling. The result is an asymptomatic carrier state, allowing $>10^5$ CFU of bacteria per ml to persist without evoking a host response.

Without step 2, neutrophils accumulate in the tissues and cause an exaggerated inflammatory state with tissue destruction. Bacterial killing is also impaired. In the mouse, step 2 depends on the expression of the mIL-8Rh receptor, and we have evidence that CXCR1 mutations may disarm the host defense and cause severe disease also in humans.

These findings illustrate the importance of the innate host response in the defense against mucosal infection.

ACKNOWLEDGMENTS
This study was supported by grants from the Swedish Medical Research Council (07934, 14577, 14578); the Crafoord, Wallenberg (97.123), Lundberg, and Österlund Foundations; and the Royal Physiographic Society. C.S. is the recipient of an unrestricted grant from Bristol-Myers Squibb.

REFERENCES

Agace, W. W., S. R. Hedges, M. Ceska, and C. Svanborg. 1993a. Interleukin-8 and the neutrophil response to mucosal gram-negative infection. *J. Clin. Invest.* **92:**780–781.

Agace, W., S. Hedges, U. Andersson, J. Andersson, M. Ceska, and C. Svanborg. 1993b. Selective cytokine production by epithelial cells following exposure to *Escherichia coli. Infect. Immun.* **61:**602–609.

Ahuja, S. K., T. Ozcelik, A. Milatovitch, U. Francke, and P. M. Murphy. 1992. Molecular evolution of the human interleukin-8 receptor gene cluster. *Nat. Genet.* **2:**31–36.

Bergstén, G., M. Samuelsson, B. Wullt, I. Leijonhofvud, H. Fischer, and C. Svanborg. PapG-dependent adhesion breaks mucosal inertia and triggers the innate response. *J. Infect. Dis.*, in press.

Beutler, B. 2000. Tlr4: central component of the sole mammalian LPS sensor. *Curr. Opin. Immunol.* **12:**20–26.

Bonecchi, R., G. Bianchi, P. P. Bordignon, D. D'Ambrosio, R. Lang, A. Borsatti, S. Sozzani, P. Allavena, P. A. Gray, A. Mantovani, and F. Sinigaglia. 1998. Differential expression of chemokine receptors and chemotactic responsiveness of type 1 T helper cells (Th1s) and Th2s. *J. Exp. Med.* **187:**129–134.

Cacalano, G., J. Lee, K. Kikly, A. M. Ryan, S. Pitts-Meek, B. Hultgren, W. I. Wood, and M. W. Moore. 1994. Neutrophil and B cell expansion in mice that lack the murine IL-8 receptor homolog. *Science* **265:**682–684.

Eden, C. S., and H. Leffler. 1980. Glycosphingolipids of human urinary tract epithelial cells as possible receptors for adhering Escherichia coli bacteria. *Scand. J. Infect. Dis.* **24**(Suppl.):144–147.

Frendeus, B., G. Godaly, L. Hang, D. Karpman, A. C. Lundstedt, and C. Svanborg. 2000. Interleukin 8 receptor deficiency confers susceptibility to acute experimental pyelonephritis and may have a human counterpart. *J. Exp. Med.* **192:**881–890.

Frendeus, B., C. Wachtler, M. Hedlund, H. Fischer, P. Samuelsson, M. Svensson, and C. Svanborg. 2001a. Escherichia coli P fimbriae utilize the Toll-like receptor 4 pathway for cell activation. *Mol. Microbiol.* **40:**37–51.

Frendeus, B., G. Godaly, L. Hang, D. Karpman, and C. Svanborg. 2001b. Interleukin-8 receptor deficiency confers susceptibility to acute pyelonephritis. *J. Infect. Dis.* **183**(Suppl.):S56–S60.

Freter, R. 1972. Parameters affecting the association of vibrios with the intestinal surface in experimental cholera. *Infect. Immun.* **6:**134–141.

Ganz, T. 2001. Defensins in the urinary tract and other tissues. *J. Infect. Dis.* **183**(Suppl.):S41–S42.

Godaly, G., A. E. Proudfoot, R. E. Offord, C. Svanborg, and W. W. Agace. 1997. Role of epithelial interleukin-8 (IL-8) and neutrophil IL-8 receptor A in Escherichia coli-induced transuroepithelial neutrophil migration. *Infect. Immun.* **65:**3451–3456.

Godaly, G., B. Frendeus, A. Proudfoot, M. Svensson, P. Klemm, and C. Svanborg. 1998. Role of fimbriae-mediated adherence for neutrophil migration across Escherichia coli-infected epithelial cell layers. *Mol. Microbiol.* **30:**725–735.

Godaly, G., L. Hang, B. Frendeus, and C. Svanborg. 2000. Transepithelial neutrophil migration is CXCR1 dependent in vitro and is defective in IL-8 receptor knockout mice. *J. Immunol.* **165:**5287–5294.

Godaly, G., G. Bergsten, L. Hang, H. Fischer, B. Frendeus, A. C. Lundstedt, M. Samuelsson, P. Samuelsson, and C. Svanborg. 2001. Neutrophil recruitment, chemokine receptors, and resistance to mucosal infection. *J. Leukoc. Biol.* **69:**899–906.

Green, S. P., A. Chuntharapai, and J. T. Curnutte. 1996. Interleukin-8 (IL-8), melanoma growth-stimulatory activity, and neutrophil-activating peptide selectively mediate priming of the neutrophil NADPH oxidase through the type A or type B IL-8 receptor. *J. Biol. Chem.* **271:**25400–25405.

Hagberg, L., U. Jodal, T. K. Korhonen, G. Lidin-Janson, U. Lindberg, and C. Svanborg-Eden. 1981. Adhesion, hemagglutination, and virulence of Escherichia coli causing urinary tract infections. *Infect. Immun.* **31:**564–570.

Hagberg, L., I. Engberg, R. Freter, J. Lam, S. Olling, and C. Svanborg-Eden. 1983. Ascending, unobstructed urinary tract infection in mice caused by pyelonephritogenic Escherichia coli of human origin. *Infect. Immun.* **40:**273–283.

Hagberg, L., R. Hull, S. Hull, J. R. McGhee, S. M. Michalek, and C. Svanborg-Eden. 1984. Difference in susceptibility to gram-negative urinary tract infection between C3H/HeJ and C3H/HeN mice. *Infect. Immun.* **46:**839–844.

Hammond, M. E., G. R. Lapointe, P. H. Feucht, S. Hilt, C. A. Gallegos, C. A. Gordon, M. A. Giedlin, G. Mullenbach, and P. Tekamp-Olson. 1995. IL-8 induces neutrophil chemotaxis predominantly via type I IL-8 receptors. *J. Immunol.* **155:**1428–1433.

Hang, L., B. Wullt, Z. Shen, D. Karpman, and C. Svanborg. 1998. Cytokine repertoire of epithelial cells lining the human urinary tract. *J. Urol.* **159:**2185–2192.

Hang, L., B. Frendeus, G. Godaly, and C. Svanborg. 2000. Interleukin-8 receptor knockout mice have subepithelial neutrophil entrapment and renal scarring following acute pyelonephritis. *J. Infect. Dis.* **182:**1738–1748.

Haraoka, M., L. Hang, B. Frendeus, G. Godaly, M. Burdick, R. Strieter, and C. Svanborg. 1999. Neutrophil recruitment and resistance to urinary tract infection. *J. Infect. Dis.* **180:**1220–1229.

Hedges, S., M. Svensson, and C. Svanborg. 1992. Interleukin-6 response of epithelial cell lines to bacterial stimulation in vitro. *Infect. Immun.* **60:**1295–1301.

Hedlund, M., M. Svensson, A. Nilsson, R. D. Duan, and C. Svanborg. 1996. Role of the ceramide-signaling pathway in cytokine responses to P-fimbriated Escherichia coli. *J. Exp. Med.* **183:**1037–1044.

Hedlund, M., R. D. Duan, A. Nilsson, and C. Svanborg. 1998. Sphingomyelin, glycosphingolipids and ceramide signalling in cells exposed to P-fimbriated Escherichia coli. *Mol. Microbiol.* **29:**1297–1306.

Hedlund, M., C. Wachtler, E. Johansson, L. Hang, J. E. Somerville, R. P. Darveau, and C. Svanborg. 1999. P fimbriae-dependent, lipopolysaccharide-independent activation of epithelial cytokine responses. *Mol. Microbiol.* **33:**693–703.

Hedlund, M., B. Frendeus, C. Wachtler, L. Hang, H. Fischer, and C. Svanborg. 2001. Type 1 fimbriae deliver an LPS- and TLR4-dependent activation signal to CD14-negative cells. *Mol. Microbiol.* **39:**542–552.

Kunin, C. 1987. *Detection, Prevention and Management of Urinary Tract Infections.* Lea and Febiger, Philadelphia, Pa.

Kunin, C. M., Q. F. Chin, and S. Chambers. 1987. Morbidity and morality associated with indwelling urinary catheters in elderly patients in a nursing home—confounding due to the presence of associated diseases. *J. Am. Geriatr. Soc.* **35:**1001–1006.

Lamm, M. E., J. G. Nedrud, C. S. Kaetzel, and M. B. Mazanec. 1995. IgA and mucosal defense. *APMIS* 103:241–246.

Lee, J., G. Cacalano, T. Camerato, K. Toy, M. W. Moore, and W. I. Wood. 1995. Chemokine binding and activities mediated by the mouse IL-8 receptor. *J. Immunol.* 155:2158–2164.

Leffler, H., and C. Svanborg-Eden. 1980. Chemical identification of a glycosphingolipid receptor for *Escherichia coli* attaching to human urinary tract epithelial cells and agglutinating human erythrocytes. *FEMS Microbiol. Lett.* 24:144–147.

Leffler, H., and C. Svanborg-Eden. 1981. Glycolipid receptors for uropathogenic *Escherichia coli* on human erythrocytes and uroepithelial cells. *Infect. Immun.* 34:920–929.

Lindberg, F., B. Lund, L. Johansson, and S. Normark. 1987. Localization of the receptor-binding protein adhesin at the tip of the bacterial pilus. *Nature* 328:84–87.

Linder, H., I. Engberg, I. M. Baltzer, K. Jann, and C. Svanborg-Eden. 1988. Induction of inflammation by *Escherichia coli* on the mucosal level: requirement for adherence and endotoxin. *Infect. Immun.* 56:1309–1313.

Lippert, U., M. Artuc, A. Grutzkau, A. Moller, A. Kenderessy-Szabo, D. Schadendorf, J. Norgauer, K. Hartmann, R. Schweitzer-Stenner, T. Zuberbier, B. M. Henz, and S. Kruger-Krasagakes. 1998. Expression and functional activity of the IL-8 receptor type CXCR1 and CXCR2 on human mast cells. *J. Immunol.* 161:2600–2608.

Lloyd, A., W. Modi, H. Sprenger, S. Cevario, J. Oppenheim, and D. Kelvin. 1993. Assignment of genes for interleukin-8 receptors (IL8R) A and B to human chromosome band 2q35. *Cytogenet. Cell Genet.* 63:238–240.

Middendorf, B., G. Blum-Oehler, U. Dobrindt, I. Muhldorfer, S. Salge, and J. Hacker. 2001. The pathogenicity islands (PAIs) of the uropathogenic *Escherichia coli* strain 536: island probing of PAI II536. *J. Infect. Dis.* 183(Suppl.):S17–S20.

Middleton, J., S. Neil, J. Wintle, I. Clark-Lewis, H. Moore, C. Lam, M. Auer, E. Hub, and A. Rot. 1997. Transcytosis and surface presentation of IL-8 by venular endothelial cells. *Cell* 91:385–395.

Ochensberger, B., L. Tassera, D. Bifrare, S. Rihs, and C. A. Dahinden. 1999. Regulation of cytokine expression and leukotriene formation in human basophils by growth factors, chemokines and chemotactic agonists. *Eur. J. Immunol.* 29:11–22.

Ogra, P., L. M., Bienenstock, J. Mestecky, W. Strober, and J. McGhee. 2003. *Mucosal Immunology*, 3rd ed. Academic Press, San Diego, Calif.

Petering, H., O. Gotze, D. Kimmig, R. Smolarski, A. Kapp, and J. Elsner. 1999. The biologic role of interleukin-8: functional analysis and expression of CXCR1 and CXCR2 on human eosinophils. *Blood* 93:694–702.

Plos, K., H. Connell, U. Jodal, B. I. Marklund, S. Marild, B. Wettergren, and C. Svanborg. 1995. Intestinal carriage of P. fimbriated *Escherichia coli* and the susceptibility to urinary tract infection in young children. *J. Infect. Dis.* 171:625–631.

Poltorak, A., X. He, I. Smirnova, M. Y. Liu, C. Van Huffel, X. Du, D. Birdwell, E. Alejos, M. Silva, C. Galanos, M. Freudenberg, P. Ricciardi-Castagnoli, B. Layton, and B. Beutler. 1998. Defective LPS signaling in C3H/HeJ and C57BL/10ScCr mice: mutations in Tlr4 gene. *Science* 282: 2085–2088.

Quan, J. M., T. R. Martin, G. B. Rosenberg, D. C. Foster, T. Whitmore, and R. B. Goodman. 1996. Antibodies against the N-terminus of IL-8 receptor A inhibit neutrophil chemotaxis. *Biochem. Biophys. Res. Commun.* 219:405–411.

Sallusto, F., P. Schaerli, P. Loetscher, C. Schaniel, D. Lenig, C. R. Mackay, S. Qin, and A. Lanzavecchia. 1998. Rapid and coordinated switch in chemokine receptor expression during dendritic cell maturation. *Eur. J. Immunol.* 28:2760–2769.

Sansonetti, P. J. 2001. Rupture, invasion and inflammatory destruction of the intestinal barrier by Shigella, making sense of prokaryote-eukaryote cross-talks. *FEMS Microbiol. Rev.* 25:3–14.

Shahin, R. D., I. Engberg, L. Hagberg, and C. Svanborg Eden. 1987. Neutrophil recruitment and bacterial clearance correlated with LPS responsiveness in local gram-negative infection. *J. Immunol.* 138: 3475–3480.

Svanborg, C., et al. 1985. P. 385–398. *In* E. Skamene (ed.), *Genetic Control of Host Resistance to Infection and Malignancy.* Wiley-Liss, New York, N.Y.

Sung, M. A., K. Fleming, H. A. Chen, and S. Matthews. 2001. The solution structure of PapGII from uropathogenic *Escherichia coli* and its recognition of glycolipid receptors. *EMBO Rep.* 2:621–627.

Svanborg, C., G. Godaly, and M. Hedlund. 1999. Cytokine responses during mucosal infections: role in disease pathogenesis and host defence. *Curr. Opin. Microbiol.* 2:99–105.

Svanborg, C., G. Bergsten, H. Fischer, B. Frendéus, G. Godaly, E. Gustafsson, L. Hang, M. Hedlund, A. C. Lundstedt, M. Samuelsson, P. Samuelsson, M. Svensson, and B. Wullt. 2002. Adhesion, signal transduction and mucosal inflammation, p. 223–246. *In* M. Wilson (ed.), *Bacterial Adhesion to Host Tissues—Mechanisms and Consequences*, vol. 1. Cambridge University Press, Cambridge, United Kingdom.

Svanborg-Eden, C., L. A. Hanson, U. Jodal, U. Lindberg, and A. S. Akerlund. 1976. Variable adherence to normal human urinary-tract epithelial cells of *Escherichia coli* strains associated with various forms of urinary-tract infection. *Lancet* 1:490–492.

Svensson, M., R. Lindstedt, N. S. Radin, and C. Svanborg. 1994. Epithelial glucosphingolipid expression as a determinant of bacterial adherence and cytokine production. *Infect. Immun.* **62:**4404–4410.

Svensson, M., B. Frendeus, T. Butters, F. Platt, R. Dwek, and C. Svanborg. 2003. Glycolipid depletion in antimicrobial therapy. *Mol. Microbiol.* **47:**453–461.

Warren, J. W., H. L. Mobley, and A. L. Trifillis. 1988. Internalization of *Escherichia coli* into human renal tubular epithelial cells. *J. Infect. Dis.* **158:**221–223.

Wold, A. E., M. Thorssen, S. Hull, and C. S. Eden. 1988. Attachment of *Escherichia coli* via mannose- or Gal alpha 1→Gal-beta-containing receptors to human colonic epithelial cells. *Infect. Immun.* **56:**2531–2537.

Wullt, B., G. Bergsten, M. Samuelsson, N. Gebretsadik, R. Hull, and C. Svanborg. 2001. The role of P fimbriae for colonization and host response induction in the human urinary tract. *J. Infect. Dis.* **183**(Suppl. 1)**:**S43–S46.

PANETH CELLS IN INNATE IMMUNITY AND INTESTINAL INFLAMMATION

Satish Keshav

9

INTRODUCTION

Paneth cells are specialized intestinal epithelial cells found mainly in the crypts of the small intestine. They were first reported in the literature in 1872 (Schwalbe, 1872), and Paneth described their microscopic appearance more extensively in 1888 (Paneth, 1888). They are present in all of the mammals regularly used in biomedical research, such as mice, rats, guinea pigs, hamsters, rabbits, and monkeys, as well as in pigs and horses, and Paneth cell–like cells are also found in frogs (Porter et al., 2002; Reilly et al., 1994). Using standard histochemical staining, some reports suggest that Paneth cells are absent from the small intestine of cats and dogs, although this has not been settled (Sheahan and Jervis, 1976). Early reports suggesting that the intestines of cows, sheep, ostriches, crocodiles, and snakes do not contain Paneth cells should be viewed as provisional until they can be confirmed by more specific markers. Their function remained entirely unknown for many years until the localization of various gene products implicated them in

antimicrobial host defense and other processes (de Sauvage et al., 1992; Ghoos and Vantrappen, 1971; Keshav et al., 1990; Ouellette et al., 1989; Porter et al., 2002).

The presence of antimicrobial proteins in Paneth cells, which are secreted in response to bacterial products, implicates these cells in host defense against infection as part of the innate immune system (Bevins et al., 1999; Ganz, 1999; Porter et al., 2002). They may also influence the growth and differentiation of other cells in the intestinal wall and participate in inflammation (Porter et al., 2002). There are striking parallels between the secretory repertoire of Paneth cells and leukocytes, and both cell types, which are normally required for host defense, apparently have the potential to cause harm to the host by promoting self-destructive inflammation. Thus it is important to understand their function and regulation, partly because it may be feasible to modify their behavior for therapeutic ends.

Origin and Location within the Intestinal Epithelium

Paneth cells are located at the bases of the crypts of Lieberkühn, which are invaginations of the surface epithelium in the mucosa of the small intestine. The openings of the crypts

Satish Keshav, Centre for Gastroenterology, Department of Medicine, Royal Free & University College Medical School, University College London, Rowland Hill Street, London NW3 2PF, United Kingdom.

The Innate Immune Response to Infection
Ed. by S. H. E. Kaufmann, R. Medzhitov, and S. Gordon
©2004 ASM Press, Washington, D.C.

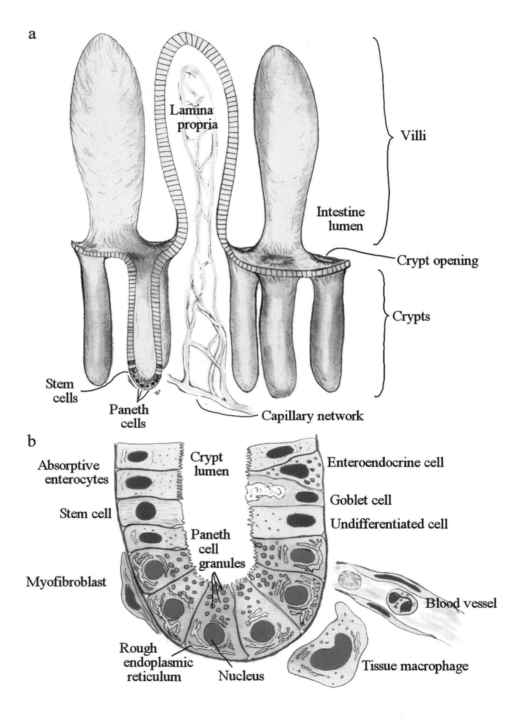

a

Lamina propria

Villi

Intestine lumen

Crypt opening

Crypts

Stem cells

Paneth cells

Capillary network

b

Absorptive enterocytes

Crypt lumen

Enteroendocrine cell

Stem cell

Goblet cell

Undifferentiated cell

Paneth cell granules

Myofibroblast

Blood vessel

Rough endoplasmic reticulum

Nucleus

Tissue macrophage

onto the intestinal surface lie at the bases of the villi, which are fingerlike projections of the mucosa that serve to increase the absorptive surface area (Fig. 1a). Crypts vary in size and composition along the length of the intestine and are deepest in the proximal small intestine (duodenum and jejunum) and shorter distally in the terminal ileum (Bjerknes and Cheng, 1981). There are approximately 10 to 15 Paneth cells at the base of each intestinal crypt, with the lowest numbers in the duodenum and jejunum and the highest numbers in the ileum (Kamal et al., 2002) (S. Keshav, personal observation). In humans, scattered Paneth cells can also be seen in the proximal large intestine (cecum and ascending colon) (Stamp et al., 1992; Tanaka et al., 2001). There are no Paneth cells in the normal esophagus or stomach, nor in the biliary tract or outside the gastrointestinal system. Nonetheless, metaplastic Paneth cells are frequently noted in the large intestine in inflammatory bowel disease (IBD) and in colorectal cancer, and metaplastic intestinal mucosa in the stomach and esophagus may contain Paneth cells (Dieckgraefe et al., 2002; Haapamaki et al., 1999; Lewin, 1969; Stamp et al., 1992; Takubo et al., 1995; Tanaka et al., 2001). Curiously, tumors of the biliary tract, urothelium, and female reproductive tract have been reported to contain Paneth cells (Adlakha and Bostwick, 1994; Lee and Trainer, 1990; Soga et al., 1995).

Intestinal crypts contain the stem cells from which all intestinal epithelial cells are constantly and rapidly renewed, and Paneth cells occupy an intriguing position adjacent to the stem cell zone (Fig. 1b) (Bjerknes and Cheng,

2001; Booth and Potten, 2000; Mills and Gordon, 2001). The three non–Paneth cell lineages derived from the division of intestinal stem cells—absorptive enterocytes, mucus-producing goblet cells, and hormone-secreting enteroendocrine cells—continue to proliferate, differentiate, and migrate toward the opening of the crypt and the surface of the intestinal lumen. Paneth cells, however, migrate toward the crypt base, cease to divide, and remain in situ for approximately 20 days. In contrast, absorptive enterocytes mature and die in 2 to 3 days and are shed from the tips of the villi. Interspersed among the Paneth cells in the base of the crypt are undifferentiated cells, which replace senescent Paneth cells, and a few enteroendocrine cells. Paneth cells are present in the fetal intestine, although numbers are low at birth and increase postnatally, independently of the presence of intestinal microorganisms (Bry et al., 1994; Dinsdale and Biles, 1986).

There are apparently strong signals promoting the differentiation and retention of Paneth cells in the crypt base as chemical ablation of Paneth cells is followed by rapid repopulation, and genetic targeting of a cytotoxin to these cells causes only a partial phenotype (see below) (Garabedian et al., 1997; Sawada et al., 1991). Genetic deletion of ephrin B and its receptors EphB2 and EphB3 in transgenic mice demonstrates that these cell surface molecules, which are downstream targets of the intracellular β-catenin/WNT signal transduction system, are critically important in maintaining the normal position of Paneth cells at the base of the intestinal crypt (Batlle et al., 2002). Ectopic

FIGURE 1 Paneth cells in the small intestinal epithelium. (a) Schematic diagram showing the relationship of crypts to villi and the position of Paneth cells in the base of the crypts. Numerous crypts supply absorptive enterocytes to each villus, which is the major surface for digestion and absorption of nutrients. (b) Cross-sectional diagram showing the relationship of Paneth cells to other cells in the crypt epithelium. Paneth cells occupy the most basal position and migrate toward the base as they differentiate and mature. Stem cells are probably located immediately adjacent to the Paneth cells, and the other intestinal epithelial cell types differentiate and migrate toward the lumen of the intestine and the opening of the crypt. The ultrastructure of Paneth cells is also depicted diagrammatically, showing the prominent rough endoplasmic reticulum, nucleus, Golgi apparatus, and secretory vesicles.

Paneth cells in EphB2- and EphB3-deficient mice display the typical morphology and gene expression profile of Paneth cells, arguing against microenvironment-induced expression of these genes in the crypt base.

Genetic inactivation of the 5-hydroxytryptamine 2A (5-HT$_{2A}$) receptor in transgenic mice causes an approximately 50% reduction in the number of Paneth cells (Fiorica-Howells et al., 2002). This suggests that 5-HT$_{2A}$ receptors, which are expressed on the basolateral surface of Paneth cells, transduce a trophic signal. However, ablation of 5-HT$_{2A}$ receptors also reduces enteric smooth muscle bulk and the number of enteric neurons and enterocytes, so that indirect effects on enteric neuronal function or a more general effect may be operating. Genetic manipulation of rac1 function in the intestinal epithelium demonstrates that this intracellular signaling molecule regulates the rate of Paneth cell and enterocyte differentiation and migration from the crypt, without altering the position or number of these cells within the crypt and villus unit (Stappenbeck and Gordon, 2000).

Paneth Cell Structure

Ultrastructurally, Paneth cells resemble other exocrine secretory cells, such as acinar cells of the pancreas (Mathan et al., 1987; Satoh et al., 1990). They have a pyramidal shape, with a broad base located on the basement membrane of the crypt epithelium, and the apex facing the crypt lumen. They contain an extensive network of rough endoplasmic reticulum that is located in the basal and lateral portion of the cell and a large centrally placed nucleus with a preponderance of transcriptionally active euchromatin. The Golgi apparatus and secretory granules are located in the apical region, which is filled with many large secretory granules. The luminal surface of Paneth cells usually demonstrates a few microvilli, testifying to their origin from intestinal epithelial stem cells rather than from an extraintestinal source, such as circulating lymphohemopoietic precursors. In standard hematoxylin and eosin-stained sections, the secretory granules are intensely eosinophilic, clearly marking out the Paneth cells. The granules can also be specifically stained with dyes such as phloxine-tartrazine, periodic acid-Schiff, and Blancofor BA, as well as pokeweed (*Phytolacca americana*) lectin, so that Paneth cells can be identified and quantitated histochemically (Evans et al., 1994; Porter et al., 2002).

Immunochemical staining for Paneth cell gene products, such as lysozyme and secretory phospholipase A2 (sPLA$_2$), allows more precise identification and quantification (Nevalainen and Haapanen, 1993; Scott and Brandtzaeg, 1981). Although typical Paneth cells are easily recognized morphologically, prominent granules and standard histochemical staining may be lacking in cells that nonetheless have a similar pattern of gene expression and possibly equivalent physiological and pathophysiological roles (Scott and Brandtzaeg, 1981). For example, in mice in which a Paneth cell-specific promoter was used to target expression of the simian virus 40 T antigen, driving continuous proliferation and inhibiting maturation, the number of differentiated Paneth cells was reduced, and intermediate cells appeared with characteristics of both goblet cells and Paneth cells expressing lysozyme and sPLA$_2$ (Garabedian et al., 1997). Similarly, although morphologically distinct Paneth cells are normally not found in the mouse large intestine, basal colonocytes in the crypts express the sPLA$_2$ gene (Keshav et al., 1997). Thus the use of specific markers may reveal that Paneth cells or their equivalents are more widely present than previously appreciated.

Paneth Cell Function

The functions of Paneth cells are largely surmised from their repertoire of expressed genes, while direct experimentation has also confirmed a definite role in protection against enteric bacterial infection (Hooper et al., 2003; Wilson et al., 1999). The main difficulty in determining the functions of Paneth cells lies in the lack of adequate models in which the cells are successfully ablated or augmented and the lack of in vitro culture models of primary cells or transformed lines with Paneth cell-like features.

PANETH CELL-SPECIFIC GENE EXPRESSION

Over 30 different genes with potential roles in antimicrobial defense, growth regulation, inflammation, digestion, and regulation of metal transport and storage have been localized to Paneth cells by a variety of techniques, including immunohistochemistry and in situ hybridization (Table 1). Based on the expression of these genes, Paneth cells are thought to contribute to host defense against bacteria, digestion of microbial products and possibly food substances, regulation of stem cell and progenitor cell growth and differentiation, regulation of inflammation and immune reactivity, regulation of salt and water secretion by enterocytes, and regulation of metal ion absorption, storage, and dispersal, and to respond to a variety of hormonal and microbial signals. A schematic view of how Paneth cell products may function in the intestine is shown in Fig. 2. The earliest products localized to Paneth cells included antimicrobial proteins such as lysozyme and defensins and the cytokine tumor necrosis factor α (TNF-α), which suggested functional homology between Paneth cells in the intestine, and macrophages and neutrophils, which also express antibacterial proteins and inflammatory cytokines and have an established and important role in innate immunity and inflammation (Chung et al., 1988; Ghoos and Vantrappen, 1971; Keshav et al., 1990; Ouellette et al., 1989).

Unfortunately, the list of products in Table 1 is neither definitive nor exhaustive, as some products have only been demonstrated in single reports without independent confirmation; undoubtedly there will be many other granule, cytoplasmic, and cell surface molecules discovered in Paneth cells. Early reports suggested that Paneth cells contained phagocytic vacuoles enclosing bacterial debris (Erlandsen and Chase, 1972a, 1972b). However, these observations, which are apparently inconsistent with the mainly exocrine character of Paneth cells, have not been replicated more recently, despite numerous studies focusing on the interaction of bacteria with intestinal epithelial cells (Ayabe et al., 2000; Garabedian et al., 1997; A. Ouellette, personal communication). Thus, it is unclear if Paneth cells can or do phagocytose microorganisms, although in one report, osteopontin immunoreactivity was noted in structures resembling phagolysosomes within the cytoplasm of Paneth cells (Qu and Dvorak, 1997).

It has been suggested that the unique composition of proteins in Paneth cell granules may cause nonspecific binding of nucleic acid probes, so that in situ hybridization is unreliable for demonstrating gene expression by these cells (Garrett et al., 1992). In our experience, and that of many other investigators, this potential nonspecific interaction does not cause appreciable difficulties; provided that the correct controls are used, in situ hybridization remains a reliable and powerful means of demonstrating specific gene expression. Modern nonisotopic methods of detection allow precise subcellular localization of the RNA signal in the basolateral cytoplasm, away from the protein-rich granules, reducing the risk of misinterpreting artifactual binding of nucleic acid probes to granule proteins (Color Plate 3). There is clearly a need to define the secretory and gene expression repertoire of Paneth cells, and powerful modern technologies such as laser capture microdissection, gene array analysis, and proteomics could help to achieve this (Emmert-Buck et al., 1996; Hooper et al., 2001).

Defensins

Antimicrobial products, such as lysozyme, sPLA$_2$, and defensins, are readily and reproducibly demonstrated in Paneth cell granules from many species, and there is little doubt that Paneth cell secretion of active antimicrobials, and most prominently of defensins, is important in host defense (Ouellette and Bevins, 2001; Porter et al., 2002). The defensins are short, cysteine-rich peptides with a conserved

TABLE 1 Paneth cell gene expression[a]

Gene product	Proposed function	Leukocyte equivalent?	References
Granule products and putative secretion products			
Antimicrobial products			
Lysozyme	Breakdown of peptidoglycan in bacterial cell walls	Macrophages, neutrophils	Chung et al. (1988), Ghoos and Vantrappen (1971)
α–Defensins (cryptdins)	Bacterial killing	Mainly neutrophils	Ouellette and Bevins (2001), Ouellette et al. (1989)
sPLA$_2$ (type IIa)	Breakdown of bacterial cell membranes, possible roles in systemic inflammation	No	Keshav et al. (1997), Kiyohara et al. (1992), Nevalainen and Haapanen (1993)
Angiogenin 4	Antibacterial, ? angiogenic		Hooper et al. (2003)
Secretory immunoglobulin A	Antibacterial		Erlandsen et al. (1976), Satoh et al. (1986a)
Proteolytic enzymes and inhibitors			
Matrilysin (MMP7)	Posttranslational modification and activation of defensins, extracellular matrix modeling, modulates tumor growth		Wilson et al. (1995)
Trypsin	Posttranslational modification and activation of defensins, digestion	No	Bohe et al. (1986), Ghosh et al. (2002)
Secretory leukocyte protease inhibitor	Protease inhibitor, necessary for wound healing, anti-inflammatory	Various cells	Bergenfeldt et al. (1996)
α-1 Antitrypsin	Protease inhibitor	Various cells, macrophages	Molmenti et al. (1993)
Pancreatic secretory trypsin inhibitor	Protease inhibitor		Bohe et al. (1988)
Mpgc60	Homology to protease inhibitors	No	Krause et al. (1998)
Other enzymes			
Phospholipase B/lipase	? Digestive; ? antimicrobial	No	Takemori et al. (1998)
DNase I	? Digestive; ? antimicrobial	No	Shimada et al. (1998)
Xanthine oxidase	Unknown		Morita et al. (2001)
Other products			
TNF-α	Regulation of inflammation, potential role in promoting apoptosis	Mainly macrophages, lymphocytes	Keshav et al. (1990), Schmauder-Chock et al. (1994), Tan et al. (1993)
EGF	Regulation of epithelial cell proliferation and differentiation	No	Poulsen et al. (1986)

Molecule	Function	Cell type	Reference
Guanylin	Regulation of salt and water secretion	No	Cohen et al. (1998), de Sauvage et al. (1992)
Intelectin	Secreted C-type lectin, binds bacterial sugars		Komiya et al. (1998), Tsuji et al. (2001)
HIP/PAP, also regenerating gene III (RegIII) and related Reglα	Unknown, first identified in regenerating pancreatic islets and also found in Paneth cells and in colonic adenomas	No	Dieckgraefe et al. (2002), Masciotra et al. (1995)
Osteopontin	Various. Regulation of bone mineralization, inflammation, tumor metastases	Macrophages	Qu and Dvorak (1997)
CSF-1, macrophage CSF	Macrophage growth factor	Various	Ryan et al. (2001)
Cytoplasmic proteins and other products			
Metallothionein	Sequestration of metals, mainly zinc	Macrophages	Szczurek et al. (2001)
Zinc	Cofactor for enzymes, transcription factors, ?antimicrobial	No	Elmes and Jones (1981), Szczurek et al. (2001)
Rab3D	Regulation of degranulation and secretion		Ohnishi et al. (1996)
Calcium-regulated heat-stable protein (CRHSP28)	Regulation of degranulation and secretion		Groblewski et al. (1999)
NOD2/CARD15	Intracellular interaction with microbial products, mediation of responses to microbial products, mutated in small intestinal Crohn's disease	Monocytes, possibly other leukocytes	Lala et al. (2003)
Membrane molecules and cell surface receptors			
Fas ligand	Induction of apoptosis in Fas-expressing cells	Various	Lee et al. (1999), Moller et al. (1996)
CD1 (murine)	Antigen presentation to major histocompatibility complex class I-restricted T lymphocytes	Various	Lacasse and Martin (1992)
CD15	Phagocytic receptor	Neutrophils	Ariza et al. (1996)
CD44 variant 6	Interaction with epithelial cells, lymphocytes, and other leukocytes	Various	Mirecka et al. (1995)
Serotonin (5-HT$_{2A}$) receptor	Responses to 5-HT, the ubiquitous mediator of intestinal neuroendocrine responses		Fiorica-Howells et al. (2002)

(continued)

TABLE 1 Paneth cell gene expression*ᵃ* *(continued)*

Gene product	Proposed function	Leukocyte equivalent?	References
Vasoactive intestinal peptide receptor	Regulation of secretion		Tsumura et al. (1998)
Prolactin receptor	?Trophic response to prolactin		Garcia-Caballero et al. (1996)
α1E voltage–gated calcium channel	Regulation of secretion		Grabsch et al. (1999)
AE2 anion exchanger	Chloride and bicarbonate secretion		Alper et al. (1999)
MRP	Transport of metals and xenobiotics into and out of cells	Various, including B cells	Peng et al. (1999)
EphB2 and EphB3	Transduction of ephrin B-mediated signaling, positioning of cells in the crypt epithelium		Batlle et al. (2002)

ᵃGenes, proteins, and elements localized specifically to Paneth cells are shown, together with their putative function. Products are grouped according to their subcellular localization and likely function. The contents of the table are not exhaustive, nor definitive, for reasons that are explained in the text.

structure that were first identified as major components of the antibacterial repertoire of neutrophils (Eisenhauer et al., 1992; Lehrer and Ganz, 1992). The two major families, α- and β-defensins, share sequence homology and antibacterial activity and differ in the arrangement of their intramolecular disulfide bonds, tertiary structure, and tissue distribution, with β-defensins more widely distributed in various epithelia (Bevins et al., 1999). There are 19 different Paneth cell-specific α-defensins in mice, where they are also known as cryptdins; there are two in humans, human defensins 5 and 6 (HD5 and HD6) (Ouellette and Bevins, 2001). Mature α-defensins are derived from a larger precursor by proteolytic cleavage, which is catalyzed by matrilysin (matrix metalloproteinase 7 [MMP7]) in mice and trypsin in humans, which are also synthesized and secreted by Paneth cells (Ghosh et al., 2002; Wilson et al., 1995). Paneth cell defensins from mice and humans are active against a number of known pathogens, including *Escherichia coli*, *Salmonella enterica* serovar Typhimurium, *Listeria monocytogenes*, *Candida albicans*, and *Giardia lamblia*, although there is variation in the antimicrobial spectrum of different defensins (Aley et al., 1994; Porter et al., 1997). A further layer of complexity is added by differential regional expression of various defensins in the intestine (Darmoul and Ouellette, 1996). Genetic inactivation of matrilysin causes a measurable defect in host resistance to bacterial infection, clearly suggesting a nonredundant role for Paneth cell defensins in enteric host defense (see below) (Wilson et al., 1999).

sPLA₂

sPLA₂ enzymes comprise a large and diverse group, including intracellular forms that are required for arachidonic acid release and eicosanoid synthesis, and a digestive enzyme secreted by the pancreas (Balsinde et al., 1999). Paneth cell-derived sPLA₂ is distinct from these enzymes and is most similar to bee and snake venom enzymes, with which it shares antimicrobial activity (Harwig et al., 1995;

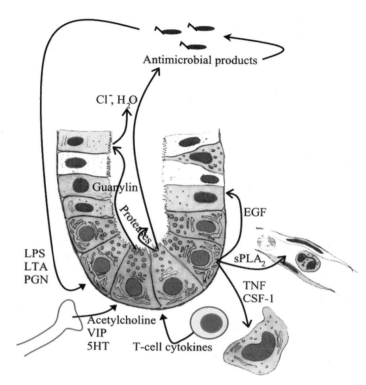

FIGURE 2 Schematic view of Paneth cell gene expression. The putative functions of various Paneth cell products are depicted. Antibacterial products are secreted apically, where they function to regulate the population of microorganisms in the intestinal lumen. Guanylin released apically may stimulate secretion of chloride ions and water from crypt enterocytes, which express guanylin receptors on their luminal surface. Cytokines and growth factors may be released apically or basolaterally and probably act on adjacent cells in the epithelium and lamina propria. Products such as $sPLA_2$ may be released both apically and basolaterally, and they may be secreted in sufficient amounts to enter the circulation. Cell surface receptors on the Paneth cell membrane may mediate interactions with the products of enteric neurons, inflammatory and immune cells, and bacterial products. PGN, peptidoglycan; 5HT, 5-hydroxy tryptamine; LTA, lipoteichoic acid; VIP, vasoactive intestinal peptide.

Laine et al., 2000). Although $sPLA_2$ is not produced by leukocytes, it is found in the circulation, where it behaves as an acute-phase reactant. The origin of circulating $sPLA_2$, which is induced by a variety of inflammatory conditions not necessarily involving the intestine, is probably the liver, which synthesizes the other major acute-phase proteins (Gronroos et al., 2002; Nyman et al., 1996). In addition to its antimicrobial action, $sPLA_2$ may have direct proinflammatory actions and may contribute to atheroma formation by its action on circulating lipoprotein-bound lipids, which may partly account for the increased risk of atherogenesis in chronic inflammation (Ivandic et al., 1999; Leitinger et al., 1999). Inactivation of the $sPLA_2$ gene by an insertion mutation occurs in a number of mouse strains, including C57BL/6, against a background of many other genetic variations and produces no gross defect in host defense, although interestingly the host immune response to duodenal infection with *Helicobacter felis* is altered, and tumor

formation is altered in $apc^{MIN/+}$ mice, which model human familial adenomatous polyposis (see below) (Dietrich et al., 1993; Wang et al., 1998).

Lysozyme

Lysozyme, one of the earliest endogenous antimicrobial proteins described, is secreted in large quantities by Paneth cells and macrophages and is present in neutrophil granules as well as in secretions such as saliva and tears (Chung et al., 1988; Fleming, 1922; Ghoos and Vantrappen, 1971; Gordon et al., 1974). Despite being secreted in large quantities, its in vitro antimicrobial activity appears limited; to resolve this paradox, Fleming suggested that no successful pathogen could exist that was susceptible to this ubiquitously distributed bacteriolytic enzyme. Although its role in host defense has not been formally tested, recent experiments suggest that lysozyme is an important antibacterial component in the lung (Cole et al., 2002). In mice, separate genes direct lysozyme production in myelomonocytic cells and Paneth cells (Cross et al., 1988), and genetic deletion of the myelomonocytic (M) gene produces an interesting phenotype, suggesting that a major function of the enzyme is to limit inflammation by degrading the immunostimulatory peptidoglycan component of bacterial cell walls (Ganz et al., 2003). It would be interesting to determine whether the Paneth cell (P) gene can play a similar role in the intestine, particularly as peptidoglycan-derived muramyl dipeptide is considered the most likely natural ligand for the Crohn's disease-associated *NOD2* gene, which is also present in Paneth cells (see below) (Inohara et al., 2003; Lala et al., 2003; Ogura et al., 2001a).

Angiogenin

The most recently identified antimicrobial peptide secreted by Paneth cells is mouse angiogenin 4, whose expression is greatly increased by intestinal colonization with the commensal organism *Bacteroides thetaiotaomicron* (Hooper et al., 2003). Angiogenin 4 secretion is stimulated by bacterial lipopolysaccharide (LPS) in vitro, and the peptide kills potential pathogens such as *Enterococcus faecalis* and *L. monocytogenes* without affecting the growth of commensals such as *E. coli* K-12 and *B. thetaiotaomicron*. Thus, secretion of angiogenin 4 by Paneth cells, which is regulated by commensal flora, may in turn restrict the growth of pathogens in the intestine and simultaneously allow normal commensals to establish themselves. Human angiogenin also has antimicrobial activity against some pathogens, although the exact spectrum of activity differs from that of murine angiogenin 4 (Hooper et al., 2003). These exciting findings clearly have far-reaching implications for how Paneth cells could maintain a healthy microenvironment within the intestine and potentially influence the development of diseases associated with an abnormal response to bacteria, such as IBD and colorectal cancer (Elson, 2002; Jass et al., 2002; Sohn et al., 2001).

Zinc and Metallothionein

The presence of high concentrations of zinc and metallothionein in Paneth cells is intriguing and unexplained. In zinc deficiency, Paneth cell morphology is altered, and although metallothionein declines to undetectable levels in most epithelial cells, it can still be detected in the cytoplasm of Paneth cells (Elmes and Jones, 1980; Szczurek et al., 2001). Zinc in Paneth cells may represent a store of the metal from which circulating levels can be maintained, and Paneth cells may also regulate uptake and release of this essential but potentially toxic element by neighboring epithelial cells. Zinc may be critical for Paneth cell function itself. For example, a number of Paneth cell proteins bind zinc, and it is required for the functioning of matrilysin, which in mice is essential for processing defensins (Morita et al., 2001).

Guanylin

Guanylin is the endogenous homologue of a bacterial enterotoxin (*E. coli* heat-stable toxin STa) that causes severe watery diarrhea, and ligand binding to its receptor on the cell surface of enterocytes and renal tubular cells stimulates an intrinsic guanyl cyclase activity, increasing intracellular cyclic GTP concentration and consequent chloride and water efflux (de Sauvage et al., 1992). Guanylin could therefore regulate salt and water secretion in the intestine and kidney, and although Paneth cells are not the only, nor the major, source of guanylin, they may play a critical regulatory role (Cohen et al., 1998). In the intestinal crypt, local secretion of guanylin may contribute to defense by promoting net flow out of the crypt, flushing out microorganisms and transporting antimicrobial products to the lumen of the intestine.

Secreted Intercellular Signaling Molecules

Paneth cells express a number of genes encoding secretory products that could mediate intercellular signaling, such as TNF-α, epidermal growth factor (EGF), colony stimulation factor 1 (CSF-1), osteopontin, and angiogenin 4 (Table 1). It is not known if these products are found only in secretory granules, destined for exocytosis at the apical cell surface, or if they are also directed to the basolateral space, from where they may diffuse in the lamina propria and interact with leukocytes and endothelial cells, which are plausible targets (Trahair et al., 1989). Multidrug resistance-associated protein (MRP), which is an ATP-binding cassette protein that could transport endogenous and exogenous compounds across cell membranes, is concentrated in the basolateral membrane of Paneth cells, although it is unlikely to account for the secretion of proteins such as TNF-α and EGF (Peng et al., 1999).

Cell Surface Signaling Molecules

Our knowledge of the signaling molecules present on the cell surface of Paneth cells remains rudimentary. Paneth cell granules are secreted in response to cholinergic agonists, neuroendocrine hormones, and bacterial products, but not fungal or protozoal products (Ayabe et al., 2000; Hooper et al., 2003; Satoh, 1988a, 1988b; Satoh et al., 1992, 1989). Expression of the putative receptors and signaling transduction molecules listed in Table 1 (vasoactive intestinal peptide receptor, 5-HT$_{2A}$ receptor, voltage-gated calcium channel) suggests responsiveness to neurotransmitters; other cell surface signaling molecules involved in microbial recognition, such as Toll-like receptor 4 (TLR4) and CD14, are absent or expressed at low levels (Hausmann et al., 2002; Keshav et al., 1990). The cholinergic receptors mediating secretion have not yet been identified. It will be interesting to identify specific agonists and antagonists that could modify Paneth cell responses.

The presence of membrane molecules that could mediate interaction with leukocytes and other cells is intriguing and suggests that Paneth cell function is coordinated and integrated with that of other cells of the innate and adaptive immune system. Fas ligand, for example, may promote apoptosis of lymphocytes and other cells bearing Fas, whereas CD44 could mediate cell-cell adhesion with subsets of leukocytes (Lee et al., 1999; Mirecka et al., 1995; Moller et al., 1996). Expression of CD1 by murine Paneth cells suggests that they could present glycolipid microbial antigens to intestinal T cells (Lacasse and Martin, 1992). However, expression of CD1 molecules in Paneth cells has not been widely reported, even though it is well recognized that intestinal epithelial cell lines can use these molecules to present antigen in vitro (Blumberg, 2001); further work is necessary to characterize their physiological and pathophysiological significance in Paneth cells.

NOD2 and CARD15

Mutations in the *NOD2* gene are strongly associated with susceptibility to Crohn's disease of the terminal ileum (Ahmad et al., 2002; Ogura et al., 2001a), and the recent demonstration that Paneth cells strongly express both the RNA and the protein for *NOD2* is particularly interesting because it is the first definite link between these cells and a common and important human gastrointestinal disease (Lala et al., 2003). The NOD2 protein is thought to mediate the interaction of mammalian cells with bacterial products, especially peptidoglycan (Inohara et al., 2003; Ogura et al., 2001b). Crohn's disease-associated mutations are clustered in the N-terminal domains, which are homologous to the leucine-rich region domains of TLRs and plant R proteins, which bind microbial components; therefore, NOD2 in Paneth cells, which apparently lack TLR4 and CD14 (Hausmann et al., 2002; Keshav et al., 1990), could be essential for mediating responses to bacterial products. Further mechanistic data are eagerly awaited to determine exactly how the expression of NOD2 in Paneth cells may lead to Crohn's disease, although the localization of NOD2-associated Crohn's disease to the terminal ileum, which has the highest density of Paneth cells, is suggestive of a functional link.

EXPERIMENTAL APPROACHES TO INVESTIGATING PANETH CELL FUNCTION

Paneth cells have not been successfully cultured in vitro, and none of the generally available immortalized intestinal epithelial cell lines display the highly differentiated features of Paneth cells, such as apical secretion and production of highly restricted products such as the α-defensins (Bernet-Camard et al., 1996; Wehkamp et al., 2002). However, many cell lines express genes such as lysozyme genes, which are abundantly expressed in Paneth cells and also in other epithelial lineages such as Brunner's glands and the ulceration-associated cell lineage (Chung et al., 1988; Stamp et al., 1992). For this reason, Paneth cell gene expression has mainly been studied in situ and in vivo. Gene expression studies using in situ hybridization and immunohistochemistry have yielded the greatest amount of information, albeit of a descriptive nature (see Table 1).

Functional data supporting a role for Paneth cells in innate immunity and other functions have come from attempts to determine the effect of gene and cell ablation or by determining the effect of various treatments on Paneth cell numbers, morphology, and secretion. These studies, taken with gene expression data, provide varying degrees of support for a role for Paneth cells in antibacterial defense, intestinal inflammation, intestinal epithelial cell growth and differentiation, intestinal tumorigenesis, salt and water secretion, and metal ion homeostasis and are summarized in Table 2. Evidence from genetically modified animals and the study of naturally occurring mutants have contributed to our understanding of Paneth cell morphogenesis and positioning in the crypt epithelium (Batlle et al., 2002; Wilson et al., 1999; Darmoul and Ouellette, 1996; Fiorica-Howells et al., 2002; Stappenbeck and Gordon, 2000). Attempts to ablate Paneth cells by using the specific cryptdin 2 promoter have been only partly and transiently successful, and they demonstrate that the expression of Paneth cell-specific genes may be maintained even when the formation of morphologically typical Paneth cells is inhibited (Garabedian et al., 1997), which is an important reminder that morphology may be an unreliable guide to the presence and extent of Paneth cells.

Gene and Cell Ablation

The clearest demonstration of an important in vitro role for Paneth cell-derived products in antibacterial defense comes from experimental ablation of the matrilysin *MMP7* gene, which in the mouse intestine is expressed exclusively in Paneth cells and is necessary and sufficient for the posttranslational cleavage and activation of antimicrobial α-defensins (Wilson et al., 1999). Mice lacking matrilysin cannot therefore produce mature enteric α-defensins and as a result are susceptible to infection with bacteria such as *S. enterica* serovar Typhimurium at doses that are nonlethal in wild-type littermates. Matrilysin-deficient mice also develop fewer intestinal adenomas in the *apc*MIN/+ genetic background (Wilson et al., 1997), suggesting that Paneth cells and their products influence the development of neoplasia in the intestine (see below).

Lack of *s*PLA$_2$ occurs spontaneously in murine strains such as C57BL/6, which allowed the identification of *s*PLA$_2$ as the *MOM-1* locus gene, which modifies the phenotypic expression of the *apc*MIN gene (hence MOM for modifier of min) (Dietrich et al., 1993). Absence of *s*PLA$_2$ in the intestine also alters the character of the host immune response to duodenal *H. felis* infection, which may have implications for pathogenesis of *Helicobacter pylori* infection in humans, although a more global defect in antibacterial immunity is not apparent (Wang et al., 1998).

Paneth cells can be selectively killed by injecting the zinc-chelating compound diphenylthiocarbazone (dithizone) into rats, which rapidly depopulates the crypt base (Sawada et al., 1991). The Paneth cell niche, however, is rapidly repopulated within 24 h by accelerated differentiation of progenitor cells in the adjacent epithelium in a process that requires TNF-α production by Paneth cells

TABLE 2 Putative Paneth cell functions[a]

Function	Mediating gene(s)	Supporting evidence	Counterevidence	Conclusion
Antibacterial defense, innate immunity, maintenance of normal commensal microbial species in intestine, preventing colonization by pathogens	Lysozyme, $sPLA_2$, α-defensins, angiogenin 4, metallothionein and zinc, MRP, matrilysin, trypsin, NOD2	Matrilysin knockout is susceptible to intestinal infection; Paneth cell secretion in vivo and in vitro in response to microbial products; Paneth cell hyperplasia in response to intestinal bacterial overgrowth and helminthic infection; increased angiogenin 4 expression in response to bacterial colonization; angiogenin 4 is selectively microbicidal to pathogens and not to normal commensal organisms; Crohn's disease associated with inherited mutations in NOD2 gene that is expressed in Paneth cells	No discernible phenotype in partial Paneth cell ablation model (CR2-Tox mice)	Likely and proven. Extent, specificity, regulation, and abnormalities associated with human disease yet to be investigated in detail.
Inflammation	TNF-α, CSF-1, CD1, CD44, Fas ligand, NOD2	TNF-α in Paneth cells is induced in inflammatory diseases in humans (necrotizing enterocolitis, Crohn's disease) and in rats (hypoxia-reperfusion injury); TNF-α overexpression in TNFΔARE mice causes terminal ileal inflammation; NOD2 mutations associated with terminal ileal Crohn's disease; Paneth cell metaplasia occurs in the colon in inflammatory bowel disease; enteric helminth infection and T-cell proliferation cause transient Paneth cell hyperplasia	Expression of TNF-α is widespread in many cells; CSF-1, CD1, CD44, expression not yet confirmed independently; no discernible inflammatory phenotype in CR2-Tox, matrilysin knockout, or naturally occurring $sPLA_2$-deficient mice	Likely. Direct experimental demonstration required, and relevance to human disease to be determined.

(continued)

TABLE 2 Putative Paneth cell functions[a] (*continued*)

Function	Mediating gene(s)	Supporting evidence	Counterevidence	Conclusion
Influence on epithelial cell growth and differentiation, maintenance of stem cell niche	EGF, TNF-α, Fas ligand	Proximity of Paneth cells to stem cells	No effect of CR2-tox gene on crypt-villus morphology; genetic deletion of EphB2 and EphB3 proteins causes ectopic distribution of Paneth cells with no apparent effect on overall crypt-villus morphology; no Paneth cells adjacent to stem cells in the large intestine	Unproven and seems increasingly unlikely
Effect on intestinal neoplasia	sPLA$_2$, matrilysin, Fas ligand, TNF-α, HIP/PAP (*REG1α* gene)	sPLA$_2$ deficiency increases number of adenomas in $apc^{MIN/+}$ mice; matrilysin knockout causes 60% fewer tumors in $apc^{MIN/+}$ mice; Paneth cell metaplasia expressing HIP/PAP (*reg*) gene is widespread in human colorectal cancer; intestinal tumors very common in the colon (no Paneth cells) and exceedingly rare in the small intestine (abundant Paneth cells)	No mechanism demonstrated for sPLA$_2$ or matrilysin effect on $apc^{MIN/+}$ mice; Paneth cell metaplasia is considered a response to injury in IBD and colorectal cancer	Possible. Plausible mechanistic model lacking. Given that colon cancer is the second leading cause of cancer-related death, may be highly important
Salt and water homeostasis	Guanylin	Constitutive expression of guanylin in Paneth cells	Guanylin and uroguanylin highly expressed by other cells, particularly in the large intestine	Unproven; may yet prove to be important
Heavy metal homeostasis	Metallothionein	High zinc concentrations in Paneth cells; zinc deficiency causes morphological abnormalities in Paneth cells; dietary zinc supplementation augments host defense		Unproven; may yet prove to be important

[a]The major putative functions of Paneth cells are shown, with a comparison of the case for and against each function. Some functions, given the present balance of evidence, are more plausible than others.

and is accompanied by altered patterns of secretion of transforming growth factors α and β-1 (TGF-α and TGF-β1) in the crypt (Seno et al., 2001, 2002).

Targeting an attenuated version of the diphtheria toxin A chain or simian virus 40 T antigen to Paneth cells using the cryptdin-2 promoter potentially allows precise and limited deletion of Paneth cells, and, indeed, neonatal mice born with the targeted transgenes (CR2-tox and CR2-TAg) lack visible Paneth cells (Garabedian et al., 1997). However, Paneth cells repopulate the intestinal crypts in the early neonatal period, suggesting either that transgene expression is suppressed, that crypts in which the transgene is extinguished have a survival advantage, or that strong differentiation factors operating in the crypt promote Paneth cell differentiation despite the local expression of a potent cytotoxin. In fact, despite the lack of morphologically identifiable Paneth cells in the crypts of CR2-TAg transgenic mice, Paneth cell products such as lysozyme and sPLA$_2$ are expressed in cells that are morphologically intermediate between Paneth cells and goblet cells. These data therefore argue in favor of a local influence promoting Paneth cell differentiation in the crypt base in the small intestine (Garabedian et al., 1997).

Initial analysis of CR2-Tox and CR2-TAg mice did not reveal any defect in growth and development of the transgenic animals, nor in the morphology of the intestine, suggesting that Paneth cells are not essential for the normal morphogenesis of the small intestinal epithelium (Garabedian et al., 1997). However, the mice have so far not been subject to an infectious or inflammatory stimulus to determine if they respond abnormally under these circumstances, and the full implications of this particular mouse model may only become apparent after further study (Lencer, 1998). For example, detailed morphological observation of the vasculature of the small intestine in CR2-Tox mice suggests that Paneth cell ablation is associated with an attenuated capillary network in the lamina propria around the crypt and in the villus, which is altered by the presence of enteric bacteria (Stappenbeck et al., 2002).

In Vitro Secretion Assays

Although it has been known for many years that enteric microbial colonization and systemic administration of cholinergic agonists stimulate Paneth cell degranulation (Satoh, 1988a, 1988b; Satoh et al., 1989), this was most conclusively and elegantly demonstrated by Ayabe and colleagues (2000), who reproduced the secretory response of Paneth cells in vitro using isolated intestinal crypts from the small intestine of mice. Secretion was dose and time dependent, and up to 20% of the total cellular content of α-defensins could be released on maximal stimulation. The amount of α-defensin released was sufficient to kill susceptible bacteria in vitro, and the calculated concentrations in the crypt lumen are predicted to be microbicidal. The isolated crypts responded to cholinergic agonists, LPS, lipid A, lipoteichoic acid, and muramyl dipeptide, as well as to whole gram–positive and gram–negative bacteria, although *Cryptococcus neoformans*, *C. albicans*, and *G. lamblia* did not elicit secretion. This powerful methodology can now be used to determine the physiological and pharmacological control of Paneth cell secretion with much greater speed and accuracy than was previously possible. The technique can also be applied to human intestinal crypts obtained endoscopically or surgically, which secrete lysozyme in response to cholinomimetics and bacterial LPS (A. Bromfield and S. Keshav, unpublished results).

In Vivo Infection and Secretory Responses

Paneth cells are present in the intestine independent of microbial colonization, although bacterial overgrowth, for example following the formation of an isolated intestinal loop, causes Paneth cell hyperplasia (Keren et al., 1975). In germfree mice, a change in Paneth cell granule numbers and size is seen following bacterial colonization (Satoh et al., 1986b;

Satoh and Vollrath, 1986). This model has been used to measure secretory responses in response to microbial products, cholinergic agonists, and peptide hormones (Satoh, 1988a, 1988b; Satoh et al., 1989). Recently, using both the CR2-Tox transgenic mouse model and germfree mice whose enteric flora was reconstituted with a single commensal organism (*B. thetaiotaomicron*), Hooper and colleagues (2003) demonstrated regulation of Paneth cell gene expression by bacterial colonization, independent of any changes in Paneth cell numbers. These exciting results suggest a previously unexpected level of complexity in the response of Paneth cells to infection, which may be critically important in host defense.

In mice infected with nematodes, Paneth cell hyperplasia accompanies the successful elimination of parasites, suggesting that Paneth cells play a role in antiparasite immunity (Kamal et al., 2002). This response has been studied in mouse strains lacking various T-cell subsets, and it is apparent that the Paneth cell hyperplasia observed at the peak of infection is dependent on the presence of functional T cells and that intestinal intraepithelial T cells can support this response even in athymic nude mice (Kamal et al., 2001). Paneth cell hyperplasia by itself, however, may be insufficient to ensure parasite expulsion in athymic nude mice (Kamal et al., 2002). Although the exact mechanism by which T cells stimulate Paneth cell proliferation is unknown, cytokines that are essential for immunity to parasites, such as interleukin-4, may be involved, and their role should now be investigated in detail.

Paneth Cells, Stem Cells, and Cancer

The location of Paneth cells adjacent to the stem cell zone of the small intestinal crypts has led to speculation that they play some role in maintaining stem cell function. This has not been proved, and indeed, Paneth cells are absent from the majority of colonic crypts, so that this function seems unlikely. Furthermore, crypt and villus development in *ephB2* and

ephB3 knockout mice is apparently normal, despite the aberrant positioning of Paneth cells in the epithelium (Batlle et al., 2002).

Nonetheless, it is intriguing that carcinoma is frequent in the large intestine and virtually absent from the small intestine. Enteric microorganisms and their products, which include a number of potential carcinogens, could play a role in intestinal carcinogenesis, suggesting that Paneth cells, which maintain the relative sterility of the small intestine, may also be important (Jass et al., 2002; Sohn et al., 2001). Absence of the $sPLA_2$ gene is associated with increased numbers of tumors in $apc^{MIN/+}$ mice, and introduction of a functional $sPLA_2$ gene reverses this phenotype (Cormier et al., 1997; Dietrich et al., 1993). This modifying effect on the apc^{MIN} gene requires local production of $sPLA_2$ in the intestine, although the exact mechanism of how $sPLA_2$ reduces intestinal adenoma formation is still unknown (Dove et al., 1998). Unfortunately, functional $sPLA_2$ polymorphisms have not been found in humans, and so far there is no evidence to suggest that genetic changes in $sPLA_2$ expression affect the risk of inherited or sporadic colorectal cancer in humans (Praml et al., 1998; Tomlinson et al., 1996).

Genetic ablation of matrilysin results in 60% fewer adenomas in $apc^{MIN/+}$ mice (Wilson et al., 1997). However, human Paneth cells do not express the matrilysin gene, although it is expressed in epithelial cells in pancreatitis, gastric, and colonic cancers, where expression is associated with a worse prognosis (Nakamura et al., 2002; Newell et al., 2002). Metaplastic Paneth cells expressing the hepatocarcinoma-intestine-pancreas/pancreatitis-associated protein (HIP/PAP)-related *REG1α* gene, which may be mitogenic, are also noted in a large proportion of colonic tumors (Dieckgraefe et al., 2002; Fukui et al., 1998). Thus, although there are a number of circumstantial observations implicating Paneth cells in intestinal cancer, the mechanistic evidence remains sketchy. For example, are the apparent effects of $sPLA_2$ and matrilysin exerted directly on an aspect of cellular transformation and proliferation, or are they mediated indirectly through effects on microbial flora and/or inflammatory and immune cells?

Paneth Cells in Inflammation

Although infection and inflammation are closely linked pathophysiologically, the role of Paneth cells in inflammatory processes is not yet established. Although Paneth cells are largely absent from the large intestine in health, Paneth cell metaplasia, that is, the appearance of scattered Paneth cells in a proportion of crypts, occurs in the inflamed segment of intestine in IBD (Lewin, 1969; Tanaka et al., 2001). It is unknown whether this response is simply an epiphenomenon related to the various other changes occurring in the inflamed mucosa or is more directly involved in the pathogenesis of IBD, nor if it is beneficial or harmful. The extent of Paneth cell metaplasia may be underestimated by simply using morphological criteria and is usually more apparent when specific markers of Paneth cell-specific gene expression such as lysozyme or $sPLA_2$ are used (Haapamaki et al., 1999; C. Osborne and S. Keshav, unpublished observations). The mechanisms responsible for Paneth cell metaplasia are unknown, although cytokines similar to those that are presumed to stimulate Paneth cell proliferation in response to parasitic infection may be involved (Kamal et al., 2002). The potential role of Paneth cells in IBD is discussed further in the next section.

POTENTIAL RELEVANCE IN HUMAN HEALTH AND DISEASE

Paneth cells present a highly specific, regionally restricted target for therapy in any disease process in which they are implicated. Acute infectious diarrhea remains the single largest cause of infant death in the world, with a disproportionate effect among the poor. The global human immunodeficiency virus/AIDS pandemic exacerbates this situation, as previously relatively harmless organisms opportunistically cause intractable infection (Guerrant et al., 2002). Although most infectious diarrhea can be eliminated by improved sanitation and nutrition, such progress may actually contribute to the increasing incidence of atopic and immune-mediated illnesses in regions where common childhood infections are eliminated—the so-called "hygiene hypothesis" (Strachan, 2000). Similarly, the irritable bowel syndrome, which may affect up to 25% of the population in the West, is associated with abnormalities in the enteric flora in a proportion of patients (Madden and Hunter, 2002). Other common diseases associated with disturbance of the host relationship with enteric bacteria include antibiotic-associated diarrhea and, in severely ill patients, bacterial translocation across the intestinal epithelium, which is implicated in the life-threatening systemic inflammatory response syndrome (Hurley and Nguyen, 2002). Thus, regulation of the interaction of the innate immune system with enteric pathogens is critical for health, and understanding this relationship may allow it to be manipulated to prevent infection and maintain essential functions such as tolerization to environmental antigens.

Intestinal Infection and Necrotizing Enterocolitis

Diarrhea is a standard host response to intestinal infection, and it probably serves to reduce the enteric load of pathogenic microorganisms while simultaneously assisting the dissemination of the same organisms to the rest of the susceptible population via fecal-oral transmission. Guanylin, which is a potent secretagogue, is expressed in Paneth cells throughout the small intestine and also in colonocytes on the surface of the large intestine and may contribute to the secretory diarrheal response following enteric infection (Cohen et al., 1998; de Sauvage et al., 1992). Guanylin may also have a local role in crypts in the small intestine, and the systemic effect of guanylin, which is to stimulate natriuresis, may be mediated by guanylin produced elsewhere (Fonteles et al., 1998; Kita et al., 1999).

Morphological and histochemical studies of Paneth cells do not show any consistent abnormalities in infectious diarrhea, or in chronic intestinal infestations, although these studies may need to be repeated using more specific and sensitive markers and new assays to measure Paneth cell secretory function in vitro. Necrotizing enterocolitis (NEC) is a severe illness affecting premature neonates that are enterally fed with artificial formula feeds rather than breast milk (Kliegman, 2003). NEC is probably triggered by intestinal infection, and inflammation and ischemia localized to the terminal ileum are prominent pathological features (Kliegman, 1990). Although the condition is relatively infrequent, it is the most common serious gastrointestinal disease in neonates and carries a high mortality. Various abnormalities in Paneth cells have been identified in NEC, including overexpression of TNF-α and possibly a deficiency of antibacterial products such as lysozyme and α-defensins, although the data are inconsistent on this point (Coutinho et al., 1998; Salzman et al., 1998; Tan et al., 1993; S. Lala and S. Keshav, unpublished data). Further research is needed to determine if the primary defect in this condition does indeed lie in Paneth cell function, possibly as a result of gestational prematurity and developmental delay.

Zinc Deficiency and Acrodermatitis Enteropathica

Metallothionein and zinc are abundant in Paneth cells, and metallothionein can be detected in Paneth cells even with zinc deprivation, which causes a reduction in metallothionein levels elsewhere (Szczurek et al., 2001). Zinc deficiency causes ultrastructural abnormalities in Paneth cells, and it seems likely that metallothionein and zinc play an important role in Paneth cell function (Kury et al., 2002; Prasad, 1995). Acrodermatitis enteropathica is a rare autosomal recessively inherited condition characterized by the reduced ability to absorb dietary zinc and is linked to mutations in the *SLC39A4* gene, which belongs to a family of zinc-transporting proteins (Kury et al., 2002). The gene is expressed in the kidney and the intestine and most abundantly in the duodenum. In addition to skin lesions and hair loss, patients with acrodermatitis enteropathica develop diarrhea, and ultrastructural examination demonstrates inclusion bodies in Paneth cells. Correcting the zinc deficiency reverses these abnormalities, which mirror those associated with dietary zinc deficiency (Prasad, 1995). Interestingly, zinc supplementation in children augments host defense against enteric pathogens that cause diarrhea, as well against respiratory infection (Baqui et al., 2002; Sazawal et al., 1995). Could the effect of zinc supplementation be mediated by an effect on Paneth cell function?

IBD

Paneth cell metaplasia in the large intestine, associated with IBD and colon cancer, has already been mentioned. TNF-α is critically important in the pathogenesis of Crohn's disease (Papadakis and Targan, 2000), and although Paneth cells in mice constitutively express TNF-α RNA, this is evidently not translated into protein under normal circumstances (Keshav et al., 1990). The TNF-α gene is not constitutively expressed by Paneth cells in humans and rats, although it is induced by inflammation and is readily detected in Crohn's disease-affected tissue (Lala et al., 2003; Tan et al., 1993; Tani et al., 2000). Interestingly, transgenic mice overexpressing endogenous TNF-α, due to the deletion of the 3' untranslated region AU-rich regulatory element (TNFΔARE mice), spontaneously develop inflammation of the terminal ileum, which is the region of the intestine with the greatest concentration of Paneth cells, modeling human Crohn's disease (Kontoyiannis et al., 1999). Thus the TNFΔARE mouse could represent a "Paneth cell-driven" model of intestinal inflammation, although this hypothesis has not yet received experimental support. Bone marrow-derived cells expressing the TNFΔARE transgene can apparently transfer inflammation to recipients expressing the normal TNF-α gene in stromal tissues (including the intestine) (Kontoyiannis et al., 2002). However, Paneth cell-derived TNF-α overproduction may still contribute to the overall pathology, and this possibility could be tested by using a promoter such as cryptdin-2 to target the TNFΔARE construct specifically to Paneth cells.

The expression of NOD2 mRNA and protein in Paneth cells was unexpected (Lala et al., 2003), as circulating monocytes were originally shown to express the gene most abundantly (Ogura et al., 2001b). Nonetheless, as *NOD2* mutations are almost exclusively associated with Crohn's disease of the terminal ileum (Ahmad et al., 2002), it is plausible that the effect of the mutations is expressed through a cell that is particularly abundant in this region of the intestine.

The current working model of Crohn's disease is that an aberrant, genetically programmed response to one or many environmental factors, of which enteric bacteria are the principal candidates, results in chronic granulomatous inflammation, which is amplified and maintained by the recruitment of activated lymphocytes and macrophages (Jewell, 1998; Van Heel et al., 2001). Although Crohn's disease is characterized by extensive local activation of NF-κB, and binding of LPS and muramyl dipeptide to NOD2 activates NF-κB, disease-causing mutations in *NOD2* reduce this response (Inohara et al., 2003; Ogura et al., 2001a; Schreiber et al., 1998). A hypothetical model in which the primary defect in NOD2-mediated signaling is expressed in Paneth cells could resolve this apparent contradiction.

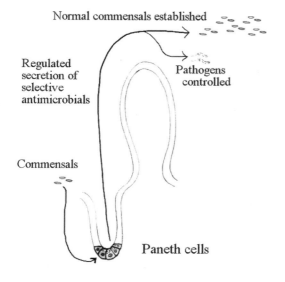
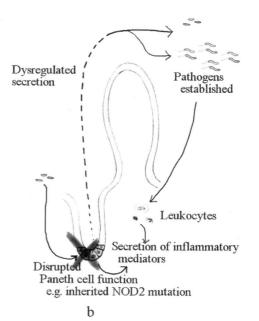

a   b

FIGURE 3 Hypothetical model for the pathogenesis of NOD2-mediated Crohn's disease. (a) In the normal intestinal epithelium, Paneth cells respond to microbial stimulation by secreting antibacterial substances that promote a normal balance of intestinal commensals and suppress the growth of pathogens. (b) Defects in the ability of Paneth cells to respond to bacterial stimulation (for example, caused by inherited mutations in the *NOD2* gene) may allow pathogenic bacteria to establish themselves in the intestine. Such bacteria, in turn, may induce inflammation by interaction with epithelial cells and leukocytes, and Paneth cells may exacerbate the resulting pathology by secreting proinflammatory mediators.

Inherited mutations in the *NOD2* gene might abrogate the appropriate responses of Paneth cells to enteric microorganisms, resulting in dysregulated secretion of antimicrobial peptides and the synthesis and secretion of inflammatory mediators. Dysregulated secretion of antimicrobials might allow the proliferation of previously controlled and restricted potential pathogens, such as the LF82 strain of adhesive-invasive *E. coli*, isolated from patients with Crohn's disease (Glasser et al., 2001). These bacteria might induce inflammation by direct interaction with epithelial cells and leukocytes, stimulating the release of inflammatory mediators and the recruitment of more inflammatory cells, and Paneth cells might exacerbate this process by secreting inflammatory mediators such as TNF-α (Fig. 3). Furthermore, Paneth cell-derived lysozyme may be critically important in degrading and inactivating bacterial peptidoglycan, so that a relative defect in the production of lysozyme could also exacerbate inflammation.

SUMMARY

Paneth cells are a major cellular component of the crypts of the small intestine, and their position, distinctive morphology, and extensive secretory repertoire suggest that they may perform important functions. Expression of antimicrobial genes, and experimental studies showing that Paneth cells respond to bacterial products and are required for enteric host defense, establish them as a significant component of innate immunity in the intestine. Other putative functions, including a role in regulating inflammation in the intestine, modifying the behavior of neighboring epithelial cells, and influencing the course of neoplasia, remain plausible and are supported by circumstantial evidence, largely gained from the study of gene expression and the effects of naturally occurring or genetically engineered mutations in key genes. In addition, they may be involved in many other roles, including the regulation of salt and water secretion in the intestine and heavy metal ion homeostasis. The possibility that Paneth cells play a role in important human diseases, including infectious diarrhea, NEC, and IBD, is also supported by circumstantial data, such as their expression of the Crohn's disease susceptibility gene, *NOD2*. Important further work remains to be done to define the pathophysiological role of Paneth cells and to determine how their function is regulated physiologically and how it may be manipulated to achieve therapeutic aims.

REFERENCES

Adlakha, H., and D. G. Bostwick. 1994. Paneth cell-like change in prostatic adenocarcinoma represents neuroendocrine differentiation: report of 30 cases. *Hum. Pathol.* **25:**135–139.

Ahmad, T., A. Armuzzi, M. Bunce, K. Mulcahy-Hawes, S. E. Marshall, T. R. Orchard, J. Crawshaw, O. Large, A. de Silva, J. T. Cook, M. Barnardo, S. Cullen, K. I. Welsh, and D. P. Jewell. 2002. The molecular classification of the clinical manifestations of Crohn's disease. *Gastroenterology* **122:**854–866.

Aley, S. B., M. Zimmerman, M. Hetsko, M. E. Selsted, and F. D. Gillin. 1994. Killing of *Giardia lamblia* by cryptdins and cationic neutrophil peptides. *Infect. Immun.* **62:**5397–5403.

Alper, S. L., H. Rossmann, S. Wilhelm, A. K. Stuart-Tilley, B. E. Shmukler, and U. Seidler. 1999. Expression of AE2 anion exchanger in mouse intestine. *Am. J. Physiol.* **277**(Part 1)**:**G321–G332.

Ariza, A., D. Lopez, E. M. Castella, C. Munoz, M. J. Zujar, and J. L. Mate. 1996. Expression of CD15 in normal and metaplastic Paneth cells of the digestive tract. *J. Clin. Pathol.* **49:**474–477.

Ayabe, T., D. P. Satchell, C. L. Wilson, W. C. Parks, M. E. Selsted, and A. J. Ouellette. 2000. Secretion of microbicidal alpha-defensins by intestinal Paneth cells in response to bacteria. *Nat. Immunol.* **1:**113–118.

Balsinde, J., M. A. Balboa, P. A. Insel, and E. A. Dennis. 1999. Regulation and inhibition of phospholipase A2. *Annu. Rev. Pharmacol. Toxicol.* **39:**175–189.

Baqui, A. H., R. E. Black, S. El Arifeen, M. Yunus, J. Chakraborty, S. Ahmed, and J. P. Vaughan. 2002. Effect of zinc supplementation started during diarrhoea on morbidity and mortality in Bangladeshi children: community randomised trial. *BMJ* **325:**1059.

Batlle, E., J. T. Henderson, H. Beghtel, M. M. van den Born, E. Sancho, G. Huls, J. Meeldijk, J. Robertson, M. van de Wetering, T. Pawson, and H. Clevers. 2002. Beta-catenin and TCF mediate cell positioning in the intestinal epithelium by controlling the expression of EphB/ephrinB. *Cell* **111:**251–263.

Bergenfeldt, M., M. Nystrom, M. Bohe, C. Lindstrom, A. Polling, and K. Ohlsson. 1996. Localization of immunoreactive secretory leukocyte protease inhibitor (SLPI) in intestinal mucosa. *J. Gastroenterol.* **31**:18–23.

Bernet-Camard, M. F., M. H. Coconnier, S. Hudault, and A. L. Servin. 1996. Differentiation-associated antimicrobial functions in human colon adenocarcinoma cell lines. *Exp. Cell Res.* **226**:80–89.

Bevins, C. L., E. Martin-Porter, and T. Ganz. 1999. Defensins and innate host defence of the gastrointestinal tract. *Gut* **45**:911–915.

Bjerknes, M., and H. Cheng. 1981. Methods for the isolation of intact epithelium from the mouse intestine. *Anat. Rec.* **199**:565–574.

Bjerknes, M., and H. Cheng. 2001. Modulation of specific intestinal epithelial progenitors by enteric neurons. *Proc. Natl. Acad. Sci. USA* **98**:12497–12502.

Blumberg, R. S. 2001. Characterization of CD1d in mucosal immune function: an immunotherapeutic target for inflammatory bowel disease. *Keio J. Med.* **50**:39–44.

Bohe, M., C. Lindstrom, and K. Ohlsson. 1986. Immunohistochemical demonstration of pancreatic secretory proteins in human paneth cells. *Scand. J. Gastroenterol.* **126**(Supp.):65–68.

Bohe, M., C. Lindstrom, and K. Ohlsson. 1988. Immunoreactive pancreatic secretory trypsin inhibitor in gastrointestinal mucosa. *Adv. Exp. Med. Biol.* **240**:101–105.

Booth, C., and C. S. Potten. 2000. Gut instincts: thoughts on intestinal epithelial stem cells. *J. Clin. Invest.* **105**:1493–1499.

Bry, L., P. Falk, K. Huttner, A. Ouellette, T. Midtvedt, and J. I. Gordon. 1994. Paneth cell differentiation in the developing intestine of normal and transgenic mice. *Proc. Natl. Acad. Sci. USA* **91**:10335–10339.

Chung, L. P., S. Keshav, and S. Gordon. 1988. Cloning the human lysozyme cDNA: inverted Alu repeat in the mRNA and in situ hybridization for macrophages and Paneth cells. *Proc. Natl. Acad. Sci. USA* **85**:6227–6231.

Cohen, M. B., J. A. Hawkins, and D. P. Witte. 1998. Guanylin mRNA expression in human intestine and colorectal adenocarcinoma. *Lab. Invest.* **78**:101–108.

Cole, A. M., H. I. Liao, O. Stuchlik, J. Tilan, J. Pohl, and T. Ganz. 2002. Cationic polypeptides are required for antibacterial activity of human airway fluid. *J. Immunol.* **169**:6985–6991.

Cormier, R. T., K. H. Hong, R. B. Halberg, T. L. Hawkins, P. Richardson, R. Mulherkar, W. F. Dove, and E. S. Lander. 1997. Secretory phospholipase Pla2g2a confers resistance to intestinal tumorigenesis. *Nat. Genet.* **17**:88–91.

Coutinho, H. B., H. C. da Mota, V. B. Coutinho, T. I. Robalinho, A. F. Furtado, E. Walker, G.

King, Y. R. Mahida, H. F. Sewell, and D. Wakelin. 1998. Absence of lysozyme (muramidase) in the intestinal Paneth cells of newborn infants with necrotising enterocolitis. *J. Clin. Pathol.* **51**:512–514.

Cross, M., I. Mangelsdorf, A. Wedel, and R. Renkawitz. 1988. Mouse lysozyme M gene: isolation, characterization, and expression studies. *Proc. Natl. Acad. Sci. USA* **85**:6232–6236.

Darmoul, D., and A. J. Ouellette. 1996. Positional specificity of defensin gene expression reveals Paneth cell heterogeneity in mouse small intestine. *Am. J. Physiol.* **271**(Part 1):G68–G74.

de Sauvage, F. J., S. Keshav, W. J. Kuang, N. Gillett, W. Henzel, and D. V. Goeddel. 1992. Precursor structure, expression, and tissue distribution of human guanylin. *Proc. Natl. Acad. Sci. USA* **89**:9089–9093.

Dieckgraefe, B. K., D. L. Crimmins, V. Landt, C. Houchen, S. Anant, R. Porche-Sorbet, and J. H. Ladenson. 2002. Expression of the regenerating gene family in inflammatory bowel disease mucosa: Reg Ialpha upregulation, processing, and antiapoptotic activity. *J. Invest. Med.* **50**:421–434.

Dietrich, W. F., E. S. Lander, J. S. Smith, A. R. Moser, K. A. Gould, C. Luongo, N. Borenstein, and W. Dove. 1993. Genetic identification of Mom-1, a major modifier locus affecting Min-induced intestinal neoplasia in the mouse. *Cell* **75**:631–639.

Dinsdale, D., and B. Biles. 1986. Postnatal changes in the distribution and elemental composition of Paneth cells in normal and corticosteroid-treated rats. *Cell Tissue Res.* **246**:183–187.

Dove, W. F., R. T. Cormier, K. A. Gould, R. B. Halberg, A. J. Merritt, M. A. Newton, and A. R. Shoemaker. 1998. The intestinal epithelium and its neoplasms: genetic, cellular and tissue interactions. *Philos. Trans. R. Soc. London Ser. B* **353**:915–923.

Eisenhauer, P. B., S. S. Harwig, and R. I. Lehrer. 1992. Cryptdins: antimicrobial defensins of the murine small intestine. *Infect. Immun.* **60**:3556–3565.

Elmes, M. E., and J. G. Jones. 1980. Ultrastructural studies on Paneth cell apoptosis in zinc deficient rats. *Cell Tissue Res.* **208**:57–63.

Elmes, M. E., and J. G. Jones. 1981. Paneth cell zinc: a comparison of histochemical and microanalytical techniques. *Histochem. J.* **13**:335–337.

Elson, C. O. 2002. Genes, microbes, and T cells—new therapeutic targets in Crohn's disease. *N. Engl. J. Med.* **346**:614–616.

Emmert-Buck, M. R., R. F. Bonner, P. D. Smith, R. F. Chuaqui, Z. Zhuang, S. R. Goldstein, R. A. Weiss, and L. A. Liotta. 1996. Laser capture microdissection. *Science* **274**:998–1001.

Erlandsen, S. L., and D. G. Chase. 1972a. Paneth cell function: phagocytosis and intracellular digestion of intestinal microorganisms. I. Hexamita muris. *J. Ultrastruct. Res.* **41**:296–318.

Erlandsen, S. L., and D. G. Chase. 1972b. Paneth cell function: phagocytosis and intracellular digestion of intestinal microorganisms. II. Spiral microorganism. *J. Ultrastruct. Res.* **41:**319–333.

Erlandsen, S. L., C. B. Rodning, C. Montero, J. A. Parsons, E. A. Lewis, and I. D. Wilson. 1976. Immunocytochemical identification and localization of immunoglobulin A within Paneth cells of the rat small intestine. *J. Histochem. Cytochem.* **24:**1085–1092.

Evans, G. S., S. Chwalinski, G. Owen, C. Booth, A. Singh, and C. S. Potten. 1994. Expression of pokeweed lectin binding in murine intestinal Paneth cells. *Epithelial. Cell Biol.* **3:**7–15.

Fiorica-Howells, E., R. Hen, J. Gingrich, Z. Li, and M. D. Gershon. 2002. 5-HT(2A) receptors: location and functional analysis in intestines of wild-type and 5-HT(2A) knockout mice. *Am. J. Physiol. Gastrointest. Liver Physiol.* **282:**G877–G893.

Fleming, A. 1922. On a remarkable bacteriolytic element found in tissues and secretions. *Proc. R. Soc. London B. Ser.* **93:**306–317.

Fonteles, M. C., R. N. Greenberg, H. S. Monteiro, M. G. Currie, and L. R. Forte. 1998. Natriuretic and kaliuretic activities of guanylin and uroguanylin in the isolated perfused rat kidney. *Am. J. Physiol.* **275**(Part 2):F191–F197.

Fukui, H., Y. Kinoshita, T. Maekawa, A. Okada, S. Waki, S. Hassan, H. Okamoto, and T. Chiba. 1998. Regenerating gene protein may mediate gastric mucosal proliferation induced by hypergastrinemia in rats. *Gastroenterology* **115:**1483–1493.

Ganz, T. 1999. Defensins and host defense. *Science* **286:**420–421.

Ganz, T., V. Gabayan, H. I. Liao, L. Liu, A. Oren, T. Graf, and A. M. Cole. 2003. Increased inflammation in lysozyme M-deficient mice in response to *Micrococcus luteus* and its peptidoglycan. *Blood* **101:**2388–2392.

Garabedian, E. M., L. J. Roberts, M. S. McNevin, and J. I. Gordon. 1997. Examining the role of Paneth cells in the small intestine by lineage ablation in transgenic mice. *J. Biol. Chem.* **272:**23729–23740.

Garcia-Caballero, T., G. Morel, R. Gallego, M. Fraga, E. Pintos, D. Gago, B. K. Vonderhaar, and A. Beiras. 1996. Cellular distribution of prolactin receptors in human digestive tissues. *J. Clin. Endocrinol. Metab.* **81:**1861–1866.

Garrett, K. L., M. D. Grounds, and M. W. Beilharz. 1992. Nonspecific binding of nucleic acid probes to Paneth cells in the gastrointestinal tract with in situ hybridization. *J. Histochem. Cytochem.* **40:**1613–1618.

Ghoos, Y., and G. Vantrappen. 1971. The cytochemical localization of lysozyme in Paneth cell granules. *Histochem. J.* **3:**175–178.

Ghosh, D., E. Porter, B. Shen, S. K. Lee, D. Wilk, J. Drazba, S. P. Yadav, J. W. Crabb, T. Ganz, and C. L. Bevins. 2002. Paneth cell trypsin is the processing enzyme for human defensin-5. *Nat. Immunol.* **3:**583–590.

Glasser, A. L., J. Boudeau, N. Barnich, M. H. Perruchot, J. F. Colombel, and A. Darfeuille-Michaud. 2001. Adherent invasive *Escherichia coli* strains from patients with Crohn's disease survive and replicate within macrophages without inducing host cell death. *Infect. Immun.* **69:**5529–5537.

Gordon, S., J. Todd, and Z. A. Cohn. 1974. In vitro synthesis and secretion of lysozyme by mononuclear phagocytes. *J. Exp. Med.* **139:**1228–1248.

Grabsch, H., A. Pereverzev, M. Weiergraber, M. Schramm, M. Henry, R. Vajna, R. E. Beattie, S. G. Volsen, U. Klockner, J. Hescheler, and T. Schneider. 1999. Immunohistochemical detection of alpha1E voltage-gated Ca(2+) channel isoforms in cerebellum, INS-1 cells, and neuroendocrine cells of the digestive system. *J. Histochem. Cytochem.* **47:**981–994.

Groblewski, G. E., M. Yoshida, H. Yao, J. A. Williams, and S. A. Ernst. 1999. Immunolocalization of CRHSP28 in exocrine digestive glands and gastrointestinal tissues of the rat. *Am. J. Physiol.* **276**(Part 1):G219–G226.

Gronroos, J. O., V. J. Laine, and T. J. Nevalainen. 2002. Bactericidal group IIA phospholipase A2 in serum of patients with bacterial infections. *J. Infect. Dis.* **185:**1767–1772.

Guerrant, R. L., M. Kosek, S. Moore, B. Lorntz, R. Brantley, and A. A. Lima. 2002. Magnitude and impact of diarrheal diseases. *Arch. Med. Res.* **33:**351–355.

Haapamaki, M. M., J. M. Gronroos, H. Nurmi, K. Alanen, and T. J. Nevalainen. 1999. Gene expression of group II phospholipase A2 in intestine in Crohn's disease. *Am. J. Gastroenterol.* **94:**713–720.

Harwig, S. S., L. Tan, X. D. Qu, Y. Cho, P. B. Eisenhauer, and R. I. Lehrer. 1995. Bactericidal properties of murine intestinal phospholipase A2. *J. Clin. Invest.* **95:**603–610.

Hausmann, M., S. Kiessling, S. Mestermann, G. Webb, T. Spottl, T. Andus, J. Scholmerich, H. Herfarth, K. Ray, W. Falk, and G. Rogler. 2002. Toll-like receptors 2 and 4 are up-regulated during intestinal inflammation. *Gastroenterology* **122:**1987–2000.

Hooper, L. V., M. H. Wong, A. Thelin, L. Hansson, P. G. Falk, and J. I. Gordon. 2001. Molecular analysis of commensal host-microbial relationships in the intestine. *Science* **291:**881–884.

Hooper, L. V., T. S. Stappenbeck, C. V. Hong, and J. I. Gordon. 2003. Angiogenins: a new class of microbicidal proteins involved in innate immunity. *Nat. Immunol.* **4:**269–273.

Hurley, B. W., and C. C. Nguyen. 2002. The spectrum of pseudomembranous enterocolitis and antibiotic-associated diarrhea. *Arch. Intern. Med.* **162:** 2177–2184.

Inohara, N., Y. Ogura, A. Fontalba, O. Gutierrez, F. Pons, J. Crespo, K. Fukase, S. Inamura, S. Kusumoto, M. Hashimoto, S. J. Foster, A. P. Moran, J. L. Fernandez-Luna, and G. Nunez. 2003. Host recognition of bacterial muramyl dipeptide mediated through NOD2. Implications for Crohn's disease. *J. Biol. Chem.* **278:**5509–5512.

Ivandic, B., L. W. Castellani, X. P. Wang, J. H. Qiao, M. Mehrabian, M. Navab, A. M. Fogelman, D. S. Grass, M. E. Swanson, M. C. de Beer, F. de Beer, and A. J. Lusis. 1999. Role of group II secretory phospholipase A2 in atherosclerosis: 1. Increased atherogenesis and altered lipoproteins in transgenic mice expressing group IIa phospholipase A2. *Arterioscler. Thromb. Vasc. Biol.* **19:**1284–1290.

Jass, J. R., V. L. Whitehall, J. Young, and B. A. Leggett. 2002. Emerging concepts in colorectal neoplasia. *Gastroenterology* **123:**862–876.

Jewell, D. P. 1998. Ulcerative colitis and Crohn's disease—susceptibility genes and clinical patterns. *J. Gastroenterol.* **33:**458–462.

Kamal, M., M. S. Dehlawi, L. R. Brunet, and D. Wakelin. 2002. Paneth and intermediate cell hyperplasia induced in mice by helminth infections. *Parasitology* **125**(Part 3):275–281.

Kamal, M., D. Wakelin, and Y. Mahida. 2001. Mucosal responses to infection with Trichinella spiralis in mice. *Parasite J. Soc. Francaise Parasitol.* **8**(Suppl.): S110–S113.

Keren, D. F., H. L. Elliott, G. D. Brown, and J. H. Yardley. 1975. Atrophy of villi with hypertrophy and hyperplasia of Paneth cells in isolated (thiry-Vella) ileal loops in rabbits. Light-microscopic studies. *Gastroenterology* **68:**83–93.

Keshav, S., L. Lawson, L. P. Chung, M. Stein, V. H. Perry, and S. Gordon. 1990. Tumor necrosis factor mRNA localized to Paneth cells of normal murine intestinal epithelium by in situ hybridization. *J. Exp. Med.* **171:**327–332.

Keshav, S., A. J. McKnight, R. Arora, and S. Gordon. 1997. Cloning of intestinal phospholipase A2 from intestinal epithelial RNA by differential display PCR. *Cell Prolif.* **30:**369–383.

Kita, T., K. Kitamura, J. Sakata, and T. Eto. 1999. Marked increase of guanylin secretion in response to salt loading in the rat small intestine. *Am. J. Physiol.* **277**(Part 1):G960–G966.

Kiyohara, H., H. Egami, Y. Shibata, K. Murata, S. Ohshima, and M. Ogawa. 1992. Light microscopic immunohistochemical analysis of the distribution of group II phospholipase A2 in human digestive organs. *J. Histochem. Cytochem.* **40:**1659–1664.

Kliegman, R. M. 1990. Models of the pathogenesis of necrotizing enterocolitis. *J. Pediatr.* **117**(Part 2):S2–S5.

Kliegman, R. M. 2003. The relationship of neonatal feeding practices and the pathogenesis and prevention of necrotizing enterocolitis. *Pediatrics* **111:**671–672.

Komiya, T., Y. Tanigawa, and S. Hirohashi. 1998. Cloning of the novel gene intelectin, which is expressed in intestinal paneth cells in mice. *Biochem. Biophys. Res. Commun.* **251:**759–762.

Kontoyiannis, D., M. Pasparakis, T. T. Pizarro, F. Cominelli, and G. Kollias. 1999. Impaired on/off regulation of TNF biosynthesis in mice lacking TNF AU-rich elements: implications for joint and gut-associated immunopathologies. *Immunity* **10:**387–398.

Kontoyiannis, D., G. Boulougouris, M. Manoloukos, M. Armaka, M. Apostolaki, T. Pizarro, A. Kotlyarov, I. Forster, R. Flavell, M. Gaestel, P. Tsichlis, F. Cominelli, and G. Kollias. 2002. Genetic dissection of the cellular pathways and signaling mechanisms in modeled tumor necrosis factor-induced Crohn's-like inflammatory bowel disease. *J. Exp. Med.* **196:**1563–1574.

Krause, R., M. Hemberger, M. Messerschmid, W. Mayer, R. Kothary, C. Dixkens, and R. Fundele. 1998. Molecular cloning and characterization of murine Mpgc60, a gene predominantly expressed in the intestinal tract. *Differentiation* **63:**285–294.

Kury, S., B. Dreno, S. Bezieau, S. Giraudet, M. Kharfi, R. Kamoun, and J. P. Moisan. 2002. Identification of SLC39A4, a gene involved in acrodermatitis enteropathica. *Nat. Genet.* **31:**239–240.

Lacasse, J., and L. H. Martin. 1992. Detection of CD1 mRNA in Paneth cells of the mouse intestine by in situ hybridization. *J. Histochem. Cytochem.* **40:**1527–1534.

Laine, V. J., D. S. Grass, and T. J. Nevalainen. 2000. Resistance of transgenic mice expressing human group II phospholipase A2 to *Escherichia coli* infection. *Infect. Immun.* **68:**87–92.

Lala, S., Y. Ogura, C. Osborne, S.-Y. Hor, A. Bromfield, S. Davies, O. Ogunbiyi, G. Nuñez, and S. Keshav. 2003. Crohn's disease and the NOD2 gene: a role for Paneth cells. *Gastroenterology* **125:**47–57.

Lee, K. R., and T. D. Trainer. 1990. Adenocarcinoma of the uterine cervix of small intestinal type containing numerous Paneth cells. *Arch. Pathol. Lab. Med.* **114:**731–733.

Lee, S. H., M. S. Shin, W. S. Park, S. Y. Kim, S. M. Dong, H. K. Lee, J. Y. Park, R. R. Oh, J. J. Jang, J. Y. Lee, and N. J. Yoo. 1999. Immunohistochemical analysis of Fas ligand expression in normal human tissues. *APMIS* **107:**1013–1019.

Lehrer, R. I., and T. Ganz. 1992. Defensins: endogenous antibiotic peptides from human leukocytes. *Ciba Found. Symp.* **171:**276–290.

Leitinger, N., A. D. Watson, S. Y. Hama, B. Ivandic, J. H. Qiao, J. Huber, K. F. Faull, D. S.

Grass, M. Navab, A. M. Fogelman, F. C. de Beer, A. J. Lusis, and J. A. Berliner. 1999. Role of group II secretory phospholipase A2 in atherosclerosis: 2. Potential involvement of biologically active oxidized phospholipids. *Arterioscler. Thromb. Vasc. Biol.* **19**:1291–1298.

Lencer, W. I. 1998. Paneth cells: on the front line or in the backfield? *Gastroenterology* **114**:1343–1345.

Lewin, K. 1969. The Paneth cell in disease. *Gut* **10**:804–811.

Madden, J. A., and J. O. Hunter. 2002. A review of the role of the gut microflora in irritable bowel syndrome and the effects of probiotics. *Br. J. Nutr.* **88**(Suppl. 1):S67–S72.

Masciotra, L., P. Lechene de la Porte, J. M. Frigerio, N. J. Dusetti, J. C. Dagorn, and J. L. Iovanna. 1995. Immunocytochemical localization of pancreatitis-associated protein in human small intestine. *Dig. Dis. Sci.* **40**:519–524.

Mathan, M., J. Hughes, and R. Whitehead. 1987. The morphogenesis of the human Paneth cell. An immunocytochemical ultrastructural study. *Histochemistry* **87**:91–96.

Mills, J. C., and J. I. Gordon. 2001. The intestinal stem cell niche: there grows the neighborhood. *Proc. Natl. Acad. Sci. USA* **98**:12334–12336.

Mirecka, J., D. Marx, and A. Schauer. 1995. Immunohistochemical localization of CD44 variants 5 and 6 in human gastric mucosa and gastric cancer. *Anticancer Res.* **15**:1459–1465.

Moller, P., H. Walczak, S. Reidl, J. Strater, and P. H. Krammer. 1996. Paneth cells express high levels of CD95 ligand transcripts: a unique property among gastrointestinal epithelia. *Am. J. Pathol.* **149**:9–13.

Molmenti, E. P., D. H. Perlmutter, and D. C. Rubin. 1993. Cell-specific expression of alpha 1-antitrypsin in human intestinal epithelium. *J. Clin. Invest.* **92**:2022–2034.

Morita, Y., M. Sawada, H. Seno, S. Takaishi, H. Fukuzawa, N. Miyake, H. Hiai, and T. Chiba. 2001. Identification of xanthine dehydrogenase/xanthine oxidase as a rat Paneth cell zinc-binding protein. *Biochim. Biophys. Acta* **1540**:43–49.

Nakamura, H., S. Horita, N. Senmaru, Y. Miyasaka, T. Gohda, Y. Inoue, M. Fujita, T. Meguro, T. Morita, and K. Nagashima. 2002. Association of matrilysin expression with progression and poor prognosis in human pancreatic adenocarcinoma. *Oncol. Rep.* **9**:751–755.

Nevalainen, T. J., and T. J. Haapanen. 1993. Distribution of pancreatic (group I) and synovial-type (group II) phospholipases A2 in human tissues. *Inflammation* **17**:453–464.

Newell, K. J., L. M. Matrisian, and D. K. Driman. 2002. Matrilysin (matrix metalloproteinase-7) expression in ulcerative colitis-related tumorigenesis. *Mol. Carcinog.* **34**:59–63.

Nyman, K. M., W. Uhl, J. Forsstrom, M. Buchler, H. G. Beger, and T. J. Nevalainen. 1996. Serum phospholipase A2 in patients with multiple organ failure. *J. Surg. Res.* **60**:7–14.

Ogura, Y., D. K. Bonen, N. Inohara, D. L. Nicolae, F. F. Chen, R. Ramos, H. Britton, T. Moran, R. Karaliuskas, R. H. Duerr, J. P. Achkar, S. R. Brant, T. M. Bayless, B. S. Kirschner, S. B. Hanauer, G. Nunez, and J. H. Cho. 2001a. A frameshift mutation in NOD2 associated with susceptibility to Crohn's disease. *Nature* **411**:603–606.

Ogura, Y., N. Inohara, A. Benito, F. F. Chen, S. Yamaoka, and G. Nunez. 2001b. Nod2, a Nod1/Apaf-1 family member that is restricted to monocytes and activates NF-kappaB. *J. Biol. Chem.* **276**:4812–4818.

Ohnishi, H., S. A. Ernst, N. Wys, M. McNiven, and J. A. Williams. 1996. Rab3D localizes to zymogen granules in rat pancreatic acini and other exocrine glands. *Am. J. Physiol.* **271**(Part 1):G531–G538.

Ouellette, A. J., and C. L. Bevins. 2001. Paneth cell defensins and innate immunity of the small bowel. *Inflamm. Bowel Dis.* **7**:43–50.

Ouellette, A. J., R. M. Greco, M. James, D. Frederick, J. Naftilan, and J. T. Fallon. 1989. Developmental regulation of cryptdin, a corticostatin/defensin precursor mRNA in mouse small intestinal crypt epithelium. *J. Cell Biol.* **108**:1687–1695.

Paneth, J. 1888. Ueber die secernirenden Zellen des Dunndarm-Epithels. *Arch. Mikroskop. Anat.* **31**:113–191.

Papadakis, K. A., and S. R. Targan. 2000. Tumor necrosis factor: biology and therapeutic inhibitors. *Gastroenterology* **119**:1148–1157.

Peng, K. C., F. Cluzeaud, M. Bens, J. P. Van Huyen, M. A. Wioland, R. Lacave, and A. Vandewalle. 1999. Tissue and cell distribution of the multidrug resistance-associated protein (MRP) in mouse intestine and kidney. *J. Histochem. Cytochem.* **47**:757–768.

Porter, E. M., E. van Dam, E. V. Valore, and T. Ganz. 1997. Broad-spectrum antimicrobial activity of human intestinal defensin 5. *Infect. Immun.* **65**:2396–2401.

Porter, E. M., C. L. Bevins, D. Ghosh, and T. Ganz. 2002. The multifaceted Paneth cell. *Cell. Mol. Life Sci.* **59**:156–170.

Poulsen, S. S., E. Nexo, P. S. Olsen, J. Hess, and P. Kirkegaard. 1986. Immunohistochemical localization of epidermal growth factor in rat and man. *Histochemistry* **85**:389–394.

Praml, C., L. C. Amler, S. Dihlmann, L. H. Finke, P. Schlag, and M. Schwab. 1998. Secretory type II phospholipase A2 (PLA2G2A) expression status in colorectal carcinoma derived cell lines and in normal colonic mucosa. *Oncogene* **17**:2009–2012.

Prasad, A. S. 1995. Zinc: an overview. *Nutrition* **11**(Suppl. 1):93–99.

Qu, H., and A. M. Dvorak. 1997. Ultrastructural localization of osteopontin immunoreactivity in phagolysosomes and secretory granules of cells in human intestine. *Histochem. J.* **29**:801–812.

Reilly, D. S., N. Tomassini, C. L. Bevins, and M. Zasloff. 1994. A Paneth cell analogue in Xenopus small intestine expresses antimicrobial peptide genes: conservation of an intestinal host-defense system. *J. Histochem. Cytochem.* **42**:697–704.

Ryan, G. R., X. M. Dai, M. G. Dominguez, W. Tong, F. Chuan, O. Chisholm, R. G. Russell, J. W. Pollard, and E. R. Stanley. 2001. Rescue of the colony-stimulating factor 1 (CSF-1)-nullizygous mouse (Csf1(op)/Csf1(op)) phenotype with a CSF-1 transgene and identification of sites of local CSF-1 synthesis. *Blood* **98**:74–84.

Salzman, N. H., R. A. Polin, M. C. Harris, E. Ruchelli, A. Hebra, S. Zirin-Butler, A. Jawad, E. Martin Porter, and C. L. Bevins. 1998. Enteric defensin expression in necrotizing enterocolitis. *Pediatr. Res.* **44**:20–26.

Satoh, Y. 1988a. Atropine inhibits the degranulation of Paneth cells in ex-germ-free mice. *Cell Tissue Res.* **253**:397–402.

Satoh, Y. 1988b. Effect of live and heat-killed bacteria on the secretory activity of Paneth cells in germ-free mice. *Cell Tissue Res.* **251**:87–93.

Satoh, Y., and L. Vollrath. 1986. Quantitative electron microscopic observations on Paneth cells of germfree and ex-germfree Wistar rats. *Anat. Embryol.* **173**:317–322.

Satoh, Y., K. Ishikawa, H. Tanaka, and K. Ono. 1986a. Immunohistochemical observations of immunoglobulin A in the Paneth cells of germ-free and formerly-germ-free rats. *Histochemistry* **85**:197–201.

Satoh, Y., K. Ishikawa, K. Ono, and L. Vollrath. 1986b. Quantitative light microscopic observations on Paneth cells of germ-free and ex-germ-free Wistar rats. *Digestion* **34**:115–121.

Satoh, Y., K. Ishikawa, Y. Oomori, M. Yamano, and K. Ono. 1989. Effects of cholecystokinin and carbamylcholine on Paneth cell secretion in mice: a comparison with pancreatic acinar cells. *Anat. Rec.* **225**:124–132.

Satoh, Y., M. Yamano, M. Matsuda, and K. Ono. 1990. Ultrastructure of Paneth cells in the intestine of various mammals. *J. Electron. Microsc. Tech.* **16**:69–80.

Satoh, Y., K. Ishikawa, Y. Oomori, S. Takeda, and K. Ono. 1992. Bethanechol and a G-protein activator, NaF/AlCl3, induce secretory response in Paneth cells of mouse intestine. *Cell Tissue Res.* **269**:213–220.

Sawada, M., K. Takahashi, S. Sawada, and O. Midorikawa. 1991. Selective killing of Paneth cells by intravenous administration of dithizone in rats. *Int. J. Exp. Pathol.* **72**:407–421.

Sazawal, S., R. E. Black, M. K. Bhan, N. Bhandari, A. Sinha, and S. Jalla. 1995. Zinc supplementation in young children with acute diarrhea in India. *N. Engl. J. Med.* **333**:839–844.

Schmauder-Chock, E. A., S. P. Chock, and M. L. Patchen. 1994. Ultrastructural localization of tumour necrosis factor-alpha. *Histochem. J.* **26**:142–151.

Schreiber, S., S. Nikolaus, and J. Hampe. 1998. Activation of nuclear factor kappa B inflammatory bowel disease. *Gut* **42**:477–484.

Schwalbe, G. 1872. Beitrage zur Kenntnis der Drusen in den Darmwandungen, in's Besondere der Brunner'schen Drusen. *Arch. Mikroskop. Anat.* **8**:92–140.

Scott, H., and P. Brandtzaeg. 1981. Enumeration of Paneth cells in coeliac disease: comparison of conventional light microscopy and immunofluorescence staining for lysozyme. *Gut* **22**:812–816.

Seno, H., M. Sawada, H. Fukuzawa, Y. Morita, S. Takaishi, H. Hiai, and T. Chiba. 2001. Enhanced expression of transforming growth factor (TGF)-alpha precursor and TGF-beta1 during Paneth cell regeneration. *Dig. Dis. Sci.* **46**:1004–1010.

Seno, H., M. Sawada, H. Fukuzawa, Y. Morita-Fujisawa, S. Takaishi, H. Hiai, and T. Chiba. 2002. Involvement of tumor necrosis factor alpha in intestinal epithelial cell proliferation following Paneth cell destruction. *Scand. J. Gastroenterol.* **37**:154–160.

Sheahan, D. G., and H. R. Jervis. 1976. Comparative histochemistry of gastrointestinal mucosubstances. *Am. J. Anat.* **146**:103–131.

Shimada, O., H. Ishikawa, H. Tosaka-Shimada, T. Yasuda, K. Kishi, and S. Suzuki. 1998. Detection of deoxyribonuclease I along the secretory pathway in Paneth cells of human small intestine. *J. Histochem. Cytochem.* **46**:833–840.

Soga, N., R. Suzuki, and Y. Komeda. 1995. [A case report of prostate cancer with Paneth cell-like change]. *Hinyokika Kiyo* **41**:891–894.

Sohn, K. J., S. A. Shah, S. Reid, M. Choi, J. Carrier, M. Comiskey, C. Terhorst, and Y. I. Kim. 2001. Molecular genetics of ulcerative colitis-associated colon cancer in the interleukin 2- and beta(2)-microglobulin-deficient mouse. *Cancer Res.* **61**:6912–6917.

Stamp, G. W., R. Poulsom, L. P. Chung, S. Keshav, R. E. Jeffery, J. A. Longcroft, M. Pignatelli, and N. A. Wright. 1992. Lysozyme gene expression in inflammatory bowel disease. *Gastroenterology* **103**:532–538.

Stappenbeck, T. S., and J. I. Gordon. 2000. Rac1 mutations produce aberrant epithelial differentiation in the developing and adult mouse small intestine. *Development* **127**:2629–2642.

Stappenbeck, T. S., L. V. Hooper, and J. I. Gordon. 2002. Developmental regulation of intestinal angiogenesis by indigenous microbes via Paneth cells. *Proc. Natl. Acad. Sci. USA* **99**:15451–15455.

Strachan, D. P. 2000. Family size, infection and atopy: the first decade of the "hygiene hypothesis." *Thorax* 55(Suppl. 1):S2–S10.

Szczurek, E. I., C. S. Bjornsson, and C. G. Taylor. 2001. Dietary zinc deficiency and repletion modulate metallothionein immunolocalization and concentration in small intestine and liver of rats. *J. Nutr.* 131:2132–2138.

Takemori, H., F. N. Zolotaryov, L. Ting, T. Urbain, T. Komatsubara, O. Hatano, M. Okamoto, and H. Tojo. 1998. Identification of functional domains of rat intestinal phospholipase B/lipase. Its cDNA cloning, expression, and tissue distribution. *J. Biol. Chem.* 273:2222–2231.

Takubo, K., J. M. Nixon, and J. R. Jass. 1995. Ducts of esophageal glands proper and paneth cells in Barrett's esophagus: frequency in biopsy specimens. *Pathology* 27:315–317.

Tan, X., W. Hsueh, and F. Gonzalez-Crussi. 1993. Cellular localization of tumor necrosis factor (TNF)-alpha transcripts in normal bowel and in necrotizing enterocolitis. TNF gene expression by Paneth cells, intestinal eosinophils, and macrophages. *Am. J. Pathol.* 142:1858–1865.

Tanaka, M., H. Saito, T. Kusumi, S. Fukuda, T. Shimoyama, Y. Sasaki, K. Suto, A. Munakata, and H. Kudo. 2001. Spatial distribution and histogenesis of colorectal Paneth cell metaplasia in idiopathic inflammatory bowel disease. *J. Gastroenterol. Hepatol.* 16:1353–1359.

Tani, T., M. Fujino, K. Hanasawa, T. Shimizu, Y. Endo, and M. Kodama. 2000. Bacterial translocation and tumor necrosis factor-alpha gene expression in experimental hemorrhagic shock. *Crit. Care Med.* 28:3705–3709.

Tomlinson, I. P., N. E. Beck, K. Neale, and W. F. Bodmer. 1996. Variants at the secretory phospholipase A2 (PLA2G2A) locus: analysis of associations with familial adenomatous polyposis and sporadic colorectal tumours. *Ann. Hum. Genet.* 60(Part 5):369–376.

Trahair, J. F., M. R. Neutra, and J. I. Gordon. 1989. Use of transgenic mice to study the routing of secretory proteins in intestinal epithelial cells: analysis of human growth hormone compartmentalization as a function of cell type and differentiation. *J. Cell. Biol.* 109(Part 2):3231–3242.

Tsuji, S., J. Uehori, M. Matsumoto, Y. Suzuki, A. Matsuhisa, K. Toyoshima, and T. Seya. 2001. Human intelectin is a novel soluble lectin that recognizes galactofuranose in carbohydrate chains of bacterial cell wall. *J. Biol. Chem.* 276:23456–23463.

Tsumura, T., A. Hazama, T. Miyoshi, S. Ueda, and Y. Okada. 1998. Activation of cAMP-dependent Cl-currents in guinea-pig paneth cells without relevant evidence for CFTR expression. *J. Physiol.* 512(Part 3):765–777.

Van Heel, D. A., D. P. McGovern, and D. P. Jewell. 2001. Crohn's disease: genetic susceptibility, bacteria, and innate immunity. *Lancet* 357:1902–1904.

Wang, T. C., J. R. Goldenring, C. Dangler, S. Ito, A. Mueller, W. K. Jeon, T. J. Koh, and J. G. Fox. 1998. Mice lacking secretory phospholipase A2 show altered apoptosis and differentiation with *Helicobacter felis* infection. *Gastroenterology* 114:675–689.

Wehkamp, J., B. Schwind, K. R. Herrlinger, S. Baxmann, K. Schmidt, M. Duchrow, C. Wohlschlager, A. C. Feller, E. F. Stange, and K. Fellermann. 2002. Innate immunity and colonic inflammation: enhanced expression of epithelial alpha-defensins. *Dig. Dis. Sci.* 47:1349–1355.

Wilson, C. L., K. J. Heppner, L. A. Rudolph, and L. M. Matrisian. 1995. The metalloproteinase matrilysin is preferentially expressed by epithelial cells in a tissue-restricted pattern in the mouse. *Mol. Biol. Cell* 6:851–869.

Wilson, C. L., K. J. Heppner, P. A. Labosky, B. L. Hogan, and L. M. Matrisian. 1997. Intestinal tumorigenesis is suppressed in mice lacking the metalloproteinase matrilysin. *Proc. Natl. Acad. Sci. USA* 94:1402–1407.

Wilson, C. L., A. J. Ouellette, D. P. Satchell, T. Ayabe, Y. S. Lopez-Boado, J. L. Stratman, S. J. Hultgren, L. M. Matrisian, and W. C. Parks. 1999. Regulation of intestinal alpha-defensin activation by the metalloproteinase matrilysin in innate host defense. *Science* 286:113–117.

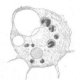

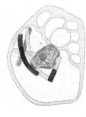

Fig. 1. Eine mit 1%igem Neutralrot behandelte Amöbe.

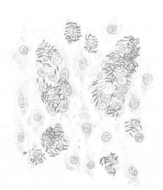

Fig. 21. Reaktion der Taubenphagocyten gegen die Tuberkelbacillen des Menschen.

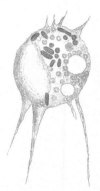

Fig. 38. Colibacillus im Innern eines Makrophagen aus der Meerschweinchenbauchhöhle (Färbung mit Neutralrot).

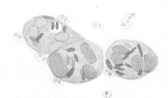

Fig. 23. Makrophag der Leber einer an Milzbrand gestorbenen Ratte mit Milzbrandbacillen.

Fig. 36. Peritonealexsudat eines Meerschweinchens mit freien Streptokokken und mit Proteusbacillen, welche im Innern von Mikrophagen liegen.

Fig. 44. In einem Meerschweinchenmakrophagen befindliche Pestbacillen, welche aus demselben auszutreten beginnen.

COLOR PLATE P (Preface)

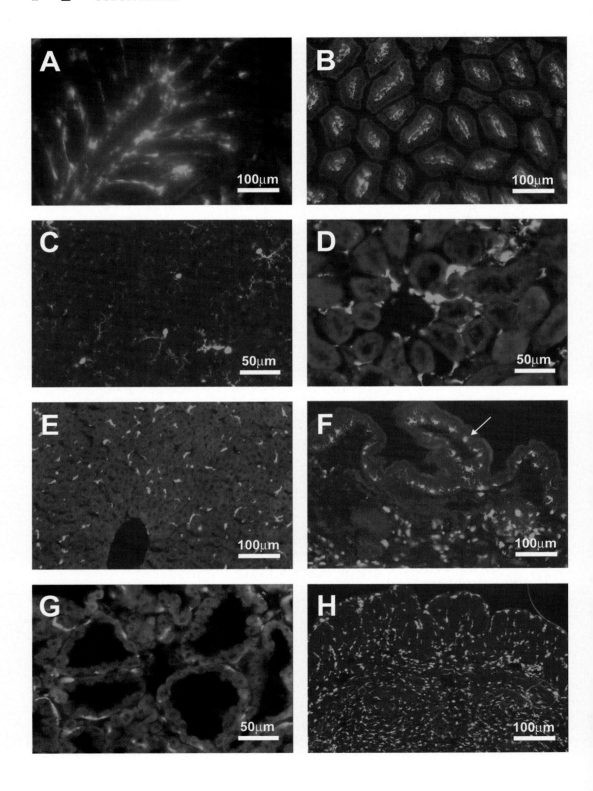

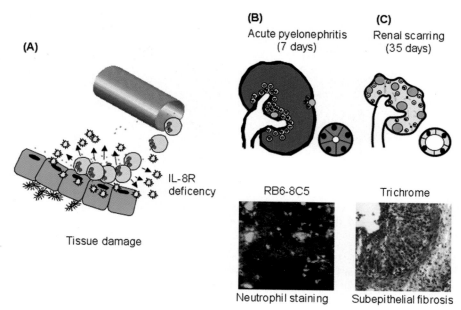

(A)

IL-8R deficency

Tissue damage

(B)
Acute pyelonephritis
(7 days)

(C)
Renal scarring
(35 days)

RB6-8C5

Trichrome

Neutrophil staining

Subepithelial fibrosis

COLOR PLATE 2 (chapter 8)   Renal scarring and tissue damage in mIL–8Rh KO mice. (A) The infected mice develop acute pyelonephritis, with bacteremia and enlarged edematous kidneys. After several weeks, there is renal scarring with abscesses and small pale kidneys. (B) Tissue neutrophil aggregates visualized by the antineutrophil antibody RB6-8C5. (C) Renal scarring with fibrosis, as shown by trichrome staining.

COLOR PLATE 1 (chapter 4)   Expression of a c-*fms* EGFP transgene in *MacGreen* mice. A 7.2-kb c-*fms* promoter plus enhancer directs the expression of the EGFP reporter gene into cells of the MPS of the mice. These examples illustrate the abundance of macrophages in all of the tissues of the mouse, as well as their characteristic stellate morphology and association with epithelia. Panels A and B illustrate the abundance of macrophages in the intestine; the EGFP+ marker is expressed specifically in lamina propria macrophages, as shown in the longitudinal section of colon's crypts (A) and in the cross section of small intestine villi (B). (C) The remarkably ramified morphology of microglia, the macrophages of the brain-expressing EGFP. (D) Transgenic EGFP expression in the macrophages that occupy the kidney interstitium aligned along basement membranes of kidney tubules. (E) Note the uneven distribution of Kupffer cells, the liver macrophages, within liver lobules. Within the skin, dermal macrophages express EGFP, as do Langerhans cells, the immature antigen-presenting DCs within the epidermis, as shown in (F), which is a cross section of the skin (arrow). Macrophage numbers change substantially in many organs of the female reproductive system during estrous cycle and pregnancy. (G) EGFP expression in macrophages lining the epithelial cells of alveoli of lactating mammary gland. (H) Numerous EGFP+ macrophages within the uterine endometrium.

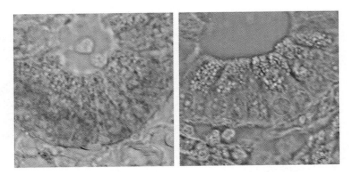

COLOR PLATE 3 In situ hybridization showing expression of NOD2 in human Paneth cells. Digoxigenin-labeled NOD2 antisense riboprobe was hybridized to a section of normal human terminal ileum and detected immunohistochemically using an antibody to digoxigenin and a peroxidase-labeled secondary antibody. The brown peroxidase reaction product is seen in the basolateral portion of the cells, while the apically located secretory vesicles are unstained. A control section hybridized to a sense-strand NOD2 riboprobe is shown on the right. The sections were counterstained with hematoxylin and viewed under a 40× phase-contrast objective to demonstrate the granules.

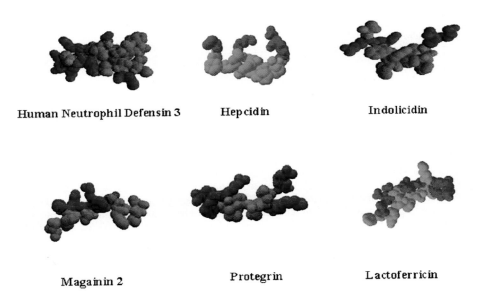

COLOR PLATE 4 (chapter 17) Amphipathic distribution of cationic hydrophilic and hydrophobic amino acids in antimicrobial peptides of different structural classes. Red, basic (positively charged) amino acids; green, hydrophobic amino acids. Other amino acids are not shown. Magainin is depicted in its α-helical configuration.

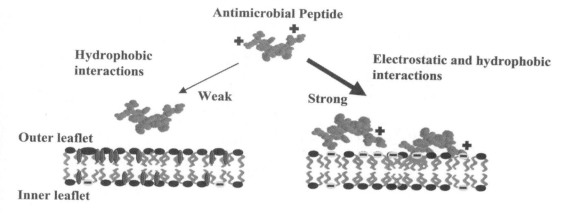

Antimicrobial Peptide

Hydrophobic interactions

Electrostatic and hydrophobic interactions

Weak

Strong

Outer leaflet

Inner leaflet

Prototypic plasma membrane of a multicellular organism (erythrocyte)

Bacterial cytoplasmic membrane

Cholesterol

Zwitterionic phospholipid

Anionic phospholipids

COLOR PLATE 5 (chapter 17)   The membrane target of antimicrobial peptides of multicellular organisms and the basis of specificity. Protegrin is depicted as a prototype; colors as in Fig. 1 (from Zasloff, 2002).

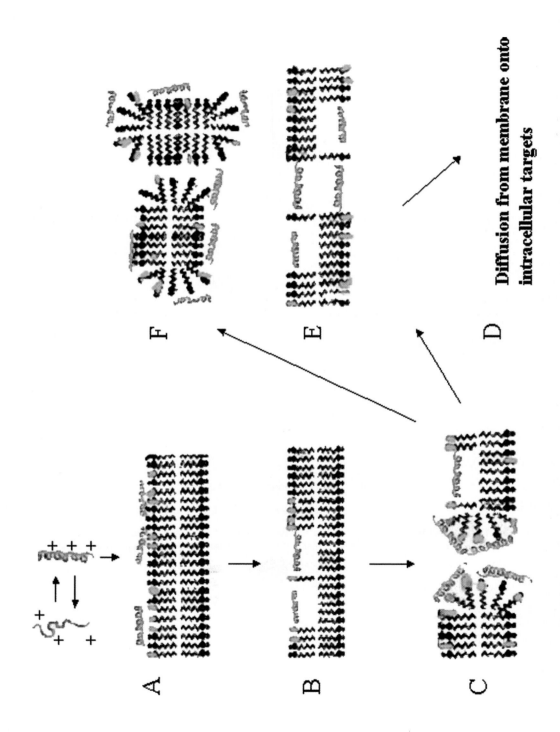

Diffusion from membrane onto intracellular targets

COLOR PLATE 6 (chapter 17) The SMH mechanism of action of an antimicrobial peptide. An α-helical peptide is depicted. (A) Carpeting of the outer leaflet with peptides. (B) Integration of the peptide into the membrane and thinning of the outer leaflet. (C) Phase transition and "wormhole" formation. Transient "pores" form at this stage. (D) Transport of lipids and peptides into the inner leaflet. (E) Diffusion of peptides onto intracellular targets (in some cases). (F) Collapse of the membrane into fragments and physical disruption of the target cell's membrane. Lipids with yellow head groups are acidic, or negatively charged. Lipids with black head groups have no net charge.

HUMORAL FACTORS

COLLECTINS AND THE ACUTE-PHASE RESPONSE

Howard Clark, Thilo Stehle, Alan Ezekowitz, and Kenneth Reid

10

The innate immune system in mammals provides a phylogenetically conserved first line of defense against infection. Recent understanding reveals that the mammalian innate immune system relies on a variety of antimicrobial and antiviral molecules that conspire to limit infection. It is also clear that the innate immune system is a necessary antecedent for the development of a sustained adaptive immune response. In this chapter we focus on one essential component of the innate immune system, that is, non–antibody-mediated pathogen recognition and opsonization. In particular our focus is the collectin subgroup of the superfamily of lectins, known as the C-type lectins (Ezekowitz, 1991). The collectins appear to play an important role as pattern recognition molecules in the protection of mammals from viral, fungal, and bacterial infection.

COLLECTINS: C-TYPE (CALCIUM-DEPENDENT) CARBOHYDRATE-BINDING PROTEINS WITH COLLAGEN DOMAINS

Collectins are members of the C-type lectin superfamily (see Fig. 1). Lectins are proteins capable of recognizing and binding carbohydrates, and in mammals three major classes of lectins have been characterized: the P-type (pentraxins), the S-type (galectins), and the C-type (calcium-dependent) lectins. The C-type lectin superfamily consists of proteins sharing a common structural module known as a carbohydrate recognition domain (CRD) (Drickamer, 1989) (Fig. 1).

CRDs vary in length from 115 to 130 amino acids, but all contain 18 invariant and 14 additional conservatively substituted amino acids, including four cysteines contributing to two conserved intrachain disulfide bonds (Drickamer, 1989). This pattern of conserved residues and the need for calcium for carbohydrate recognition serves to define the C-type CRDs. With a few exceptions, CRDs in the C-type lectin superfamily are linked to multiple other non-CRD protein domains. Many different arrangements are found in the superfamily, including linkage of the CRD to

Howard Clark and Kenneth Reid, MRC Immunochemistry Unit, Department of Biochemistry, University of Oxford, Oxford OX1 3QU, United Kingdom. *Thilo Stehle and Alan Ezekowitz*, Laboratory of Developmental Immunology, Harvard Department of Paediatrics, Massachusetts General Hospital, 15 Parkman St., Boston, MA 02114.

The Innate Immune Response to Infection
Ed. by S. H. E. Kaufmann, R. Medzhitov, and S. Gordon
©2004 ASM Press, Washington, D.C.

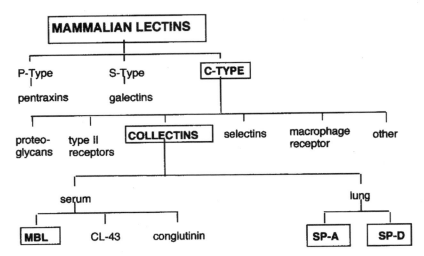

FIGURE 1 Mammalian lectins. The collectins form a subgroup of the C-type lectin superfamily. The lung collectins SP-A and SP-D, with the serum collectin MBL, are the only secreted collectins so far described in humans.

transmembrane domains; epidermal growth factor-like domains; complement-like domains; fibronectin-like domains; glycosaminoglycan attachment domains; and, in the case of the collectins, to collagen-like domains (Drickamer, 1989).

Collectins are the only soluble, cell-free, C-type lectins found in humans. In humans and rodents, mannose-binding lectin (MBL) is the only major serum collectin, although low levels of both surfactant protein A (SP-A) and surfactant protein D (SP-D) are also found in serum. Three additional serum collectins, conglutinin, CL-43, and CL-46, have been identified in the cow but not yet in other species (Hoppe and Reid, 1994). SP-A and SP-D are expressed in the alveolar and airway lining fluid, but their expression is not limited to the surfactant system. SP-D is in fact widely expressed at human mucosal surfaces (Madsen et al., 2000), and SP-A has also been found at extrapulmonary sites, such as the middle ear and small and large intestine in some species (Bourbon and Chailley-Heu, 2001; Paananen et al., 2001).

COLLECTIN STRUCTURE

All collectins follow the same principle of construction (Hoppe and Reid, 1994) (Fig. 2). Three polypeptide chains form a fiberlike trimer (13, 20, and 46 nm in length for MBL, SP-A, and SP-D, respectively) that features an elongated tail and a globular head. This trimeric building block then assembles further into multimers of trimers, where the precise number of trimers present in a multimer varies from protein to protein. The trimer can be subdivided into four distinct regions: a short N terminus, an extended collagenlike helix, an alpha-helical coiled-coil region, and a C-terminal CRD. Each of these four regions serves a specific function. Residues at the N terminus mediate covalent interactions between the three chains. The collagen helix mediates trimer formation as well as the assembly of the trimers into higher-order multimers. The alpha-helical coiled coil also mediates trimer formation, and in the case of SP-D it confers asymmetry onto the protein (Hakansson et al., 1999). It alone can mediate the formation of a stable trimer even in the absence of the

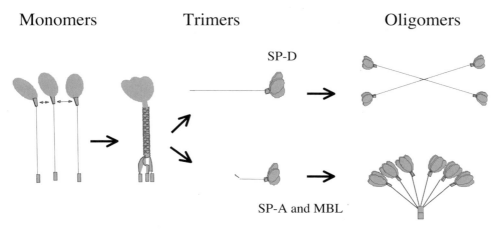

FIGURE 2 MBL, SP-A, and SP-D are collectins with collagenous and carbohydrate-binding domains. Oligomerization of the trimeric building blocks greatly enhances the avidity of binding to carbohydrate targets via the CRDs.

N-terminal residues and the collagen helix (Hoppe et al., 1994; Zhang et al., 2001). Each globular CRD contains a binding site for monosaccharides and is responsible for recognition of carbohydrates. This modular design is typical of fiberlike proteins with receptor-binding and oligomerization domains. As with many other such proteins, sequences linking the regions introduce flexibility at defined positions into the protein, and it is likely that these "hinges" are critical for the function of the collectins. Flexibility between the alpha-helical coiled coil and the CRD, which has been observed experimentally by comparing the structure of the same MBL trimer in different crystal forms (Sheriff et al., 1994), is thought to facilitate the engagement of carbohydrate receptors by allowing the CRDs to move with respect to the fibrous tail structure. Sequence irregularities and lack of conservation also indicate that a region of flexibility exists between the coiled-coil region and the collagen helix. This hinge region may also help to engage ligands and may also be required to allow for formation of the bouquetlike multimeric structures. The MBL-associated serine proteases (MASPs) probably bind to MBL near the N terminus in the collagenlike domain

(Wallis and Drickamer, 1999). In human MBL three separate mutations have been described in the collagenous domain, which are associated with immunodeficiency and a reduced ability to activate complement (Wallis and Cheng, 1999). The structural changes induced by the mutations lead to reduced complement activation either because of the generation of smaller oligomeric forms due to adventitious disulfide bond formation or because of their reduced ability to bind associated MASPs (Wallis and Dodd, 2000).

Crystal structures of wild-type and mutant MBL in the presence and absence of carbohydrates (Sheriff et al., 1994; Weis and Drickamer, 1994; Ng et al., 1996, 2002) have established the specificity of MBL for its ligands, and these studies can serve as a model for carbohydrate recognition by the collectin family members. Each MBL CRD recognizes a minimal structural motif of a pair of adjacent equatorial monosaccharide hydroxyl groups. This "micropattern" is present in mannose or fucose but not, for example, in sialic acid. Binding to the micropattern occurs in a metal-dependent fashion, via a protein-bound calcium ion that directly contacts both carbohydrate hydroxyls. Additional contacts involve a small set of conserved amino acid side chains surrounding the calcium (Fig. 3).

The crystal structures of trimeric MBL show that the individual monosaccharide-binding sites are about 0.5 nm apart (Weis and Drickamer, 1994; Sheriff et al., 1994). This allows carbohydrate chains of a length of greater than 50 nm to engage more than one binding site on the oligomeric protein, thereby producing a higher-affinity multivalent interaction. A shorter chain would not be able to engage the MBL trimer in this fashion, and

thus the spacing between the CRDs defines a macropattern present only in longer carbohydrate chains (Fig. 2). The affinity of a single CRD for a single carbohydrate is only in the millimolar range (Lee et al., 1991). It is tempting to speculate that the combination of micro- and macropattern allows for high-avidity binding to the longer sugar chains on the cell surfaces of the pathogen. Mammalian cells generally have shorter carbohydrate chains, and each chain would be unable to interact with more than one CRD and thus not fit the

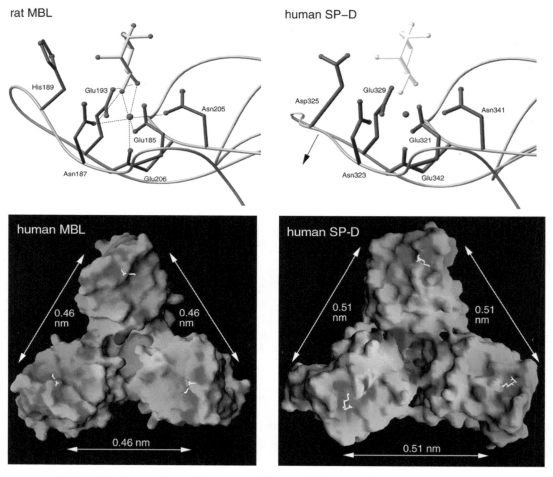

FIGURE 3 Comparison of the structural features of the CRDs from MBL and SP-D. Both MBL and SP-D trimers are very similar in structure. A striking feature of the SP-D trimer structure is the central area containing positively charged residues (indicated in dark gray) that may facilitate its interaction with negatively charged residues on pathogen targets such as LPS.

macropattern of MBL. The other collectin family members have somewhat different specificities for individual carbohydrates; however, the principles of recognition of larger chains are likely to be very similar. The crystal structure of SP-D has shown that its arrangement of CRDs in the trimer is very similar to that of MBL (Hakansson et al., 1999). Thus the recognition of "patterns" probably underlies the ability of the collectins to distinguish potential pathogens that require an immune response from innocuous substances including self-antigens (Ezekowitz, 1991; Hoffmann et al., 1999).

In vitro, the collectins recognize a broad range of pathogens including bacteria, viruses, and fungi (Tables 1, 2, and 3), but the affinity of binding to different microbes differs between collectins. Subtle structural differences among the collectins are likely responsible for these differences, which can be classified into three groups: variations in micropattern speci-

TABLE 1 Microbial targets of SP-A

Microbial target	Reference(s)
Escherichia coli J5	Pikaar et al. (1995)
Staphylococcus aureus	Geertsma et al. (1994)
Streptococcus pneumoniae	McNeely and Coonrod (1993)
Group A Streptococcus	Tino and Wright (1996)
Group B Streptococcus	LeVine et al. (1997, 1999a)
Haemophilus influenzae type a	McNeely and Coonrod (1994), Tino and Wright (1996)
Klebsiella pneumoniae	Kabha et al. (1997)
Pseudomonas aeruginosa	LeVine et al. (1998)
Mycoplasma pulmonis	Hickman-Davis et al. (1999)
Mycobacterium tuberculosis	Downing et al. (1995)
Influenza virus type A	Hartshorn et al. (1997)
Herpes simplex virus	van Iwaarden et al. (1991)
Respiratory syncytial virus	LeVine et al. (1999b)
Aspergillus fumigatus	Strong et al. (2002)
Pneumocystis carinii	Phelps and Rose (1991)
Cryptococcus neoformans	Schelenz et al. (1995)

TABLE 2 Microbial targets of SP-D

Microbial target	Reference
Escherichia coli	Kuan et al. (1992)
Salmonella minnesota	Kuan et al. (1992)
Haemophilus influenzae	Tino and Wright (1996)
Klebsiella pneumoniae	Lim et al. (1994)
Pseudomonas aeruginosa	Restrepo et al. (1999)
Influenza virus type A	Hartshorn et al. (1994)
Respiratory syncytial virus	Hickling et al. (1999)
Pneumocystis carinii	O'Riordan et al. (1995)
Aspergillus fumigatus	Strong et al. (2002)
Cryptococcus neoformans	Schelenz et al. (1995)

ficity within each CRD, variations in macropattern (the trimeric structure and arrangement of CRDs with respect to each other), and variations in multimeric assembly of trimers.

Micropattern

To date, only the structure of MBL has been determined in complex with ligands. Although SP-D was crystallized as an unliganded trimer, it does contain a (weakly bound) calcium ion, and inspection of structural features and the sequence in the vicinity of this ion shows that the MBL residues recognizing the micropattern are absolutely conserved in SP-D (Fig. 3). Thus it can be concluded that SP-D engages a micropattern that is very similar, if

TABLE 3 Microbial targets of MBL

Microbial target	Reference
Salmonella montevideo	Kuhlman et al. (1989)
Neisseria meningitidis	Drogari-Apiranthitou et al. (1997)
Neisseria gonorrhoeae	Gulati et al. (2002)
HIV	Ezekowitz et al. (1989)
Influenza virus type A	Kase et al. (1999)
Saccharomyces cerevisiae	Super et al. (1989)
Pneumocystis carinii	Ezekowitz et al. (1991)
Plasmodium falciparum	Klabunde et al. (2002)

not identical, to the adjacent equatorial hydroxyl groups recognized by MBL. Small differences in surface loops surrounding the ligand-binding site may alter the overall specificity of the CRD somewhat beyond the micropattern. For example, His189 of rat MBL is located at the edge of the carbohydrate-binding pocket, and the histidine side chain packs against the bound monosaccharide ring. The corresponding residue in SP-D is Asp325, and the different side chain structure and negative charge may influence the orientation of the bound ligand and also impart new selective properties onto the binding pocket. It was indeed shown earlier that substitutions at this position influence the orientation of bound ligands in rat MBL (Ng et al., 2002)

Macropattern

Although the overall structure of the SP-D trimer is similar to that of MBL, there are subtle differences. The SP-D trimer is somewhat asymmetric, with a tyrosine residue from one chain perturbing the alpha-helical coiled-coil structure such that the distances between the three CRDs are no longer exactly equal. The SP-D trimer also has a large electropositive potential near the trimer center, and this has led to speculation that this feature might facilitate the interaction with negative charges on lipopolysaccharide (LPS) moieties of microbial carbohydrates or phospholipids of pulmonary surfactant. The MBL trimer does not have a similar feature; its central cavity is more or less electroneutral.

Multimeric Assembly

The collectin trimers assemble into oligomers in one of two higher-order geometries. In the case of SP-A and MBL, the fibrillar stalks of collagen orient the CRDs into a conformation that resembles a bouquet of flowers and contains hexamers of trimers. By contrast, in the case of SP-D and bovine conglutinin, the individual trimers are arranged as a cruciform that is formed from four trimers (Hoppe and Reid, 1994) (Fig. 2). These different geo-metries presumably allow the massive cross-linking or agglutination of bound pathogens characteristic of the collectins and confer the advantage of broadening the range of potential microbial targets bound by the collectins. The fibrillar stalks may have additional properties including receptor or cofactor-binding sites (Malhotra et al., 1994).

COLLECTINS ARE PRESENT AT SITES THAT SUPPORT THEIR ROLE IN INNATE IMMUNITY

A key feature of pattern recognition molecules such as collectins is that they should be present at physiologically appropriate sites to facilitate their role in first-line host defense. The three collectin genes are developmentally regulated, with a marked increase in expression late in gestation. SP-A mRNA is detected in human fetal lung as early as 24 weeks gestation (Ballard et al., 1986). SP-A can be readily detected by immunoassay in tracheal aspirates (range, 1 to 2 μg/ml, not corrected for extracellular lung fluid volume) from both preterm and term infants (Chida et al., 1988), but a detailed developmental profile after premature birth has not been reported. Miyamura et al. (1994) reported low levels of SP-A and SP-D in amniotic fluid from preterm births. Both SP-A and SP-D were detectable immunochemically in amniotic fluid as early as 26 weeks gestation, and SP-A levels rose sharply from 32 weeks toward term. By contrast, SP-D levels in the same samples rose only moderately. SP-D levels in tracheal lavage samples from premature infants are low and do not correlate with gestational age, but are related to infection status (H. Clark et al., unpublished data). Levels of SP-D in samples from infants with chorioamnionitis are also increased (Curley et al., unpublished results).

In humans, SP-A levels are increased with acute pneumonic infections, including pneumocystis pneumonia (Phelps and Rose, 1991), but are decreased in chronic inflammatory diseases such as idiopathic fibrosis (McCormack et al., 1991). Complex cytokine networks likely regulate both cell numbers and transcription rates during these conditions so that collectin levels will likely be variable with both the stage and the type of disease. There is rapid upregulation of SP-A and SP-D in mice following intratracheal endotoxin administration (McIntosh et al., 1996), and it has been shown that SP-D acts as a rapid scavenger of endotoxin in vivo (van Rozendaal et al., 1999). There are rapid rises in SP-A and SP-D levels after intrapulmonary challenge with LPS, fungal allergens (Strong et al., 2002), or intra-amniotic endotoxin (Bachurski et al., 2001). Thus the levels of SP-A and SP-D are modulated in response to challenge with infectious agents or their components, consistent with their proposed role in first-line host defense.

Several studies of serum MBL levels in humans report levels between 0.07 and 6.4 μg/ml in children (3 years and older) and adults (Terai et al., 1993) and a level of 1 μg/ml in term infants (Terai and Kobayashi, 1993). Interestingly, MBL levels rose in the first 5 days after delivery at term to values equal to or greater than adult values (Terai et al., 1993). Using different antibodies, Lipscombe and colleagues (1992) found a median concentration of 0.99 μg/ml (range, 0.64 to 1.41 μg/ml). MBL has been characterized as an acute-phase protein on the basis of increased levels of hepatic mRNA after trauma (Ezekowitz et al., 1988) and circulating protein during infection (Tabona et al., 1995). Relative to major acute-phase reactants such as C-reactive protein and serum amyloid protein, the MBL response is both modest and delayed, with a peak response (1.5- to 2-fold increase) at approximately 72 h (Tabona et al., 1995). The presence of a consensus heat shock element in the 5′ upstream region of the human MBL gene (Sastry et al., 1989; Arai et al., 1993), similar to that found in the C-reactive protein gene and other acute-phase genes, is consistent with the idea that the collectin genes are primed to respond rapidly but nonspecifically to stress and infection. In vitro the MBL gene is regulated by mediators of the acute-phase response including interleukin-1 (IL-1), IL-6, dexamethasone, and heat shock proteins (Arai et al., 1993).

COLLECTINS PLAY A ROLE AS PATTERN RECOGNITION MOLECULES IN FIRST-LINE HOST DEFENSE

A consensus opinion is that collectins play a key role in innate immunity (Tables 1, 2, and 3). For the surfactant apoproteins SP-A and SP-D, their domain is predominantly the lung, although SP-D in particular may also be an important part of mucosal immunity. For MBL as a serum protein, its role appears to be as an ante-antibody as it acts like a broad-spectrum antibody and is able to activate complement via a novel mechanism. In this section we explore the experimental evidence that supports these contentions.

SP-A and SP-D

SP-A and SP-D have overlapping and distinct roles in defending the lung against noxious agents. The spread of influenza virus beyond the upper airways into the lung would bring the virus into contact with both SP-A and SP-D. However, Crouch and colleagues (2000) reported SP-D to be 1 log order more effective than MBL, SP-A, or conglutinin in binding to influenza virus. The target specificities of individual collectins for bacteria overlap only partially, and the precise modes of interaction can differ markedly. For example, it was shown that SP-A preferentially interacts with the lipid A moiety of the LPS of gram-negative bacteria (Van Iwaarden et al., 1994), whereas SP-D interacts with the core oligosaccharides (Kuan et al., 1992).

The multimeric structure of SP-A and SP-D facilitates massive microbial agglutination in vitro (Kuan et al., 1992). However, it appears that agglutination is not an essential prerequisite for the collectins to promote phagocytosis, nor is phagocytosis of agglutinated bacteria always enhanced by collectins (Pikaar et al., 1995). Higher-order multimers promote aggregation of pathogens more effectively than dodecamers or trimers, which are poorly effective in this regard. For example, truncated forms of human SP-D lacking the collagen domain have been reported to cause dose-dependent agglutination of *Escherichia coli* Y1088, although it was much less effective than the native form (Eda et al., 1997). In some cases, aggregation may facilitate phagocytosis, although the importance of such interactions for phagocytosis and killing of microbes is immune cell and organism specific. For example, SP-D agglutinates *Mycobacterium tuberculosis* but inhibits phagocytosis (Ferguson et al., 1999). By contrast, phagocytosis of mucoid *Pseudomonas aeruginosa* is enhanced without the need for agglutination (Restrepo et al., 1999). Interestingly, a truncated trimeric recombinant rat SP-D lacking the collagen domain failed to agglutinate *M. tuberculosis*, while still inhibiting its phagocytosis by human macrophages in a dose-dependent manner, demonstrating that this protective effect of SP-D is independent of agglutination (Ferguson et al., 2002).

It is becoming clear that the effect of SP-A or SP-D on specific pathogens may involve both acting as a direct opsonin (e.g., Geertsma et al., 1994) and also in some circumstances modulating macrophage function, perhaps by increasing the activity of the macrophage mannose receptor (Kabha et al., 1997). Direct binding of SP-A or SP-D to the microorganism is also not always essential to trigger microbicidal activity: specific prior interaction between SP-A and interferon-activated macrophages was found to be essential for SP-A-mediated mycoplasmal killing. Coating of *Mycoplasma pulmonis* with SP-A before the addition of macrophages did not result in significant killing (Hickman-Davis et al., 1999). Similarly, human neutrophils that were preincubated with SP-D were more effective at phagocytosis of *E. coli* than untreated neutrophils presented with *E. coli* that had been preincubated with SP-D (Hartshorn et al., 1998). Thus, the consequences to the host of collectin binding may vary depending on the microbe and the cellular environment.

The MBL as an Ante-Antibody

The MBL is a prototypic pattern recognition molecule that is able to recognize a wide range of microorganisms. This group includes certain gram-positive and gram-negative organisms, yeasts, parasites, and mycobacteria; *Trypanosoma cruzi*; and viruses such as influenza virus, herpes simplex virus, respiratory syncytial virus, and the human immunodeficiency virus (HIV) (Epstein et al., 1996). Importantly, MBL can distinguish species self or altered self from nonself by recognizing the patterns that decorate the surfaces of microorganisms, virally infected cells, and transformed cells from normal host cells. A key question therefore is how the MBL is able to recognize a wide range of apparently disparate carbohydrate structures, yet still retain the ability to distinguish species self from nonself. The answer lies in recent structural studies that begin to define the specificity of pattern recognition as discussed above.

MBL can act as an opsonin and has the ability to interact with the complement cascades (Ikeda et al., 1987). The initial studies evaluating the interactions between MBL and the complement cascades focused on the known pathways. Human MBL was first shown to substitute for C1q and interact directly with two serine proteases, C1r and C1s, in vitro (Lu et al., 1990). This MBL-C1r-C1s complex is able to activate the classical complement pathway convertase. Once bound to a ligand, MBL was shown to initiate the alternative complement pathway. However, in 1994, Fujita and his colleagues discovered the MBL pathway of complement activation when they demonstrated that MBL is able to activate the classical complement by a novel serine protease, MASP-1, independent of antibodies, C1q, C1r, and C1s. It now appears that three novel serine proteases, MASP-1, MASP-2, and the alternative splice form of MASP-1, MASP-3, and a nonprotease (Map19) associate with MBL in a calcium-dependent manner (Dahl et al., 2001). The MASP domain structure is very similar to that of C1r and C1s. Comparative studies in deuterostomes, chordates, and vertebrates indicate that the MASP1/3 gene most likely gave rise to MASP-2, and gene duplication events led to C1r and C1s. Recent evidence indicates that MBL and MASP-2 ligand complexes activate the classical pathway convertase (Dahl et al., 2001). It also appears that MASP-3 plays a regulatory role, as it is able to downregulate the C4 and C2 cleaving activity of MASP-2 (Dahl et al., 2001). Lower MBL oligomers result in MBL–MASP-1–Map19 complexes that directly cleave C3 (Dahl et al., 2001). This latter pathway links the MBL pathway with the alternative pathway that seems to act as an amplification loop.

Despite the striking structural similarity between MBL and the lung collectins, especially SP-A, there is no evidence that SP-A or SP-D can activate complement. However, SP-A binds to C1q, and recently investigators have found evidence that SP-A may regulate complement activation by affecting C1q-mediated complement activation (Watford et al., 2001).

Effects on Chemotaxis, Phagocytosis, and Killing of Pathogens. SP-A is a chemoattractant for alveolar macrophages (Wright and Youmans, 1993). SP-D stimulates directional actin polymerization and is chemotactic for alveolar macrophages (Tino and Wright, 1999), neutrophils, and monocytes (Crouch et al., 1995). Trimeric recombinant rat SP-D mutants retained their ability to elicit chemotaxis of neutrophils in vitro (Cai et al., 1999), suggesting that the essential element for this in vitro effect is the CRD. The phagocytosis of bound bacteria (Kuan et al., 1992) and fungi (Madan et al., 1997) by monocytes and macrophages is enhanced by collectins. In some, but not all, experimental settings intracellular killing is also enhanced (Clark et al., 2000). In contrast, MBL-coated *Pneumocystis carinii* are taken up less well by alveolar macrophages, presumably by shielding the microbial sugars normally recognized by the macrophage mannose receptor (Ezekowitz et al., 1991). *P. carinii* isolated from bronchoalveolar lavage of human patients with HIV are densely coated with SP-A (Phelps and Rose, 1991). The possibility that collectin binding to microbes may not always be beneficial should also be considered in that some (e.g., intracellular) pathogens may exploit collectin interaction as a means of infecting cells.

Interaction with Viruses. MBL, SP-A, and SP-D all bind glycoconjugates on some viruses such as influenza A (Hartshorn et al., 1994) and HIV (Ezekowitz et al., 1989). In both cases, the consequence of collectin binding appears to be the inhibition of viral infectivity by the shielding of viral cell receptor binding sites on hemagglutinin of influenza virus and gp120 of HIV. As with bacteria, the agglutinated viruses are actively taken up by phagocytic cells (van Iwaarden et al., 1991; Hartshorn et al., 1994). Oligomerization may be essential for effective inhibitory activity against some viruses. For example, a truncated trimeric recombinant form of SP-D was able to inhibit respiratory syncytial virus infectivity in vitro and in vivo (Hickling et al., 1999), whereas in the case of influenza virus, despite the ability of the trimeric protein to bind (Hartshorn et al., 2000), enhanced internalization of viral particles required multimerization of trimeric subunits into dodecamers (Crouch et al., 2000).

Collectin Receptors. Although MBL can activate complement and effect microbial killing via the lectin pathway, the precise mechanism whereby the lung collectins interact with phagocytic cells in host defense remains uncertain. Some evidence exists that the collectins are able to utilize the same receptor as C1q, at least on polymorphonuclear leukocytes and monocytes (Malhotra et al., 1990, 1992). However, there is some controversy as to exactly which cell surface molecules, having transmembrane and cytoplasmic domains, can serve as receptors for C1q and mediate intracellular signaling upon the binding of C1q (Lu et al., 2002). The receptor recognition site in C1q is thought to be in the collagenous region, but this has not been convincingly demonstrated with the collectins. Also, the finding that truncated forms of SP-D, lacking the greater part of the collagenous region, maintain certain functions both in vitro and in vivo (Clark and Reid, 2002) indicates that many of the cellular effects of SP-D may be mediated via the neck region and CRDs. A putative receptor expressed on the surface of macrophage gp340 has been cloned and identified as belonging to the scavenger receptor family (Holmskov, 2000), and SP-D binds this molecule, in a non–carbohydrate-dependent fashion via the CRD. SP-A has been shown to interact with CD14, the LPS receptor, as well as the Toll-like receptor 4, and a number of molecules have been proposed as putative SP-A receptors (Holmskov, 2000). It seems possible that a family of collectin-specific receptors may be present on phagocytic and perhaps other inflammatory cells through which they exert their effects. Indeed, it has been proposed, based on a variety of in vitro and in vivo experiments, that the $\alpha 2$ macroglobulin receptor (CD91), in association with cell surface calreticulin (a protein normally found in the endoplasmic reticulum and that has, in the past, been defined as cC1qR), can act as a receptor for the clearance of apoptotic cells, after binding of these cells by SP-A, SP-D, or C1q (Ogden et al., 2001; Vandivier et al., 2002). The possible physiological importance of this clearance pathway is highlighted, as discussed below, by the observation that SP-D-deficient mice show an accumulation of apoptotic and necrotic macrophages in the lungs.

Elucidation of the In Vivo Role of the Collectins: Phenotypes of Collectin-Deficient Mice. The generation of collectin gene knockout mice has allowed an investigation of the relative importance of these in vitro collectin-microbe and collectin-immune cell interactions in the host defense of the whole organism. SP-A knockout mice have been demonstrated to be susceptibile to infectious challenge with a range of bacteria and viruses, including group B *Streptococcus* spp., *Pseudomonas* spp., and respiratory syncytial virus (LeVine and Whitsett, 2001). However, it has been more difficult to assess the specific in vivo contribution of SP-D to host defense in infectious models using SP-D knockout mice because of their having a more complicated lung phenotype. The SP-D-deficient mouse develops chronic low-

grade pulmonary inflammation, characterized by an excess of alveolar pulmonary surfactant phospholipid, hyperplastic type II cells, and a peribronchial lymphocytic infiltrate with an excessive number of alveolar macrophages (Botas et al., 1998). The alveolar macrophages show increased expression of reactive oxygen species and matrix metalloproteinases, and the mice develop features of emphysematous change with dilated air spaces and pulmonary fibrosis (Wert et al., 2000). This phenotype clearly reveals a critical role for SP-D in regulating lung inflammation, even in the nonchallenged, noninfected lung.

LeVine has demonstrated that SP-D knockout mice have an enhanced inflammatory reaction and defective phagocytosis in response to challenge with group B *Streptococcus* spp. and *Haemophilus influenzae* (LeVine et al., 2000). Despite defective phagocytosis, clearance of the bacterial challenge was normal, perhaps compensated for by enhanced bacterial killing in the setting of enhanced production of reactive oxygen species (LeVine et al., 2000). In our own studies of challenge with pneumococci, however, in addition to the enhanced inflammatory response after bacterial challenge, the microbes persisted longer in the upper respiratory tract in the SP-D-deficient animals (Jounblat et al., unpublished). These and other studies using SP-A and SP-D knockout mice have clearly demonstrated that the lung collectins act in first-line defense and modulate the inflammatory response to pulmonary infection.

Collectins at the Interface Between Innate and Adaptive Immunity. In vitro studies suggest that SP-A and SP-D might instruct the acquired response by influencing antigen presentation and lymphocyte proliferation. Studies using the knockout mouse models have provided further evidence of the interplay between innate and adaptive immunity influenced by collectin effects on immune cell proliferation, activation, and removal. In this way the collectins are able to influence both innate and adaptive immune systems (Wright et al., 2001).

Enhanced Antigen Presentation. SP-D has recently been shown to enhance the presentation of *E. coli* antigens to dendritic cells (Brinker et al., 2001). Whole-length recombinant rat SP-D bound preferentially to immature rather than mature dendritic cells and enhanced presentation (as measured by IL-2 production) of an *E. coli* antigen to a major histocompatibility complex class II-restricted T-cell hybridoma at concentrations from 0.1 to 1 μg/ml. This interaction with dendritic cells was carbohydrate mediated and calcium dependent and has also been observed with a truncated trimeric recombinant human SP-D CRD (S. Desai, M.S.c thesis, University of Oxford). This important finding implies that collectins are involved in antigen presentation and in instructing secondary immune responses.

Effects on Lymphocyte Proliferation. Both SP-A and SP-D function in the inhibition of IL-2-dependent T-lymphocyte proliferation (Borron et al., 1998a, 1998b). Wang et al. (1998) have also reported that SP-A and SP-D as well as a recombinant human SP-D lacking the collagenous and N-terminal domains showed an inhibitory effect on allergen-induced lymphocyte proliferation and histamine release in children with asthma. These observations are consistent with the peribronchial lymphocytic proliferation seen in the absence of SP-D in the lungs of SP-D knockout mice.

Clearance of Apoptotic Immune Cells. Rapid removal of apoptotic cells is recognized as a centrally important mechanism for maintenance of immune homeostasis and the resolution of inflammation (Fadok and Chimini, 2001). C1q is known to be important in the recognition of apoptotic cells, and failure of clearance of apoptotic cells may trigger inflammation (Taylor et al., 2000). Both MBL and C1q bind apoptotic Jurkat T cells in vitro

and enhance their clearance by monocyte-derived macrophages (Ogden et al., 2001). This suggests that the collectins might act as opsonins for apoptotic and/or necrotic cells. Schagat et al. (2001) demonstrated preferential binding of SP-A and SP-D to the surface of apoptotic neutrophils and the promotion of their phagocytosis by alveolar macrophages. Supportive of this view, a high proportion of resident macrophages in the SP-D-deficient lung are apoptotic (Clark et al., 2002), and SP-D knockout mice are deficient in clearing apoptotic neutrophils from the alveolar space (Vandivier et al., 2002).

MBL HAPLOTYPES AND SUSCEPTIBILITY TO SYSTEMIC DISEASE

One central tenet of innate immunity is that molecules of the innate immune system are hard wired in the genome compared with antigen receptors on T cells and B cells. This view of pattern recognition molecules may be too absolute, as it appears that molecules like MBL, although fundamentally similar in all humans, display a number of variations that define MBL serum levels in individuals. To begin with, MBL has three replacement single nucleotide polymorphisms (SNPs) in exon 1 of the MBL gene: D52C, G54D, and G57E (Turner and Hamvas, 2000). These SNPs disrupt the collagen helix and hence the assembly of trimers and therefore act as dominant mutations resulting in profound reductions in high-order MBL oligomers. The presence of these low-producing coding alleles is termed O. Thus, O/A individuals might have one-eighth the level of some A/A individuals. In addition, SNPs located in the 5′ regulatory region of the MBL gene at −550g/c (alleles H/L), −221c/g (alleles X/Y), and +4c/t (alleles P/Q) are found to have linkage disequilibrium with exon 1 SNPs. The 52C allele is always in *cis* with −550/−221 H/Y alleles, and 54D and 57E are always in *cis* with L/Y. Even wild-type alleles are regulated. When A or wild-type alleles are in *cis* with −550/−221 promoter haplotypes HY, LY, and LX, MBL serum levels are high, intermediate, and low, respectively. It should be noted that LPX A/A individuals have very low levels that are less than 500 ng/ml (normal range is 1 to 5 μg/ml). It is interesting to note that median MBL serum levels appear to differ in distinct population groups and that this correlates with the prevalence of high-, medium-, and low-producing alleles. On average, levels decrease from Eskimos to Chinese to Caucasians to Africans.

Several studies have demonstrated an association with low-coding MBL alleles and increased risk of infection. The hypothesis would predict that low or undetectable levels of MBL predispose the host to infections. The initial idea was that an opsonic defect in serum that correlated with a broad phenotype of recurrent infection was due to a lack of MBL in young children. Later, Turner modified this concept and suggested that the phenotype of susceptibility to infection was more obvious if there was an associated defect in adaptive or innate immunity. One example would be that an antibody isotype deficiency in conjunction with low MBL levels would collectively present the host with an increased risk to infection. Garred and colleagues (1999) demonstrated that patients with cystic fibrosis who also inherit low-secretor MBL haplotypes have a reduction in life expectancy of 5 to 8 years. Although the exact mechanism is not clear, one plausible explanation is that these patients' lungs are colonized earlier with *Burkholderia cepacia* and *Pseudomonas aeruginosa*. Once this occurs, a refractory cycle of lung injury begins that ultimately results in the demise of the patient.

The importance of the innate immune system as an antecedent to adaptive immunity is well illustrated when innate immunity is disrupted as a consequence of cancer chemotherapy. The risk of infection in febrile neutropenic cancer patients undergoing chemotherapy has been recognized since 1966. Although there have been many thoughtful studies that stratify patients according to risk, it was not until recently that attention was paid

to assessing patients' premorbid genetic susceptibility to infection. Two recent studies have addressed this question with MBL as a paradigm. Neth and colleagues (2001) found that children with febrile neutropenia postchemotherapy who had low-secretor haplotypes had hospital stays that were on average 2 days longer than those patients who were MBL sufficient. Peterslund and colleagues (2001) showed that of 54 adult patients with cancer, 16 with clinically significant events, as defined, such as bacteremia and pneumonia, had low levels of MBL. Taken together, these preliminary studies indicate that there is a threshold level of MBL that correlates with increased risk of infection.

The similarity between C1q and MBL has led investigators to examine whether deficiency in MBL, like that of C1q, might predispose the host to autoimmunity. Several studies demonstrate an association of low-producing MBL alleles and autoimmunity. This point is best illustrated in one study where the relationship between MBL allele and time of diagnosis in 163 patients' common variable immunodeficiency is compared with 100 controls. The mean age of onset of infections was 6.8 years in patients with low-producing MBL alleles (LXPA haploype) compared with 29.3 years in those patients who had high-producing haplotypes (HYPA). Furthermore, MBL low-producing alleles were significantly associated with autoimmunity in this group (P = 0.0003).

Other independent studies have indicated an association between low-producing MBL haplotypes and systemic lupus erythematosus (SLE) (Ip et al., 1998; Tsutsumi et al., 2001; Villarreal et al., 2001). This association is of particular interest as homozygous deficiencies in classical complement proteins are associated with increased susceptibility to SLE (Bowness et al., 1994; Naves et al., 1998; Walport et al., 1998). It is important to place these observations in context with what is currently known about the pathophysiology of SLE. SLE is a multisystem autoimmune disease that is characterized by the production of numerous autoantibodies against a variety of nuclear and cytoplasmic antigens such as DNA, histones, ribonuclear proteins, calreticulin, and phospholipids (Mills, 1994). The disease is heterogeneous in humans and may involve skin, blood vessels, joints, brain, serosal surfaces, the heart, and lungs. SLE is considered the prototypic systemic autoimmune disease that appears to result from B-cell hyperactivity (Mamula et al., 1994; Odendahl et al., 2000). The pathways that initiate B-cell activation are multiple and complex. Studies in humans and lupus-prone mice indicate genetic abnormalities where many genes influence B-cell function and predispose to SLE (Hirose et al., 2000; Morel et al., 2000, 2001). It appears that these polygenetic traits directly or indirectly influence B-cell function. It appears that C1q is involved in the clearance of DNA. C1q binds directly to the surface blebs of apoptotic cells that contain nuclear proteins and nuclear acids that are lupus autoantigens (Bowness et al., 1994). It is interesting to note that mice that lack the serum amyloid protein, a protein that also binds nuclear material, spontaneously develop SLE, adding further support to the "clearance" hypothesis (Bickerstaff et al., 1999). Accordingly, failure to clear nuclear debris that is mediated by these two serum proteins fails to downregulate autoreactive B cells, and this leads to B-cell activation and autoantibody production. In this regard, a recent study by Ogden et al. (2001) is of particular relevance as it demonstrates that human MBL, like C1q, is able to bind apoptotic cells selectively and that these cells are cleared by macrophages in vitro. This study goes on to demonstrate that clearance of MBL and C1q apoptotic complexes by macrophages is mediated via calreticulin (cC1q receptor) and CD91 (α2-macroglobulin receptor), but not by other putative collectin receptors. This carefully conducted study indicates that both C1q and MBL may have overlapping roles. This raises the question as to whether MBL null mice spontaneously develop SLE-like features as has been demonstrated in C1qa null mice. In addition, it would be interesting to evaluate the relative risk of developing autoimmunity in patients who lack both C1q and MBL.

SP-A AND SP-D HAPLOTYPES AND SYSTEMIC DISEASE

To date, no mutations of the translated portions of the SP-A or SP-D genes have been reported, but no systematic search for human SP-A or SP-D deficiency has so far been undertaken. Considerable allelic polymorphism in the nontranslated region of the human SP-A and SP-D genes has been found. SP-A polymorphisms associated with increased severity of respiratory distress syndrome have been identified (Kala et al., 1998), and at least one study has linked these as susceptibility factors in the development of neonatal chronic lung disease (Weber et al., 2000). Certain SP-A and SP-D alleles have been linked to possible susceptibilities to chronic obstructive pulmonary disease in a Mexican population (Guo et al., 2001), and both SP-A and SP-D polymorphisms are associated with increased severity of childhood infection with respiratory syncytial virus (Haataja et al., 2001; Lofgren et al., 2002).

THERAPEUTIC POTENTIAL OF RECOMBINANT MBL

Aside from the now well-characterized mutations of the MBL genes associated with low MBL levels and susceptibility to infection, variant alleles have been associated with a more severe clinical course in cystic fibrosis (Garred et al., 1999), and at least one cystic fibrosis patient has been treated with some success with MBL purified from human serum (Garred et al., 2002). MBL deficiency has been associated with a predisposition to infection with meningococcus (Bax et al., 1999) and *Aspergillus* (Crosdale et al., 2001), and there is evidence that immunosuppressed patients undergoing chemotherapy for malignancy may be especially vulnerable if they are MBL deficient (Mullighan et al., 2000, 2002; Peterslund et al., 2001). Neth et al. (2001) have suggested that this patient population could benefit from treatment with MBL infusions.

THERAPEUTIC POTENTIAL OF RECOMBINANT SP-A AND SP-D

The findings that SP-A and SP-D play a pivotal role in the regulation of macrophage-mediated inflammation in the lung, in the defense against invasion by pathogens, and in modulating inflammatory responses to infection and allergenic stimuli have intriguing clinical implications for a range of lung diseases. The demonstration of activity in infectious, allergic, and inflammatory mouse models of truncated recombinant forms of SP-D that can be produced artificially in large amounts raises the prospects of their use as novel therapeutic agents.

Replacement of whole-length human SP-D dodecamers corrected a defect in clearance of influenza A virus from the respiratory tract of SP-D-deficient mice (LeVine et al., 2001). Truncated recombinant forms of SP-D have not been widely tested in infectious models, so the structural requirements for SP-D function in host defense in vivo have not been extensively investigated. Transgenic overexpression of a trimeric neck/CRD recombinant SP-A in the SP-A-deficient background failed to correct the structural and functional defects of the surfactant system characteristic of the SP-A null mouse—namely, the lack of tubular myelin and decreased surface activity (Ikegami et al., 2001)—but did correct the susceptibility to infection with group B streptococci (F. McCormack, presented at the meeting of the American Thoracic Society, 2001). This suggests that a truncated trimeric SP-A maintains some host defense function in vivo. Two studies have demonstrated that truncated trimeric forms of SP-D neck/CRD maintain significant host defense function in vivo against respiratory syncytial virus (Hickling et al., 1999) and the fungal pathogen *Aspergillus fumigatus* (Madan et al., 2001).

CONCLUSIONS

Innate immunity relies on the coordinate action of a wide variety of antimicrobial and antiviral molecules that attempt to limit an infectious challenge. It is clear that the collectins play a key part of this armory. A great deal of progress has been made in defining the role for collectins as first-line host defense molecules. The exciting possibility exists that this knowledge may be harnessed and translated into novel adjuvant therapies.

REFERENCES

Arai, T., P. Tabona, and J. A. Summerfield. 1993. Human mannose-binding protein gene is regulated by interleukins, dexamethasone and heat shock. *Q. J. Med.* **86:**575–582.

Bachurski, C. J., G. F. Ross, M. Ikegami, B. W. Kramer, and A. H. Jobe. 2001. Intra-amniotic endotoxin increases pulmonary surfactant proteins and induces SP-B processing in fetal sheep. *Am. J. Physiol. Lung Cell. Mol. Physiol.* **280:**L279–L285.

Ballard, P. L., S. Hawgood, H. Liley, G. Wellenstein, L. W. Gonzales, B. Benson, B. Cordell, and R. T. White. 1986. Regulation of pulmonary surfactant apoprotein SP 28-36 gene in fetal human lung. *Proc. Natl. Acad. Sci. USA* **83:**9527–9531.

Bax, W. A., O. J. Cluysenaer, A. K. Bartelink, P. C. Aerts, R. A. Ezekowitz, and H. van Dijk. 1999. Association of familial deficiency of mannose-binding lectin and meningococcal disease. *Lancet* **354:**1094–1095.

Bickerstaff, M. C., M. Botto, W. L. Hutchinson, J. Herbert, G. A. Tennent, A. Bybee, D. A. Mitchell, H. T. Cook, P. J. Butler, M. J. Walport, and M. B. Pepys. 1999. Serum amyloid P component controls chromatin degradation and prevents antinuclear autoimmunity. *Nat. Med.* **5:**694–697.

Borron, P. J., E. C. Crouch, J. F. Lewis, J. R. Wright, F. Possmayer, and L. J. Fraher. 1998a. Recombinant rat surfactant-associated protein D inhibits human T lymphocyte proliferation and IL-2 production. *J. Immunol.* **161:**4599–4603.

Borron, P., F. X. McCormack, B. M. Elhalwagi, Z. C. Chroneos, J. F. Lewis, S. Zhu, J. R. Wright, V. L. Shepherd, F. Possmayer, K. Inchley, and L. J. Fraher. 1998b. Surfactant protein A inhibits T cell proliferation via its collagen-like tail and a 210-kDa receptor. *Am. J. Physiol.* **275:**L679–L686.

Botas, C., F. Poulain, J. Akiyama, C. Brown, L. Allen, J. Goerke, J. Clements, E. Carlson, A. M. Gillespie, C. Epstein, and S. Hawgood. 1998. Altered surfactant homeostasis and alveolar type II cell morphology in mice lacking surfactant protein D. *Proc. Natl. Acad. Sci. USA* **95:**11869–11874.

Bourbon, J. R., and B. Chailley-Heu. 2001. Surfactant proteins in the digestive tract, mesentery, and other organs: evolutionary significance. *Comp. Biochem. Physiol. A Mol. Integr. Physiol.* **129:**151–161.

Bowness, P., K. A. Davies, P. J. Norsworthy, P. Athanassiou, J. Taylor-Wiedeman, L. K. Borysiewicz, P. A. Meyer, and M. J. Walport. 1994. Hereditary C1q deficiency and systemic lupus erythematosus. *Q. J. Med.* **87:**455–464.

Brinker, K. G., E. Martin, P. Borron, E. Mostaghel, C. Doyle, C. V. Harding, and J. R. Wright. 2001. Surfactant protein D enhances bacterial antigen presentation by bone marrow–derived dendritic cells. *Am. J. Physiol. Lung Cell. Mol. Physiol.* **281:**L1453–L1463.

Cai, G. Z., G. L. Griffin, R. M. Senior, W. J. Longmore, and M. A. Moxley. 1999. Recombinant SP-D carbohydrate recognition domain is a chemoattractant for human neutrophils. *Am. J. Physiol.* **276:** L131–L136.

Chida, S., D. S. Phelps, C. Cordle, R. Soll, J. Floros, and H. W. Taeusch. 1988. Surfactant-associated proteins in tracheal aspirates of infants with respiratory distress syndrome after surfactant therapy. *Am. Rev. Respir. Dis.* **137:**943–947.

Clark, H., and K. B. Reid. 2002. Structural requirements for surfactant protein D function in vitro and in vivo: therapeutic potential of recombinant SP-D. *Immunobiology* **205:**619–631.

Clark, H. W., K. B. Reid, and R. B. Sim. 2000. Collectins and innate immunity in the lung. *Microbes Infect.* **2:**273-278.

Clark, H., N. Palaniyar, P. Strong, J. Edmondson, S. Hawgood, and K. B. Reid. 2002. Surfactant protein d reduces alveolar macrophage apoptosis in vivo. *J. Immunol.* **169:**2892–2899.

Crosdale, D. J., K. V. Poulton, W. E. Ollier, W. Thomson, and D. W. Denning. 2001. Mannose-binding lectin gene polymorphisms as a susceptibility factor for chronic necrotizing pulmonary aspergillosis. *J. Infect. Dis.* **184:**653–656.

Crouch, E. C., A. Persson, G. L. Griffin, D. Chang, and R. M. Senior. 1995. Interactions of pulmonary surfactant protein D (SP-D) with human blood leukocytes. *Am. J. Respir. Cell Mol. Biol.* **12:**410–415.

Crouch, E., K. Hartshorn, and I. Ofek. 2000. Collectins and pulmonary innate immunity. *Immunol. Rev.* **173:**52–65.

Dahl, M. R., S. Thiel, M. Matsushita, T. Fujita, A. C. Willis, T. Christensen, T. Vorup-Jensen, and J. C. Jensenius. 2001. MASP-3 and its association with distinct complexes of the mannan-binding lectin complement activation pathway. *Immunity* **15:**127–135.

Downing, J. F., R. Pasula, J. R. Wright, H. L. D. Twigg, and W. J. D. Martin. 1995. Surfactant protein a promotes attachment of *Mycobacterium tuberculosis* to alveolar macrophages during infection with human immunodeficiency virus. *Proc. Natl. Acad. Sci. USA* **92:**4848–4852.

Drickamer, K. 1989. Demonstration of carbohydrate-recognition activity in diverse proteins which share a common primary structure motif. 627th meeting , Nottingham **17:**13–15.

Drogari-Apiranthitou, M., C. A. Fijen, S. Thiel, A. Platonov, L. Jensen, J. Dankert, and E. J. Kuijper. 1997. The effect of mannan-binding lectin on opsonophagocytosis of *Neisseria meningitidis*. *Immunopharmacology* **38:**93–99.

Eda, S., Y. Suzuki, T. Kawai, K. Ohtani, T. Kase, Y. Fujinaga, T. Sakamoto, T. Kurimura, and N. Wakamiya. 1997. Structure of a truncated human surfactant protein D is less effective in agglutinating bacteria than the native structure and fails to inhibit haemagglutination by influenza A virus. *Biochem. J.* **323:**393–399.

Epstein, J., Q. Eichbaum, S. Sheriff, and R. A. Ezekowitz. 1996. The collectins in innate immunity. *Curr. Opin. Immunol.* **8:**29–35.

Ezekowitz, A. B. 1991. Ante-antibody immunity. *Curr. Biol.* **1:**60–62.

Ezekowitz, R. A., L. E. Day, and G. A. Herman. 1988. A human mannose-binding protein is an acute-phase reactant that shares sequence homology with other vertebrate lectins. *J. Exp. Med.* **167:**1034–1046. (Erratum **174:**753, 1991.)

Ezekowitz, R. A., M. Kuhlman, J. E. Groopman, and R. A. Byrn. 1989. A human serum mannose-binding protein inhibits in vitro infection by the human immunodeficiency virus. *J. Exp. Med.* **169:** 185–196.

Ezekowitz, R. A., D. J. Williams, H. Koziel, M. Y. Armstrong, A. Warner, F. F. Richards, and R. M. Rose. 1991. Uptake of *Pneumocystis carinii* mediated by the macrophage mannose receptor. *Nature* **351:** 155–158.

Fadok, V. A., and G. Chimini. 2001. The phagocytosis of apoptotic cells. *Semin. Immunol.* **13:**365–372.

Ferguson, J. S., D. R. Voelker, F. X. McCormack, and L. S. Schlesinger. 1999. Surfactant protein D binds to *Mycobacterium tuberculosis* bacilli and lipoarabinomannan via carbohydrate-lectin interactions resulting in reduced phagocytosis of the bacteria by macrophages. *J. Immunol.* **163:**312–321.

Ferguson, J. S., D. R. Voelker, J. A. Ufnar, A. J. Dawson, and L. S. Schlesinger. 2002. Surfactant protein D inhibition of human macrophage uptake of *Mycobacterium tuberculosis* is independent of bacterial agglutination. *J. Immunol.* **168:**1309–1314.

Garred, P., T. Pressler, H. O. Madsen, B. Frederiksen, A. Svejgaard, N. Hoiby, M. Schwartz, and C. Koch. 1999. Association of mannose-binding lectin gene heterogeneity with severity of lung disease and survival in cystic fibrosis. *J. Clin. Invest.* **104:**431–437.

Garred, P., T. Pressler, S. Lanng, H. O. Madsen, C. Moser, I. Laursen, F. Balstrup, and C. Koch.

2002. Mannose-binding lectin (MBL) therapy in an MBL-deficient patient with severe cystic fibrosis lung disease. *Pediatr. Pulmonol.* **33**:201–207.

Geertsma, M. F., P. H. Nibbering, H. P. Haagsman, M. R. Daha, and R. van Furth. 1994. Binding of surfactant protein A to C1q receptors mediates phagocytosis of *Staphylococcus aureus* by monocytes. *Am. J. Physiol.* **267**:L578–L584.

Gulati, S., K. Sastry, J. C. Jensenius, P. A. Rice, and S. Ram. 2002. Regulation of the mannan-binding lectin pathway of complement on *Neisseria gonorrhoeae* by C1-inhibitor and alpha 2-macroglobulin. *J. Immunol.* **168**:4078–4086.

Guo, X., H. M. Lin, Z. Lin, M. Montano, R. Sansores, G. Wang, S. DiAngelo, A. Pardo, M. Selman, and J. Floros. 2001. Surfactant protein gene A, B, and D marker alleles in chronic obstructive pulmonary disease of a Mexican population. *Eur. Respir. J.* **18**:482–490.

Haataja, R., R. Marttila, P. Uimari, J. Lofgren, M. Ramet, and M. Hallman. 2001. Respiratory distress syndrome: evaluation of genetic susceptibility and protection by transmission disequilibrium test. *Hum. Genet.* **109**:351–355.

Hakansson, K., N. K. Lim, H. J. Hoppe, and K. B. Reid. 1999. Crystal structure of the trimeric alpha-helical coiled-coil and the three lectin domains of human lung surfactant protein D. *Struct. Fold. Des.* **7**:255–264.

Hartshorn, K. L., E. C. Crouch, M. R. White, P. Eggleton, A. I. Tauber, D. Chang, and K. Sastry. 1994. Evidence for a protective role of pulmonary surfactant protein D (SP-D) against influenza A viruses. *J. Clin. Invest.* **94**:311–319.

Hartshorn, K. L., M. R. White, V. Shepherd, K. Reid, J. C. Jensenius, and E. C. Crouch. 1997. Mechanisms of anti-influenza activity of surfactant proteins A and D: comparison with serum collectins. *Am. J. Physiol.* **273**:L1156–L1166.

Hartshorn, K. L., E. Crouch, M. R. White, M. L. Colamussi, A. Kakkanatt, B. Tauber, V. Shepherd, and K. N. Sastry. 1998. Pulmonary surfactant proteins A and D enhance neutrophil uptake of bacteria. *Am. J. Physiol.* **274**:L958–L969.

Hartshorn, K. L., M. R. White, D. R. Voelker, J. Coburn, K. Zaner, and E. C. Crouch. 2000. Mechanism of binding of surfactant protein D to influenza A viruses: importance of binding to haemagglutinin to antiviral activity. *Biochem. J.* **351**:449–458.

Hickling, T. P., H. Bright, K. Wing, D. Gower, S. L. Martin, R. B. Sim, and R. Malhotra. 1999. A recombinant trimeric surfactant protein D carbohydrate recognition domain inhibits respiratory syncytial virus infection in vitro and in vivo. *Eur. J. Immunol.* **29**:3478–3484.

Hickman-Davis, J., J. Gibbs-Erwin, J. R. Lindsey, and S. Matalon. 1999. Surfactant protein A mediates mycoplasmacidal activity of alveolar macrophages by production of peroxynitrite. *Proc. Natl. Acad. Sci. USA* **96**:4953–4958.

Hirose, S., Y. Jiang, Y. Hamano, and T. Shirai. 2000. Genetic aspects of inherent B-cell abnormalities associated with SLE and B-cell malignancy: lessons from New Zealand mouse models. *Int. Rev. Immunol.* **19**:389–421.

Hoffmann, J. A., F. C. Kafatos, C. A. Janeway, and R. A. Ezekowitz. 1999. Phylogenetic perspectives in innate immunity. *Science* **284**:1313–1318.

Holmskov, U. L. 2000. Collectins and collectin receptors in innate immunity. *APMIS* **100**(Suppl.):1–59.

Hoppe, H. J., and K. B. Reid. 1994. Collectins— soluble proteins containing collagenous regions and lectin domains—and their roles in innate immunity. *Protein Sci.* **3**:1143–1158.

Hoppe, H. J., P. N. Barlow, and K. B. Reid. 1994. A parallel three stranded alpha-helical bundle at the nucleation site of collagen triple-helix formation. *FEBS Lett.* **344**:191–195.

Ikeda, K., T. Sannoh, N. Kawasaki, T. Kawasaki, and I. Yamashina. 1987. Serum lectin with known structure activates complement through the classical pathway. *J. Biol. Chem.* **262**:7451–7454.

Ikegami, M., B. M. Elhalwagi, N. Palaniyar, K. Dienger, T. Korfhagen, J. A. Whitsett, and F. X. McCormack. 2001. The collagen-like region of surfactant protein A (SP-A) is required for correction of surfactant structural and functional defects in the SP-A null mouse. *J. Biol. Chem.* **276**:38542–38548.

Ip, W. K., S. Y. Chan, C. S. Lau, and Y. L. Lau. 1998. Association of systemic lupus erythematosus with promoter polymorphisms of the mannose-binding lectin gene. *Arthritis Rheum.* **41**:1663–1668.

Kabha, K., J. Schmegner, Y. Keisari, H. Parolis, J. Schlepper-Schaeffer, and I. Ofek. 1997. SP-A enhances phagocytosis of Klebsiella by interaction with capsular polysaccharides and alveolar macrophages. *Am. J. Physiol.* **272**:L344–L352.

Kala, P., T. Ten Have, H. Nielsen, M. Dunn, and J. Floros. 1998. Association of pulmonary surfactant protein A (SP-A) gene and respiratory distress syndrome: interaction with SP-B. *Pediatr. Res.* **43**:169–177.

Kase, T., Y. Suzuki, T. Kawai, T. Sakamoto, K. Ohtani, S. Eda, A. Maeda, Y. Okuno, T. Kurimura, and N. Wakamiya. 1999. Human mannan-binding lectin inhibits the infection of influenza A virus without complement. *Immunology* **97**:385–392.

Klabunde, J., A. C. Uhlemann, A. E. Tebo, J. Kimmel, R. T. Schwarz, P. G. Kremsner, and J. F. Kun. 2002. Recognition of *Plasmodium falciparum* proteins by mannan-binding lectin, a component of the human innate immune system. *Parasitol. Res.* **88**: 113–117.

Kuan, S. F., K. Rust, and E. Crouch. 1992. Interactions of surfactant protein D with bacterial lipopolysaccharides. Surfactant protein D is an *Escherichia coli*-binding protein in bronchoalveolar lavage. *J. Clin. Invest.* **90:**97–106.

Kuhlman, M., K. Joiner, and R. A. Ezekowitz. 1989. The human mannose-binding protein functions as an opsonin. *J. Exp. Med.* **169:**1733–1745.

Lee, R. T., Y. Ichikawa, M. Fay, K. Drickamer, M. C. Shao, and Y. C. Lee. 1991. Ligand-binding characteristics of rat serum-type mannose-binding protein (MBP-A). Homology of binding site architecture with mammalian and chicken hepatic lectins. *J. Biol. Chem.* **266:**4810–4815.

LeVine, A. M., and J. A. Whitsett. 2001. Pulmonary collectins and innate host defense of the lung. *Microbes Infect.* **3:**161–166.

LeVine, A. M., M. D. Bruno, K. M. Huelsman, G. F. Ross, J. A. Whitsett, and T. R. Korfhagen. 1997. Surfactant protein A-deficient mice are susceptible to group B streptococcal infection. *J. Immunol.* **158:**4336–4340.

LeVine, A. M., K. E. Kurak, M. D. Bruno, J. M. Stark, J. A. Whitsett, and T. R. Korfhagen. 1998. Surfactant protein-A-deficient mice are susceptible to *Pseudomonas aeruginosa* infection. *Am. J. Respir. Cell Mol. Biol.* **19:**700–708.

LeVine, A. M., K. E. Kurak, J. R. Wright, W. T. Watford, M. D. Bruno, G. F. Ross, J. A. Whitsett, and T. R. Korfhagen. 1999a. Surfactant protein-A binds group B streptococcus enhancing phagocytosis and clearance from lungs of surfactant protein-A-deficient mice. *Am. J. Respir. Cell Mol. Biol.* **20:**279–286.

LeVine, A. M., J. Gwozdz, J. Stark, M. Bruno, J. Whitsett, and T. Korfhagen. 1999b. Surfactant protein-A enhances respiratory syncytial virus clearance in vivo. *J. Clin. Invest.* **103:**1015–1021.

LeVine, A. M., J. A. Whitsett, J. A. Gwozdz, T. R. Richardson, J. H. Fisher, M. S. Burhans, and T. R. Korfhagen. 2000. Distinct effects of surfactant protein A or D deficiency during bacterial infection on the lung. *J. Immunol.* **165:**3934–3940.

LeVine, A. M., J. A. Whitsett, K. L. Hartshorn, E. C. Crouch, and T. R. Korfhagen. 2001. Surfactant protein D enhances clearance of influenza A virus from the lung in vivo. *J. Immunol.* **167:**5868–5873.

Lim, B. L., J. Y. Wang, U. Holmskov, H. J. Hoppe, and K. B. Reid. 1994. Expression of the carbohydrate recognition domain of lung surfactant protein D and demonstration of its binding to lipopolysaccharides of gram-negative bacteria. *Biochem. Biophys. Res. Commun.* **202:**1674–1680.

Lipscombe, R. J., Y. L. Lau, R. J. Levinsky, S. M., J. A. Summerfield, and M. W. Turner. 1992. Identical point mutation leading to low levels of man-nose binding protein and poor C3b mediated opsoni-sation in Chinese and Causasian populations. *Immunol. Lett.* **32:**253–258.

Lofgren, J., M. Ramet, M. Renko, R. Marttila, and M. Hallman. 2002. Association between surfactant protein A gene locus and severe respiratory syncytial virus infection in infants. *J. Infect. Dis.* **185:**283–289.

Lu, J. H., S. Thiel, H. Wiedemann, R. Timpl, and K. B. Reid. 1990. Binding of the pentamer/hexamer forms of mannan-binding protein to zymosan activates the proenzyme C1r2C1s2 complex, of the classical pathway of complement, without involvement of C1q. *J. Immunol.* **144:**2287–2294.

Lu, J., C. Teh, U. Kishore, and K. B. Reid. 2002. Collectins and ficolins: sugar pattern recognition molecules of the mammalian innate immune system. *Biochim. Biophys. Acta* **1572:**387–400.

Madan, T., P. Eggleton, U. Kishore, P. Strong, S. S. Aggrawal, P. U. Sarma, and K. B. Reid. 1997. Binding of pulmonary surfactant proteins A and D to *Aspergillus fumigatus* conidia enhances phagocytosis and killing by human neutrophils and alveolar macrophages. *Infect. Immun.* **65:**3171–3179.

Madan, T., U. Kishore, M. Singh, P. Strong, E. M. Hussain, K. B. Reid, and P. U. Sarma. 2001. Protective role of lung surfactant protein D in a murine model of invasive pulmonary aspergillosis. *Infect. Immun.* **69:**2728–2731.

Madsen, J., A. Kliem, I. Tornoe, K. Skjodt, C. Koch, and U. Holmskov. 2000. Localization of lung surfactant protein D on mucosal surfaces in human tissues. *J. Immunol.* **164:**5866–5870.

Malhotra, R., S. Thiel, K. B. Reid, and R. B. Sim. 1990. Human leukocyte C1q receptor binds other soluble proteins with collagen domains. *J. Exp. Med.* **172:**955–959.

Malhotra, R., J. Haurum, S. Thiel, and R. B. Sim. 1992. Interaction of C1q receptor with lung surfactant protein A. *Eur. J. Immunol.* **22:**1437–1445.

Malhotra, R., J. Lu, U. Holmskov, and R. B. Sim. 1994. Collectins, collectin receptors and the lectin pathway of complement activation. *Clin. Exp. Immunol.* **97**(Suppl. 2):4–9.

Mamula, M. J., S. Fatenejad, and J. Craft. 1994. B cells process and present lupus autoantigens that initiate autoimmune T cell responses. *J. Immunol.* **152:**1453–1461.

McCormack, F. X., T. E. King, Jr., D. R. Voelker, P. C. Robinson, and R. J. Mason. 1991. Idiopathic pulmonary fibrosis. Abnormalities in the bronchoalveolar lavage content of surfactant protein A. *Am. Rev. Respir. Dis.* **144:**160–166.

McIntosh, J. C., A. H. Swyers, J. H. Fisher, and J. R. Wright. 1996. Surfactant proteins A and D increase in response to intratracheal lipopolysaccharide. *Am. J. Respir. Cell Mol. Biol.* **15:**509–519.

McNeely, T. B., and J. D. Coonrod. 1993. Comparison of the opsonic activity of human surfactant protein A for *Staphylococcus aureus* and *Streptococcus pneumoniae* with rabbit and human macrophages. *J. Infect. Dis.* **167**:91–97.

McNeely, T. B., and J. D. Coonrod. 1994. Aggregation and opsonization of type A but not type B *Haemophilus influenzae* by surfactant protein A. *Am. J. Respir. Cell Mol. Biol.* **11**:114–122.

Mills, J. A. 1994. Systemic lupus erythematosus. *N. Engl. J. Med.* **330**:1871–1879.

Miyamura, K., R. Malhotra, H. J. Hoppe, K. B. Reid, P. J. Phizackerley, P. Macpherson, and A. Lopez Bernal. 1994. Surfactant proteins A (SP-A) and D (SP-D): levels in human amniotic fluid and localization in the fetal membranes. *Biochim. Biophys. Acta* **1210**:303–307.

Morel, L., B. P. Croker, K. R. Blenman, C. Mohan, G. Huang, G. Gilkeson, and E. K. Wakeland. 2000. Genetic reconstitution of systemic lupus erythematosus immunopathology with polycongenic murine strains. *Proc. Natl. Acad. Sci. USA* **97**:6670–6675.

Morel, L., K. R. Blenman, B. P. Croker, and E. K. Wakeland. 2001. The major murine systemic lupus erythematosus susceptibility locus, Sle1, is a cluster of functionally related genes. *Proc. Natl. Acad. Sci. USA* **98**:1787–1792.

Mullighan, C. G., S. E. Marshall, and K. I. Welsh. 2000. Mannose binding lectin polymorphisms are associated with early age of disease onset and autoimmunity in common variable immunodeficiency. *Scand. J. Immunol.* **51**:111–122.

Mullighan, C. G., S. Heatley, K. Doherty, F. Szabo, A. Grigg, T. P. Hughes, A. P. Schwarer, J. Szer, B. D. Tait, L. Bik To, and P. G. Bardy. 2002. Mannose-binding lectin gene polymorphisms are associated with major infection following allogeneic hemopoietic stem cell transplantation. *Blood* **99**:3524–3529.

Naves, M., A. H. Hajeer, L. S. Teh, E. J. Davies, J. Ordi-Ros, P. Perez-Pemen, M. Vilardel-Tarres, W. Thomson, J. Worthington, and W. E. Ollier. 1998. Complement C4B null allele status confers risk for systemic lupus erythematosus in a Spanish population. *Eur. J. Immunogenet.* **25**:317–320.

Neth, O., I. Hann, M. W. Turner, and N. J. Klein. 2001. Deficiency of mannose-binding lectin and burden of infection in children with malignancy: a prospective study. *Lancet* **358**:614–618.

Ng, K. K., K. Drickamer, and W. I. Weis. 1996. Structural analysis of monosaccharide recognition by rat liver mannose-binding protein. *J. Biol. Chem.* **271**:663–674.

Ng, K. K., A. R. Kolatkar, S. Park-Snyder, H. Feinberg, D. A. Clark, K. Drickamer, and W. I. Weis. 2002. Orientation of bound ligands in mannose-binding proteins. Implications for multivalent ligand recognition. *J. Biol. Chem.* **277**:16088–16095.

Odendahl, M., A. Jacobi, A. Hansen, E. Feist, F. Hiepe, G. R. Burmester, P. E. Lipsky, A. Radbruch, and T. Dorner. 2000. Disturbed peripheral B lymphocyte homeostasis in systemic lupus erythematosus. *J. Immunol.* **165**:5970–5979.

Ogden, C. A., A. deCathelineau, P. R. Hoffmann, D. Bratton, B. Ghebrehiwet, V. A. Fadok, and P. M. Henson. 2001. C1q and mannose binding lectin engagement of cell surface calreticulin and CD91 initiates macropinocytosis and uptake of apoptotic cells. *J. Exp. Med.* **194**:781–795.

O'Riordan, D. M., J. E. Standing, K. Y. Kwon, D. Chang, E. C. Crouch, and A. H. Limper. 1995. Surfactant protein D interacts with *Pneumocystis carinii* and mediates organism adherence to alveolar macrophages. *J. Clin. Invest.* **95**:2699–2710.

Paananen, R., V. Glumoff, R. Sormunen, W. Voorhout, and M. Hallman. 2001. Expression and localization of lung surfactant protein B in Eustachian tube epithelium. *Am. J. Physiol. Lung Cell. Mol. Physiol.* **280**:L214–L220.

Peterslund, N. A., C. Koch, J. C. Jensenius, and S. Thiel. 2001. Association between deficiency of mannose-binding lectin and severe infections after chemotherapy. *Lancet* **358**:637–638.

Phelps, D. S., and R. M. Rose. 1991. Increased recovery of surfactant protein A in AIDS-related pneumonia. *Am. Rev. Respir. Dis.* **143**:1072–1075.

Pikaar, J. C., W. F. Voorhout, L. M. van Golde, J. Verhoef, J. A. Van Strijp, and J. F. van Iwaarden. 1995. Opsonic activities of surfactant proteins A and D in phagocytosis of gram-negative bacteria by alveolar macrophages. *J. Infect. Dis.* **172**:481–489.

Restrepo, C. I., Q. Dong, J. Savov, W. I. Mariencheck, and J. R. Wright. 1999. Surfactant protein D stimulates phagocytosis of *Pseudomonas aeruginosa* by alveolar macrophages. *Am. J. Respir. Cell Mol. Biol.* **21**:576–585.

Sastry, K., G. A. Herman, L. Day, E. Deignan, G. Bruns, C. C. Morton, and R. A. Ezekowitz. 1989. The human mannose-binding protein gene. Exon structure reveals its evolutionary relationship to a human pulmonary surfactant gene and localization to chromosome 10. *J. Exp. Med.* **170**:1175–1189.

Schagat, T. L., J. A. Wofford, and J. R. Wright. 2001. Surfactant protein A enhances alveolar macrophage phagocytosis of apoptotic neutrophils. *J. Immunol.* **166**:2727–2733.

Schelenz, S., R. Malhotra, R. B. Sim, U. Holmskov, and G. J. Bancroft. 1995. Binding of host collectins to the pathogenic yeast *Cryptococcus neoformans*: human surfactant protein D acts as an agglutinin for acapsular yeast cells. *Infect. Immun.* **63**:3360–3366.

Sheriff, S., C. Y. Chang, and R. A. Ezekowitz. 1994. Human mannose-binding protein carbohydrate recognition domain trimerizes through a triple alpha-helical coiled-coil. *Nat. Struct. Biol.* **1:**789–794.

Strong, P., K. B. Reid, and H. Clark. 2002. Intranasal delivery of a truncated recombinant human SP-D is effective at down regulating allergic hypersensitivity in mice sensitised to allergens of Aspergillus fumigatus. *Clin. Exp. Immunol.* **130:**19–24.

Super, M., S. Thiel, J. Lu, R. J. Levinsky, and M. W. Turner. 1989. Association of low levels of mannan-binding protein with a common defect of opsonisation. *Lancet* **2:**1236–1239.

Tabona, P., A. Mellor, and J. A. Summerfield. 1995. Mannose binding protein is involved in first-line host defence: evidence from transgenic mice. *Immunology* **85:**153–159.

Taylor, P. R., A. Carugati, V. A. Fadok, H. T. Cook, M. Andrews, M. C. Carroll, J. S. Savill, P. M. Henson, M. Botto, and M. J. Walport. 2000. A hierarchical role for classical pathway complement proteins in the clearance of apoptotic cells in vivo. *J. Exp. Med.* **192:**359–366.

Terai, I., and K. Kobayashi. 1993. Perinatal changes in serum mannose-binding protein (MBP) levels. *Immunol. Lett.* **38:**185–187.

Terai, I., K. Kobayashi, T. Fujita, and K. Hagiwara. 1993. Human serum mannose binding protein (MBP): development of an enzyme-linked immunosorbent assay (ELISA) and determination of levels in serum from 1085 normal Japanese and in some body fluids. *Biochem. Med. Metab. Biol.* **50:**111–119.

Tino, M. J., and J. R. Wright. 1996. Surfactant protein A stimulates phagocytosis of specific pulmonary pathogens by alveolar macrophages. *Am. J. Physiol.* **270:**L677–L688.

Tino, M. J., and J. R. Wright. 1999. Surfactant proteins A and D specifically stimulate directed actin-based responses in alveolar macrophages. *Am. J. Physiol.* **276:**L164–L174.

Tsutsumi, A., K. Sasaki, N. Wakamiya, K. Ichikawa, T. Atsumi, K. Ohtani, Y. Suzuki, T. Koike, and T. Sumida. 2001. Mannose-binding lectin gene: polymorphisms in Japanese patients with systemic lupus erythematosus, rheumatoid arthritis and Sjogren's syndrome. *Genes Immun.* **2:**99–104.

Turner, M. W., and R. M. Hamvas. 2000. Mannose-binding lectin: structure, function, genetics and disease associations. *Rev. Immunogenet.* **2:**305–322.

Vandivier, R. W., C. A. Ogden, V. A. Fadok, P. R. Hoffmann, K. K. Brown, M. Botto, M. J. Walport, J. H. Fisher, P. M. Henson, and K. E. Greene. 2002. Role of surfactant proteins A, D, and C1q in the clearance of apoptotic cells in vivo and in vitro: calreticulin and CD91 as a common collectin receptor complex. *J. Immunol.* **169:**3978–3986.

van Iwaarden, J. F., J. A. van Strijp, M. J. Ebskamp, A. C. Welmers, J. Verhoef, and L. M. van Golde. 1991. Surfactant protein A is opsonin in phagocytosis of herpes simplex virus type 1 by rat alveolar macrophages. *Am. J. Physiol. Lung Cell. Mol. Physiol.* **261:**L204–L209.

Van Iwaarden, J. F., J. C. Pikaar, J. Storm, E. Brouwer, J. Verhoef, R. S. Oosting, L. M. van Golde, and J. A. van Strijp. 1994. Binding of surfactant protein A to the lipid A moiety of bacterial lipopolysaccharides. *Biochem. J.* **303:**407–411.

van Rozendaal, B. A., C. H. van de Lest, M. van Eijk, L. M. van Golde, W. F. Voorhout, H. P. van Helden, and H. P. Haagsman. 1999. Aerosolized endotoxin is immediately bound by pulmonary surfactant protein D in vivo. *Biochim. Biophys. Acta* **1454:**261–269.

Villarreal, J., D. Crosdale, W. Ollier, A. Hajeer, W. Thomson, J. Ordi, E. Balada, M. Villardell, L. S. Teh, and K. Poulton. 2001. Mannose binding lectin and FcgammaRIIa (CD32) polymorphism in Spanish systemic lupus erythematosus patients. *Rheumatology* (Oxford) **40:**1009–1012.

Wallis, R., and J. Y. Cheng. 1999. Molecular defects in variant forms of mannose-binding protein associated with immunodeficiency. *J. Immunol.* **163:**4953–4959.

Wallis, R., and R. B. Dodd. 2000. Interaction of mannose-binding protein with associated serine proteases: effects of naturally occurring mutations. *J. Biol. Chem.* **275:**30962–30969.

Wallis, R., and K. Drickamer. 1999. Molecular determinants of oligomer formation and complement fixation in mannose-binding proteins. *J. Biol. Chem.* **274:**3580–3589.

Walport, M. J., K. A. Davies, and M. Botto. 1998. C1q and systemic lupus erythematosus. *Immunobiology* **199:**265–285.

Wang, J. Y., C. C. Shieh, P. F. You, H. Y. Lei, and K. B. Reid. 1998. Inhibitory effect of pulmonary surfactant proteins A and D on allergen-induced lymphocyte proliferation and histamine release in children with asthma. *Am. J. Respir. Crit. Care Med.* **158:**510–518.

Watford, W. T., J. R. Wright, C. G. Hester, H. Jiang, and M. M. Frank. 2001. Surfactant protein A regulates complement activation. *J. Immunol.* **167:**6593–6600.

Weber, B., A. Borkhardt, S. Stoll-Becker, I. Reiss, and L. Gortner. 2000. Polymorphisms of surfactant protein A genes and the risk of bronchopulmonary dysplasia in preterm infants. *Turk. J. Pediatr.* **42:**181–185.

Weis, W. I., and K. Drickamer. 1994. Trimeric structure of a C-type mannose-binding protein. *Structure* **2:**1227–1240.

Wert, S. E., M. Yoshida, A. M. LeVine, M. Ikegami, T. Jones, G. F. Ross, J. H. Fisher, T. R. Korfhagen, and J. A. Whitsett. 2000. Increased metalloproteinase activity, oxidant production, and emphysema in surfactant protein D gene-inactivated mice. *Proc. Natl. Acad. Sci. USA* **97:**5972–5977.

Wright, J. R., and D. C. Youmans. 1993. Pulmonary surfactant protein A stimulates chemotaxis of alveolar macrophage. *Am. J. Physiol.* **264:**L338–L344.

Wright, J. R., P. Borron, K. G. Brinker, and R. J. Folz. 2001. Surfactant Protein A. Regulation of innate and adaptive immune responses in lung inflammation. *Am. J. Respir. Cell Mol. Biol.* **24:**513–517.

Zhang, P., A. McAlinden, S. Li, T. Schumacher, H. Wang, S. Hu, L. Sandell, and E. Crouch. 2001. The amino-terminal heptad repeats of the coiled-coil neck domain of pulmonary surfactant protein d are necessary for the assembly of trimeric subunits and dodecamers. *J. Biol. Chem.* **276:**19862–19870.

COMPLEMENT AND ITS RECEPTORS IN INFECTION

Admar Verschoor and Michael C. Carroll

‖

COMPLEMENT: AN INTRODUCTION

Elements of the complement system are found in a wide array of species, ranging from primitive arthropods to modern humans. The complement system's pervasiveness and its highly conserved biochemical features hint at the considerable advantages it offers its host.

Early characterizations of the complement system pointed out its role as an immediate, nonadaptive line of defense to infectious agents. At the same time, it is involved in the induction of the inflammatory response. However, additional strengths of the complement system outside these long-recognized features of innate immunity are still being revealed. More recently established, for instance, is the role complement plays in clearance of apoptotic bodies from the circulation. Through targeting apoptotic cells to the liver and spleen for destruction, complement receptors on erythrocytes help remove self-antigens that are linked to autoimmune disorders. Another recognition regarding complement's wide range of functions is its instructive role on the adaptive arm of immunity. Humoral and memory responses, as well as certain cytotoxic and helper responses to infection, appear highly dependent on complement and its site of synthesis.

Conditions associated with complement's deregulation also underline the immunological potency of the complement system. Apart from increased susceptibility to infection in the absence of certain complement factors, increased or reduced complement levels have been implicated in the pathogenesis of a number of immune diseases. For example, deficiencies in complement components C1, C2 or C4 predispose humans to autoimmune diseases, such as systemic lupus erythematosus (Walport, 2001b). This disease is clinically characterized by the formation of DNA-specific autoantibodies and decreased serum levels for major complement components. Conversely, long-term clinical studies recently confirmed a positive correlation between elevated serum levels of the classical pathway initiating C-reactive protein and the risk of heart attack, a condition that is increasingly understood in terms of chronic inflammation. This correlation appears to be a stronger indicator of disease risk than others, such as high- and low-density lipoprotein levels (Ridker et al., 2002).

Admar Verschoor and Michael C. Carroll, Departments of Pathology and Pediatrics, Harvard Medical School, The CBR Institute for Biomedical Research, 800 Huntington Ave., Boston, MA 02115-5701.

The Innate Immune Response to Infection
Ed. by S. H. E. Kaufmann, R. Medzhitov, and S. Gordon
©2004 ASM Press, Washington, D.C.

In this chapter we focus on the general modus operandi of complement and its receptors in infection. We discuss the various pathways of complement activation and their microbial triggers and highlight some of the mechanisms and strategies pathogens have evolved to counteract or "hijack" the complement system. Finally, we devote a significant portion of the chapter to examining how the source of complement affects adaptive immunity to infectious agents.

COMPLEMENT FACTORS AND ACTIVATION PATHWAYS

Complement activation is induced by a variety of triggers and proceeds through a series of enzymatic, proteolytic, and complex-forming steps. Defined by the mode of activation and the subsequent proteolytic cascade in which activation occurs, three activation pathways are recognized: classical, mannan-binding lectin (MBL), and alternative. Although each pathway has unique combinations of initiating proteins, all converge into a common lytic pathway. The resulting lytic pathway protein cluster, the membrane attack complex (MAC), ultimately destroys the structural integrity of bacteria or enveloped viruses (see The Lytic Pathway, below). The pathways are schematically represented in Fig. 1. Invading agents also become covalently decorated with complement activation products that are recognized and bound by an array of complement receptors. We discuss this process of antigen (Ag) opsonization and subsequent complement receptor-mediated binding and phagocytosis of the complex in more detail in Complement Receptors and Infection, below.

The Classical Pathway

The classical pathway of complement was the first activation pathway described, and it is purely this historical fact that lends it the designation "classical." In fact, evolutionary data suggest that this pathway is the most recently evolved. Although the classical pathway utilizes aspects of the complement system that appear early in evolution, precursors of the immunoglobulin (Ig) superfamily required for its initiation did not emerge until the advent of vertebrates (see also Complement and Adaptive Immunity in an Evolutionary Context, below). Also noteworthy in an etymological sense is that it was the observation of a labile serum protein fraction "complementing" stable antibody (Ab) in the process of opsonizing and killing bacteria that led to the designation "complement." We discuss below, however, how the alternative pathway activates complement, independent of Ig (see The Alternative Pathway, below).

Human IgM and IgG isotypes are strong activators of the classical pathway, the former 1,000-fold more potent (Cooper, 1985). IgM and most IgG allotypes (except IgG4) activate classical complement after forming an antibody–antigen complex. Only Ag-bound Ab meets the conformational requirements necessary to initiate complement activation by allowing the first component of the classical complement cascade (C1) to bind. The C1 complex is comprised of subunits C1q, C1r, and C1s, which interact in a calcium-dependent manner and are present mostly in their associated form (Ziccardi and Cooper, 1977). C1 inhibitor (C1-inh) associates with the unbound C1 complex, thus preventing its tendency to initiate the classical pathway acciden-

FIGURE 1 Schematic overview of the complement cascade. Classical, MBL, and alternative pathways commence from the left side of the figure, leading to the converging point of C3 activation (top right). In every subsequent proteolytic step, the position of the new addition to the antigen complex is shown in black for clarity. From the central C3 activation step downwards, the C3 amplification loop through the alternative pathway is indicated by asterisks. The lytic pathway is initiated with the formation of C5 convertase and leads to the assembly of the C5,6,7,8,(n)9 MAC that interferes with the target's structural integrity by penetrating the cellular membrane (bottom right).

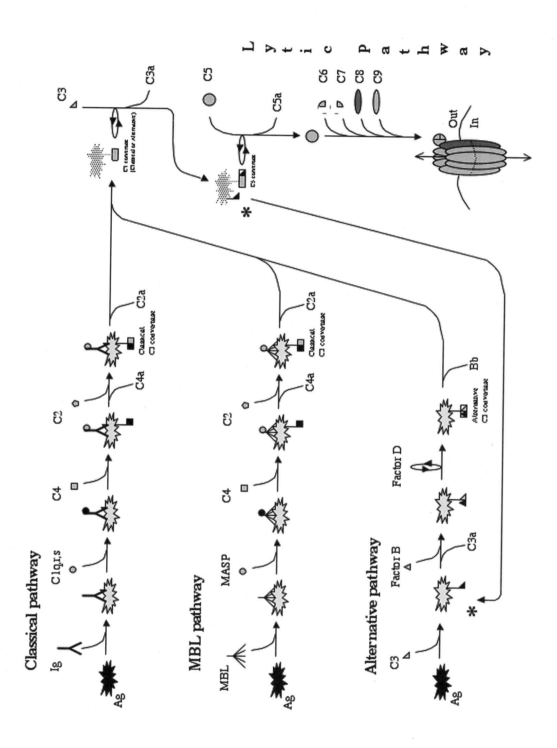

tally, independent of Ig. However, when the C1q portion does bind an Ig-Ag complex, the inhibition is undone and activation of the remainder of the classical pathway can occur. In certain cases, as described for human immunodeficiency virus (HIV), C1q is known to directly bind Ag and activate the classical pathway (Ebenbichler et al., 1991).

C1r and C1s, subunits in the C1 complex, expose a serine protease that activates components C4 and C2. In this process, C4 splits into C4a and C4b and a highly reactive thioester becomes exposed within the latter. Using this thioester, C4b opsonizes Ag whenever a suitable acceptor group is available, i.e., hydroxyl or amino groups. When these groups are unavailable in the immediate proximity, the unstable thioester quickly hydrolyzes and C4b becomes nonreactive C4bi. This swift hydrolysis process limits the scope of damage close to the site of activation. During C4 activation, the smaller C4a peptide is released and diffuses, acting as a weak anaphylatoxin (see also Anaphylatoxin Receptors below).

The C1s subunit also splits C2 into fragments C2a and C2b. Some confusion in the nomenclature arises here, as the general practice to refer to the smaller activation product as C#a and the larger as C#b is not followed in all publications. For purposes of uniformity we refer to the small, 34-kDa product as C2a and the 74-kDa product as C2b. C2b provides the serine protease that in association with C4b forms the classical pathway C3 convertase. C3 convertase can enzymatically generate great quantities of C3a and C3b from native C3. Reminiscent of the C4 activation products, C3a functions as a powerful anaphylatoxin, and C3b is an efficient opsonin.

In addition to cleaving C3, the C3 convertase can bind C3b to form the C5 convertase. C5 convertase generates C5a and C5b from C5. C5b initiates the lytic pathway (see The Lytic Pathway below), whereas C5a acts as the classical pathway's strongest anaphylatoxin inflammatory mediator. Like C3a, and to a lesser extent C4a, C5b activates phagocytic

cells and stimulates smooth muscle contraction, vasodilatation, and chemoattraction of leukocytes (reviewed by Ember et al., 1998).

In summary, (i) Ag interaction with certain Ig, especially IgM, leads to covalent deposition of C4b and increasing amounts of C3b through C3 convertase onto that Ag; (ii) building on C3 convertase, C5 convertase is generated, initiating the lytic pathway; and (iii) anaphylatoxins C4a, C3a, and C5a (in order of increasing potency) are generated to induce inflammatory responses.

The MBL Pathway

The key difference between the MBL and classical pathways is their mode of initiation. Instead of antibody interacting with C1q, the activating role is met by a mannan-binding collagenous lectin (collectin), MBL for short. MBL specifically binds mannose-containing carbohydrates (and to a lesser extent other polymeric carbohydrates that contain residues such as glucose or fructose) primarily accessible on viral and bacterial membranes. Although MBL and C1q do not share sequence homology, their structure and functionality are remarkably similar. Upon binding to the specific polysaccharide residues, MBL can bind and activate MBL-associated serine proteases (MASPs) 1, 2, and 3, not unlike Ab-associated C1q binds C1r and C1s. The similarity is further stressed by reports of Ag-bound MBL activating the C1r and C1s proenzyme complex directly, without C1q involvement (Lu et al., 1990). C1 inhibitor has an inactivating influence on MASPs, similar to its influence on C1r and C1s. This complex is also a potent activator of C4 and C2, and the MBL and classical pathways converge here to identical downstream events. Thus, the main distinction between classical and MBL pathways lies in their Ab dependence or independence, respectively. It has been suggested, however, that MBL–MASP-1 can omit C2 and C4 activation to activate C3 directly (Matsushita et al., 1998).

Genetic defects in MBL predispose primarily to recurrent childhood infections. This tendency suggests that the MBL pathway plays an important role in complement activation in early life when levels of maternal Ab (chiefly IgG allotypes, capable of activating the classical pathway) diminish and the child's own immune repertoire is still developing (Walport, 2001a).

The Alternative Pathway

The alternative pathway of complement activation can be initiated in the absence of Ag-specific Ab. This important feature allows complement to assert its protective functions in the host, before Ag-driven adaptive responses have developed. Typically, it takes a few days to a week for IgM and Ag-specific IgG, respectively, to reach titers significant enough to trigger the classical pathway. Arguably, it is during this low-Ig period that the alternative pathway is especially important. Moreover, the alternative pathway can amplify the effects of the classical or MBL pathways.

Omitting C2 and C4, which mark the MBL and classical pathways, spontaneous hydrolysis of C3 or direct activation through specific sugar groups on pathogen surfaces starts the self-sustaining cycle of C3 activation. This positive-amplification loop, whereby C3 activation products are capable of initiating further C3 activation, is an important and defining characteristic of the alternative pathway. Research on this mode of complement activation was pioneered by Pillemer using yeast cell wall extracts, also known as zymosan. Zymosan is a mannose-rich sugar, but we now know that the alternative pathway-activating polysaccharides include lipopolysaccharides (LPSs) found on bacterial cell walls (Gewurz et al., 1968) and those of fungal, viral, or even plant origin, such as inulin. The alternative pathway shows a remarkable ability to recognize "foreignness" in, and specifically respond to, a wide range of nonself substances, despite its inability to utilize the flexibility of Ag-specific Ab for its activation. This capacity can be partially understood through its tight regulation on self-surfaces by host regulatory pro-

teins (see Complement Inhibitors, Regulators, and Mimicry, below). However, most of the molecular aspects of the alternative pathway's highly efficient activation toward nonself agents remain poorly understood.

Upon encounter with a directly activating agent, or through spontaneous conformational change, C3's thioester becomes exposed. This allows covalent binding to acceptor sites, i.e., hydroxyl or amino groups, provided activation occurs in close proximity to a suitable surface. If not, the thioester rapidly reacts with water or other serum components. Once activated and covalently bound to a surface, activated C3 can noncovalently interact with serum-borne factor B. At this point, serum protease factor D cleaves factor B to generate protease Bb and a small peptide Ba. Ba quickly diffuses, its function unknown. The surface-bound C3,Bb complex can now serve as C3 convertase. This complex, stabilized by factor P, is reminiscent of the classical pathway's C4b,2b complex. Because C4b and C3b, as well as C2b and factor Bb, are homologous proteins, it is not surprising that their functional properties are similar. In further analogy to the classical pathway, C5 convertase is generated through coupling of C3b to C3 convertase of the alternative pathway.

The Lytic Pathway

One defining characteristic of the complement cascade is its ability to lyse bodies surrounded by a lipid membrane, i.e., whole cells, bacteria, or enveloped viruses such as herpes-, myxo-, paramyxo-, or retroviruses. Ehrlich recognized this trait at the dawn of the 20th century, coining the term "complement" when he observed how heat-labile serum components "complemented" Ab in bacterial lysis. However, it took many more years of research before the underlying nature of the lysing capability was understood in detail and ascribed to components C5 through C9. Although the alternative, classical, and MBL pathways are initiated and proceed in different manners, they converge with the formation of

C5 convertases that generate C5b. The latter component signals the start of the lytic pathway and becomes part of the MAC. It is this complex that is ultimately responsible for the lysing ability of the complement system. The MAC is a rather large protein aggregate, with a molecular mass upward of 1.600 kDa. Its spatial conformation creates a pore within the lipid membrane allowing for free diffusion between "in" and "out." This process effectively kills the target by osmosis, now that it can no longer maintain the cross-membrane nutrient, pH, salt, or voltage gradients needed for proper functioning.

After C5b has been generated through classical or alternative C5 convertases, it binds C6 from the serum. This still soluble complex can now recruit C7, allowing the aggregate of three molecules to insert itself into a nearby bilipid layer by virtue of the hydrophobic regions generated when C7 joins the C5bC6 complex (C5b-7). Once this complex is inserted into the target membrane, C8 can bind. To effectively induce lysis, however, insertion of one or more C9 molecules is required. The complex generated by virtue of one C9 molecule creates a pore of minimal size and can offer protection to simple, non-metabolizing structures, such as lipid-enveloped viruses. Oligomerization of C9 causes the pore to widen far enough to kill living cells or bacteria, structures that can, to a certain level, actively respond to and fight membrane damage and gradient loss.

COMPLEMENT INHIBITORS, REGULATORS, AND MIMICRY

Complement is a powerful and broad first line of defense. Not only does it provide a means to directly destruct invading microbes, its activation also induces inflammation and aids in the formation of adaptive memory responses (see Complement and Adaptive Immunity, below). One obvious consequence of these abilities of complement is the need to keep its potentially self-harming force in check. Harnessing the self-destructive power of complement is achieved in a number of ways. The inherent instability of many intermediate protein complexes limits their activity proximal to the site of intended activation. The presence of additional molecules capable of promoting or counteracting specific stages of complement activation, depending on the location, also helps to reign in complement. These regulatory proteins can be either serum borne or membrane bound and have either a stabilizing or destabilizing effect on various complement activation products.

Intended microbial targets have also evolved ways to control and evade complement. Evolutionary pressure or "gene snatching" has led to modes of complement regulation that are remarkably similar between distinct species. In other cases no clear connection can be drawn. Certain species do not encode their own regulatory proteins, but use their host's proteins instead. Simply physical features will in other cases still prevent complement from damaging the target organism.

Here we describe host complement regulatory proteins as well as several microbial answers to complement attack.

Regulation of the Early Classical Pathway

The classical pathway is under control in the early stage where the proenzymatic C1 complex forms from its C1q, C1r, and C1s subcomponents. Only upon binding the constant heavy-chain moieties of an Ab-Ag complex does C1 inhibitor loose its limiting grip on C1, thus initiating the classical pathway. Deficiencies in C1-inh, a serine protease inhibitor or serpin, have been associated with uncontrolled and continuous activation of C2 and C4, leading to functional deficiency in these factors. Hereditary angioneurotic edema, associated with C1-inh deficiency, is most likely due to excess C2 activation and dysregulated activation of the intrinsic coagulation pathway and bradykinin release (Donaldson et al., 1977).

Acting at this same early stage of classical activation, *Escherichia coli* expresses C1q-binding protein that interferes with C1q's association to C1r and C1s (van den Berg et al., 1996). Without C1s serine protease, no cleaving of C2 or C4 can occur, and the classical pathway is inhibited.

Regulation and Modulation on the C3 Level

From the host point of view, the need to tightly control complement is evident at the C3 level. C3 is the central component in all three complement activation pathways. The broad range of covalent binding preferences of activated C3 to hydroxyl and amino residues cannot absolutely prevent the formation of C3 convertases on self-surfaces. Its capacity for spontaneous activation, as well as the highly efficient and self-sustaining C3 amplification loop through the alternative pathway, makes control at the C3 level a necessity. Without regulating proteins, constant activation would be limited only by C3 depletion. Because C3 is a highly abundant serum protein, at concentrations of over 1 mg/ml, depletion would probably not occur before significant host damage is inflicted. The potency of complement C3 explains not only why many regulating proteins act on the C3 level to protect the host, but also why invading agents use this approach extensively.

As for the host, C3 activation, through alternative or classical C3 convertases, is arguably most effectively achieved by controlling C3 deposition on cell surfaces. To this end, soluble C4-binding protein (C4bp), membrane cofactor protein (MCP or CD46), and membrane-bound complement receptor 1 (CR1 or CD35) act as cofactors in C4b to iC4b (part of the classical C3 convertase complex) by serum factor I. MCP and CR1 also extend this so-called cofactor activity to the C3b portion of the alternative C3 convertase. Factor H is a serum protein that utilizes factor I to destabilize the alternative C3 convertase.

Apart from their cofactor activity, factor H, C4bp, and CR1 also offer a direct way to interfere with the stability of C3 convertases, called decay-accelerating activity. Although C4bp limits its activity to the classical C3 con-

vertase, factor H, CR1, and decay-accelerating factor (DAF or CD55) dissociate classical and alternative C3 convertases. C4bp and factor H are plasma borne, whereas CR1, DAF, and MCP offer the host protection from potential complement damage in a membrane-bound fashion.

Many microbes have evolved similar strategies to elude host complement responses to their presence. For example, Epstein-Barr virus, a member of the gammaherpesvirus family responsible for causing mononucleosis in humans, has its own decay-accelerating activity for alternative C3 convertase (Mold et al., 1988). The virus works in a fashion similar to MCP, CR1, and factor H, utilizing a yet unknown cofactor with an affinity for factor I. Another gammaherpesvirus, *Herpesvirus saimiri*, which is associated with lymphomas and leukemia in certain primates, utilizes a complement control protein with homology to MCP and DAF (Albrecht and Fleckenstein, 1992). Other microbial homologs of DAF are found during certain life cycle stages of the *Trypanosoma cruzi* parasite that is responsible for Chagas' disease. The parasite expresses a 160-kDa glycoprotein called gp160 (Norris et al., 1991) and T-DAF (Kipnis et al., 1988) before it enters the human cell and is effectively protected from complement attack. Vaccinia virus, a member of the *Poxviridae*, achieves decay-accelerating activity through its expression of complement control protein (VCP) (Kotwal and Moss, 1988). VCP resembles C4bp, but extends its destabilizing activity to both alternative and classical C3 convertases. The alphaherpesviruses herpes simplex virus type 1 (HSV-1) and HSV-2 encode glycoprotein C (gC) to avert C3-mediated complement attack. HSV-1 gC (gC-1) is best understood in its mode of action; its association with C3b in the alternative C3 convertase prevents factor P from stabilizing the complex, promoting its dissociation (Hung et al., 1994). Recently, murine gammaherpesvirus 68 protein was found to protect the virus from C3 during acute infection. Various other gammaherpesviruses encode homologs of this regulator of complement activation, but their effects have not yet been studied in detail (Kapadia et al., 2002).

HIV, a member of the retrovirus family, encodes glycoproteins that enable it to control complement damage. Its host cell-derived lipid membrane is decorated with glycoproteins gp41 and gp120 (Pinter et al., 1995a, 1995b). These glycoproteins have the remarkable ability to bind host factor H from the serum and mediate resistance to complement lysis. The effectiveness of this unorthodox method of complement mediation is accentuated by the observation that protection is lost when anti-gp41 Ab is used to block factor H association with the glycoprotein (Stoiber et al., 1996). In addition to the endogenous glycoproteins, HIV uses membrane-associated host complement regulatory proteins to protect itself. During the budding process from their host cell, new HIV virions acquire membrane-bound host complement regulatory proteins DAF (Marschang et al., 1995) and CD59 (Saifuddin et al., 1995) (see Regulation of and Protection from MAC Lysis, below), together with the lipid membrane. Apart from encoding or deriving complement modulation proteins from the host, physical properties that protect host cells from complement damage may be transferred to the microbe. For example, schistosomes apply an effective strategy by acquiring sialic acid residues from their host (Simpson and Smithers, 1980). Sialic acids reduce binding of C3b fragments, thus limiting the associated alternative pathway amplification loop.

Regulation of and Protection from MAC Lysis

Purely physical properties can also help microorganisms avoid MAC-induced damage. When bacterial strains are divided on the basis of their Gram staining, two patterns of resistance to complement-mediated lysis emerge. Gram-positive bacteria, such as *Streptococcus* sp., resist MAC complexes from penetrating their membrane by protecting it with the peptidoglycan cell wall. Peptidoglycan, a highly cross-linked polymer of *N*-acetylglucosamine and muramic acid, provides a physical barrier up to 30 nm thick that protects from complement-mediated lysis. Certain lysis-resistant gram-positive species actually promote complement activation. For example, *Staphylococcus aureus* expresses IgG-binding proteins on its surface (Zhang et al., 1998) that effectively activate complement in the bacteria's vicinity (Stalen-heim and Castensson, 1971). IgG binding is common among clinical strains of *S. aureus*, suggesting that host tissue damage from excessive complement activation creates a suitable environment for the bacterium's maintenance.

In comparison, the cell wall of gram-negative bacteria, not more than 2 to 4 nm thick, does little to prevent insertion of the MAC complex into the membrane. The gram-negative cell wall generally supports LPSs, molecular structures that potently induce the alternative pathway (see The Alternative Pathway above). Induction occurs at some distance from the bacterium because LPS is supported by multimeric carbohydrate structures, known as O-Ags (Nikaido and Nakae, 1979). Long O-Ags, such as those of *E. coli*, *Klebsiella*, and *Salmonella* spp., help "neutralize" C3 at a safe distance from the otherwise vulnerable cellular membrane. Activated C3's inherently labile thioester and slowed diffusion through the outer layer effectively shield the bacterial membrane from MAC formation.

Both membrane-bound and soluble MAC inhibitors protect human cells from complement-mediated autolysis. One membrane-bound MAC formation inhibitor molecule is CD59. Anchored into the lipid bilayer through its phosphoinositol glycolipid tail, CD59 prevents activation of C9 molecules, restricting C9 from joining the C5b-8 complex. Host CD59 becomes incorporated into the viral membrane of budding HIV particles, also extending CD59-mediated avoidance from complement lysis to the virion (Saifuddin et al., 1995). Homologous restriction factor (HRF) is another membrane-linked MAC inhibitor. Found on platelets, erythrocytes, and lymphoid and myeloid lineage cells, HRF inhibits channel formation of the MAC complex. HRF has a high affinity for C9, but its exact mode of action is not yet determined (Zalman et al., 1986).

Two other host proteins known to control MAC formation are not membrane bound. S protein and SP40,40 both use the soluble form of C5b-7 as a substrate. S protein prevents C9 polymerization onto the C5b-7 complex and occupies its membrane-binding site (Podack et al., 1984). SP40,40 operates similarly, neutralizing the lipophilicity of the C5b-7 complex (Choi et al., 1989). Both proteins seem to confine MAC's range of action to its induction site.

COMPLEMENT RECEPTORS AND INFECTION

Apart from direct lysis, the complement system mediates its effects on the immune response through specific receptors for its activation products. Complement receptors play an important role in the uptake and clearance of opsonized Ag, enhancing adaptive and innate cellular responses, and inducing inflammatory responses. However, microorganisms also utilize certain complement receptors to their advantage.

CR1

CR1 (or CD35) functions as a complement control protein, as described in Regulation and Modulation on the C3 Level, above, and as an important receptor for activation products of C3 (C3b and iC3b) and C4 (C4b), as well as for C1q and MBL. Multiple allotypes of CR1 have been described in humans, all of which possess a 25-amino-acid (aa) transmembrane portion and a 43-aa cytoplasmic tail, but with a varying number of so-called short consensus repeats for the extracytoplasmic domain varies. The q32 band of human chromosome 1 houses CR1 and many other coding sequences for related complement control and receptor proteins, including those for C4bp, CR2, DAF, factor H, and MCP.

On human erythrocytes, CR1 plays an important role in clearing immune complexes by targeting them to the liver and spleen. Kupffer cells, phagocytic cells that permanently reside in great numbers within the liver, form the main means of immune complex disposal through uptake of erythrocyte-borne immune complexes. In the spleen, phagocytic Ag-presenting cells extract complexed Ag, for processing and presentation to lymphocytes. In this process, CR1 also fulfills a notable function by aiding monocyte phagocytosis of complement-opsonized Ag. On follicular dendritic cells (FDCs), CR1 helps retain Ag in its native form on the germinal center (GC) reaction (for a more detailed discussion, see Molecular Basis of Complement Enhancement of the Humoral Response, below).

In addition to its involvement in complement processes, CR1 has been reported to provide a mode of cell entry for malaria-causing *Plasmodium falciparum* through its surface protein PfEMP1 (Krych-Goldberg et al., 2002).

CR2

CR2 (or CD21) fulfills a key function in directly linking adaptive and innate immunity. Like CR1, it maps to the q32 band of human chromosome 1. In mice, CR1 is actually a shorter alternative splicing product of CR2 (Kurtz et al., 1990). Two allotypes of human CR2 have been described, both possessing a 24-aa transmembrane region and 43-aa cytoplasmic tail. These CR2 allotypes are differentiated by the number of short consensus repeats in the extracellular domains, 15 (CD21 short) or 16 (CD21 long) (Liu et al., 1997). CR2 has a binding specificity for C3d, C3dg, and iC3b, each a downstream activation product of C3b. CR2 affects the adaptive immune response through two different but related ways. First, on B cells, CR2 works in conjunction with CD19 and CD81 to form a coreceptor for the Ag-specific B-cell receptor (BCR) (Sato et al., 1997). Once the complement-opsonized Ag engages the BCR and coreceptor, coligation lowers the activation threshold of the B cell by as much as 10,000-fold when compared with the Ag alone (Dempsey et al., 1996) (see Molecular Basis of

Complement Enhancement of the Humoral Response, below). In addition, CR2 expression on FDCs (Reynes et al., 1985) plays a role reminiscent of CR1s in trapping Ag (Fang et al., 1998; Qin et al., 1998).

A well-known example of an infectious agent using CR2 as a means of cell entry is the Epstein-Barr virus, a B-cell-tropic virus of the betaherpesvirus family (Martin et al., 1994).

CR3 and CR4

CR3 (Mac-1 or CD11b, CD18) and CR4 (or CD11c, CD18) are heterodimers that consist of two noncovalently associated type I transmembrane glycoproteins, referred to as subunits alpha (CD11b or -c, respectively) and beta (CD18). Both CRs belong to the leukocyte-restricted integrin family, which includes the closely related lymphocyte function-associated antigen 1 (LFA-1), and share considerable structural homology. The gene for their common CD18 beta subunit is located on human chromosome 21 and encodes a 747-aa product (including the signal peptide) of 95 kDa. The coding sequences for the alpha subunits CD11b and -c are found in a cluster on chromosome 16. These subunits are structurally related (with a 67% aa similarity) and have a molecular mass of 165 and 150 kDa, respectively.

Expression of CR3 and CR4 is detected mostly on cells of the myeloid lineage. High expression levels of CR3, compared with CR4, are found on monocytic phagocytes. CR4 expression is detected in greater amounts than CR3 on tissue macrophages. However, high levels of CR4 are also found on dendritic cells of mice, whereas lower levels are observed on human dendritic cells and activated B lymphocytes. Other nonmyeloid cells positive for CR3 primarily include NK cells and CD5[+] B lymphocytes.

Both CR3 and CR4 fulfill an important role as integrin on phagocytes, aiding migration through vascular endothelium into sites of inflammation. To this effect, integrins bind their specific counterreceptors, referred to as cellular adhesion molecules, on the endothelium (reviewed by von Andrian and Mackay,

2000). NK cell activation is aided when surface CR3 recognizes Ag opsonized with C3 activation products (Ramos et al., 1989). However, the phagocytosis-aiding and -activating functions of C3 breakdown products, through CR3 on mononuclear cells (Ohkuro et al., 1995; Takizawa et al., 1996), are the most notable features in the context of this chapter. Both CR3 and CR4 bind iC3b, a proteolytic product of Ag-bound C3b formed upon interaction with factor I, and to a lesser degree C3b and C3dg.

C1q Receptor

C1q is an obvious target for complement receptors on Ag-processing cells because it becomes attached to immune complexes in the earliest stages of classical pathway activation through interaction with Ab (mainly multivalent IgM). Various receptor molecules are known to bind C1q, of which C1qRp has been studied most extensively (reviewed by McGreal and Gasque, 2001). C1qRp is a 66.5-kDa type I membrane glycoprotein, found on B cells, macrophages, monocytes, platelets, and endothelial cells. This receptor consists of a calcium-dependent (C-type) carbohydrate recognition domain, five epidermal growth factor-like domains, and a cytoplasmic tyrosine phosphorylation site involved in signaling. In addition to its function in complement-mediated phagocytosis of immune complexes, C1qRp has also been shown to have a similar affinity for MBL and pulmonary surfactant protein A-containing complexes (Malhotra et al., 1990). MBL and surfactant protein A are structurally related to C1q.

Anaphylatoxin Receptors

One important result of complement system activation, in addition to the various effects resulting from lysis and opsonization, is the induction of inflammation. Inflammation is mainly achieved through the generation of the C3a, C4a, and C5a anaphylatoxins. The effect of these soluble peptides is achieved through specific receptors on particular cell surfaces. On immune tissue, anaphylatoxin-specific receptors are mainly found on myeloid lineage cells such as neutrophils, monocytes and macrophages, basophils, eosinophils, and mast cells. Anaphylatoxin receptors are also found on many other tissues, including heart, lung, spleen, spinal cord, and brain as reviewed by Kohl (2001).

With their wide distribution, anaphylatoxins can exert effects through a great variety of cells. Their proinflammatory effects can be thought of in concerted chemotactic, vasoactive, and activating terms. Generally speaking, the overall potency of the anaphylatoxins decreases in the order C5a > C3a >> C4a. Complement activation and the consequent release of C5a potently stimulate migration of leukocytes (especially neutrophils and eosinophils) toward the site of infection (Hugli and Muller-Eberhard, 1978). C3a and C5a are also strong spasmogens, which induce smooth muscle contraction. The capillary narrowing that results, combined with the direct increasing effect of anaphylatoxins on the permeability of capillary-lining endothelial cells, aids extravasation.

Anaphylatoxins also induce upregulation of adhesion molecules on endothelium. These combined effects result in an influx of serum proteins (including complement) and inflammatory cells (including cells capable of complement production) into the site of infection. The cycle of inflammation that was set in motion by localized complement activation is further enhanced indirectly by degranulation of mast cells and granulocytes. Anaphylatoxin receptor binding on mast cells promotes their release of potent inflammatory mediators, such as histamine and serotonin, and induces their general activation (Cochrane and Muller-Eberhard, 1968; Dias Da Silva and Lepow, 1967).

In short, the direct and indirect effects of anaphylatoxins on activation, degranulation, chemotaxis, vasoactivity, and adhesion in a wide variety of cells and tissues make them potent mediators of inflammation. This potency is well illustrated in studies revealing that mice with a disrupted C3a receptor (C3aR) are protected from the pathogenic effects of bronchial asthma, a hyperresponsive inflamma-

tory state traditionally thought to be chiefly associated with allergen-specific IgE-triggering mast cells (Humbles et al., 2000).

The role of anaphylatoxin receptors becomes more complicated when we consider relatively recent work describing an *attenuating* effect of C3aR on inflammation induced by LPS in an in vivo endotoxic shock model (Kildsgaard et al., 2000). Future work should clarify whether anaphylatoxins and their receptors should be seen as inflammation modulatory molecules, rather than the more traditional and restricted proinflammatory designation.

COMPLEMENT AND ADAPTIVE IMMUNITY

At first sight, innate and adaptive immunity seem quite distinct systems: the innate system is broad, fast acting, and evolutionarily primitive; the adaptive system is specific, slower to develop, and further evolved. A strong correlation between the presence or absence of innate complement components and the development of an effective adaptive response, however, has been recognized for many years. Over the past decade, the nature of cooperation between these two systems has become clearer. The classical pathway has an especially strong enhancing effect on Ab and memory responses to various Ags. The absence of one or more classical complement components also predisposes to various Ig-dependent autoimmune diseases.

Complement and Adaptive Immunity in an Evolutionary Context

It is interesting to theorize how this intricate cooperation between two systems arose, as the adaptive and innate complement immunity branches seem to have developed quite separately in distinct evolutionary stages. In fact, early complement components of the alternative pathway have been identified in arthropods (which include, among others, modern-day insects and date back approximately 500 million years) and other invertebrates and were determined to have mainly opsonizing, nonlytic capacities (Al-Sharif et al.,

1998; Nonaka et al., 1999). Until the emergence of the earliest vertebrates, i.e., jawless fish approximately 400 million years ago, that possess hemolytic activity, opsonization remained the only form of complement immunity in evidence. Subsequently, within a short time frame in evolutionary history, cartilaginous and bony fish appear that have not only classical and lytic pathway complement molecules, but also the first hallmarks of a modern adaptive immune system (Hashimoto et al., 1992; Hinds and Litman, 1986). In addition to their specialized immune tissues (B and T lymphocytes), cartilaginous fish also developed the first highly organized adaptive immune organs (thymus and spleen).

The simultaneous appearance of classical pathway complement and adaptive immunity could possibly account for the intimate relationship that has developed between the two. Indeed, in modern evolutionary forms, such as the higher vertebrates including humans and mice, the influence of complement on the adaptive immune response (and certain autoimmune disorders [Walport, 2002]) is largely due to the components of the classical pathway. An additional factor that might have promoted cooperation between adaptive immunity and classical complement is the close linkage of some of their hallmark genes on the mammalian genome. Key classical pathway molecules, such as C2 and C4, share their location on the genome with adaptive immunity genes of the major histocompatibility complex (MHC). Taken together, these arguments indicate that, although portions of the complement system are phylogenically much older than adaptive immunity, the part most influential in adaptive responses appears to have evolved alongside it.

Recognizing the Role of Complement in Adaptive Immunity

Knowledge of complement's role in the general immune response stems from observations made around the start of the 20th century. Nonetheless, another half-century passed before the first indications were found that complement has a role beyond innate immunity, fulfilling a crucial task in instructing adaptive responses. In 1968 Lay and Nussenzweig first reported the existence of complement receptors on murine lymphocytes, and in a 1971 report they described C3 receptors on B lymphocytes in more detail (Bianco et al., 1970; Eden et al., 1971). One year later, Pepys (1972) reported that transient depletion of C3 results in impaired humoral responses to both T-dependent and T-independent Ags. By 1975 he had identified the involvement of complement in localizing Ag to the GC and, in so doing, uncovered what was later recognized as one of the underlying mechanisms of complement's humoral response-enhancing potential (Papamichail et al., 1975). In 1983, Thorbecke's group reported that the highly specialized GC microenvironment in secondary lymphoid organs contained great numbers of memory B lymphocytes (Coico et al., 1983), whereas more recently Kelsoe and coworkers contributed greatly to our understanding of GC architecture and its dynamics of selection, mutation, and class switching so important to highly specific memory formation (Kelsoe, 1996). The fact that FDCs are responsible for Ag trapping and retention within the GC became well established in the early 1980s (Schnizlein et al., 1984). These combined observations helped to shape our understanding of how the complement system asserts its influence over adaptive immunity.

Molecular Basis of Complement Enhancement of the Humoral Response

Modern molecular techniques made further advances possible in understanding just how complement aids adaptive immunity. Various groups, including ours, generated mice deficient in complement factors or their receptors through genetic targeting. Recombinant DNA techniques also made it possible to design and produce consistent, well-defined fusions between model Ags and complement factors that could serve as reagents. These techniques provided highly controlled alternatives to naturally deficient or transiently depleted animals or the in vitro-generated immune complexes that were used until then. Step by step, it became generally recognized that mechanistically there are two nonmutually exclusive ways in which complement exerts its effect on humoral responses and memory formation, namely, through B-cell coreceptor signaling and FDC Ag retention (Fig. 2).

First, deposition of complement factors on pathogens or other foreign surfaces facilitates Ag binding and presentation to naive Ag-specific B lymphocytes in secondary lymphoid organs, such as the spleen and lymph nodes (Carroll, 1998). As Pepys already indicated, this process occurs within the GC by means of FDCs. FDCs retain Ag on their surface for extended periods of time (Mandel et al., 1981), perhaps years. The Ag is kept in its native form to allow B lymphocytes to sample the Ag with Ag-specific BCRs. Ag retention through complement receptors allows FDCs to present an assortment of Ags in a nonspecific fashion (complement opsonized), enabling

them to accommodate B cells of various specificities. Immunization experiments revealed that mice with genetically disrupted CR1 and CR2 showed impaired Ab responses, similar to animals deficient in one or more classical complement factors (Ahearn et al., 1996; Da Costa et al., 1999; Molina et al., 1996) (Fig. 3). Comparable results were obtained by blocking CR1 and CR2 with specific monoclonal Ab (Gustavsson et al., 1995). Although these experiments do not directly attribute the entire Ab defect to complement deficiency on FDCs (complement receptors on other cell types, including B cells, could contribute as well), visible reduction in Ag retention indicated a role for FDCs. The role of CR1 and CR2 on FDCs was further examined by adoptively transferring normal bone marrow (BM) into CR1/2-deficient mice. Animals were created in which complement receptors are expressed by B lymphocytes, but not FDCs. Following immunization, the mice developed normal Ab titers, but the endurance of these responses was impaired, stressing the importance of FDCs in

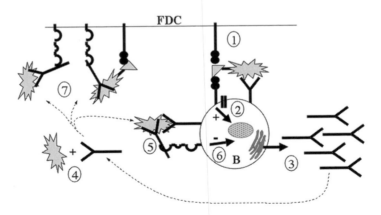

FIGURE 2 Molecular basis for complement enhancement of the humoral response. (1) Ag captured and presented on the FDC surface through CR1/2 or FcR is presented to Ag-specific B cell in the germinal center. (2) Recognition of Ag through the BCR and coligation of the CR2, CD19, CD81-signaling complex through complement leads to B-cell activation and (3) Ag-specific Ab production. (4) Specific Ab complexes with Ag result in (5 and 6) downregulation of the B-cell response by engagement of the cell surface BCR and FcR. Also, formation of Ag–Ab(-C′) complexes results in enhanced trapping of Ag onto the FDC surface through CR and FcR (7), creating a long-term Ag pool.

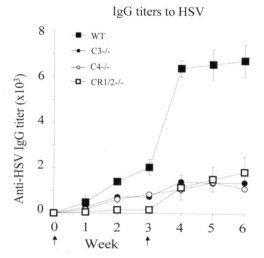

IgG titers to HSV

FIGURE 3 Impaired humoral responses in classical complement or complement receptor knockout mice. C3-, C4-, or CR1/2-deficient animals reveal impaired humoral responses upon peripheral HSV infection. Recombinant β-galactosidase-expressing HSV-1 (strain HD-2) was used for inoculation, giving essentially the same results as WT virus but also allowing assessment of the response to β-galactosidase (as reported by Da Costa et al., 1999). The results mirror, in a well-controlled way, early immunization experiments with animals that were transiently depleted or naturally deficient in one or more complement factors.

Ag retention to allow long-term memory development (Fang et al., 1998). It should be noted that FDCs utilize Fc receptors in addition to complement receptors to retain complement (Radoux et al., 1985). However, recent immunization experiments by Barrington et al. (2002), using knockout mice deficient in complement and/or Fc receptors, reveal that complement plays a critical role in the maintenance of long-term B-lymphocyte memory.

Complement's influence on humoral responses and memory formation is also evidenced by the Ab response-enhancing effect that its activation products have on the B lymphocyte. There, the enhancing effect is achieved by engaging coreceptors on the cell surface, in combination with the Ag-specific BCR. Arguably, this process occurs most effi-

ciently within the highly specialized microenvironment of the GC through Ag retained on the surface of FDCs. Fearon and colleagues performed one of the more elegant and definitive experiments showing a strong effect of complement-opsonized Ag on B cells. By producing a fusion protein between model Ag hen egg lysozyme and varying numbers of complement C3d, they established that the amount of hen egg lysozyme required to trigger B-cell activation was 10,000-fold less when three copies of C3d were attached (Dempsey et al., 1996). The effect on the B cell is transferred by Ag-C3d-mediated coligation of the BCR and the coreceptor complex, which includes CR2, CD81, and the signal-transducing CD19 (Fearon, 1993). In vivo experiments utilizing similar constructs now include C3d fusion proteins with influenza A virus hemagglutinin (Ross et al., 2000), measles hemagglutinin (Green et al., 2001), and HIV gp120 (Ross et al., 2001). Most groups report enhancement of neutralizing Abs, avidity maturation, and accelerated protection when using these fusion constructs. These results correlate with Fearon's in vitro data and the extensive in vivo data obtained with complement and complement receptor knockout mice. One notable exception to these combined studies is a report by Suradhat et al. describing an inhibited immune response following immunization with their bovine rotavirus VP7 or bovine herpesvirus type 1 glycoprotein D C3d-fusion DNA vaccines (Suradhat et al., 2001).

Complement and T Lymphocytes

In addition to influence on the humoral response, studies from several groups have implicated complement in modifying the T-cell response. Complement's mode of action, however, is much less clear than that on B cells. Complement receptors are expressed on subgroups of human T cells (CR1 [Wilson et al., 1983], CR2 [Fischer et al., 1991], and CR4 [Miller et al., 1986]) and potentially have a role in connecting adaptive and innate immunity. In mice, where most of complement's effects on T cells have been reported, the presence of complement receptors on T cells has also been suggested (Erdei et al., 1984; Kerekes et al., 1998; Pratt et al., 2002). Defective T-cell activation has been described in various infection, disease, and transplant models using C3-deficient mice and organs. For example, diminished T-cell responses and prolonged graft survival are observed when C3-deficient kidneys are transplanted (Pratt et al., 2002). A model using C3$^{-/-}$ mice in influenza virus infection reports a role for C3 in T-cell priming (Kopf et al., 2002), as does another pulmonary model investigating C3 in asthma pathogenesis (Drouin et al., 2001). However, in other immunization models using infectious HSV or bacteriophage φX174, the absence of C3 did not affect T-cell response (Da Costa et al., 1999; Fischer et al., 1996). The seeming discrepancy between these results suggests that the role of complement in T-cell responses is dependent on the nature, dose, and/or location of Ag. Whether complement has a direct effect on T-cell priming and activation, transmitted through complement receptors, has not been conclusively demonstrated and remains a subject of debate (Lakkis, 2002). Some in vitro evidence exists for a model in which complement aides T-cell activation indirectly through enhanced Ag uptake and subsequent presentation by B cells (Thornton et al., 1994). Although B cells synthesize only Ig when the BCR is engaged in an Ag-specific way (Thornton et al., 1996), Ag processing and MHC-restricted presentation to stimulate T cells can be mediated by complement in a non-BCR-specific manner (Boackle et al., 1997, 1998).

LOCAL COMPLEMENT SYNTHESIS AND ITS EFFECTS

The liver synthesizes a large variety and quantity of many complement components. For example, the vast majority of C3 in the circulation is hepatic cell derived. Although the liver provides a constitutive level of many serum complement proteins, components such as MBL, factor B, C9, C4, and C3 are considered acute-phase proteins whose levels of production go up quickly in response to inflammatory stimuli. The typical C3 concentration in the blood is around 1 mg/ml, whereas total complement accounts for about 3.5 mg/ml among 60 to 78 mg of total plasma proteins per ml. With these high circulating concentrations, the complement system is often regarded and referred to as a plasma-borne system.

However, various nonhepatic local sources of complement have been described. In certain cases, these sources contribute substantial quantities of complement to the circulation. A recent study showed that wild-type (WT) bone marrow (BM) engraftment into C1q-deficient mice restored serum C1q levels, and therewith the hemolytic activity of the serum in vitro (Petry et al., 2001). In humans, C7 has been shown to have substantial extrahepatic sources that contribute measurably to the circulating complement pool (Naughton et al., 1996b). In rats, between 30 and 40% of systemic C6 was determined to be extrahepatic, including 5% BM derived (Brauer et al., 1994). Renal contribution to the circulating C3 pool has been shown to be up to 4.5% of total serum C3 (Tang et al., 1999).

Other extrahepatic complement sources have a more modest influence on circulating complement levels. Their level of synthesis is likely regulated and local. For example, there is negligible long-term BM contribution to the circulating C3 pool in patients that received BM transplants for hematological malignancies. It should be mentioned, however, that in a number of patients the level of BM-derived C3 transiently rose from 0.1 to 1.5% (2.6% in extreme cases) following BM transplant (Naughton et al., 1996a). These data show that, although BM-derived cells are capable of producing detectable levels of C3, such levels occur only immediately following transplantation. This period is, arguably, atypical and clinical and characterized by the presence of inflammatory stimuli, including graft-versus-host response. When similar BM transfer experiments are carried out under well-controlled laboratory conditions using inbred

a

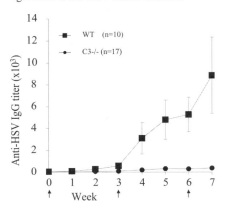

IgG titers to i.d. HSV in non-chimeras

b

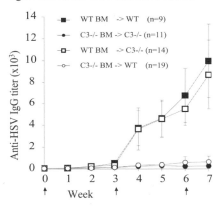

IgG titers to i.d. HSV in BM-chimeras

c

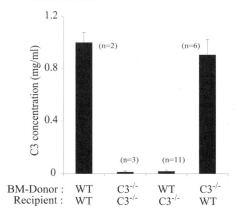

Serum C3 titers

mouse strains, negligible levels of C3 are found in the circulation (Fischer et al., 1998). In addition to BM-derived cells, other local, low-level C3-producing tissues include skin fibroblasts (Katz et al., 1989), epidermal keratinocytes (Terui et al., 1997), astroglioma cells (Barnum et al., 1993), and various endothelial (Brooimans et al., 1990) and epithelial cells (Brooimans et al., 1991; Strunk et al., 1988; Varsano et al., 2000). These tissues contribute C3 to the circulation at undetermined levels that are probably quite low.

The relative large quantities and ease with which serum complement can be determined focused attention on complement in the circulation. Observations regarding its function were related to serum levels. Even with the advent of more modern techniques and recognition of extrahepatic sources, knowledge of C3's effects and regulation in vivo remains limited. Available information is extracted largely from in situ hybridization and cell culture studies. Simultaneous synthesis of complement by multiple sources, as well as a highly mobile serum fraction, complicates attempts to isolate and study the role of any particular source. Therefore, in vivo studies typically underestimate not only the contribution of extrahepatic production to the total complement content, but also its biological potential.

In certain cases, transplantation experiments can offer a solution to this problem. For example, a study looking at the role of renal C3 in mice determined tempered rejection of MHC-mismatched renal grafts if it concerns

FIGURE 4 Local myeloid C3 synthesis is essential for humoral responses to peripheral HSV infection. (a) Peripheral HSV infection leads to robust humoral responses in WT but not $C3^{-/-}$ animals. (b) Local BM-derived myeloid C3 synthesis can rescue this defect in WT BM $\rightarrow$ $C3^{-/-}$ animals. Upon further investigation, local C3 synthesis appears essential, as evidenced by infection of $C3^{-/-}$ BM $\rightarrow$ WT animals. (c) $C3^{-/-}$ BM $\rightarrow$ WT animals show WT-like levels of circulating C3, but do not respond to HSV. In contrast, WT BM $\rightarrow$ $C3^{-/-}$ animals have essentially $C3^{-/-}$ serum levels, but respond with WT-like humoral responses. i.d., intradermally.

a C3-deficient donor (Pratt et al., 2002). Although the mechanism that is proposed in the report (i.e., direct effect of complement on T-cell activation) remains a subject of discussion (see Complement and T Lymphocytes, above), the transplantation approach clearly shows how extrahepatic C3 can contribute to accelerated graft rejection. Similarly, in rats it was found that the combined extrahepatic fraction of the C6 pool contributes to hypera-

cute rejection of cardiac xenografts (Brauer et al., 1995). As, in addition, it has been established that circulating C1q levels in C1q$^{-/-}$ mice become fully restored through a WT BM transplant (Petry et al., 2001), it might be expected that its biological effects in experimental C1q models such as nephrotoxic nephritis also become restored (Robson et al., 2001). However, this has not yet been formally shown.

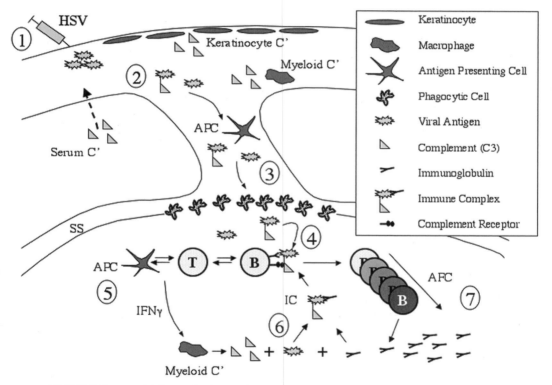

FIGURE 5. Model for myeloid C3 enhancement of the humoral response in the periphery. Upon HSV infection (1), viral Ag in the skin encounters complement from various sources, including those that are serum, keratinocyte, or myeloid derived (2). Although serum or keratinocyte C3 is clearly present, C3$^{-/-}$ BM → WT animals suggest that these sources of C3 do not result in enhancement of the humoral response. Carried by the afferent lymphatics (3), Ag reaches the peripheral lymph nodes in free, complement-complexed or antigen–presenting cell (APC)-processed form. There it is recognized by Ag-specific B- cells (4) that receive T-cell help generated though MHC-restricted APC interaction (5). Gamma interferon (IFNγ) is generated in this process and has been shown to stimulate macrophages to produce complement factors, which then can opsonize drained Ag (6). Opsonized Ag can enhance the B-cell response significantly (7), increasing the amount of specific Ab produced. Specific Ab aids the formation of Ag, Ab, C' immune complexes, structures that are especially immunogenic. SS, subcapsular sinus; IC, immune complex; AFC, antibody-forming cell.

Myeloid C3 and the Humoral Response

Previous studies by our laboratory underlined the Ab-enhancing capacities of localized production of complement factor C3 in an intravenous immunization model, as well as a cutaneous HSV infection model (Fischer et al., 1998; Verschoor et al., 2001). These studies showed that, in the absence of circulating C3, local production by BM-derived myeloid cells is sufficient and necessary to initiate a full humoral response to peripheral HSV infection (Fig. 4). C3 in the circulation appeared to access peripheral lymph nodes or the site of infection insufficiently to enhance B-cell responses. By contrast, C3 in the circulation or produced locally can enhance humoral immunity to an intravenously introduced Ag. Because of the intimate connection between the skin and draining lymph nodes, through the lymphatics, an innovative approach will be required to conclusively show how myeloid C3 plays its role.

The finding that local synthesis of C3 by myeloid cells is not only sufficient, but necessary, for an effective humoral response to peripheral infection by HSV raises a general question regarding the source of complement proteins required in C3 activation, i.e., C1 (C1q, C1r, C1s), C2, and C4. Macrophages are a major source of C1q (Petry et al., 2001) and are known to produce other early classical pathway components (McPhaden and Whaley, 1993). In particular, macrophages are a sufficient C4 source to restore the humoral response to Ags administered intravenously in $C4^{-/-}$ mice (Gadjeva et al., 2002). Therefore, a developing model is that, on activation by inflammatory cytokines, such as gamma interferon, macrophages secrete C1, C2, C4, and C3 in levels sufficient to ensure efficient coupling of C3 to pathogens (Fig. 5). This autonomous role for macrophages might be critical in sites, such as peripheral lymph nodes, where complement proteins within the circulation are not readily available for activation and binding of C3 to foreign Ags.

These experiments have established myeloid C3's unique qualities in inducing a robust humoral response in peripheral infection. To date, it is the only known source with a site-restricted complement function that does not overlap with alternative sources. Its fundamental importance in adaptive immunity in the periphery might make it a factor of consideration in vaccine development or possibly part of standard clinical analyses where serum complement is measured now.

ACKNOWLEDGMENTS

We express our thanks to Michelle Ottaviano for her valuable contributions in editing this manuscript. Work of M.C.C.'s laboratory described in this chapter is supported by National Institutes of Health grant AI42257.

REFERENCES

Ahearn, J. M., M. B. Fischer, D. Croix, S. Goerg, M. Ma, J. Xia, X. Zhou, R. G. Howard, T. L. Rothstein, and M. C. Carroll. 1996. Disruption of the Cr2 locus results in a reduction in B-1a cells and in an impaired B cell response to T-dependent antigen. *Immunity* **4:**251–262.

Albrecht, J. C., and B. Fleckenstein. 1992. New member of the multigene family of complement control proteins in herpesvirus saimiri. *J. Virol.* **66:**3937–3940.

Al-Sharif, W. Z., J. O. Sunyer, J. D. Lambris, and L. C. Smith. 1998. Sea urchin coelomocytes specifically express a homologue of the complement component C3. *J. Immunol.* **160:**2983–2997.

Barnum, S. R., J. L. Jones, and E. N. Benveniste. 1993. Interleukin-1 and tumor necrosis factor-mediated regulation of C3 gene expression in human astroglioma cells. *Glia* **7:**225–236.

Barrington, R. A., O. Pozdnyakova, M. R. Zafari, C. D. Benjamin, and M. C. Carroll. 2002. B lymphocyte memory: role of stromal cell complement and FcgammaRIIB receptors. *J. Exp. Med.* **196:**1189–1199.

Bianco, C., R. Patrick, and V. Nussenzweig. 1970. A population of lymphocytes bearing a membrane receptor for antigen-antibody-complement complexes. I. Separation and characterization. *J. Exp. Med.* **132:**702–720.

Boackle, S. A., V. M. Holers, and D. R. Karp. 1997. CD21 augments antigen presentation in immune individuals. *Eur. J. Immunol.* **27:**122–129.

Boackle, S. A., M. A. Morris, V. M. Holers, and D. R. Karp. 1998. Complement opsonization is required for presentation of immune complexes by resting peripheral blood B cells. *J. Immunol.* **161:**6537–6543.

Brauer, R. B., T. T. Lam, D. Wang, L. R. Horwitz, A. D. Hess, A. S. Klein, F. Sanfilippo, and W. M. Baldwin, III. 1995. Extrahepatic synthesis of C6 in the rat is sufficient for complement-mediated hyperacute rejection of a guinea pig cardiac xenograft. *Transplantation* **59:**1073–1076.

Brauer, R. B., W. M. Baldwin, III, D. Wang, L. R. Horwitz, A. D. Hess, A. S. Klein, and F. Sanfilippo. 1994. Hepatic and extrahepatic biosynthesis of complement factor C6 in the rat. *J. Immunol.* **153:**3168–3176.

Brooimans, R. A., A. A. van der Ark, W. A. Buurman, L. A. van Es, and M. R. Daha. 1990. Differential regulation of complement factor H and C3 production in human umbilical vein endothelial cells by IFN-gamma and IL-1. *J. Immunol.* **144:**3835–3840.

Brooimans, R. A., A. P. Stegmann, W. T. van Dorp, A. A. van der Ark, F. J. van der Woude, L. A. van Es, and M. R. Daha. 1991. Interleukin 2 mediates stimulation of complement C3 biosynthesis in human proximal tubular epithelial cells. *J. Clin. Invest.* **88:**379–384.

Carroll, M. C. 1998. CD21, CD35 in B cell activation. *Semin. Immunol.* **10:**279–286.

Choi, N. H., T. Mazda, and M. Tomita. 1989. A serum protein SP40,40 modulates the formation of membrane attack complex of complement on erythrocytes. *Mol. Immunol.* **26:**835–840.

Cochrane, C. G., and H. J. Muller-Eberhard. 1968. The derivation of two distinct anaphylatoxin activities from the third and fifth components of human complement. *J. Exp. Med.* **127:**371–386.

Coico, R. F., B. S. Bhogal, and G. J. Thorbecke. 1983. Relationship of germinal centers in lymphoid tissue to immunologic memory. VI. Transfer of B cell memory with lymph node cells fractionated according to their receptors for peanut agglutinin. *J. Immunol.* **131:**2254–2257.

Cooper, N. R. 1985. The classical complement pathway: activation and regulation of the first complement component. *Adv. Immunol.* **37:**151–216.

Da Costa, X. J., M. A. Brockman, E. Alicot, M. Ma, M. B. Fischer, X. Zhou, D. M. Knipe, and M. C. Carroll. 1999. Humoral response to herpes simplex virus is complement-dependent. *Proc. Natl. Acad. Sci. USA* **96:**12708–12712.

Dempsey, P. W., M. E. Allison, S. Akkaraju, C. C. Goodnow, and D. T. Fearon. 1996. C3d of complement as a molecular adjuvant: bridging innate and acquired immunity. *Science* **271:**348–350.

Dias Da Silva, W., and I. H. Lepow. 1967. Complement as a mediator of inflammation. II. Biological properties of anaphylatoxin prepared with purified components of human complement. *J. Exp. Med.* **125:**921–946.

Donaldson, V. H., F. S. Rosen, and D. H. Bing. 1977. Role of the second component of complement (C2) and plasmin in kinin release in hereditary angioneurotic edema (H.A.N.E.) plasma. *Trans. Assoc. Am. Physicians* **90:**174–183.

Drouin, S. M., D. B. Corry, J. Kildsgaard, and R. A. Wetsel. 2001. Cutting edge: the absence of C3 demonstrates a role for complement in Th2 effector functions in a murine model of pulmonary allergy. *J. Immunol.* **167:**4141–4145.

Ebenbichler, C. F., N. M. Thielens, R. Vornhagen, P. Marschang, G. J. Arlaud, and M. P. Dierich. 1991. Human immunodeficiency virus type 1 activates the classical pathway of complement by direct C1 binding through specific sites in the transmembrane glycoprotein gp41. *J. Exp. Med.* **174:**1417–1424.

Eden, A., C. Bianco, and V. Nussenzweig. 1971. A population of lymphocytes bearing a membrane receptor antigen-antibody-complement complexes. II. Specific isolation. *Cell. Immunol.* **2:**658–669.

Ember, J., M. Jagels, and T. Hugli. 1998. Characterization of complement anaphylatoxins and their biological responses, p. 241–284. *In* J. Volanakis and M. Frank (ed.), *The Human Complement System in Health and Disease.* Marcel Dekker, Inc., New York, N.Y.

Erdei, A., E. Spaeth, J. Alsenz, E. Rude, T. Schulz, J. Gergely, and M. P. Dierich. 1984. Role of C3b receptors in the enhancement of interleukin-2-dependent T-cell proliferation. *Mol. Immunol.* **21:**1215–1221.

Fang, Y., C. Xu, Y. X. Fu, V. M. Holers, and H. Molina. 1998. Expression of complement receptors 1 and 2 on follicular dendritic cells is necessary for the generation of a strong antigen-specific IgG response. *J. Immunol.* **160:**5273–5279.

Fearon, D. T. 1993. The CD19-CR2-TAPA-1 complex, CD45 and signaling by the antigen receptor of B lymphocytes. *Curr. Opin. Immunol.* **5:**341–348.

Fischer, E., C. Delibrias, and M. D. Kazatchkine. 1991. Expression of CR2 (the C3dg, EBV receptor, CD21) on normal human peripheral blood T lymphocytes. *J. Immunol.* **146:**865–869.

Fischer, M. B., M. Ma, S. Goerg, X. Zhou, J. Xia, O. Finco, S. Han, G. Kelsoe, R. G. Howard, T. L. Rothstein, E. Kremmer, F. S. Rosen, and M. C. Carroll. 1996. Regulation of the B cell response to T-dependent antigens by classical pathway complement. *J. Immunol.* **157:**549–556.

Fischer, M. B., M. Ma, N. C. Hsu, and M. C. Carroll. 1998. Local synthesis of C3 within the splenic lymphoid compartment can reconstitute the impaired immune response in C3-deficient mice. *J. Immunol.* **160:**2619–2625.

Gadjeva, M., A. Verschoor, M. A. Brockman, H. Jezak, L. M. Shen, D. M. Knipe, and M. C. Carroll. 2002. Macrophage-derived complement component C4 can restore humoral immunity in C4-deficient mice. *J. Immunol.* **169:**5489–5495.

Gewurz, H., H. S. Shin, and S. E. Mergenhagen. 1968. Interactions of the complement system with endotoxic lipopolysaccharide: consumption of each of the six terminal complement components. *J. Exp. Med.* **128:**1049–1057.

Green, T. D., B. R. Newton, P. A. Rota, Y. Xu, H. L. Robinson, and T. M. Ross. 2001. C3d enhancement of neutralizing antibodies to measles hemagglutinin. *Vaccine* **20:**242–248.

Gustavsson, S., T. Kinoshita, and B. Heyman. 1995. Antibodies to murine complement receptor 1 and 2 can inhibit the antibody response in vivo without inhibiting T helper cell induction. *J. Immunol.* **154:**6524–6528.

Hashimoto, K., T. Nakanishi, and Y. Kurosawa. 1992. Identification of a shark sequence resembling the major histocompatibility complex class I alpha 3 domain. *Proc. Natl. Acad. Sci. USA* **89:**2209–2212.

Hinds, K. R., and G. W. Litman. 1986. Major reorganization of immunoglobulin VH segmental elements during vertebrate evolution. *Nature* **320:**546–549.

Hugli, T. E., and H. J. Muller-Eberhard. 1978. Anaphylatoxins: C3a and C5a. *Adv. Immunol.* **26:**1–53.

Humbles, A. A., B. Lu, C. A. Nilsson, C. Lilly, E. Israel, Y. Fujiwara, N. P. Gerard, and C. Gerard. 2000. A role for the C3a anaphylatoxin receptor in the effector phase of asthma. *Nature* **406:**998–1001.

Hung, S. L., C. Peng, I. Kostavasili, H. M. Friedman, J. D. Lambris, R. J. Eisenberg, and G. H. Cohen. 1994. The interaction of glycoprotein C of herpes simplex virus types 1 and 2 with the alternative complement pathway. *Virology* **203:**299–312.

Kapadia, S. B., B. Levine, S. H. Speck, and H. W. T. Virgin. 2002. Critical role of complement and viral evasion of complement in acute, persistent, and latent gamma-herpesvirus infection. *Immunity* **17:**143–155.

Katz, Y., M. Revel, and R. C. Strunk. 1989. Interleukin 6 stimulates synthesis of complement proteins factor B and C3 in human skin fibroblasts. *Eur. J. Immunol.* **19:**983–988.

Kelsoe, G. 1996. The germinal center: a crucible for lymphocyte selection. *Semin. Immunol.* **8:**179–184.

Kerekes, K., J. Prechl, Z. Bajtay, M. Jozsi, and A. Erdei. 1998. A further link between innate and adaptive immunity: C3 deposition on antigen-presenting cells enhances the proliferation of antigen-specific T cells. *Int. Immunol.* **10:**1923–1930.

Kildsgaard, J., T. J. Hollmann, K. W. Matthews, K. Bian, F. Murad, and R. A. Wetsel. 2000. Cutting edge: targeted disruption of the C3a receptor gene demonstrates a novel protective anti-inflammatory role for C3a in endotoxin-shock. *J. Immunol.* **165:**5406–5409.

Kipnis, T. L., K. A. Joiner, W. D. da Silva, M. T. Rimoldi, C. H. Hammer, and A. Sher. 1988. Identification of membrane components of *Trypanosoma cruzi* modulators of complement system. *Mem. Inst. Oswaldo Cruz* **83**(Suppl. 1):571–575.

Kohl, J. 2001. Anaphylatoxins and infectious and noninfectious inflammatory diseases. *Mol. Immunol.* **38:**175–187.

Kopf, M., B. Abel, A. Gallimore, M. Carroll, and M. F. Bachmann. 2002. Complement component C3 promotes T-cell priming and lung migration to control acute influenza virus infection. *Nat. Med.* **8:**373–378.

Kotwal, G. J., and B. Moss. 1988. Vaccinia virus encodes a secretory polypeptide structurally related to complement control proteins. *Nature* **335:**176–178.

Krych-Goldberg, M., J. M. Moulds, and J. P. Atkinson. 2002. Human complement receptor type 1 (CR1) binds to a major malarial adhesin. *Trends Mol. Med.* **8:**531–537.

Kurtz, C. B., E. O'Toole, S. M. Christensen, and J. H. Weis. 1990. The murine complement receptor gene family. IV. Alternative splicing of Cr2 gene transcripts predicts two distinct gene products that share homologous domains with both human CR2 and CR1. *J. Immunol.* **144:**3581–3591.

Lakkis, F. G. 2002. Transplant rejection: mind your T-cell language. *Nat. Med.* **8:**1043; author reply 1043–1044.

Lay, W. H., and V. Nussenzweig. 1968. Receptors for complement of leukocytes. *J. Exp. Med.* **128:**991–1009.

Liu, Y. J., J. Xu, O. de Bouteiller, C. L. Parham, G. Grouard, O. Djossou, B. de Saint-Vis, S. Lebecque, J. Banchereau, and K. W. Moore. 1997. Follicular dendritic cells specifically express the long CR2/CD21 isoform. *J. Exp. Med.* **185:**165–170.

Lu, J. H., S. Thiel, H. Wiedemann, R. Timpl, and K. B. Reid. 1990. Binding of the pentamer/hexamer forms of mannan-binding protein to zymosan activates the proenzyme C1r2C1s2 complex, of the classical pathway of complement, without involvement of C1q. *J. Immunol.* **144:**2287–2294.

Malhotra, R., S. Thiel, K. B. Reid, and R. B. Sim. 1990. Human leukocyte C1q receptor binds other soluble proteins with collagen domains. *J. Exp. Med.* **172:**955–959.

Mandel, T. E., R. P. Phipps, A. P. Abbot, and J. G. Tew. 1981. Long-term antigen retention by dendritic cells in the popliteal lymph node of immunized mice. *Immunology* **43:**353–362.

Marschang, P., J. Sodroski, R. Wurzner, and M. P. Dierich. 1995. Decay-accelerating factor (CD55) protects human immunodeficiency virus type 1 from inactivation by human complement. *Eur. J. Immunol.* **25:**285–290.

Martin, D. R., R. L. Marlowe, and J. M. Ahearn. 1994. Determination of the role for CD21 during Epstein-Barr virus infection of B-lymphoblastoid cells. *J. Virol.* **68:**4716–4726.

Matsushita, M., Y. Endo, M. Nonaka, and T. Fujita. 1998. Complement-related serine proteases in tunicates and vertebrates. *Curr. Opin. Immunol.* **10:**29–35.

McGreal, E., and P. Gasque. 2001. Structure-function studies of the receptors for complement C1q. *Biochem. Soc. Trans.* **30:**1010–1014.

McPhaden, A. R., and K. Whaley. 1993. Complement biosynthesis by mononuclear phagocytes. *Immunol. Res.* **12:**213–232.

Miller, L. J., R. Schwarting, and T. A. Springer. 1986. Regulated expression of the Mac-1, LFA-1, p150,95 glycoprotein family during leukocyte differentiation. *J. Immunol.* **137:**2891–2900.

Mold, C., B. M. Bradt, G. R. Nemerow, and N. R. Cooper. 1988. Epstein-Barr virus regulates activation and processing of the third component of complement. *J. Exp. Med.* **168:**949–969.

Molina, H., V. M. Holers, B. Li, Y. Fung, S. Mariathasan, J. Goellner, J. Strauss-Schoenberger, R. W. Karr, and D. D. Chaplin. 1996. Markedly impaired humoral immune response in mice deficient in complement receptors 1 and 2. *Proc. Natl. Acad. Sci. USA* **93:**3357–3361.

Naughton, M. A., M. Botto, M. J. Carter, G. J. Alexander, J. M. Goldman, and M. J. Walport. 1996a. Extrahepatic secreted complement C3 contributes to circulating C3 levels in humans. *J. Immunol.* **156:**3051–3056.

Naughton, M. A., M. J. Walport, R. Wurzner, M. J. Carter, G. J. Alexander, J. M. Goldman, and M. Botto. 1996b. Organ-specific contribution to circulating C7 levels by the bone marrow and liver in humans. *Eur. J. Immunol.* **26:**2108–2112.

Nikaido, H., and T. Nakae. 1979. The outer membrane of Gram-negative bacteria. *Adv. Microb. Physiol.* **20:**163–250.

Nonaka, M., K. Azumi, X. Ji, C. Namikawa-Yamada, M. Sasaki, H. Saiga, A. W. Dodds, H. Sekine, M. K. Homma, M. Matsushita, Y. Endo, and T. Fujita. 1999. Opsonic complement component C3 in the solitary ascidian, *Halocynthia roretzi*. *J. Immunol.* **162:**387–391.

Norris, K. A., B. Bradt, N. R. Cooper, and M. So. 1991. Characterization of a *Trypanosoma cruzi* C3 binding protein with functional and genetic similarities to the human complement regulatory protein, decay-accelerating factor. *J. Immunol.* **147:**2240–2247.

Ohkuro, M., M. Ogura-Masaki, K. Kobayashi, M. Sakai, K. Takahashi, and S. Nagasawa. 1995. Effect of iC3b binding to immune complexes upon the phagocytic response of human neutrophils: synergistic functions between Fc gamma R and CR3. *FEBS Lett* **373:**189–192.

Papamichail, M., C. Gutierrez, P. Embling, P. Johnson, E. J. Holborow, and M. B. Pepys. 1975. Complement dependence of localisation of aggregated IgG in germinal centres. *Scand. J. Immunol.* **4:**343–347.

Pepys, M. B. 1972. Role of complement in induction of the allergic response. *Nat. New Biol.* **237:**157–159.

Petry, F., M. Botto, R. Holtappels, M. J. Walport, and M. Loos. 2001. Reconstitution of the complement function in C1q-deficient (C1qa$^{-/-}$) mice with wild-type bone marrow cells. *J. Immunol.* **167:**4033–4037.

Pinter, C., A. G. Siccardi, R. Longhi, and A. Clivio. 1995a. Direct interaction of complement factor H with the C1 domain of HIV type 1 glycoprotein 120. *AIDS Res. Hum. Retrovir.* **11:**577–588.

Pinter, C., A. G. Siccardi, L. Lopalco, R. Longhi, and A. Clivio. 1995b. HIV glycoprotein 41 and complement factor H interact with each other and share functional as well as antigenic homology. *AIDS Res. Hum. Retrovir.* **11:**971–980.

Podack, E. R., K. T. Preissner, and H. J. Muller-Eberhard. 1984. Inhibition of C9 polymerization within the SC5b-9 complex of complement by S-protein. *Acta Pathol. Microbiol. Immunol. Scand. Suppl.* **284:**89–96.

Pratt, J. R., S. A. Basheer, and S. H. Sacks. 2002. Local synthesis of complement component C3 regulates acute renal transplant rejection. *Nat. Med.* **8:**582–587.

Qin, D., J. Wu, M. C. Carroll, G. F. Burton, A. K. Szakal, and J. G. Tew. 1998. Evidence for an important interaction between a complement-derived CD21 ligand on follicular dendritic cells and CD21 on B cells in the initiation of IgG responses. *J. Immunol.* **161:**4549–4554.

Radoux, D., C. Kinet-Denoel, E. Heinen, M. Moeremans, J. De Mey, and L. J. Simar. 1985. Retention of immune complexes by Fc receptors on mouse follicular dendritic cells. *Scand. J. Immunol.* **21:**345–353.

Ramos, O. F., M. Patarroyo, E. Yefenof, and E. Klein. 1989. Requirement of leukocytic cell adhesion molecules (CD11a-c/CD18) in the enhanced NK lysis of iC3b-opsonized targets. *J. Immunol.* **142:**4100–4104.

Reynes, M., J. P. Aubert, J. H. Cohen, J. Audouin, V. Tricottet, J. Diebold, and M. D. Kazatchkine. 1985. Human follicular dendritic cells express CR1, CR2, and CR3 complement receptor antigens. *J. Immunol.* **135:**2687–2694.

Ridker, P. M., N. Rifai, L. Rose, J. E. Buring, and N. R. Cook. 2002. Comparison of C-reactive protein and low-density lipoprotein cholesterol levels in the prediction of first cardiovascular events. *N. Engl. J. Med.* **347:**1557–1565.

Robson, M. G., H. T. Cook, M. Botto, P. R. Taylor, N. Busso, R. Salvi, C. D. Pusey, M. J. Walport, and K. A. Davies. 2001. Accelerated nephrotoxic nephritis is exacerbated in C1q-deficient mice. *J. Immunol.* **166:**6820–6828.

Ross, T. M., Y. Xu, R. A. Bright, and H. L. Robinson. 2000. C3d enhancement of antibodies to hemagglutinin accelerates protection against influenza virus challenge. *Nat. Immunol.* **1:**127–131.

Ross, T. M., Y. Xu, T. D. Green, D. C. Montefiori, and H. L. Robinson. 2001. Enhanced avidity maturation of antibody to human immunodeficiency virus envelope: DNA vaccination with gp120-C3d fusion proteins. *AIDS Res. Hum. Retrovir.* **17:**829–835.

Saifuddin, M., C. J. Parker, M. E. Peeples, M. K. Gorny, S. Zolla-Pazner, M. Ghassemi, I. A. Rooney, J. P. Atkinson, and G. T. Spear. 1995. Role of virion-associated glycosylphosphatidylinositol-linked proteins CD55 and CD59 in complement resistance of cell line-derived and primary isolates of HIV-1. *J. Exp. Med.* **182:**501–509.

Sato, S., A. S. Miller, M. C. Howard, and T. F. Tedder. 1997. Regulation of B lymphocyte development and activation by the CD19/CD21/CD81/Leu 13 complex requires the cytoplasmic domain of CD19. *J. Immunol.* **159:**3278–3287.

Schnizlein, C. T., A. K. Szakal, and J. G. Tew. 1984. Follicular dendritic cells in the regulation and maintenance of immune responses. *Immunobiology* **168:**391–402.

Simpson, A. J., and S. R. Smithers. 1980. Characterization of the exposed carbohydrates on the surface membrane of adult *Schistosoma mansoni* by analysis of lectin binding. *Parasitology* **81:**1–15.

Stalenheim, G., and S. Castensson. 1971. Protein A from *Staphylococcus aureus* conversion of complement factor C3 by aggregates between IgG and protein A. *FEBS Lett.* **14:**79–81.

Stoiber, H., C. Pinter, A. G. Siccardi, A. Clivio, and M. P. Dierich. 1996. Efficient destruction of human immunodeficiency virus in human serum by inhibiting the protective action of complement factor H and decay accelerating factor (DAF, CD55). *J. Exp. Med.* **183:**307–310.

Strunk, R. C., D. M. Eidlen, and R. J. Mason. 1988. Pulmonary alveolar type II epithelial cells synthesize and secrete proteins of the classical and alternative complement pathways. *J. Clin. Invest.* **81:**1419–1426.

Suradhat, S., R. P. Braun, P. J. Lewis, L. A. Babiuk, S. van Drunen Littel-van den Hurk, P. J. Griebel, and M. E. Baca-Estrada. 2001. Fusion of C3d molecule with bovine rotavirus VP7 or bovine herpesvirus type 1 glycoprotein D inhibits immune responses following DNA immunization. *Vet. Immunol. Immunopathol.* **83:**79–92.

Takizawa, F., S. Tsuji, and S. Nagasawa. 1996. Enhancement of macrophage phagocytosis upon iC3b deposition on apoptotic cells. *FEBS Lett.* **397:**269–272.

Tang, S., W. Zhou, N. S. Sheerin, R. W. Vaughan, and S. H. Sacks. 1999. Contribution of renal secreted complement C3 to the circulating pool in humans. *J. Immunol.* **162:**4336–4341.

Terui, T., K. Ishii, M. Ozawa, N. Tabata, T. Kato, and H. Tagami. 1997. C3 production of cultured human epidermal keratinocytes is enhanced by IFNgamma and TNFalpha through different pathways. *J. Invest. Dermatol.* **108:**62–67.

Thornton, B. P., V. Vetvicka, and G. D. Ross. 1994. Natural antibody and complement-mediated antigen processing and presentation by B lymphocytes. *J. Immunol.* **152:**1727–1737.

Thornton, B. P., V. Vetvicka, and G. D. Ross. 1996. Function of C3 in a humoral response: iC3b/C3dg bound to an immune complex generated with natural antibody and a primary antigen promotes antigen uptake and the expression of co-stimulatory molecules by all B cells, but only stimulates immunoglobulin synthesis by antigen-specific B cells. *Clin. Exp. Immunol.* **104:**531–537.

van den Berg, R. H., M. C. Faber-Krol, J. A. van de Klundert, L. A. van Es, and M. R. Daha. 1996. Inhibition of the hemolytic activity of the first component of complement C1 by an *Escherichia coli* C1q binding protein. *J. Immunol.* **156:**4466–4473.

Varsano, S., M. Kaminsky, M. Kaiser, and L. Rashkovsky. 2000. Generation of complement C3 and expression of cell membrane complement inhibitory proteins by human bronchial epithelium cell line. *Thorax* **55:**364–369.

Verschoor, A., M. A. Brockman, D. M. Knipe, and M. C. Carroll. 2001. Cutting edge: myeloid complement C3 enhances the humoral response to peripheral viral infection. *J. Immunol.* **167:**2446–2451.

von Andrian, U. H., and C. R. Mackay. 2000. T-cell function and migration. Two sides of the same coin. *N. Engl. J. Med.* **343:**1020–1034.

Walport, M. J. 2001a. Complement. First of two parts. *N. Engl. J. Med.* **344:**1058–1066.

Walport, M. J. 2001b. Complement. Second of two parts. *N. Engl. J. Med.* **344:**1140–1144.

Walport, M. J. 2002. Complement and systemic lupus erythematosus. *Arthritis Res.* **4**(Suppl. 3):S279–S293.

Wilson, J. G., T. F. Tedder, and D. T. Fearon. 1983. Characterization of human T lymphocytes that express the C3b receptor. *J. Immunol.* **131:**684–689.

Zalman, L. S., L. M. Wood, and H. J. Muller-Eberhard. 1986. Isolation of a human erythrocyte membrane protein capable of inhibiting expression of homologous complement transmembrane channels. *Proc. Natl. Acad. Sci. USA* **83:**6975–6979.

Zhang, L., K. Jacobsson, J. Vasi, M. Lindberg, and L. Frykberg. 1998. A second IgG-binding protein in *Staphylococcus aureus*. *Microbiology* **144**(Pt. 4):985–991.

Ziccardi, R. J., and N. R. Cooper. 1977. The subunit composition and sedimentation properties of human C1. *J. Immunol.* **118:**2047–2052.

COAGULATION AND INNATE IMMUNITY

Charles T. Esmon

12

Triggering the innate immune system has long been recognized to result in potential stimulation of the blood coagulation system. More recently, the highly integrated interactions of these two systems have begun to become apparent. Inflammation triggered by the innate immune system not only initiates the blood clotting process, but the natural anticoagulant pathways, components of which are consumed or downregulated by the inflammatory mediators, play an important role in limiting the inflammatory response. In this chapter I summarize the current information on the linkage between the regulation of the coagulation and inflammatory responses to infection.

THE IMPACT OF INFLAMMATION ON COAGULATION

Bacterial pathogens lead to the generation of inflammatory cytokines such as tumor necrosis factor alpha (TNF-α) and interleukin-1β (IL-1β). These mediators, or the endotoxin itself, induce formation synthesis and expres-

sion of tissue factor, primarily on monocytes and macrophages (Walsh, 1987; Edgington et al., 1991). Once the tissue factor is exposed to the blood, it will trigger a coagulation response (Fig. 1). Under normal circumstances, the tissue factor is found almost exclusively on extravascular cells, where it is strategically located to initiate coagulation when the blood vessels are injured (Drake et al., 1989). Once the tissue factor is exposed to blood, it binds factor VII (VIIa), and the tissue factor-factor VIIa complex then catalyzes the activation of either factor X or factor IX. Factor Xa binds to factor Va to form a complex that rapidly converts prothrombin to thrombin. Alternatively, the factor IXa-factor VIIIa complex provides an alternative mechanism for activating factor X (second row, Fig. 1). This "bypass" mechanism seems to be important because of the rapid inactivation of the tissue factor-factor VIIa complex by the tissue factor pathway inhibitor (TFPI), a high-affinity, reversible Kunitz-type protease inhibitor.

As depicted in Fig. 1, both the initiation and the amplification phases of coagulation occur on membrane surfaces. Functional surfaces require negatively charged phospholipids, particularly phosphatidylserine. Potent cell agonists are required to expose these surfaces

Charles T. Esmon, Cardiovascular Biology Research Program, Oklahoma Medical Research Foundation; Departments of Pathology, and Biochemistry and Molecular Biology, University of Oklahoma Health Sciences Center; and Howard Hughes Medical Institute, Oklahoma City, OK 73104.

The Innate Immune Response to Infection
Ed. by S. H. E. Kaufmann, R. Medzhitov, and S. Gordon
©2004 ASM Press, Washington, D.C.

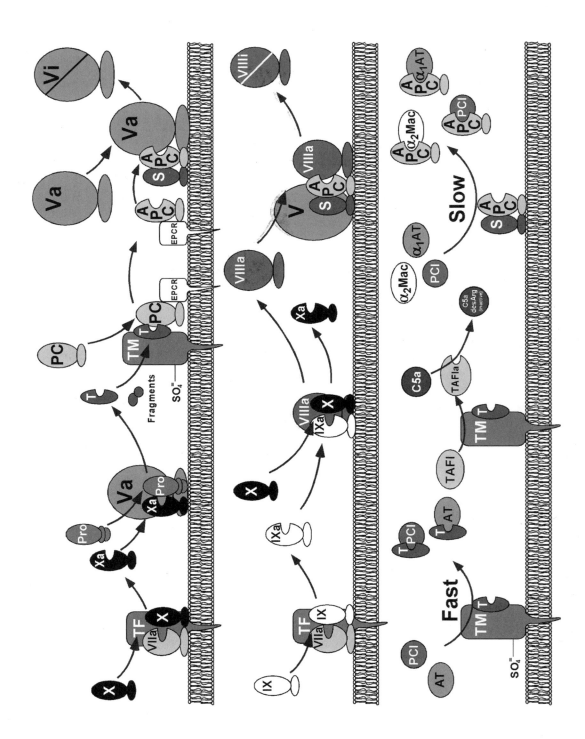

optimally. Physiologically, these include a combination of thrombin plus collagen (Bevers et al., 1991; Alberio et al., 2000) or the membrane attack complex of complement C5b-9 (Sims et al., 1988). Complement involvement in amplifying the coagulant response is made more likely by the observation that the acute-phase protein, C-reactive protein, appears to augment complement activation during sepsis (Wolbink et al., 1998). Although the critical regulatory role of this membrane surface exposure is often overlooked, it is clear that this is a major regulatory event controlling physiological and pathological clotting. For example, infusion of factor Xa at relatively high concentrations has little thrombotic effect unless the factor is coinfused with negatively charged phospholipids (a mimic of the activated cell surface or cellular microparticles released following treatment with potent cell agonists) (Giles et al., 1988). Furthermore, with a simple proinflammatory stimulus such as TNF-α, infusion of negatively charged phospholipid vesicles can amplify the response to lead to significant fibrin formation when neither the TNF nor the lipid alone has a significant effect (Taylor et al., 1996). Thus, inflammation can contribute directly to two critical events in coagulation: the synthesis and expression of intravascular tissue factor and the generation of membrane surfaces capable of augmenting the initiation and propagation of the coagulant response.

Assembly of the prothrombin activation complex results in thrombin generation. Thrombin, however, impacts both its own generation and the inflammatory response (Fig. 2). In addition to its well-known functions in clotting fibrinogen and activated platelets, thrombin plays a major role in leukocyte activation. Thrombin leads to expression of adhesion molecules on the endothelial cell surface such as P-selectin (Lorant et al., 1991) and also leads to formation of platelet-activating factor, a potent neutrophil agonist (Bar-Shavit et al., 1986). Neutrophil activation is potentiated by adhesion to P-selectin, further augmenting the inflammatory response. P-selectin itself plays an important role in thrombus formation. Under both flow (Palabrica et al., 1992) and stasis conditions (Wakefield et al., 2000), interfering with P-selectin interaction with its ligand, PSGL-1, diminishes thrombus formation. P-selectin is found in both endothelium and platelets, and after platelet activation, neutrophils will adhere and their activation will be augmented by the interaction with P-selectin.

Inflammation can affect coagulation status in less overt fashions. Inflammatory mediators such as IL-6 can not only increase platelet production, but the platelets that are generated are

FIGURE 1 A simplified view of the regulation of blood coagulation by the protein C pathway. Factor VIIa binds to tissue factor (TF) to activate factor X, generating factor Xa. Factor Xa then binds to factor Va. The complex of factors Xa and V converts prothrombin (Pro) to thrombin (T). Thrombin can then either bind to TM or carry out procoagulant reactions like fibrin formation or platelet activation. When bound to TM, thrombin can activate protein C (PC) to APC. This process is enhanced when protein C is bound to EPCR. APC bound to EPCR cleaves substrates other than factor Va. APC dissociates from EPCR and can then interact with protein S to inactivate factor Va. The middle row shows inactivation of the factor IXa (IXa)-factor VIIIa complex by APC. In this case, factor V participates with APC and protein S in the inactivation of factor VIIIa. In the bottom row, the plasma proteinase inhibitors that regulate the protein C activation complex and the anticoagulant complex of APC and protein S are illustrated. α_1-AT, α_1-antitrypsin; α_2-Mac, α_2-macroglobulin; PCI, protein C inhibitor; and AT, antithrombin. TAFI is activated (TAFIa) by the thrombin-TM complex. TAFIa then inactivates C5a. For simplicity, the activation of factors VII, V, and VIII is not shown. Figure modified with permission from Esmon, 1999, copyright F. K. Schattauer.

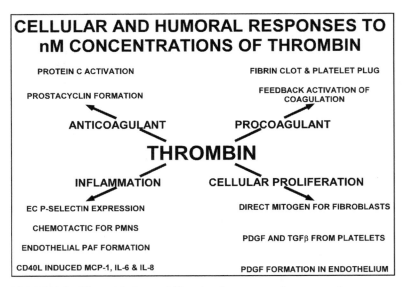

FIGURE 2 Thrombin is a multifunctional enzyme and generates the procoagulant, anticoagulant, inflammatory, and mitogenic responses. These responses serve to shift the hemostatic balance. EC, endothelial cell; PMNs, polymorphonucleocytes; PAF, platelet-activating factor; PDGF, platelet-derived growth factor; TGF-β, transforming growth factor β; CD40L, CD40 ligand; MCP-1, macrophage chemotactic protein-1. (From Esmon, 1993, with permission from the *Annual Review of Cell Biology,* vol. 9, copyright by Annual Reviews.)

more thrombogenic, demonstrating an increased sensitivity to platelet agonists like thrombin (Burstein, 1997). Once platelets are activated, they are a rich source of the proinflammatory mediator CD40 ligand. This protein can induce tissue factor formation (Pendurthi et al., 1997; Miller et al., 1998) and increase inflammatory cytokines like IL-6 and IL-8 (André et al., 2002; Henn et al., 1998).

THE IMPACT OF INFLAMMATION ON NATURAL ANTICOAGULANT PATHWAYS

Opposing this inflammation-mediated augmentation of the coagulation response are the natural anticoagulant pathways. Several of these pathways not only prevent excess clotting, but also feed back to dampen the inflammatory response. However, during severe sepsis, some of the key negative regulatory pathways are downregulated.

Regulation of Tissue Factor–Factor VIIa

Two major mechanisms regulate tissue factor–factor VIIa activity: TFPI and antithrombin and heparin. Both function by inhibiting the protease, factor VIIa bound to the tissue factor. TFPI has an unusual mechanism of action (Broze et al., 1990). Structurally, TFPI is composed of three Kunitz inhibitory domains. During the inhibitory process, TFPI first binds to factor Xa through a distinct protease inhibitory domain. The factor Xa–TFPI complex then binds to negatively charged membrane surfaces, increasing the local concentration and favoring relatively stable, reversible inhibition of factor VII bound to the tissue factor (Broze et al., 1990). The physiological importance of TFPI is demonstrated by the observation that gene deletion results in an embryonic lethal phenotype caused by a consumptive coagulopathy (Huang et al., 1997). It is difficult to assess the impact of inflammation on the TFPI function because the majority of TFPI is vessel associated (Broze et al., 1990) and much of this is stored in agonist–releasable endothelial cell granules (Lupu et al., 1995).

Although the relative importance of antithrombin inhibition of tissue factor is less clear because of its multiple other interactions, it is clear that antithrombin activities decrease markedly during severe sepsis, often to 50% or more (Levi and ten Cate, 1999). Because the rate of inhibition is strongly dependent on the inhibitor concentration, this decrease in antithrombin would contribute to increased stability of the tissue factor–factor VIIa complex and hence favor intravascular coagulation.

Antithrombin Regulation of the Amplification Reactions

Antithrombin inhibition of the factor VIIa–tissue factor complex, factor IXa, factor Xa, and thrombin is all thought to be accelerated by vascular heparinlike proteoglycans. There is evidence that these heparinlike molecules may be inactivated during severe sepsis (Klein et al., 1996), further diminishing the natural anticoagulant potential, especially when the antithrombin level has been reduced by consumption.

ZPI-Protein Z Complex Regulation of Factor Xa

In the case of factor Xa, a novel and apparently important inhibitory pathway also plays a significant role. Protein Z protease inhibitor (ZPI) binds tightly to the vitamin K-dependent protein Z. The ZPI-protein Z complex binds to negatively charged membrane surfaces, and this complex then inactivates factor Xa (Han et al., 2000). In mice, deficiency of protein Z exacerbates the thrombotic response caused by other coagulation abnormalities (Yin et al., 2000), but is not itself overtly prothrombotic. In humans, low protein Z levels appear to be associated with an increased risk of stroke (Vasse et al., 2001). Inflammation may impact this system because protein Z appears to be a negative acute-phase reactant (Raczkowski et al., 1987).

The Protein C Anticoagulant Pathway

Among the major anticoagulant mechanisms, the protein C anticoagulant pathway is the most complex and appears to be the most impacted by acute inflammatory responses. The pathway is illustrated in Fig. 1 (far right). Protein C, an inactive zymogen, circulates at about 4 μg/ml of plasma. It is activated proteolytically on the surface of the endothelium by a complex between thrombin and thrombomodulin (TM) to generate activated protein C (APC). The protein C activation rate is increased when protein C is bound to the endothelial cell protein C receptor (EPCR) (Stearns-Kurosawa et al., 1996). Since EPCR is found primarily on the endothelium of larger vessels, it may be particularly important in preventing large vessel thrombosis (Laszik et al., 1997). Protein C and APC bind to EPCR with comparable affinity ($\approx$30 nM). The APC–EPCR complex does not appear to have anticoagulant activity (Liaw et al., 2000) and appears to interact with alternative substrates and receptors (Shu et al., 2000; Riewald et al., 2002). This would be consistent with the observed ability of APC to dampen cellular responses to inflammatory agents and decrease the generation of inflammatory cytokines (Grey et al., 1993; Joyce et al., 2001). When APC dissociates from EPCR it can bind to protein S and catalyze the selective proteolytic inactivation of factors Va and VIIIa (Esmon, 2001). APC not only inhibits coagulation, but also enhances fibrinolysis. APC forms a tight 1:1 complex with plasminogen activator inhibitor 1 (PAI-1), inactivating this major inhibitor of fibrinolysis. Normally, APC reacts slowly with PAI-1, but the reaction becomes quite rapid in the presence of vitronectin (Rezaie, 2001), suggesting a dominant role for this reaction around cells releasing vitronectin.

Compared with other serine proteases or clotting factors, APC has a relatively long half-life in the blood of about 15 min before it becomes inactivated by α_1-antitrypsin (sometimes called α_1-proteinase inhibitor), protein C inhibitor, or α_2-macroglobulin (Heeb et al., 1991). The APC-inhibitor complex is then cleared relatively rapidly from the circulation. The relatively slow inactivation of APC actually allows the direct evaluation of APC levels in patients (Gruber and Griffin, 1992), which in turn allows evaluation of the functionality of the protein C activation complex in vivo.

Thrombin binding to TM not only augments protein C activation, but also results in inhibition of most of the procoagulant functions of thrombin, including fibrinogen clotting, platelet and endothelial cell activation, and factor V activation (Esmon, 2001). In addition, thrombin bound to TM is inactivated much more rapidly than free thrombin. Both antithrombin and protein C inhibitor play major roles in inactivating TM-bound thrombin, resulting in a half-life for the bound thrombin of about 1 to 2 s (Rezaie et al., 1995). In severe sepsis, downregulation of TM would result in both decreased protein C activation and decreased thrombin clearance. Results from such studies indicate that the activation complex is severely impaired in a subset of patients with severe sepsis (Liaw et al., 2002; Faust et al., 2001). The complete change in thrombin functions and regulation caused by binding to TM allows TM to serve as a molecular switch in the control of hemostasis and thrombosis.

Both TM and EPCR are downregulated by inflammatory cytokines like TNF-α at the transcriptional level (Conway and Rosenberg, 1988; Fukudome and Esmon, 1994). In cell culture, about half of the activity disappears in 8 h, and unlike some other responses, a single dose of cytokine keeps the protein and mRNA levels very low for at least 24 h. Oxidants generated by adherent neutrophils can also reduce TM activity by oxidizing a highly exposed and sensitive methionine residue on TM (Glaser et al., 1992). Alternatively, activated neutrophils release elastase that readily cleaves TM, releasing it from the cell surface (Takano et al., 1990) in a form with reduced activity. Loss of the protein C

system function is particularly important because factor Xa and factor XIa are resistant to inactivation by antithrombin when they are in complex with factors Va and VIIIa, respectively (Nesheim et al., 1982; Regan et al., 1994).

The protein C pathway seems to be particularly important in the prevention of microvascular thrombosis as demonstrated by the purpura fulminans that develops in neonates with protein C deficiency (Dreyfus et al., 1991). Downregulation of TM with the loss of thrombin clearance and decreased protein C activation would therefore be expected to have a major effect on clotting in the microcirculation, a major site of thrombotic complications in sepsis.

THE ANTI-INFLAMMATORY ACTIVITIES OF NATURAL ANTICOAGULANT PATHWAYS

Natural anticoagulants have anti-inflammatory activities as well as anticoagulant functions. Antithrombin, TFPI, and APC have all been shown to protect baboons from *Escherichia coli* sepsis when given prior to the challenge (Esmon, 2000). In the baboon and several rodent models (Enkhbaatar et al., 2000) neither synthetic factor Xa inhibitors (Enkhbaatar et al., 2000) nor active site-blocked factor Xa, an effective high-affinity competitive inhibitor of prothrombin activation in vivo (Taylor et al., 1991), failed to protect the animals from death or organ failure or to downregulate cytokine elaboration. The difference in efficacy in modulating the host response to bacterial and endotoxin infusion between artificial anticoagulants and the natural anticoagulants suggests that the anti-inflammatory activities of the natural anticoagulants may be very important aspects of their physiological functions.

Antithrombin

Antithrombin has been shown to protect from septic shock (Uchiba and Okajima, 1997). Heparin appears to prevent protection despite increasing antithrombotic activity of antithrombin. A similar negative effect of heparin in combination with antithrombin was observed in clinical trials (Opal and Esmon, 2002). In vitro, high levels of antithrombin have been shown to have anti-inflammatory activity (Uchiba and Okajima, 1997). For example, antithrombin has been shown to inhibit endotoxin-induced IL-6 formation by mononuclear cells and endothelium (Souter et al., 2001). The mechanism appears to involve antithrombin-induced signaling through proteoglycans, likely syndecan-4 (Souter et al., 2001). Antithrombin binding to cell surface receptors has also been shown to block NF-κB nuclear translocation (Oelschläger et al., 2002), which would prevent subsequent release of cytokines and induction of adhesion molecules. Antithrombin also stimulates prostacyclin release from endothelial cells in culture (Yamauchi et al., 1989), a process that appears to be protective in lung injury models (Dickneite, 1998).

TFPI

TFPI can reduce leukocyte activation and decrease TNF-α in vivo (Enkhbaatar et al., 2000). Although inhibition of cytokine elaboration appears to be independent of blood coagulation, the mechanism responsible for TFPI-mediated cellular effects remains unknown.

Protein C Pathway

APC has been shown to protect nonhuman primates from *E. coli*-induced sepsis whether given before or after the *E. coli* challenge (Taylor et al., 1987). Recently, this observation was confirmed and extended in clinical studies demonstrating that APC infusion can reduce the relative risk of all-cause 28-day mortality from severe sepsis by 19.4% (Bernard et al., 2001).

The protective effects of APC appear to be receptor mediated. APC binding to monocytic cells can block agonist-induced calcium transients (Hancock et al., 1995) and inhibit NF-κB-mediated signaling (Grey et al., 1993; Yuksel et al., 2002; Taoka et al., 1998; White

et al., 2000). In endothelium, incubation of the cells with APC reduces NF-κB mRNA levels (Joyce et al., 2001). APC reduces the expression of cell surface adhesion molecules and cytokine formation and elevates levels of molecules involved in preventing apoptosis (Joyce et al., 2001). On the monocytic cell line U937, APC has been shown to dampen both basal levels and the phorbol-induced expression of tissue factor in an EPCR-dependent fashion (Shu et al., 2000). Under appropriate conditions, APC can also cleave protease-activated receptors (Riewald et al., 2002), receptors that are normally cleaved by coagulation enzymes, particularly thrombin (Coughlin, 2000). The role of cleavage of the protease-activated receptors in APC function remains to be fully elucidated. Most of the downstream events following activation of these receptors enhance inflammation (Coughlin, 1994). It is possible that activation of the protease-activated receptors is a negative side reaction occurring under the in vitro conditions.

TM has also been found to exhibit anti-inflammatory properties. Conway and coworkers (2002) have recently revealed an additional, novel anti-inflammatory activity of TM. They found that the N-terminal domain, which has homology to the lectins (Jackman et al., 1987; Wen et al., 1987), dampened activation of the mitogen-activated protein kinase and NF-κB signaling systems. This anti-inflammatory activity was imparted either by cellular TM or by the soluble lectinlike domain. Physiologically, they showed that the presence of the lectin domain, which does not participate in protein C activation, resulted in greatly reduced leukocyte adhesion to the endothelium. This finding has considerable important ramifications. TM appears to be downregulated on endothelium overlying atherosclerotic plaques, on vein bypass grafts, in diabetes, and by acute inflammatory insults like bacterial infection (Esmon, 2002). Loss of the TM would not only reduce protein C activation, but would also increase the sensitivity of the endothelium to phenotype modulation by inflammatory mediators, particularly in the case of sepsis. The net effect would be to promote leukocyte adhesion, increase permeability, and reduce the natural antithrombotic surface. An important role for TM in endothelial cell responses was suggested earlier when overexpression of TM was found to reduce thrombosis, restenosis, and leukocyte infiltration in rabbits with deep arterial injury (Waugh et al., 1999, 2000).

TM also accelerates thrombin activation of a plasma procarboxypeptidase B, often named thrombin-activatable fibrinolysis inhibitor or TAFI (Bajzar et al., 1996). TAFI removes terminal Lys residues in fibrin. Lysine residues facilitate binding of plasminogen and plasmin and the tissue plasminogen activator (TPA). Removal of these lysine residues decreases (but does not prevent) clot lysis (Bajzar et al., 1996). This was initially viewed solely as a prothrombotic mechanism. However, removal of terminal Arg residues (a function of carboxypeptidase B enzymes) is also important in the control of vasoactive peptides. For example, C5a is an anaphylatoxin generated during ·complement activation. It is inactivated by removal of the C-terminal Arg residue. Recent studies have found that TAFI is the major enzyme responsible for the inactivation of C5a (Campbell et al., 2001, 2002). Based on this observation, activation of TAFI by the thrombin–TM complex would appear to be important in preventing vascular toxicity due to C5a in conditions where complement activation was intense. These observations provide a direct link between the control of the coagulation system and the regulation of innate immunity, in this case the complement system. This aspect of the protein C pathway may be particularly important because recent data have suggested that C-reactive protein (an acute-phase reactant) contributes significantly to complement activation in sepsis (Wolbink et al., 1998).

Like TM, EPCR has recently been found to exhibit anti-inflammatory activity. Inhibition of EPCR and protein C binding resulted in amplification of both the coagulant and the cytokine responses in animals challenged with low-dose *E. coli* (Taylor et al., 2000). Leukocyte migration into the tissues was also increased substantially. The recent finding that soluble EPCR, released by a metalloproteinase in endothelium (Xu et al., 1999), binds to activated neutrophils may provide insights into some of the mechanisms involved. Soluble EPCR binds to proteinase 3, a cytosolic protein of the neutrophil that is released upon activation. Proteinase 3 binds to neutrophil integrins, particularly Mac-1 (CD11b and CD18) (Kurosawa et al., 2000), whether or not it is bound to EPCR. In vivo data suggest that this interaction reduces the tight binding of neutrophils to activated endothelium.

EPCR has recently emerged as a candidate for modulating immune functions by novel mechanisms. At the sequence (Fukudome and Esmon, 1994), gene organization (Simmonds and Lane, 1999) and crystal structure levels (Oganesyan et al., 2002), EPCR is closely related to the major histocompatibility complex class 1 and CD1 family of proteins. Surprisingly, the crystal structure demonstrated that EPCR has a tightly bound phospholipid in the "antigen-presenting groove" (Oganesyan et al., 2002). CD1 family members are lipid antigen-presenting molecules. In the case of CD1c, this antigen appears to be a lipid derived from tuberculosis (Moody et al., 2000). The CD1 series of proteins then instruct T cells and modulate the cellular and humoral response to inflammation (Hong et al., 1999). Furthermore, they appear likely candidates to be involved in autoimmunity (Hong et al., 1999). Whether EPCR plays similar roles should become clear through analysis of genetically modified mice (Gu et al., 2002).

STRUCTURES LINKING THE COAGULATION PATHWAY AND INFLAMMATION

The parallel evolution of the coagulation and inflammatory pathways is supported by the conserved structures that they share. For example, tissue factor and the cytokine receptors share structural similarities (Morrissey et al., 1987); the lectin domain of TM has homology to the selectins involved in leukocyte adhesion (Sadler, 1997); and, as mentioned above, the structures of EPCR and the major histocompatibility complex class 1 and CD1 family members are almost superimposable (Oganesyan et al., 2002). There are also functional linkages. The complement regulatory protein C4-binding protein binds to protein S, an interaction that allows the C4-binding protein to interact with the membrane at the expense of the protein S anticoagulant function (Dahlbäck, 1991). Together these structural observations and interactions suggest that the coagulation and inflammatory pathways likely evolved in parallel.

SUMMARY

The mutual regulatory functions of the inflammatory and coagulation systems are summarized in Fig. 3. The large number of interactions provides a compelling basis for understanding how inflammation triggers a hypercoaguable state. Rapidly evolving insights into the role of coagulation inhibitors in controlling inflammation may further clarify previously unrecognized risk factors and aid in assessing the transition to frank thrombosis. The involvement of the natural anticoagulants in regulating inflammation may also provide new insights into therapeutic interventions in acute inflammatory disease. The use of APC to treat severe sepsis is a first step toward this goal. We now recognize that even the statins thought originally to function by lowering

cholesterol have important anti-inflammatory effects as well. Further identification of the links between inflammation and thrombosis should provide novel approaches to new diagnostics and therapeutics.

REFERENCES

Alberio, L., O. Safa, K. J. Clemetson, C. T. Esmon, and G. L. Dale. 2000. Surface expression and functional characterization of α-granule factor V in human platelets: effects of ionophore A23187, thrombin, collagen, and convulxin. *Blood* **95:**1694–1702.

André, P., K. S. Srinivasa Prasad, C. V. Denis, M. He, J. M. Papalia, R. O. Hynes, D. R. Phillips, and D. D. Wagner. 2002. CD40L stabilizes arterial thrombi by a β_3 integrin-dependent mechanism. *Nat. Med.* **8:**247–252.

Bajzar, L., J. Morser, and M. Nesheim. 1996. TAFI, or Plasma Procarboxypeptidase B, couples the coagulation and fibrinolytic cascades through the thrombin-thrombomodulin complex. *J. Biol. Chem.* **271:**16603–16608.

Bar-Shavit, R., A. J. Kahn, K. G. Mann, and G. D. Wilner. 1986. Identification of a thrombin sequence with growth factor activity on macrophages. *Proc. Natl. Acad. Sci. USA* **83:**976–980.

Bernard, G. R., J. L. Vincent, P. F. Laterre, S. P. LaRosa, J. F. Dhainaut, A. Lopez-Rodriguez, J. S. Steingrub, G. E. Garber, J. D. Helterbrand, E. W. Ely, C. J. Fisher, Jr., and the Recombinant Human Protein C Worldwide Evaluation in Severe Sepsis (PROWESS) Study Group. 2001. Efficacy and safety of recombinant human activated protein C for severe sepsis. *N. Engl. J. Med.* **344:**699–709.

Bevers, E. M., P. Comfurius, and R. F. A. Zwaal. 1991. Platelet procoagulant activity: physiological significance and mechanisms of exposure. *Blood Rev.* **5:**146–154.

Broze, G. J., Jr., T. J. Girard, and W. F. Novotny. 1990. Regulation of coagulation by a multivalent Kunitz-type inhibitor. *Biochemistry* **29:**7539–7546.

Burstein, S. A. 1997. Cytokines, platelet production and hemostasis. *Platelets* **8:**93–104.

Campbell, W., N. Okada, and H. Okada. 2001. Carboxypeptidase R is an inactivator of complement-derived inflammatory peptides and an inhibitor of fibrinolysis. *Immunol. Rev.* **180:**162–167.

Campbell, W. D., E. Lazoura, N. Okada, and H. Okada. 2002. Inactivation of C3a and C5a octapeptides by carboxypeptidase R and carboxypeptidase N. *Microbiol. Immunol.* **46:**131–134.

Conway, E. M., and R. D. Rosenberg. 1988. Tumor necrosis factor suppresses transcription of the

Impact of Inflammation on Coagulation

Increased	Tissue Factor
	Membrane Procoagulant Lipid
	Platelet Reactivity
	Fibrinogen
Decreased	TM
	EPCR
	Shorter APC half-life (α_1-AT ⇑)
	Protein Z
	Vascular Heparin-like Molecules
	Fibrinolysis (PAI-1 ⇑)

FIGURE 3 Impact of inflammation on coagulation.

thrombomodulin gene in endothelial cells. *Mol. Cell. Biol.* **8:**5588–5592.

Conway, E. M., M. Van de Wouwer, S. Pollefeyt, K. Jurk, H. Van Aken, A. De Vriese, J. I. Weitz, H. Weiler, P. W. Hellings, P. Schaeffer, J. M. Herbert, D. Collen, and G. Theilmeier. 2002. The lectin-like domain of thrombomodulin confers protection from neutrophil-mediated tissue damage by suppressing adhesion molecule expression via nuclear factor κB and mitogen-activated protein kinase pathways. *J. Exp. Med.* **196:**565–577.

Coughlin, S. R. 1994. Thrombin receptor function and cardiovascular disease. *Trends Cardiovasc. Med.* **4:**77–83.

Coughlin, S. R. 2000. Thrombin signalling and protease-activated receptors. *Nature* **407:**258–264.

Dahlbäck, B. 1991. Protein S and C4b-binding protein: components involved in the regulation of the protein C anticoagulant system. *Thromb. Haemost.* **66:**49–61.

Dickneite, G. 1998. Antithrombin III in animal models of sepsis and organ failure. *Sem. Thromb. Hemost.* **24:**61–69.

Drake, T. A., J. H. Morrissey, and T. S. Edgington. 1989. Selective cellular expression of tissue factor in human tissues: implications for disorders of hemostasis and thrombosis. *Am. J. Pathol.* **134:**1087–1097.

Dreyfus, M., J. F. Magny, F. Bridey, H. P. Schwarz, C. Planché, M. Dehan, and G. Tchernia. 1991. Treatment of homozygous protein C deficiency and neonatal purpura fulminans with a purified protein C concentrate. *N. Engl. J. Med.* **325:**1565–1568.

Edgington, T. S., N. Mackman, K. Brand, and W. Ruf. 1991. The structural biology of expression and function of tissue factor. *Thromb. Haemost.* **66:**67–79.

Enkhbaatar, P., K. Okajima, K. Murakami, M. Uchiba, H. Okabe, K. Okabe, and Y. Yamaguchi. 2000. Recombinant tissue factor pathway inhibitor reduces lipopolysaccharide-induced pulmonary vascular injury by inhibiting leukocyte activation. *Am. J. Respir. Crit. Care Med.* **162:**1752–1759.

Esmon, C. T. 1993. Cell mediated events that control blood coagulation and vascular injury. *Annu. Rev. Cell Biol.* **9:**1–26.

Esmon, C. T. 2000. Introduction: are natural anticoagulants candidates for modulating the inflammatory response to endotoxin? *Blood* **95:**1113–1116.

Esmon, C. T. 2001. Protein C, protein S, and thrombomodulin, p. 335–353. *In* R. W. Colman, J. Hirsh, V. J. Marder, A. W. Clowes, and J. N. George (ed.), *Hemostasis and Thrombosis: Basic Principles and Clinical Practice.* Lippincott Williams & Wilkins, Philadelphia, Pa.

Esmon, C. T. 2002. New mechanisms for vascular control of inflammation mediated by natural anticoagulant proteins. *J. Exp. Med.* **196:**561–564.

Esmon, C. T., J. Xu, J. M. Gu, D. Qu, Z. Laszik, G. Ferrell, D. J. Stearns-Kurosawa, S. Kurosawa, F. B. Taylor, Jr., and N. L. Esmon. 1999. Endothelial protein C receptor. *Thromb. Haemost.* **82:**251–258.

Faust, S. N., M. Levin, O. B. Harrison, R. D. Goldin, M. S. Lockhart, S. Kondaveeti, Z. Laszik, C. T. Esmon, and R. S. Heyderman. 2001. Dysfunction of endothelial protein C activation in severe meningococcal sepsis. *N. Engl. J. Med.* **345:**408–416.

Fukudome, K., and C. T. Esmon. 1994. Identification, cloning and regulation of a novel endothelial cell protein C/activated protein C receptor. *J. Biol. Chem.* **269:**26486–26491.

Giles, A. R., K. G. Mann, and M. E. Nesheim. 1988. A combination of factor Xa and phosphatidylcholine-phosphatidylserine vesicles bypasses factor VIII *in vivo. Br. J. Haematol.* **69:**491–497.

Glaser, C. B., J. Morser, J. H. Clarke, E. Blasko, K. McLean, I. Kuhn, R.-J. Chang, J.-H. Lin, L. Vilander, W. H. Andrews, and D. R. Light. 1992. Oxidation of a specific methionine in thrombomodulin by activated neutrophil products blocks cofactor activity. *J. Clin. Invest.* **90:**2565–2573.

Grey, S., H. Hau, H. H. Salem, and W. W. Hancock. 1993. Selective effects of protein C on activation of human monocytes by lipopolysaccharide, interferon-gamma, or PMA: modulation of effects on CD11b and CD14 but not CD25 or CD54 induction. *Transplant. Proc.* **25:**2913–2914.

Gruber, A., and J. H. Griffin. 1992. Direct detection of activated protein C in blood from human subjects. *Blood* **79:**2340–2348.

Gu, J.-M., J. T. B. Crawley, G. Ferrell, F. Zhang, W. Li, N. L. Esmon, and C. T. Esmon. 2002. Disruption of the endothelial cell protein C receptor gene in mice causes placental thrombosis and early embryonic lethality. *J. Biol. Chem.* **277:**43335–43343.

Han, X., R. Fiehler, and G. J. Broze, Jr. 2000. Characterization of the protein Z-dependent protease inhibitor. *Blood* **96:**3049–3055.

Hancock, W. W., S. T. Grey, L. Hau, C. Akalin, M. H. Sayegh, and H. H. Salem. 1995. Binding of activated protein C to a specific receptor on human mononuclear phagocytes inhibits intracellular calcium signaling and monocyte-dependent proliferative responses. *Transplantation* **60:**1525–1532.

Heeb, M. J., A. Gruber, and J. H. Griffin. 1991. Identification of divalent metal ion-dependent inhibition of activated protein C by alpha$_2$-macroglobulin and alpha$_2$-antiplasmin in blood and comparisons to inhibition of factor Xa, thrombin, and plasmin. *J. Biol. Chem.* **266:**17606–17612.

Henn, V., J. R. Slupsky, M. Gräfe, I. Anagnostopoulos, R. Förster, G. Müller-Berghaus, and R. A. Kroczek. 1998. CD40 ligand on activated platelets triggers an inflammatory reaction of endothelial cells. *Nature* **391**:591–594.

Hong, S., D. C. Scherer, N. Singh, S. K. Mendiratta, I. Serizawa, Y. Koezuka, and L. Van Kaer. 1999. Lipid antigen presentation in the immune system learned from CD1d knockout mice. *Immunol. Rev.* **169**:31–44.

Huang, Z.-F., D. Higuchi, N. Lasky, and G. J. Broze, Jr. 1997. Tissue factor pathway inhibitor gene disruption produces intrauterine lethality in mice. *Blood* **90**:944–951.

Jackman, R. W., D. L. Beeler, L. Fritze, G. Soff, and R. D. Rosenberg. 1987. Human thrombomodulin gene is intron depleted: nucleic acid sequences of the cDNA and gene predict protein structure and suggest sites of regulatory control. *Proc. Natl. Acad. Sci. USA* **84**:6425–6429.

Joyce, D. E., L. Gelbert, A. Ciaccia, B. DeHoff, and B. W. Grinnell. 2001. Gene expression profile of antithrombotic protein C defines new mechanisms modulating inflammation and apoptosis. *J. Biol. Chem.* **276**:11199–11203.

Klein, N. J., C. A. Ison, M. Peakman, M. Levin, S. Hammerschmidt, M. Frosch, and R. S. Heyderman. 1996. The influence of capsulation and lipooligosaccharide structure on neutrophil adhesion molecule expression and endothelial injury by *Neisseria meningitidis. J. Infect. Dis.* **173**:172–179.

Kurosawa, S., C. T. Esmon, and D. J. Stearns-Kurosawa. 2000. The soluble endothelial protein C receptor binds to activated neutrophils: involvement of proteinase-3 and CDIIb/CDI8. *J. Immunol.* **165**:4697–4703.

Laszik, Z., A. Mitro, F. B. Taylor, Jr., G. Ferrell, and C. T. Esmon. 1997. Human protein C receptor is present primarily on endothelium of large blood vessels: implications for the control of the protein C pathway. *Circulation* **96**:3633–3640.

Levi, M., and H. ten Cate. 1999. Disseminated intravascular coagulation. *N. Engl. J. Med.* **341**:586–592.

Liaw, P. C. Y., P. F. Neuenschwander, M. D. Smirnov, and C. T. Esmon. 2000. Mechanisms by which soluble endothelial cell protein C receptor modulates protein C and activated protein C function. *J. Biol. Chem.* **275**:5447–5452.

Liaw, P. C. Y., G. L. Ferrell, and C. T. Esmon. 2002. A monoclonal antibody against activated protein C allows rapid detection of activated protein C in plasma and reveals a calcium ion dependent epitope involved in factor Va inactivation. *J. Thromb. Haemost.* **1**:662–670.

Lorant, D. E., K. D. Patel, T. M. McIntyre, R. P. McEver, S. M. Prescott, and G. A. Zimmerman. 1991. Coexpression of GMP-140 and PAF by endothelium stimulated by histamine or thrombin: a juxtacrine system for adhesion and activation of neutrophils. *J. Cell Biol.* **115**:223–234.

Lupu, C., F. Lupu, U. Dennehy, V. V. Kakkar, and M. F. Scully. 1995. Thrombin induces the redistribution and acute release of tissue factor pathway inhibitor from specific granules within human endothelial cells in culture. *Arterioscler. Thromb. Vasc. Biol.* **15**:2055–2062.

Miller, D. L., R. Yaron, and M. J. Yellin. 1998. CD40L-CD40 interactions regulate endothelial cell surface tissue factor and thrombomodulin expression. *J. Leukoc. Biol.* **63**:373–379.

Moody, D. B., T. Ulrichs, W. Mühlecker, D. C. Young, S. S. Gurcha, E. Grant, J.-P. Rosat, M. B. Brenner, C. E. Costello, G. S. Besra, and S. A. Porcelli. 2000. CD1c-mediated T-cell recognition of isoprenoid glycolipids in *Mycobacterium tuberculosis* infection. *Nature* **404**:884–888.

Morrissey, J. H., H. Fakhrai, and T. S. Edgington. 1987. Molecular cloning of the cDNA for tissue factor, the cellular receptor for the initiation of the coagulation protease cascade. *Cell* **50**:129–135.

Nesheim, M. E., W. M. Canfield, W. Kisiel, and K. G. Mann. 1982. Studies on the capacity of factor Xa to protect factor Va from inactivation by activated protein C. *J. Biol. Chem.* **257**:1443–1447.

Oelschläger, C., J. Römisch, A. Staubitz, H. Stauss, B. Leithäuser, H. Tillmanns, and H. Hölschermann. 2002. Antithrombin III inhibits nuclear factor κB activation in human monocytes and vascular endothelial cells. *Blood* **99**:4015–4020.

Oganesyan, V., N. Oganesyan, S. Terzyan, D. Qu, Z. Dauter, N. L. Esmon, and C. T. Esmon. 2002. The crystal structure of the endothelial protein C receptor and a bound phospholipid. *J. Biol. Chem.* **277**:24851–24854.

Opal, S. M., and C. T. Esmon. 2002. Bench-to-bedside review: functional relationships between coagulation and the innate immune response and their respective roles in the pathogenesis of sepsis. *Crit. Care* **7**:23–38.

Palabrica, T., R. Lobb, B. C. Furie, M. Aronovitz, C. Benjamin, Y. M. Hsu, S. A. Sajer, and B. Furie. 1992. Leukocyte accumulation promoting fibrin deposition is mediated in vivo by P-selectin on adherent platelets. *Nature* **359**:848–851.

Pendurthi, U. R., D. Alok, and L. V. M. Rao. 1997. Binding of factor VIIa to tissue factor induces alterations in gene expression in human fibroblast cells: upregulation of poly(A) polymerase. *Proc. Natl. Acad. Sci. USA* **94**:12598–12603.

Raczkowski, C. A., M. Reichlin, C. T. Esmon, and P. C. Comp. 1987. Protein Z is a negatively responding acute phase protein. *Blood* **70**:393a. (Abstract 1427.)

Regan, L. M., B. J. Lamphear, C. F. Huggins, F. J. Walker, and P. J. Fay. 1994. Factor IXa protects factor VIIIa from activated protein C. *J. Biol. Chem.* **269**:9445–9452.

Rezaie, A. R. 2001. Vitronectin functions as a cofactor for rapid inhibition of activated protein C by plasminogen activator inhibitor-1. Implications for the mechanism of profibrinolytic action of activated protein C. *J. Biol. Chem.* **276:**15567–15570.

Rezaie, A. R., S. T. Cooper, F. C. Church, and C. T. Esmon. 1995. Protein C inhibitor is a potent inhibitor of the thrombin-thrombomodulin complex. *J. Biol. Chem.* **270:**25336–25339.

Riewald, M., R. J. Petrovan, A. Donner, B. M. Mueller, and W. Ruf. 2002. Activation of endothelial cell protease activated receptor 1 by the protein C pathway. *Science* **296:**1880–1882.

Sadler, J. E. 1997. Thrombomodulin structure and function. *Thromb. Haemost.* **78:**392–395.

Shu, F., H. Kobayashi, K. Fukudome, N. Tsuneyoshi, M. Kimoto, and T. Terao. 2000. Activated protein C suppresses tissue factor expression on U937 cells in the endothelial protein C receptor-dependent manner. *FEBS Lett.* **477:**208–212.

Simmonds, R. E., and D. A. Lane. 1999. Structural and functional implications of the intron/exon organization of the human endothelial cell protein C/activated protein C receptor (EPCR) gene: comparison with the structure of CD1/major histocompatibility complex α_1 and α_2 domains. *Blood* **94:**632–641.

Sims, P. J., F. M. Faioni, T. Wiedmer, and S. J. Shattil. 1988. Complement proteins C5b-9 cause release of membrane vesicles from the platelet surface that are enriched in the membrane receptor for coagulation factor Va and express prothrombinase activity. *J. Biol. Chem.* **263:**18205–18212.

Souter, P. J., S. Thomas, A. R. Hubbard, S. Poole, J. Romisch, and E. Gray. 2001. Antithrombin inhibits lipopolysaccharide-induced tissue factor and interleukin-6 production by mononuclear cells, human umbilical vein endothelial cells, and whole blood. *Crit. Care Med.* **29:**134–139.

Stearns-Kurosawa, D. J., S. Kurosawa, J. S. Mollica, G. L. Ferrell, and C. T. Esmon. 1996. The endothelial cell protein C receptor augments protein C activation by the thrombin-thrombomodulin complex. *Proc. Natl. Acad. Sci. USA* **93:**10212–10216.

Takano, S., S. Kimura, S. Ohdama, and N. Aoki. 1990. Plasma thrombomodulin in health and diseases. *Blood* **76:**2024–2029.

Taoka, Y., K. Okajima, M. Uchiba, K. Murakami, N. Harada, M. Johno, and M. Naruo. 1998. Activated protein C reduces the severity of compression-induced spinal cord injury in rats by inhibiting activation of leukocytes. *J. Neurosci.* **18:**1393–1398.

Taylor, F. B., Jr., A. Chang, C. T. Esmon, A. D'Angelo, S. Vigano-D'Angelo, and K. E. Blick. 1987. Protein C prevents the coagulopathic and lethal effects of *E. coli* infusion in the baboon. *J. Clin. Invest.* **79:**918–925.

Taylor, F. B., Jr., A. C. K. Chang, G. T. Peer, T. Mather, K. Blick, R. Catlett, M. S. Lockhart, and C. T. Esmon. 1991. DEGR-factor Xa blocks disseminated intravascular coagulation initiated by *Escherichia coli* without preventing shock or organ damage. *Blood* **78:**364–368.

Taylor, F. B., Jr., S. E. He, A. C. K. Chang, J. Box, G. Ferrell, D. Lee, M. Lockhart, G. Peer, and C. T. Esmon. 1996. Infusion of phospholipid vesicles amplifies the local thrombotic response to TNF and anti-protein C into a consumptive response. *Thromb. Haemost.* **75:**578–584.

Taylor, F. B., Jr., D. J. Stearns-Kurosawa, S. Kurosawa, G. Ferrell, A. C. K. Chang, Z. Laszik, S. Kosanke, G. Peer, and C. T. Esmon. 2000. The endothelial cell protein C receptor aids in host defense against *Escherichia coli* sepsis. *Blood* **95:**1680–1686.

Uchiba, M., and K. Okajima. 1997. Antithrombin III (AT III) prevents LPS-induced vascular injury: novel biological activity of AT III. *Thromb. Haemost.* **23:**583–590.

Vasse, M., E. Guegan-Massardier, J.-Y. Borg, F. Woimant, and C. Soria. 2001. Frequency of protein Z deficiency in patients with ischaemic stroke. *Lancet* **357:**933–934.

Wakefield, T. W., R. M. Strieter, R. Schaub, D. D. Myers, M. R. Prince, S. K. Wrobleski, F. J. Londy, A. M. Kadell, S. L. Brown, P. K. Henke, and L. J. Greenfield. 2000. Venous thrombosis prophylaxis by inflammatory inhibition without anticoagulation therapy. *J. Vasc. Surg.* **31:**309–324.

Walsh, P. N. 1987. Platelet-mediated trigger mechanisms in the contact phase of blood coagulation. *Sem. Thromb. Hemost.* **13:**86–94.

Waugh, J. M., E. Yuksel, J. Li, M. D. Kuo, M. Kattash, R. Saxena, R. Geske, S. N. Thung, S. M. Shenaq, and S. L. Woo. 1999. Local overexpression of thrombomodulin for in vivo prevention of arterial thrombosis in a rabbit model. *Circ. Res.* **84:**84–92.

Waugh, J. M., J. Li-Hawkins, E. Yuksel, M. D. Kuo, P. N. Cifra, P. R. Hilfiker, R. Geske, M. Chawla, J. Thomas, S. M. Shenaq, M. D. Dake, and S. L. Woo. 2000. Thrombomodulin overexpression to limit neointima formation. *Circulation* **102:**332–337.

Wen, D., W. A. Dittman, R. D. Ye, L. L. Deaven, P. W. Majerus, and J. E. Sadler. 1987. Human thrombomodulin: complete cDNA sequence and chromosome localization of the gene. *Biochemistry* **26:**4350–4357.

White, B., M. Schmidt, C. Murphy, W. Livingstone, D. O'Toole, M. Lawler, L. O'Neill, D. Kelleher, H. P. Schwarz, and O. P. Smith. 2000. Activated protein C inhibits lipopolysaccharide-induced nuclear translocation of nuclear factor kappaB (NF-kappaB) and tumour necrosis factor alpha

(TNF-alpha) production in the THP-1 monocytic cell line. *Br. J. Haematol.* **110:**130–134.

Wolbink, G.-J., A. W. J. Bossink, A. B. J. Groeneveld, M. C. M. DeGroot, L. G. Thijs, and C. E. Hack. 1998. Complement activation in patients with sepsis is in part mediated by C-reactive protein. *J. Infect. Dis.* **177:**81–87.

Xu, J., D. Qu, N. L. Esmon, and C. T. Esmon. 1999. Metalloproteolytic release of endothelial cell protein C receptor. *J. Biol. Chem.* **275:**6038–6044.

Yamauchi, T., F. Umeda, T. Inoguchi, and H. Nawata. 1989. Antithrombin III stimulates prostacy-clin production by cultured aortic endothelial cells. *Biochem. Biophys. Res. Commun.* **163:**1404–1411.

Yin, Z.-F., Z.-F. Huang, J. Cui, R. Fiehler, N. Lasky, and D. Ginsburg. 2000. Prothrombotic phenotype of protein Z deficiency. *Proc. Natl. Acad. Sci. USA* **97:**6734–6738.

Yuksel, M., K. Okajima, M. Uchiba, S. Horiuchi, and H. Okabe. 2002. Activated protein C inhibits lipopolysaccharide-induced tumor necrosis factor-α production by inhibiting activation of both nuclear factor-κB and activator protein-1 in human monocytes. *Thromb. Haemost.* **88:**267–273.

RECEPTORS

TOLL-LIKE RECEPTORS: LIGANDS AND SIGNALING

Kiyoshi Takeda and Shizuo Akira

13

Innate immunity has recently been revealed to have a skillful system that detects microbial invasion by virtue of Toll-like receptors (TLRs). TLRs comprise a large family consisting of at least 10 members. Genetic studies have established that each TLR recognizes specific components of pathogens. The signaling pathway via TLRs originates from the conserved cytoplasmic Toll/interleukin-1 (IL-1) receptor (TIR) domain. The TIR domain-containing adaptor myeloid differentiation marker 88 (MyD88) is common to TLR-mediated signaling, which leads to the production of inflammatory cytokines. However, individual TLRs seem to have their own signaling cascades. In this chapter we focus on recent advances in our understanding of the function of TLRs, particularly with regard to their ligands and signaling.

TLRs DETECT MICROBIAL INVASION

Host defense is believed to be triggered by the detection of microbial invasion into the host. However, the receptors that detect pathogens remained unclear for a long time. Genetic studies in *Drosophila* indicated that Toll was a receptor that detected pathogens (Lemaitre et al., 1996). One year later, a mammalian Toll receptor (now termed TLR4) was shown to induce the expression of genes involved in inflammatory responses (Medzhitov et al., 1997). Subsequent studies revealed that there were several Toll receptors in mammals, and they were designated TLRs. TLRs bear leucine-rich repeats (LRRs) in the extracellular portion and the TIR domain in the cytoplasmic portion. The TIR domain of TLRs shows high similarity with the cytoplasmic region of the IL-1 receptor family and further similarity with several cytoplasmic adaptors, including MyD88 and the TIR adaptor protein (TIRAP). TLRs in mammals have been shown to recognize microbial components that are not present in mammals but are conserved between pathogens, and thereby to detect the invasion of microorganisms such as bacteria, fungi, protozoa, and viruses. So far, the roles of eight members of the TLR family have been established (Fig. 1).

TLRs in Bacterial Recognition

Lipopolysaccharide (LPS) is a major component of the outer membrane of gram-negative bacteria and a potent activator of innate immune cells, including macrophages and dendritic cells (DCs). Therefore, the identifica-

Kiyoshi Takeda and Shizuo Akira, Department of Host Defense, Research Institute for Microbial Diseases, Osaka University, and SORST of Japan Science and Technology Corporation, 3-1 Yamada-oka, Suita, Osaka 565-0871, Japan.

The Innate Immune Response to Infection
Ed. by S. H. E. Kaufmann, R. Medzhitov, and S. Gordon
©2004 ASM Press, Washington, D.C.

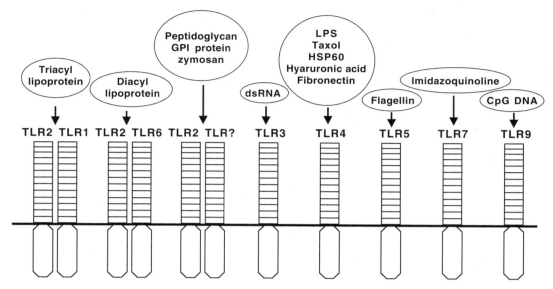

FIGURE 1 TLRs and their ligands. TLR2 is essential in the recognition of microbial lipopeptides. TLR1 and TLR6 cooperate with TLR2 to discriminate subtle differences between triacyl and diacyl lipopeptides, respectively. TLR4 is the receptor for LPS. TLR9 is essential in CpG DNA recognition, whereas TLR3 is implicated in the recognition of viral dsRNA. TLR5 recognizes flagellin. Thus, the TLR family members recognize specific patterns of bacterial components.

tion of a LPS signaling receptor has long been anticipated. It is well known that two mouse strains, C3H/HeJ and C57BL/10ScCr, are hyporesponsive to LPS and sensitive to gram-negative bacterial infection. In 1998, Beutler and colleagues identified the gene responsible for the hyporesponsiveness to LPS and found mutations in *Tlr4* in these strains (Poltorak et al., 1998). Another group also found mutations in the *Tlr4* gene in these strains (Qureshi et al., 1999). The C3H/HeJ mouse strain has a point mutation in the cytoplasmic region of the *Tlr4* gene that results in an amino acid change from proline to histidine. This mutation has been shown to result in defective TLR4-mediated signaling and to have a dominant negative effect on LPS responses (Hoshino et al., 1999). The other LPS-hyporesponsive strain, C57BL/10ScCr, has a null mutation in the *Tlr4* gene (Poltorak et al., 1998; Qureshi et al., 1999). The generation of TLR4 knockout mice further revealed the essential role of

TLR4 in LPS recognition (Hoshino et al., 1999).

TLR2 has been shown to recognize peptidoglycan, which is abundantly present in the cell walls of gram-positive bacteria (Schwandner et al., 1999; Takeuchi et al., 1999; Yoshimura et al., 1999). In addition, TLR2 recognizes lipoteichoic acids from gram-positive bacteria (Schwandner et al., 1999; Lehner et al., 2001). Accordingly, TLR2-deficient mice are highly sensitive to infection by the gram-positive bacterium *Staphylococcus aureus* (Takeuchi et al., 2000a). TLR2 is involved in the recognition of several additional bacterial components, such as lipoproteins and lipopeptides from a variety of bacteria (Takeuchi et al., 2000b), lipoarabinomannan from mycobacteria (Underhill et al., 1999a; Means et al., 1999a, 1999b), a phenol-soluble modulin from *Staphylococcus epidermidis* (Hajjar et al., 2001), glycolipids from *Treponema maltophilum* spirochetes (Opitz et al., 2001), and porins present in the outer membrane of *Neisseria* spp. (Massari et al., 2002). The mechanism by which TLR2 recognizes a variety of bacterial components is now partly explained by the fact that TLR2 associates with other TLRs, particularly TLR1 and TLR6. TLR2 ligands, such as peptidoglycan and secreted modulin from *S. epidermidis,* induced tumor necrosis factor alpha (TNF-α) production in RAW264.7 cells, which was inhibited by the expression of the dominant negative form of TLR6 (Hajjar et al., 2001; Ozinsky et al., 2000). Macrophages from TLR2-deficient mice show no inflammatory response to all the kinds of lipoproteins and lipopeptides analyzed to date. Macrophages from TLR6-deficient mice did not show any TNF-α production in response to diacyl lipopeptides from *Mycoplasma* spp., but showed a normal response to triacyl lipopeptides (Takeuchi et al., 2001). In contrast, TLR1-deficient mice were impaired in TNF-α production induced by triacyl lipopeptides, but not that induced by diacyl lipopeptides (Takeuchi et al., 2002). Thus, TLR1 and TLR6 cooperate functionally with TLR2 and participate in the discrimination of subtle structural differences among lipopeptides. TLR1 is also involved in the recognition of lipoprotein from *Mycobacterium* spp. and *Borrelia burgdorferi* (Takeuchi et al., 2002; Alexopoulou et al., 2002).

In addition to TLR2 and TLR4, several TLRs are involved in the recognition of bacterial components such as flagellin and CpG DNA. Flagellin is a protein component of the flagellum, which extends out from the outer membrane of gram-negative bacteria. Flagellin has been shown to activate immune cells via TLR5 (Hayashi et al., 2001). CpG DNA is characteristic of the genomic DNA of bacteria, in which unmethylated CpG motifs are present in the expected frequency. In the mammalian genome, CpG motifs are suppressed in frequency and are highly methylated, which causes no immunostimulatory activity. Generation of TLR9-deficient mice revealed its essential role in the recognition of CpG DNA (Hemmi et al., 2000).

TLRs in Fungal and Protozoan Recognition

TLRs recognize components of not only bacteria but also fungi and protozoa. Zymosan is a crude mixture of glucans, mannan, proteins, chitin, and glycolipids extracted from the cell walls of fungi, which activates immune cells. Zymosan has been shown to be recognized by TLR2 (Underhill et al., 1999b). The immunostimulating activity of zymosan is seemingly attributed to the presence of β glucan (Kataoka et al., 2002). Infection with the protozoan parasite *Trypanosoma cruzi* causes Chagas' disease in humans. Glycosylphosphatidylinositol (GPI) anchors that are present in the membrane of *T. cruzi* have been shown to activate the innate immune cells via TLR2 (Campos et al., 2001; Ropert et al., 2002).

TLRs in Viral Recognition

Accumulating evidence indicates that TLRs are involved in the recognition of viral invasion. TLR4 and CD14 have been shown to recognize the fusion protein of respiratory syncytial virus (Kurt-Jones et al., 2000). TLR4-mutated C3H/HeJ and C57BL/10ScCr mice were impaired in the inflammatory response to respiratory syncytial virus infection and accordingly impaired in virus clearance (Haynes et al., 2001). Mouse mammary tumor virus has been shown to activate B cells through association of that virus's envelope glycoprotein and TLR4 (Rassa et al., 2002).

Double-stranded RNA (dsRNA) is produced by many viruses during their replicative cycle and is representative of the viral components that activate immune cells mainly by inducing type I interferons (alpha/beta interferons [IFN-α/β]) and some of the IFN-inducible genes. Synthetic dsRNA, such as poly(I:C), has activity similar to that of dsRNA. TLR3-deficient mice were impaired in the response to dsRNA and poly(I:C) (Alexopoulou et al., 2001). In addition, expression of human TLR3 in the dsRNA-nonresponsive cell line 293 enabled the cells to activate NF-κB and the

IFN-β promoter in response to dsRNA and poly(I:C) (Alexopoulou et al., 2001; Matsumoto et al., 2002). These findings indicate that both TLR3 and TLR4 are involved in viral recognition.

Synthetic compounds, imidazoquinolines, exhibit potent antiviral and antitumor properties by inducing inflammatory cytokines, especially IFN-α. One of the imidazoquinoline compounds, Imiquimod, has been approved for the treatment of genital warts caused by infection with human papillomavirus. TLR7-deficient mice did not show any response to the imidazoquinolines (Hemmi et al., 2002). Therefore, TLR7 may also be involved in viral recognition. Identification of a natural ligand for TLR7 will reveal the precise role of TLRs in viral recognition.

TLRs in the Recognition of Endogenous Ligands

As described above, TLRs play a critical role in the detection of microbial invasion by recognizing specific components of pathogens. However, several reports indicate that some TLRs, particularly TLR4, are involved in the recognition of endogenous ligands regardless of infection. Heat shock proteins (HSPs) are highly conserved between bacteria and mammals. Several stressful conditions such as heat shock, radiation, and infection induce the synthesis of HSPs, which act to chaperone nascent or aberrantly folded proteins. HSPs, especially HSP60 and HSP70, activate innate immune cells such as macrophages and DCs. The immunostimulatory activity of HSP60 has been shown to be induced by TLR4 (Ohashi et al., 2000; Vabulas et al., 2001). TLR4 mutant mice were impaired in the production of inflammatory cytokines in response to HSP70 as well as HSP60 (Dybdahl et al., 2002; Vabulas et al., 2002; Asea et al., 2002). Thus, TLR4 seems to be responsible for the inflammatory responses elicited by HSPs. In addition to TLR4, TLR2 has also been shown to be required for the recognition of HSP70 (Vabulas et al., 2002; Asea et al., 2002).

Extracellular matrix components, including fibronectin, hyaluronic acid, and heparan sulfate, are produced when tissue is injured and play important roles in wound healing. The type III repeat extra domain A of fibronectin has been shown to activate immune cells through recognition by TLR4 (Okamura et al., 2001). Low-molecular-weight oligosaccharides of hyaluronic acid have been shown to be potent activators of DCs, which are mediated by TLR4 (Termeer et al., 2002). Polysaccharide fragments of heparan sulfate have been reported to induce the maturation of DCs via TLR4 (Johnson et al., 2002). Inflammatory responses to injury, immune disorders, and infection often accompany extravascular deposits of fibrin, which is generated from plasma-derived fibrinogen. Fibrinogen has also been shown to induce the production of chemokines from macrophages through recognition by TLR4 (Smiley et al., 2001). Thus, TLR4 is presumably involved in several inflammatory responses by recognizing endogenous ligands even in the absence of infection. However, all of the endogenous TLR4 ligands activate immune cells only when stimulated at very high concentrations. In addition, the ability of HSP70 to activate macrophages has recently been shown to be attributable to contaminating LPS in the HSP70 preparation (Gao and Tsan, 2003). LPS is the most powerful immunostimulator among microbial components, and the contamination will result in TLR4-dependent immune activation. Therefore, more careful experiments are required before we can conclude that TLR4 recognizes these endogenous ligands.

Molecules that Cooperate with TLRs

Although TLRs have been established to recognize specific patterns of microbial components, several additional molecules associate with some TLRs, particularly TLR4, to detect LPS. These include the LPS-binding protein (LBP), CD14, RP105, and MD-1 and -2 (Fig. 2).

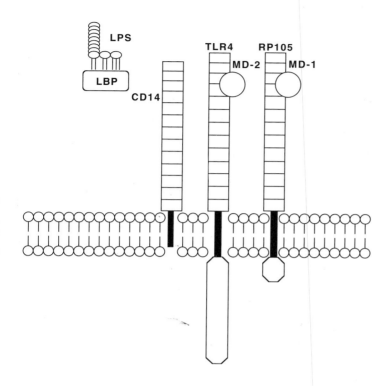

FIGURE 2 The LPS receptor complex. The LPS receptor comprises several components. TLR4 is an essential receptor component for the signal transduction via the LPS receptor complex. MD-2 associates with the extracellular portion of TLR4 and is involved in the LPS recognition. LBP is a soluble molecule that binds to the lipid A portion of LPS. The LPS–LBP complex binds to CD14 and then this complex associates with TLR4. In B cells, additional components, RP105 and MD-1, are involved in the LPS recognition.

LBP and CD14.   LBP, which was identified as a plasma protein that binds to the lipid A moiety of LPS, is a member of a family of lipid-binding proteins that act as lipid transport proteins in some cases (Tobias et al., 1986; Schumann et al., 1990). The generation of LBP-deficient mice has revealed a nonredundant role for LBP in the response to LPS (Jack et al., 1997; Wurfel et al., 1997).

The formation of LPS and LBP complexes triggers the association of this complex with another LPS-binding molecule, CD14. CD14 is a GPI-anchored protein, which is preferentially expressed on the surface of mature myeloid cells. Soluble forms of CD14 are also produced through escape from the GPI anchoring and proteolytic cleavage of the membrane-bound CD14. The importance of CD14 in the response to LPS has been demonstrated in CD14-deficient mice, which showed a reduced response to LPS (Haziot et al., 1996; Moore et al., 2000). Thus, LPS first

binds LBP, and then this complex is transferred to CD14. CD14 has no cytoplasmic region that would be required for cellular activation. Therefore, the LPS–LBP–CD14 complex requires an additional receptor that transduces the signal from the membrane into the cytoplasm, and it is TLR4 that is responsible for this signal transduction via the LPS–LBP–CD14 complex. Indeed, physical association between CD14 and TLR4 in response to LPS stimulation has been demonstrated (Jiang et al., 2000; Da Shilva Correia et al., 2001).

RP105 and MD-1.   RP105 bears an extracellular LRR domain that is structurally similar to those found in TLRs. However, unlike TLRs, RP105 has only a short cytoplasmic tail and is preferentially expressed on B cells (Miyake et al., 1995). RP105-deficient mice showed a severely impaired response to LPS in B cells, indicating that RP105 is an essential component in the recognition of LPS in B cells (Ogata et al., 2000). Miyake and colleagues (1998) also identified MD-1 as a molecule that associates with the extracellular portion of RP105. Similarly to RP105-deficient mice, MD-1-deficient mice showed impairment in LPS-induced B-cell proliferation, antibody production, and CD86 upregulation (Nagai et al., 2002). Furthermore, surface expression of RP105 was abolished in MD-1-deficient B cells, indicating that MD-1 is essential for the responsiveness to LPS and surface expression of RP105 in B cells. It remains unclear whether RP105/MD-1 is involved in the LPS recognition in other cells that express RP105/MD-1, such as DCs and macrophages.

MD-2.   Miyake and colleagues further identified MD-2, which is structurally related to MD-1 (Shimazu et al., 1999). Expression of both MD-2 and TLR4, but not TLR4 alone, conferred LPS-induced NF-κB activation in LPS-nonresponsive Ba/F3 cells, indicating that MD-2 associates functionally with TLR4. Physical association of MD-2 and TLR4 on mouse peritoneal macrophages was also shown using a monoclonal antibody against the TLR4/MD-2 complex (Akashi et al., 2000; Nomura et al., 2000). The importance of MD-2 in the LPS responsiveness was further demonstrated in genetic studies. Chinese hamster ovary cell lines that showed an impaired response to LPS have been shown to be mutated in the *MD-2* gene (Schromm et al., 2001). MD-2-deficient mice displayed severely impaired responses to LPS, and the phenotype was very similar to that of TLR4-deficient mice (Nagai et al., 2002). Analysis of the MD-2-deficient mice further demonstrated that the surface expression of TLR4 was abolished in these mice, indicating that MD-2 is required for the surface expression of TLR4 (Nagai et al., 2002).

Thus, several molecules which associate functionally with TLR4 have been identified. However, no molecules have been reported to associate with the other TLRs. It is very intriguing how TLRs, which have the conserved LRR domains in the extracellular portion, recognize quite distinct types of microbial components such as the lipid moiety, peptides, and nucleic acids. In this regard, we can hypothesize that, although molecules that associate with individual TLRs have not yet been reported, they might exist and directly recognize the microbial components. Indeed, there is a report that indicates that MD-2 directly regulates the species-specific recognition of the lipid moiety by TLR4 (Akashi et al., 2001).

SIGNALING PATHWAYS VIA TLRs

The signaling pathways via TLRs originate from the TIR domain. MyD88 harboring the TIR domain in the carboxy-terminal portion associates with the TIR domain of TLRs. Upon stimulation by TLR ligands, MyD88 recruits a family of IL-1 receptor-associated kinases (IRAKs) to TLRs. IRAKs then activate tumor receptor-associated factor 6 (TRAF6), thereby inducing activation of mitogen-activated protein (MAP) kinases and NF-κB (Fig. 3). Important roles for each molecule have been elucidated through the generation of gene-targeted mice.

MyD88 is a Common Adaptor in TLR Signaling

MyD88-deficient mice showed impaired responses to the IL-1 family of cytokines, whose receptors have the cytoplasmic TIR domain (Adachi et al., 1998). Subsequent studies of MyD88-deficient mice demonstrated that these mice did not produce any inflammatory cytokines in response to LPS, peptidoglycan, lipoproteins, CpG DNA, flagellin, dsRNA, or the imidazoquinolines (Kawai et al., 1999; Takeuchi et al., 2000b, 2000c; Hayashi et al., 2001; Alexopoulou et al., 2001; Hemmi et al., 2002; Hacker et al., 2000; Schnare et al., 2000). These findings indicate that MyD88 is an essential adaptor in the signaling pathways activated via all the TLR family members that lead to the production of inflammatory cytokines. Indeed, macrophages from MyD88-deficient mice showed no activation of NF-κB or JNK in response to

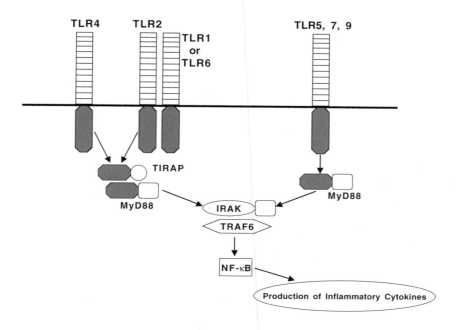

FIGURE 3 MyD88-dependent signaling pathway. A TIR domain–containing adaptor molecule, MyD88, associates with the cytoplasmic TIR domain of TLRs and recruits IRAKs to the receptor upon receptor activation. IRAKs then activate TRAF6, leading to the activation of MAP kinases and NF-κB. TIRAP, a second TIR domain–containing adaptor, is involved in the MyD88-dependent signaling pathway via TLR2 and TLR4.

peptidoglycan, lipoprotein, CpG DNA, or the imidazoquinolines.

TRAF6-deficient mice also exhibited impaired responses to both IL-1 and LPS, indicating that TRAF6 is also a critical component of both the IL-1 receptor- and the TLR4-mediated signaling pathways (Lomaga et al., 1999; Naito et al., 1999). The IRAK family has four members: IRAK-1, IRAK-2, IRAK-M, and IRAK-4 (Li et al., 2002). Physiological roles for these family members have been elucidated, except for IRAK-2. IRAK-1-deficient mice were partially impaired in their responses to IL-1 and LPS (Kanakaraj et al., 1998; Thomas et al., 1999; Swantek et al., 2000). IRAK-4-deficient mice showed almost no response to IL-1 and TLR ligands (Suzuki et al., 2002). IRAK-4 associates with IRAK-1 in response to IL-1 stimulation, and the introduction of the dominant negative form of IRAK-4 resulted in impaired IRAK-1 activa-

tion in response to IL-1. Thus, IRAK-4 presumably acts as a central mediator in the IL-1 receptor and TLR signaling, upstream of IRAK-1 (Li et al., 2002).

Additional molecules that are involved in the TLR signaling have been reported. Receptor interacting protein-2 (RIP2), harboring a carboxy-terminal CARD domain, was originally identified as a serine/threonine kinase that associates with TRAF family members and with TNF receptor family members, such as the type I TNF receptor and CD40, and induces NF-κB activation and apoptosis (McCarthy et al., 1998; Inohara et al., 1998). RIP2-deficient mice were partially impaired in their response to LPS, peptidoglycan, and dsRNA, indicating that RIP2 is involved in the TLR signaling pathways (Kobayashi et al., 2002; Chin et al., 2002). It remains to be elucidated how RIP2 is connected to the TLR signaling. Toll-interacting protein (Tollip) has been identified as a molecule present in a complex with IRAK (Burns et al., 2000). Upon stimulation with IL-1, the Tollip–IRAK complex is recruited to the IL-1R complex by the association of Tollip with IL-1RAcP. IRAK is then activated by phosphorylation, which in turn leads to dissociation of IRAK from Tollip. Tollip is seemingly involved in the negative regulation of the TLR signaling pathway because overexpression of Tollip blocked activation of NF-κB in response to TLR2 and TLR4 ligands (Bulut et al., 2002; Zhang and Ghosh, 2002). However, the physiological roles of Tollip remain to be elucidated through the generation of gene-targeted mice.

Signaling Pathways That Are Independent of MyD88

MyD88 is essential for the production of inflammatory cytokines in response to all the TLR ligands, as described above. However, unlike the case for stimulation with other TLR ligands, LPS stimulation resulted in the activation of NF-κB and JNK in MyD88-deficient macrophages, although the kinetics were delayed compared to wild-type macrophages (Kawai et al., 1999). This finding indicates that the LPS-induced inflammatory cytokine production is completely mediated by the MyD88-dependent signaling pathway, but that a pathway exists that is independent of MyD88 in the LPS response (see Fig. 4). Indeed, some LPS responses were observed in MyD88-deficient mice. DCs from MyD88-deficient, but not from TLR4-deficient, mice matured in response to LPS (Kaisho et al., 2001). Kupffer cells from MyD88-deficient mice showed caspase-1-dependent cleavage of the IL-18 precursor into the mature form after LPS stimulation (Seki et al., 2001). MyD88-deficient macrophages showed LPS-induced expression of several genes, such as those

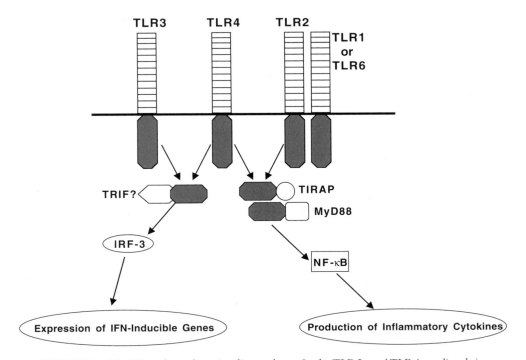

FIGURE 4 MyD88-independent signaling pathway. In the TLR3- and TLR4-mediated signaling pathways, LPS-induced activation of IRF-3 is observed in MyD88-deficient mice, indicating the presence of a MyD88-independent pathway. It remains unclear how IRF-3 is activated. Recently, a TIR domain-containing adaptor, TRIF, was found to associate with IRF-3 and TLR3, indicating a possible role for TRIF in the MyD88-independent pathway.

encoding IP-10 and GARG16, all of which are known as IFN-inducible genes (Kawai et al., 2001). In addition, MyD88-deficient macrophages showed NF-κB activation in response to dsRNA, as is the case in LPS stimulation (Alexopoulou et al., 2001). Thus, TLR4 and TLR3 utilize the MyD88-independent pathway, although it remains unclear whether the pathways activated by TLR4 and TLR3 are equivalent.

Stimulation with dsRNA or viral infection results in the activation of interferon regulatory factor 3 (IRF-3), a member of the IRF family of transcription factors, and thereby induces IFN-α/β and the IFN-inducible genes (Weaver et al., 1998; Yoneyama et al., 1998). IRF-3-deficient mice were impaired in the viral infection-induced expression of IFN-α/β, demonstrating the essential role of IRF-3 in virus-induced IFN-α/β expression (Sato et al., 2000). LPS has also been shown to activate IRF-3 (Kawai et al., 2001; Navarro and David, 1999). Thus, IRF-3 is activated in the TLR3 and TLR4 signaling pathways. Furthermore, LPS stimulation induced the activation of IRF-3 in MyD88-deficient mice, indicating that IRF-3 activation occurs in a MyD88-independent manner (Kawai et al., 2001). Subsequent studies demonstrated that LPS-induced activation of IRF-3 induced the MyD88-independent expression of IFN-β and then IFN-β induced Stat1-dependent expression of the IFN-inducible genes in macrophages and DCs (Toshchakov et al., 2002; Hoshino et al., 2002; Doyle et al., 2002). Thus, IRF-3 presumably plays an important role in the MyD88-independent pathway of TLR3 and TLR4 signaling. Analysis of the role of IRF-3 in the TLR signaling pathways would be of great interest.

IFN-α has been shown to be induced in response to the activation of TLR7 as well as TLR4 (Ito et al., 2002; Hemmi et al., 2002). However, unlike TLR4, TLR7-dependent induction of IFN-α was not observed in MyD88-deficient mice (Hemmi et al., 2002). In addition, a certain type of CpG DNA that activates TLR9 also induced IFN-α in plasmacytoid DCs (Krug et al., 2001). TLR7 and TLR9 are structurally related and presumably utilize a similar signaling cascade, thereby leading to similar biological outcomes. Therefore, we presume that an unknown signaling cascade that is dependent on MyD88 induces IFN-α in the TLR7- and TLR9-mediated signaling pathways.

TIR Domain-Containing Adaptors

In attempts to characterize the MyD88-independent signaling pathway, a second adaptor molecule containing the TIR domain was identified and designated TIRAP or MyD88-adaptor-like (Horng et al., 2001; Fitzgerald et al., 2001). The initial in vitro studies suggested that TIRAP specifically associates with TLR4 and acts as an adaptor in the MyD88-independent signaling pathway. However, TIRAP-deficient mice have recently been generated, and analysis of these mice has revealed an unexpected role for TIRAP in the TLR signaling (Yamamoto et al., 2002; Horng et al., 2002). TIRAP-deficient mice showed no production of inflammatory cytokines in response to the TLR4 ligand. However, TIRAP-deficient macrophages showed delayed activation of NF-κB and MAP kinases in response to LPS, as is the case in MyD88-deficient macrophages. Furthermore, TIRAP-deficient mice were not impaired in the LPS-induced expression of IFN-inducible genes and maturation of DCs. Even in TIRAP/MyD88 double-deficient mice, these LPS responses were normal. These findings indicate that TIRAP is essential for the TLR4-mediated MyD88-dependent, but not for the MyD88-independent, signaling pathway. In addition, although TIRAP-deficient mice showed normal responses to the TLR3, TLR7, and TLR9 ligands, they were defective in their response to the TLR2 ligands. Thus, TIRAP has been demonstrated to be essential for the MyD88-dependent signaling pathway via TLR2 and TLR4, but not for the MyD88-independent signaling. These studies further indicate that the TIR domain-containing molecules provide the specificity for individual TLR-mediated signaling pathways.

The phenotype of the TIRAP-deficient mice encouraged us to search for new TIR domain-containing adaptors, and led to the identification of a third TIR domain-containing adaptor (Yamamoto et al., 2002). Overexpression of this molecule, as well as MyD88 and TIRAP, resulted in activation of the NF-κB reporter gene in 293 cells. Furthermore, its overexpression led to the activation of the IFN-β promoter, which was not observed when MyD88 or TIRAP was overexpressed. Therefore, this molecule was named TRIF for TIR domain-containing adaptor inducing IFN-β. The dominant negative form of TRIF inhibited TLR3-dependent activation of the IFN-β promoter. Association between TRIF and IRF-3 was also shown. These findings indicate that TRIF may act in the MyD88-independent pathway leading to the induction of IFN-β. Analysis of TRIF-deficient mice will reveal its precise role in TLR signaling in the near future.

CONCLUDING REMARKS

We are now aware that innate immunity detects microbial invasion through the recognition of specific patterns of microbial components by TLRs. However, it is still elusive how TLRs recognize them. In the signaling pathways via TLRs, MyD88 is a common adaptor leading to the induction of inflammatory cytokines. However, additional adaptors, such as TIRAP and TRIF, exist that are expected to specify the TLR signaling pathway. Elucidation of the signaling pathway that is specific to each TLR will provide us with an important clue to understanding the molecular mechanisms by which innate immunity is activated and finally lead to the development of antigen-specific adaptive immunity.

ACKNOWLEDGMENTS

We thank E. Horita for excellent secretarial assistance. This work was supported by grants from the Special Coordination Funds of the Ministry of Education, Culture, Sports, Science and Technology and the Japan Research Foundation for Clinical Pharmacology.

REFERENCES

Adachi, O., T. Kawai, K. Takeda, M. Matsumoto, H. Tsutsui, M. Sakagami, K. Nakanishi, and S. Akira. 1998. Targeted disruption of the MyD88 gene results in loss of IL-1- and IL-18-mediated function. *Immunity* **9:**143–150.

Akashi, S., R. Shimazu, H. Ogata, Y. Nagai, K. Takeda, M. Kimoto, and K. Miyake. 2000. Cutting edge: cell surface expression and lipopolysaccharide signaling via the Toll-like receptor 4–MD-2 complex on mouse peritoneal macrophages. *J. Immunol.* **164:** 3471–3475.

Akashi, S., Y. Nagai, H. Ogata, M. Oikawa, K. Fukase, S. Kusumoto, K. Kawasaki, M. Nishijima, S. Hayashi, M. Kimoto, and K. Miyake. 2001. Human MD-2 confers on mouse Toll-like receptor 4 species-specific lipopolysaccharide recognition. *Int. Immunol.* **13:**1595–1599.

Alexopoulou, L., A. C. Holt, R. Medzhitov, and R. A. Flavell. 2001. Recognition of double-stranded RNA and activation of NF-κB by Toll-like receptor 3. *Nature* **413:**732–738.

Alexopoulou, L., V. Thomas, M. Schnare, Y. Lobet, J. Anguita, R. T. Schoen, R. Medzhitov, E. Fikrig, and R. A. Flavell. 2002. Hyporesponsiveness to vaccination with *Borrelia burgdorferi* OspA in humans and in TLR1- and TLR2-deficient mice. *Nat. Med.* **8:**878–884.

Asea, A., M. Rehli, E. Kabingu, J. A. Boch, O. Bare, P. E. Auron, M. A. Stevenson, and S. K. Calderwood. 2002. Novel signal transduction pathway utilized by extracellular HSP70: role of TLR2 and TLR4. *J. Biol. Chem.* **277:**15028–15034.

Bulut, Y., E. Faure, L. Thomas, O. Equils, and M. Arditi. 2002. Cooperation of Toll-like receptor 2 and 6 for cellular activation by soluble tuberculosis factor and *Borrelia burgdorferi* outer surface protein A lipoprotein: role of Toll-interacting protein and IL-1 receptor signaling molecules in Toll-like receptor 2 signaling. *J. Immunol.* **167:**987–994.

Burns, K., J. Clatworthy, L. Martin, F. Martinon, C. Plumpton, B. Maschera, A. Lewis, K. Ray, J. Tschopp, and F. Volpe. 2000. Tollip, a new component of the IL-1RI pathway, links IRAK to the IL-1 receptor. *Nat. Cell Biol.* **2:**346–351.

Campos, M. A., I. C. Almeida, O. Takeuchi, S. Akira, E. P. Valente, D. O. Procopio, L. R. Travassos, J. A. Smith, D. T. Golenbock, and R. T. Gazzinelli. 2001. Activation of Toll-like receptor-2 by glycosylphosphatidylinositol anchors from a protozoan parasite. *J. Immunol.* **167:**416–423.

Chin, A. I., P. W. Dempsey, K. Bruhn, J. F. Miller, Y. Xu, and G. Cheng. 2002. Involvement of receptor-interacting protein 2 in innate and adaptive immune responses. *Nature* **416:**190–194.

Da Shilva Correia, J., K. Soldau, U. Christen, P. S. Tobias, and R. J. Ulevitch. 2001. Lipopolysaccharide is in close proximity to each of the protein in its membrane receptor complex. *J. Biol. Chem.* **276:** 21129–21135.

Doyle, S. E., S. A. Vaidya, R. O'Connell, H. Dadgostar, P. W. Dempsey, T.-T. Wu, G. Rao, R. Sun, M. E. Haberland, R. L. Modlin, and G. Cheng. 2002. IRF3 mediates a TLR3/TLR4-specific antiviral gene program. *Immunity* **17:**251–263.

Dybdahl, B., A. Wahba, E. Lien, T. H. Flo, A. Waage, N. Qureshi, O. F. Sellevold, T. Espevik, and A. Sundan. 2002. Inflammatory response after open heart surgery: release of heat-shock protein 70 and signaling through toll-like receptor-4. *Circulation* **105:**685–690.

Fitzgerald, K. A., E. M. Palsson-McDermott, A. G. Bowie, C. Jefferies, A. S. Mansell, G. Brady, E. Brint, A. Dunne, P. Gray, M. T. Harte, D. McMurray, D. E. Smith, J. E. Sims, T. A. Bird, and L. A. J. O'Neill. 2001. Mal (MyD88-adaptor-like) is required for Toll-like receptor-4 signal transduction. *Nature* **413:**78–83.

Gao, B., and M. F. Tsan. 2003. Endotoxin contamination in recombinant human Hsp70 preparation is responsible for the induction of tumor necrosis factor α release by murine macrophages. *J. Biol. Chem.* **278:** 174–179.

Hacker, H., R. M. Vabulas, O. Takeuchi, K. Hoshino, S. Akira, and H. Wagner. 2000. Immune cell activation by bacterial CpG-DNA through myeloid differentiation marker 88 and tumor necrosis factor receptor-associated factor (TRAF)6. *J. Exp. Med.* **192:**595–600.

Hajjar, A. M., D. S. O'Mahony, A. Ozinsky, D. M. Underhill, A. Aderem, S. J. Klebanoff, and C. B. Wilson. 2001. Cutting edge: functional interactions between Toll-like receptor (TLR) 2 and TLR1 or TLR6 in response to phenol-soluble modulin. *J. Immunol.* **166:**15–19.

Hayashi, F., K. D. Smith, A. Ozinsky, T. R. Hawn, E. C. Yi, D. R. Goodlett, J. K. Eng, S. Akira, D. M. Underhill, and A. Aderem. 2001. The innate immune response to bacterial flagellin is mediated by Toll-like receptor-5. *Nature* **410:**1099–1103.

Haynes, L. M., D. D. Moore, E. A. Kurt-Jones, R. W. Finberg, L. J. Anderson, and R. A. Tripp. 2001. Involvement of Toll-like receptor 4 in innate immunity to respiratory syncytial virus. *J. Virol.* **75:** 10730–10737.

Haziot, A., E. Ferrero, F. Kontgen, N. Hijiya, S. Yamamoto, J. Silver, C. L. Stewart, and S. M. Goyert. 1996. Resistance to endotoxin shock and reduced dissemination of gram negative bacteria in CD14-deficient mice. *Immunity* **4:**407–414.

Hemmi, H., O. Takeuchi, T. Kawai, T. Kaisho, S. Sato, H. Sanjo, M. Matsumoto, K. Hoshino, H. Wagner, K. Takeda, and S. Akira. 2000. A Toll-like receptor recognizes bacterial DNA. *Nature* **408:**740–745.

Hemmi, H., T. Kaisho, O. Takeuchi, S. Sato, H. Sanjo, K. Hoshino, T. Horiuchi, H. Tomizawa, K. Takeda, and S. Akira. 2002. Small antiviral compounds activate immune cells via TLR7 MyD88-dependent signalling pathway. *Nat. Immunol.* **3:**196–200.

Horng, T., G. M. Barton, and R. Medzhitov. 2001. TIRAP: an adapter molecule in the Toll signaling pathway. *Nat. Immunol.* **2:**835–841.

Horng, T., G. M. Barton, R. A. Flavell, and R. Medzhitov. 2002. The adaptor molecule TIRAP provides signaling specificity for Toll-like receptors. *Nature* **420:**329–333.

Hoshino, K., O. Takeuchi, T. Kawai, H. Sanjo, T. Ogawa, Y. Takeda, K. Takeda, and S. Akira. 1999. Cutting edge: Toll-like receptor 4 (TLR4)-deficient mice are hyporesponsive to lipopolysaccharide: evidence for TLR4 as the *Lps* gene product. *J. Immunol.* **162:**3749–3752.

Hoshino, K., T. Kaisho, T. Iwabe, O. Takeuchi, and S. Akira. 2002. Differential involvement of IFN-β in Toll-like receptor-stimulated dendritic cell activation. *Int. Immunol.* **14:**1225–1231.

Inohara, N., L. del Peso, T. Koseki, S. Chen, and G. Nunez. 1998. RICK, a novel protein kinase containing a caspase recruitment domain, interacts with CLARP and regulates CD95-mediated apoptosis. *J. Biol. Chem.* **273:**12296–12300.

Ito, T., R. Amakawa, T. Kaisho, H. Hemmi, K. Tajima, K. Uehira, Y. Ozaki, H. Tomizawa, S. Akira, and S. Fukuhara. 2002. Interferon-α and interleukin-12 are induced differentially by Toll-like receptor 7 ligands in human blood dendritic cell subsets. *J. Exp. Med.* **195:**1507–1512.

Jack, R. S., X. Fan, M. Bernheiden, G. Rune, M. Ehlers, A. Weber, G. Kirsch, R. Mentel, B. Furll, M. Freudenberg, G. Schmitz, F. Stelter, and C. Schutt. 1997. Lipopolysaccharide-binding protein is required to combat a murine gram-negative bacterial infection. *Nature* **389:**742–745.

Jiang, Q., S. Akashi, K. Miyake, and H. R. Petty. 2000. Cutting edge: lipopolysaccharide induces physical proximity between CD14 and Toll-like receptor 4 (TLR4) prior to nuclear translocation of NF-κB. *J. Immunol.* **165:**3541–3544.

Johnson, G. B., G. J. Brunn, Y. Kodaira, and J. L. Platt. 2002. Receptor-mediated monitoring of tissue well-being via detection of soluble heparan sulfate by Toll-like receptor 4. *J. Immunol.* **168:**5233–5239.

Kaisho, T., O. Takeuchi, T. Kawai, K. Hoshino, and S. Akira. 2001. Endotoxin-induced maturation of MyD88-deficient dendritic cells. *J. Immunol.* **166:**5688–5694.

Kanakaraj, P., K. Ngo, Y. Wu, A. Angulo, P. Ghazal, C. A. Harris, J. J. Siekierka, P. A.

Peterson, and W. P. Fung-Leung. 1998. Defective interleukin (IL)-18-mediated natural killer and T helper cell type 1 responses in IL-1 receptor-associated kinase (IRAK)-deficient mice. *J. Exp. Med.* **187:** 2073–2079.

Kataoka, K., T. Muta, S. Yamazaki, and K. Takeshige. 2002. Activation of macrophages by linear (1-3)-β-D-glucans. Implications for the recognition of fungi by innate immunity. *J. Biol. Chem.* **277:**36825–36831.

Kawai, T., O. Adachi, T. Ogawa, K. Takeda, and S. Akira. 1999. Unresponsiveness of MyD88-deficient mice to endotoxin. *Immunity* **11:**115–122.

Kawai, T., O. Takeuchi, T. Fujita, J. Inoue, P. F. Muhlradt, S. Sato, K. Hoshino, and S. Akira. 2001. Lipopolysaccharide stimulates the MyD88-independent pathway and results in activation of IRF-3 and the expression of a subset of LPS-inducible genes. *J. Immunol.* **167:**5887–5894.

Kobayashi, K., N. Inohara, L. D. Hernandez, J. E. Galan, G. Nunez, C. A. Janeway, R. Medzhitov, and R. A. Flavell. 2002. RICK/Rip2/CARDIAK mediates signaling for receptors of the innate and adaptive immune systems. *Nature* **416:**194–199.

Krug, A., S, Rothenfusser, V. Hornung, B. Jahrsdorfer, S. Blackwell, Z. K. Ballas, S. Endres, A. M. Krieg, and G. Hartmann. 2001. Identification of CpG oligonucleotide sequences with high induction of IFN-α/β in plasmacytoid dendritic cells. *Eur. J. Immunol.* **31:**2154–2163.

Kurt-Jones, E. A., L. Popova, L. Kwinn, L. M. Haynes, L. P. Jones, R. A. Tripp, E. E. Walsh, M. W. Freeman, D. T. Golenbock, L. J. Anderson, and R. W. Finberg. 2000. Pattern recognition receptors TLR4 and CD14 mediate response to respiratory syncytial virus. *Nat. Immunol.* **1:**398–401.

Lehner, M. D., S. Morath, K. S. Michelsen, R. R. Schumann, and T. Hartung. 2001. Induction of cross-tolerance by lipopolysaccharide and highly purified lipoteichoic acid via different toll-like receptors independent of paracrine mediators. *J. Immunol.* **166:** 5161–5167.

Lemaitre, B., E. Nicolas, L. Michaut, J.-M. Reichhart, and J. A. Hoffmann. 1996. The dorsoventral regulatory gene cassette spatzle/Toll/cactus controls the potent antifungal response in *Drosophila* adults. *Cell* **86:**973–983.

Li, S., A. Strelow, E. J. Fontana, and H. Wesche. 2002. IRAK-4—a novel member of the IRAK family with the properties of an IRAK-kinase. *Proc. Natl. Acad. Sci. USA* **99:**5567–5572.

Lomaga, M. A., W. C. Yeh, I. Sarosi, G. S. Duncan, C. Furlonger, A. Ho, S. Morony, C. Capparelli, G. Van, S. Kaufman, A. van der Heiden, A. Itie, A. Wakeham, W. Khoo, T. Sasaki, Z. Cao, J. M. Penninger, C. J. Paige, D. L. Lacey, C. R. Dunstan, W. J. Boyle, D. V. Goeddel, and

T. W. Mak. 1999. TRAF6 deficiency results in osteopetrosis and defective interleukin-1, CD40, and LPS signaling. *Genes Dev.* **13:**1015–1024.

Massari, P., P. Henneke, Y. Ho, E. Latz, D. T. Golenbock, and L. M. Wetzler. 2002. Cutting edge: immune stimulation by neisserial porins is Toll-like receptor 2 and MyD88 dependent. *J. Immunol.* **168:** 1533–1537.

Matsumoto, M., S. Kikkawa, M. Kohase, K. Miyake, and T. Seya. 2002. Establishment of a monoclonal antibody against human Toll-like receptor 3 that blocks double-stranded RNA-mediated signaling. *Biochem. Biophys. Res. Commun.* **293:**1364–1369.

McCarthy, J. V., J. Ni, and V. M. Dixit. 1998. RIP2 is a novel NF-κB-activating and cell death-inducing kinase. *J. Biol. Chem.* **273:**16968–16975.

Means, T. K., S. Wang, E. Lien, A. Yoshimura, D. T. Golenbock, and M. J. Fenton. 1999a. Human Toll-like receptors mediate cellular activation by *Mycobacterium tuberculosis. J. Immunol.* **163:**3920–3927.

Means, T. K., E. Lien, A. Yoshimura, S. Wang, D. T. Golenbock, and M. J. Fenton. 1999b. The CD14 ligands lipoarabinomannan and lipopolysaccharide differ in their requirement for Toll-like receptors. *J. Immunol.* **163:**6748–6755.

Medzhitov, R., P. Preston-Hurlburt, and C. A. Janeway, Jr. 1997. A human homologue of the *Drosophila* Toll protein signals activation of adaptive immunity. *Nature* **388:**394–397.

Miyake, K., Y. Yamashita, M. Ogata, T. Sudo, and M. Kimoto. 1995. RP105, a novel B cell surface molecule implicated in B cell activation, is a member of the leucin-rich repeat protein family. *J. Exp. Med.* **154:**3333–3340.

Miyake, K., R. Shimazu, J. Kondo, T. Niki, S. Akashi, H. Ogata, Y. Yamashita, Y. Miura, and M. Kimoto. 1998. MD-1, a molecule that is physically associated with RP105 and positively regulates its expression. *J. Immunol.* **161:**1348–1353.

Moore, K. J., L. P. Anderson, R. R. Ingalls, B. G. Monks, R. Li, M. A. Arnaout, D. T. Golenbock, and M. W. Freeman. 2000. Divergent response to LPS and bacteria in CD14-deficient murine macrophages. *J. Immunol.* **165:**4272–4280.

Nagai, Y., S. Akashi, M. Nagafuku, M. Ogata, Y. Iwakura, S. Akira, T. Kitamura, A. Kosugi, M. Kimoto, and K. Miyake. 2002. Essential role of MD-2 in LPS responsiveness and TLR4 distribution. *Nat. Immunol.* **3:**667–672.

Naito, A., S. Azuma, S. Tanaka, T. Miyazaki, S. Takaki, K. Takatsu, K. Nakao, K. Nakamura, M. Katsuki, T. Yamamoto, and J. Inoue. 1999. Severe osteopetrosis, defective interleukin-1 signalling and lymph node organogenesis in TRAF6-deficient mice. *Genes Cells* **4:**353–362.

Navarro, L., and M. David. 1999. p38-dependent activation of interferon regulatory factor 3 by lipopolysaccharide. *J. Biol. Chem.* **274:**35535–35538.

Nomura, F., S. Akashi, Y. Sakao, S. Sato, T. Kawai, M. Matsumoto, K. Nakanishi, M. Kimoto, K. Miyake, K. Takeda, and S. Akira. 2000. Endotoxin tolerance in mouse peritoneal macrophages correlates with downregulation of surface Toll-like receptor 4 expression. *J. Immunol.* **164:**3476–3479.

Ogata, H., I. Su, K. Miyake, Y. Nagai, S. Akashi, I. Mecklenbrauker, K. Rajewski, M. Kimoto, and A. Tarakhovsky. 2000. The Toll-like receptor protein RP105 regulates lipopolysaccharide signaling in B cells. *J. Exp. Med.* **192:**23–29.

Ohashi, K., V. Burkart, S. Flohe, and H. Kolb. 2000. Cutting edge: heat shock protein 60 is a putative endogenous ligand of the toll-like receptor-4 complex. *J. Immunol.* **164:**558–561.

Okamura, Y., M. Watari, E. S. Jerud, D. W. Young, S. T. Ishizaka, J. Rose, J. C. Chow, and J. F. Strauss III. 2001. The extra domain A of fibronectin activates Toll-like receptor 4. *J. Biol. Chem.* **276:**10229–10233.

Opitz, B., N. W. Schroder, I. Spreitzer, K. S. Michelsen, C. J. Kirschning, W. Hallatschek, U. Zahringer, T. Hartung, U. B. Gobel, and R. R. Schumann. 2001. Toll-like receptor-2 mediates *Treponema* glycolipid and lipoteichoic acid-induced NF-κB translocation. *J. Biol. Chem.* **276:**22041–22047.

Ozinsky, A., D. M. Underhill, J. D. Fontenot, A. M. Hajjar, K. D. Smith, C. B. Wilson, L. Schroeder, and A. Aderem. 2000. The repertoire for pattern recognition of pathogens by the innate immune system is defined by cooperation between Toll-like receptors. *Proc. Natl. Acad. Sci. USA* **97:** 13766–13771.

Poltorak, A., X. He, I. Smirnova, M. Y. Liu, C. V. Huffel, X. Du, D. Birdwell, E. Alejos, M. Silva, C. Galanos, M. Freudenberg, P. Ricciardi-Castagnoli, B. Layton, and B. Beutler. 1998. Defective LPS signaling in C3H/HeJ and C57BL/10ScCr mice: mutation in *Tlr4* gene. *Science* **282:** 2085–2088.

Qureshi, S. T., L. Lariviere, G. Leveque, S. Clermont, K. J. Moore, P. Gros, and D. Malo. 1999. Endotoxin-tolerant mice have mutations in Toll-like receptor 4 (*Tlr4*). *J. Exp. Med.* **189:**615–625.

Rassa, J. C., J. L. Meyers, Y. Zhang, R. Kudaravalli, and S. R. Ross. 2002. Murine retroviruses activate B cells via interaction with Toll-like receptor 4. *Proc. Natl. Acad. Sci. USA* **99:**2281–2286.

Ropert, C., L. R. Ferreira, M. A. Campos, D. O. Procopio, L. R. Travassos, M. A. Ferguson, L. F. Reis, M. M. Teixeira, I. C. Almeida, and R. T. Gazzinelli. 2002. Macrophage signaling by glycosylphosphatidylinositol-anchored mucin-like glycoproteins derived from *Trypanosoma cruzi* trypomastigotes. *Microbes Infect.* **4:**1015–1025.

Sato, M., H. Suemori, N. Hata, M. Asagiri, K. Ogasawara, K. Nakao, T. Nakaya, M. Katsuki, S. Noguchi, N. Tanaka, and T. Taniguchi. 2000. Distinct and essential roles of transcription factors IRF-3 and IRF-7 in response to viruses for IFN-α/β gene induction. *Immunity* **13:**539–548.

Schnare, M., A. C. Holt, K. Takeda, S. Akira, and R. Medzhitov. 2000. Recognition of CpG DNA is mediated by signaling pathways dependent on the adaptor protein MyD88. *Curr. Biol.* **10:**1139–1142.

Schromm, A. B., E. Lien, P. Henneke, J. C. Chow, A. Yoshimura, H. Heine, E. Latz, B. G. Monks, D. A. Schwartz, K. Miyake, and D. T. Golenbock. 2001. Molecular genetic analysis of an endotoxin nonresponder mutant cell line: a point mutation in a conserved region of MD-2 abolishes endotoxin-induced signaling. *J. Exp. Med.* **194:**79–88.

Schumann, R. R., S. R. Leong, G. W. Flaggs, P. W. Gray, S. D. Wright, J. C. Mathison, P. S. Tobias, and R. Ulevitch. 1990. Structure and function of lipopolysaccharide binding protein. *Science* **249:**1429–1431.

Schwandner, R., R. Dziarski, H. Wesche, M. Rothe, and C. J. Kirschning. 1999. Peptidoglycan- and lipoteichoic acid-induced cell activation is mediated by Toll-like receptor 2. *J. Biol. Chem.* **274:**17406–17409.

Seki, E., H. Tsutsui, H. Nakano, N. Tsuji, K. Hoshino, O. Adachi, K. Adachi, S. Futatsugi, K. Kuida, O. Takeuchi, H. Okamura, J. Fujimoto, S. Akira, and K. Nakanishi. 2001. Lipopolysaccharide-induced IL-18 secretion from murine Kupffer cells independently of myeloid differentiation factor 88 that is critically involved in induction of production of IL-12 and IL-1β. *J. Immunol.* **166:**2651–2657.

Shimazu, R., S. Akashi, H. Ogata, Y. Nagai, K. Fukudome, K. Miyake, and M. Kimoto. 1999. MD-2, a molecule that confers lipopolysaccharide responsiveness on Toll-like receptor 4. *J. Exp. Med.* **189:**1777–1782.

Smiley, S. T., J. A. King, and W. W. Hancock. 2001. Fibrinogen stimulates macrophage chemokine secretion through Toll-like receptor 4. *J. Immunol.* **167:** 2887–2894.

Suzuki, N., S. Suzuki, G. S. Duncan, D. G. Millar, T. Wada, C. Mirtsos, H. Takada, A. Wakeham, A. Itie, S. Li, J. M. Penninger, H. Wesche, P. S. Ohashi, T. W. Mak, and W. C. Yeh. 2002. Severe impairment of interleukin-1 and Toll-like receptor signaling in mice lacking IRAK-4. *Nature.* **416:** 750–756.

Swantek, J. L., M. F. Tsen, M. H. Cobb, and J. A. Thomas. 2000. IL-1 receptor-associated kinase modulates host responsiveness to endotoxin. *J. Immunol.* **164:** 4301–4306.

Takeuchi, O., K. Hoshino, T. Kawai, H. Sanjo, H. Takada, T. Ogawa, K. Takeda, and S. Akira. 1999. Differential roles of TLR2 and TLR4 in recognition of Gram-negative and Gram-positive cell wall components. *Immunity* **11:**443–451.

Takeuchi, O., K. Hoshino, and S. Akira. 2000a. Cutting edge: TLR2-deficient and MyD88-deficient mice are highly susceptible to *Staphylococcus aureus* infection. *J. Immunol.* **165**:5392–5396.

Takeuchi, O., A. Kaufmann, K. Grote, T. Kawai, K. Hoshino, M. Morr, P. F. Muhlradt, and S. Akira. 2000b. Cutting edge: preferentially the R-stereoisomer of the mycoplasmal lipopeptide macrophage-activating lipopeptide-2 activates immune cells through a Toll-like receptor 2- and MyD88-dependent signaling pathway. *J. Immunol.* **164**:554–557.

Takeuchi, O., K. Takeda, K. Hoshino, O. Adachi, T. Ogawa, and S. Akira. 2000c. Cellular responses to bacterial cell wall components are mediated through MyD88-dependent signaling cascades. *Int. Immunol.* **12**:113–117.

Takeuchi, O., T. Kawai, P. F. Muhlradt, J. D. Radolf, A. Zychlinsky, K. Takeda, and S. Akira. 2001. Discrimination of bacterial lipopeptides by Toll-like receptor 6. *Int. Immunol.* **13**:933–940.

Takeuchi, O., T. Horiuchi, K. Hoshino, K. Takeda, Z. Dong, R. L. Modlin, and S. Akira. 2002. Role of TLR1 in mediating immune response to microbial lipoproteins. *J. Immunol.* **169**:10–14.

Termeer, C., F. Benedix, J. Sleeman, C. Fieber, U. Voith, T. Ahrens, K. Miyake, M. Freudenberg, C. Galanos, and J. C. Simon. 2002. Oligosaccharides of hyaluronan activate dendritic cells via Toll-like receptor 4. *J. Exp. Med.* **195**:99–111.

Thomas, J. A., J. L. Allen, M. Tsen, T. Dubnicoff, J. Danao, X. C. Liao, Z. Cao, and S. A. Wasserman. 1999. Impaired cytokine signaling in mice lacking the IL-1 receptor-associated kinase. *J. Immunol.* **163**:978–984.

Tobias, P., K. Soldau, and R. Ulevitch. 1986. Isolation of a lipopolysaccharide-binding acute phase reactant from rabbit serum. *J. Exp. Med.* **164**:777–793.

Toshchakov, V., B. W. Jones, P. Y. Perera, K. Thomas, M. J. Cody, S. Zhang, B. R. Williams, J. Major, T. A. Hamilton, M. J. Fenton, and S. N. Vogel. 2002. TLR4, but not TLR2, mediates IFN-β-induced STAT1α/β-dependent gene expression in macrophages. *Nat. Immunol.* **3**:392–398.

Underhill, D. M., A. Ozinsky, K. D. Smith, and A. Aderem. 1999a. Toll-like receptor 2 mediates mycobacteria-induced proinflammatory signaling in macrophages. *Proc. Natl. Acad. Sci. USA* **96**:14459–14463.

Underhill, D. M., A. Ozinsky, A. M. Hajjar, A. Stevens, C. B. Wilson, M. Bassetti, and A. Aderem. 1999b. The Toll-like receptor 2 is recruited to macrophage phagosomes and discriminates between pathogens. *Nature* **401**:811–815.

Vabulas, R. M., P. Ahmad-Nejad, C. da Costa, T. Miethke, C. J. Kirschning, H. Hacker, and H. Wagner. 2001. Endocytosed HSP60s use toll-like receptor 2 (TLR2) and TLR4 to activate the toll/interleukin-1 receptor signaling pathway in innate immune cells. *J. Biol. Chem.* **276**:31332–31339.

Vabulas, R. M., P. Ahmad-Nejad, S. Ghose, C. J. Kirschning, R. D. Issels, and H. Wagner. 2002. HSP70 as endogenous stimulus of toll/interleukin-1 receptor signal pathway. *J. Biol. Chem.* **277**:15107–15112.

Weaver, B. K., K. P. Kumar, and N. C. Reich. 1998. Interferon regulatory factor 3 and CREB-binding protein/p300 are subunits of double-stranded RNA-activated transcription factor DRAF1. *Mol. Cell. Biol.* **18**:1359–1368.

Wurfel, M. M., B. G. Monks, R. R. Ingalls, R. L. Dedrick, R. Delude, D. Zhou, N. Lamping, R. R. Schumann, R. Thieringer, M. J. Fenton, S. D. Wright, and D. Golenbock. 1997. Targeted deletion of the *lipopolysaccharide (LPS)-binding protein* gene leads to profound suppression of LPS responses ex vivo, whereas in vivo responses remain intact. *J. Exp. Med.* **186**:2051–2056.

Yamamoto, M., S. Sato, K. Mori, O. Takeuchi, K. Hoshino, K. Takeda, and S. Akira. 2002. A novel TIR domain-containing adaptor that preferentially activates the interferon-β promoter. *J. Immunol.* **169**:6668–6672.

Yamamoto, M., S. Sato, H. Hemmi, H. Sanjo, S. Uematsu, T. Kaisho, K. Hoshino, O. Takeuchi, M. Kobayashi, T. Fujita, K. Takeda, and S. Akira. 2002. Essential role of TIRAP/Mal for activation of the signaling cascade shared by TLR2 and TLR4. *Nature* **420**:324–329.

Yoneyama, M., W. Suhara, Y. Fukuhara, M. Fukuda, E. Nishida, and T. Fujita. 1998. Direct triggering of the type I interferon system by virus infection: activation of a transcription factor complex containing IRF-3 and CBP/p300. *EMBO J.* **17**:1087–1095.

Yoshimura, A., E. Lien, R. R. Ingalls, E. Tuomanen, R. Dziarski, and D. Golenbock. 1999. Cutting edge: recognition of Gram-positive bacterial cell wall components by the innate immune system occurs via Toll-like receptor 2. *J. Immunol.* **165**:1–5.

Zhang, G., and S. Ghosh. 2002. Negative regulation of toll-like receptor-mediated signaling by Tollip. *J. Biol. Chem.* **77**:7059–7065.

TOLL-LIKE RECEPTORS AND CONTROL OF ADAPTIVE IMMUNITY

Gregory M. Barton, Chandrashekhar Pasare, and Ruslan Medzhitov

14

BASIC PRINCIPLES OF INNATE IMMUNE RECOGNITION

The innate immune system comprises the initial line of defense to microbial infection in the host. The origins of innate immune recognition are evolutionarily ancient; many of the principles dictating how the system functions are conserved throughout metazoan organisms. Unlike the adaptive immune recognition, innate immune recognition occurs via receptors that are expressed on all cells of a given type. These receptors are directly linked with a variety of defense mechanisms. For these reasons, the innate immune response is rapid, keeping an infection in check until cells of the adaptive immune system are able to mount a response. In addition, the innate response leads to production of important mediators (soluble as well as membrane bound) that signal to other components of the immune system and help coordinate the overall immune response.

Ultimately, the goal of innate immune recognition (and of the immune system overall) is to discriminate between infectious nonself and noninfectious self (Janeway, 1989).

Infectious nonself (i.e., microbes) must be recognized and eliminated whereas self tissues must not be recognized or damaged. Failure to make this distinction can lead to destruction of host tissues and autoimmunity on the one hand or overwhelming infection on the other. Through the course of evolution, the immune systems of metazoans have developed multiple mechanisms to deal with this essential task. Conceptually, these approaches can be grouped into three general strategies: (i) pattern recognition, (ii) missing-self recognition, and (iii) induced and altered self-recognition.

Pattern recognition, mediated by pattern recognition receptors (PRRs), is based on the recognition of conserved microbial features not produced by the host (Medzhitov and Janeway, 1997). Consequently, the targets of this system are generally products of unique aspects of microbial metabolism, such as lipopolysaccharide, a component of the outer cell walls of gram-negative bacteria. PRRs are expressed on cells of the innate immune system, where they link activation of these cells to recognition of microbial infection. Over the past several years, the list of known PRRs has grown considerably, underscoring the importance of this strategy in recognition of infectious nonself.

Gregory M. Barton, Chandrashekhar Pasare, and Ruslan Medzhitov, Howard Hughes Medical Institute, Yale University School of Medicine, 300 Cedar St., TAC S660, New Haven, CT 06520.

The Innate Immune Response to Infection
Ed. by S. H. E. Kaufmann, R. Medzhitov, and S. Gordon
©2004 ASM Press, Washington, D.C.

Recognition of missing self is based on the presence of normally ubiquitous self-markers on host cells. These self-markers can serve either of two general functions. First, they can engage inhibitory receptors on innate immune cells and prevent activation of those cells. In this case, microbial infection of a host cell must be coupled with downregulation of these markers in order to release the inhibitory signal and tip the balance toward activation (Raulet et al., 2001; Ravetch and Lanier, 2000). Alternatively, the self-markers themselves prevent the activation of constitutive pathways directed toward all cells, such as the negative regulators of the C3 convertase of the alternative complement pathway. The details of these different examples are discussed in greater detail elsewhere in this book (see chapters 7 and 16). In general, though, this strategy will lead to destruction of microbial cells lacking self-markers while host cells remain protected.

Recognition of induced or altered self targets the induction of self-markers on the surface of infected cells. These markers are subsequently recognized by activating receptors expressed on innate immune cells. The mechanisms by which these self-markers are induced by infection remain unclear. Nonetheless, accumulating evidence suggests that they are used to signal the presence of infectious nonself and activate the immune system. Most notably, several families of these molecules serve as ligands for activating receptors on NK cells and some T cells (Diefenbach and Raulet, 2001). The details of these interactions are discussed in detail in chapter 7.

In this chapter, we focus on how pattern recognition is used by the innate immune system to distinguish self from nonself and how this discrimination is translated into induction of adaptive immunity. The past few years have seen significant advances in our understanding of how adaptive immune responses are controlled by the initial innate recognition of microbial infection. In particular, the identification of the Toll-like receptor (TLR) family as the critical receptor family involved in the recognition of infectious nonself has enabled researchers to examine the mechanisms by which adaptive responses are controlled by the innate immune system. Before discussing the specific mechanisms by which TLRs control adaptive immunity, we consider the general mechanisms by which self/nonself discrimination is regulated within the adaptive immune system. In the second half of the chapter we focus on how TLRs control some of these mechanisms and link microbial recognition to self and nonself discrimination by the adaptive immune system.

BASIC PRINCIPLES OF THE ADAPTIVE IMMUNE SYSTEM

The adaptive immune system provides an enormous benefit to the host as a result of the essentially limitless specificities of the antigen receptors of B and T lymphocytes. This diversity is generated by random rearrangement of gene segments within the loci of these receptors (Tonegawa, 1983). The dangerous consequence of this randomness is that some of these receptors will be self-reactive. Although the germ line-encoded receptors used by the innate immune system have evolved over millions of years to distinguish self from nonself, randomly generated receptors, by definition, cannot be subject to this selective pressure. Consequently, the antigen receptors of T and B cells must be evaluated on the basis of their specificity. These selective processes are essential for proper function of the adaptive immune system and are discussed later in this chapter.

Another key feature of lymphocyte antigen receptors is that they are expressed clonally, such that each of the millions of B and T cells expresses a receptor with a unique specificity. One consequence of this clonal expression is that the frequency of cells specific for any particular antigen is very low. If left to chance, the likelihood of the correct lymphocyte encountering its corresponding antigen during an infection would be exceedingly low. To overcome these odds, lymphocytes and antigen-presenting cells (APCs) drain from the tissues and blood into secondary lymphoid organs (i.e., lymph nodes and spleen), so that large numbers of lymphocytes can sample potential antigens efficiently (Banchereau and Steinman, 1998).

If a lymphocyte recognizes its cognate antigen during this comingling, then it becomes activated and the adaptive immune response begins. Certain critical steps in this process are controlled at the level of innate immune recognition. For example, the function of APCs is intimately linked to the innate recognition of microbes by PRRs. Engagement of these receptors on APCs leads to a series of events that collectively lead to activation of T cells. The first step is the phagocytosis and degradation of the pathogens and presentation of pathogen-derived peptide fragments on major histocompatibility complex (MHC) molecules (Cresswell et al., 1999; Mellman et al., 1998; Nakagawa and Rudensky, 1999). These peptide-MHC complexes are recognized directly by T-cell antigen receptors (TCRs). The second step is the expression of costimulatory molecules by the APC. These costimulatory molecules provide a so-called second signal to T cells. Their expression on APCs is induced by microbial products, thus assuring T cells that the peptides being recognized are microbial in origin. Conceptually, this costimulatory signal is vital to the function of the system, as T cells have no way of discerning the nature of the antigen through their randomly generated TCRs. Implicit in this arrangement is the requirement that the peptide-MHC and costimulatory molecules be expressed on the same cell in order for activation to occur, a requirement that has been demonstrated experimentally (Liu and Janeway, 1992).

Once T cells are activated by APCs exposed to pathogens, they differentiate into effector cells that perform several critical functions. Cytotoxic T cells detect their cognate peptides on infected cells and induce them to undergo apoptosis. Helper T cells (Th cells) detect the antigenic peptides presented by macrophages and B cells and induce their activation through cell surface molecules and cytokines. When activated, T cells recognize their cognate peptides presented by B cells; they deliver a costimulatory signal, such as CD40 ligand, which is required for B-cell activation and antibody class switch from immunoglobulin M (IgM) to other isotypes (Kawabe et al., 1994).

Upon activation, lymphocytes undergo a period of rapid proliferation. This expansion is necessary due to the low precursor frequency of lymphocytes with a given specificity. Consequently, it takes several days to accumulate enough lymphocytes to contain the microbial infection. The innate immune system keeps the infection in check long enough for lymphocytes to expand and eventually eliminate the microbial challenge. An important outcome of this expansion is that a small number of these lymphocytes survive as long-lived memory cells. Upon subsequent infection by the same pathogen, these cells can mount a much more rapid response that eliminates the infection more efficiently than before. This phenomenon is called "immunological memory" and provides an enormous benefit to the host (Seder and Ahmed, 2003).

In summary, the adaptive immune system generates diversity through random generation of receptors, so the specificity of these receptors is unknown a priori. Consequently, a number of mechanisms have evolved to prevent inappropriate activation of lymphocytes by self-antigens. In the next section we discuss some of these mechanisms in greater detail.

MECHANISMS OF SELF AND NONSELF DISCRIMINATION AND IMMUNE TOLERANCE

As discussed in the previous section, the antigen receptors of B and T cells must be screened on the basis of their specificities to ensure that self-reactive cells are eliminated. This screening first takes place during the development of lymphocytes in a process called central tolerance. This process is not entirely perfect and some self-reactive cells escape to the periphery. Nevertheless, these few self-reactive cells can be rendered nonfunctional even after they mature in a process called peripheral tolerance. Both of these mechanisms are essential to prevent unwanted immune responses to antigens that are derived from the tissues of the host. Failure of one or both of these processes can lead to a variety of autoimmune diseases that can be devastating to the host.

Central Tolerance

The bulk of self-reactive lymphocytes are eliminated during their development. This process, called clonal deletion, guarantees that cells possessing self-reactive TCRs or B-cell receptors do not reach the peripheral tissues. There are some differences in the way central tolerance operates for T and B cells. T cells are evaluated based on the affinity of their TCR for the millions of self-peptides bound to MHC molecules in the thymus (Starr et al., 2003). Developing T cells, or thymocytes, expressing TCRs with weak affinity for self-peptide–MHC complexes are positively selected to develop into mature T cells (Starr et al., 2003). Those thymocytes expressing TCRs with little or no affinity for self-peptide and MHC die from the lack of positive selection survival signals. Finally, the thymocytes expressing TCRs with high affinity for self-peptide–MHC complexes are eliminated in a process called negative selection (Starr et al., 2003). This process is made much more efficient by the fact that specialized cells in the thymus express proteins that would normally be found only in certain peripheral tissues (Anderson et al., 2002; Liston et al., 2003; Starr et al., 2003). These proteins are presented by MHC molecules and lead to the elimination of thymocytes that would otherwise escape negative selection. This ectopic expression of tissue-specific proteins in the thymus makes the process of negative selection much more efficient.

The general principles of B-cell selection are similar to those of T-cell selection, the goal being the elimination of B cells expressing immunoglobulin specific for self-antigens. B cells that are capable of generating a functional immunoglobulin receptor progress through development to become immature B cells, at which point they can exit the bone marrow and enter the circulation. It is at this stage that the specificity of a B-cell's immunoglobulin is evaluated. If an immature B cell recognizes soluble self-proteins, it becomes unresponsive to further stimulation, a state referred to as anergy (Goodnow et al., 1989). Anergic B cells are excluded from the follicles in the spleen and lymph node and ultimately die (Cyster et al., 1994). Immature B cells that have receptors capable of recognizing membrane-bound self-antigens receive signals leading to apoptosis of the self-reactive B lymphocytes (Hartley et al., 1991). This process is called clonal deletion. Because most B-cell responses are dependent on T-cell help, the mechanisms that suppress autoreactive T-cell responses to peptides derived from certain antigens also indirectly control B-cell responses to those antigens.

Mechanisms of Peripheral Tolerance

Control of Costimulation. In addition to the stringent developmental selection that eliminates self-reactive lymphocytes, T and B cells are subjected to additional levels of regulation in the periphery to prevent inappropriate activation. T-cell activation is dependent on signals delivered through the TCR, which recognizes peptide-MHC complexes present on APCs. In the absence of an infection, the MHC molecules on APCs are loaded with self-peptides. Interaction of TCR with such MHC molecules fails to deliver an activation signal. In general, many, but not all, TCRs with sufficiently high affinity for these self-peptide–MHC complexes will have been eliminated by negative selection. However, an additional signal is necessary for effective T-cell activation: peptide–MHC complexes on APCs need to be presented along with another set of molecules called costimulatory molecules (Jenkins and Schwartz, 1987). Induction of costimulatory molecules on APCs is tightly regulated and happens only in the presence of infection. The requirements for and consequences of induction of costimulation are discussed later in this chapter. The most important costimulatory molecules that are upregulated on APCs are B7-1 (CD80) and B7-2 (CD86) (Borriello et al., 1997). These molecules deliver activation signals through the CD28 receptor on T cells (Shahinian et al., 1993). When a T cell does not receive costimulation during activation, the resulting partial signal leads to T-cell anergy and/or apoptosis. Thus, regulation of costimulatory molecules expression on APCs is one of the mechanisms that prevent activation of self-reactive T cells.

Survival of Activated Lymphocytes. A naive T cell exists in a quiescent state until it recognizes a peptide-MHC complex with high affinity in the presence of costimulatory molecules. As we have discussed, these events will lead to the rapid expansion of that T-cell clone, increasing the number of cells with a given specificity to better fight infection. In addition, the generation of memory cells is thought to arise from this expansion. Once the infection is cleared, however, this increased number of cells becomes unnecessary and needs to be eliminated. The elimination of these activated cells protects the host from unwanted tissue damage and creates space for additional T-cell specificities.

T-cell proliferation is intimately linked to a cytokine called interleukin-2 (IL-2) (Schwartz, 2003). IL-2 is produced by activated T cells and is required for their proliferation. IL-2 binds the IL-2 receptor (IL-2R), which is upregulated on activated T cells. Signals from the IL-2R are critical for sustained division of these T cells. In seeming contrast to this role, IL-2R has also been shown to initiate signals that commit activated cells to programmed cell death (Schwartz, 2003). This is particularly evident in IL-2-deficient mice, in which accumulation of activated T cells leads to several autoimmune pathologies (Sadlack et al., 1995, 1993). This apparent contradiction can be resolved with the idea that the same signals that lead to the rapid proliferation of T cells eventually lead to upregulation of mechanisms that eliminate the cells. Indeed, activation of T

cells leads to an increase in surface levels of Fas and tumor necrosis factor (TNF) receptor. Engagement of these proteins by their respective ligands leads to induction of apoptosis of activated T cells (Brunner et al., 1995; Dhein et al., 1995; Ju et al., 1995; Zheng et al., 1995).

If all activated T cells died because of activation-related events that commit them to apoptosis, then the adaptive response would be severely compromised. Consequently, activated T cells need additional signals to rescue them from death long enough to do their job. These signals are provided by a set of cytokines that are secreted by cells of the innate immune system. Cytokines that protect T cells from death fall into two major categories: those that signal through the common gamma chain (CD122) and belong to the IL-2 family of cytokines (IL-4, IL-7, and IL-15) (Lantz et al., 2000) and type I interferons (IFNs [IFN-α and IFN-β]) (Tough et al., 1996). The cytokines that signal through the common gamma chain have been shown to upregulate expression of the anti-apoptotic protein Bcl-2. Type I IFNs appear to exert their effect on T cells through a different mechanism, although the details of this process remain unclear. In addition to these two groups of cytokines, IL-6 has been shown to protect resting T cells from death and probably has a significant role in promoting survival of activated T cells (Teague et al., 1997).

In light of their potent effect on T-cell survival, understanding the regulation of these cytokines is relevant to understanding how adaptive responses are controlled. Although IL-7 can be produced constitutively, most of the cytokines that promote T-cell survival are secreted at high levels by cells of the innate immune system following recognition of microbial infection. Therefore, when adaptive immune responses are initiated by microbial-derived antigens, activated T cells are protected from undergoing apoptosis by the cytokines that are secreted by APCs. This mechanism allows for selective survival of the expanded pool of pathogen-specific T cells. In this way, this process constitutes another checkpoint against inappropriate activation of self-reactive T cells. For example, if a self-reactive T cell escapes deletion and recognizes a self-peptide with sufficient affinity to become activated, this activation will not be accompanied by cytokine-induced survival signals. More often than not, such a response will not be sustainable and the T cells will die by activation-induced cell death, ensuring that peripheral T-cell tolerance is maintained against self-antigens. The importance of this checkpoint is evidenced by the correlation between the incidence of chronic infections and autoimmune diseases (Rose, 1998). The autoimmune responses may be driven, in part, by bystander effects due to the production of prosurvival cytokines in response to the chronic infections.

Anti-Inflammatory Mechanisms and Suppressor T Cells. Responses to self-antigens and the associated autoimmune pathology can be attributed in many cases to self-reactive T cells that have differentiated into IFN-γ-producing cells. CD4 T cells that have adopted this fate are called Th1 cells. The differentiation of Th1 cells is discussed at the end of this chapter. For this discussion, it is sufficient to note that activated self-reactive Th1 cells can directly destroy host tissues or, through their production of IFN-γ, activate macrophages, which leads to further tissue destruction. To deal with this possibility, the immune system has evolved anti-inflammatory mechanisms that act to suppress the activation of immune responses. In most cases, these mechanisms rely on the production of anti-inflammatory cytokines, such as IL-10 and transforming growth factor β (TGF-β). These cytokines suppress the proinflammatory activities of Th1 cells. The importance of these cytokines in immunosuppression is highlighted by the severe autoimmune pathology detected in mice that are genetically deficient for IL-10 or TGF-β (Kuhn et al., 1993; Shull et al., 1992). TGF-β has been shown to inhibit IL-2 production and T-cell proliferation by induction of cell cycle inhibitors, and also to prevent T-cell differentiation (Gorelik and Flavell, 2002).

A specialized class of T cells is responsible for the production of anti-inflammatory cytokines and plays a major role in controlling autoreactive T-cell responses. These T cells can be divided into two cell types based on their mechanism of action. T regulatory 1 cells (Tr1 cells) develop in a cytokine environment rich in IL-10 and then secrete high levels of IL-10 that help to subdue Th1 responses (Groux et al., 1997). Th3 cells are mucosal in origin and predominantly secrete TGF-β (Chen et al., 1994). Both IL-10 and TGF-β act in an antigen-nonspecific manner and help to suppress unwanted T-cell responses. Because inflammation and its suppression are both caused by secreted cytokines, it is possible that the balance between anti-inflammatory and proinflammatory cytokines present in the milieu determines the fate of an ongoing immune response. Infection by pathogens causes production of large quantities of proinflammatory cytokines that can override the suppressive effects of anti-inflammatory cytokines. When responses to self-antigens are inappropriately initiated, the presence of anti-inflammatory cytokines may help to inhibit such responses and maintain peripheral tolerance. Malfunction of these inhibitory mechanisms allows the self-reactive immune responses to proceed, leading to autoimmune pathology.

Another class of suppressor T cells (Treg cells) does not appear to rely on the production of anti-inflammatory cytokines. Instead, Treg cells can suppress activation of effector T cells in an antigen-specific manner. These cells constitute 5 to 10% of the total CD4 T-cell pool and can be identified by expression of both CD4 and CD25 (IL-2R alpha chain) markers (Sakaguchi et al., 1995). Treg cells develop in the thymus under the control of a specialized transcription factor, Foxp3 (Fontenot et al., 2003; Hori et al., 2003; Khattri et al., 2003). Consequently, mice that have been thymectomized on day 3 (Asano et al., 1996) or lack functional Foxp3 (Fontenot et al., 2003; Hori et al., 2003; Khattri et al., 2003) do not have Treg cells in their secondary lymphoid organs. These mice develop a severe, generalized autoimmune disease, suggesting that Treg cells play a major role in suppression of autoreactive T cells (Sakaguchi et al., 1995). Treg cells have the ability to suppress both CD4 and CD8 T-cell responses and differ from the Tr1 and Th3 cells in two ways. First, their suppressive activity depends on the physical contact with effector T cells. Second, they act in an antigen-specific manner and do not suppress bystander T-cell responses. Although production of both TGF-β and IL-10 has been implicated as a mechanism of suppression by these cells, the actual mechanism of suppression is still not known. At the molecular level they have been shown to inhibit IL-2 transcription in responding T cells (Thornton and Shevach, 1998), which prevents T-cell proliferation and clonal expansion. Existing evidence suggests that suppressor T cells act constantly to suppress immune responses in secondary lymphoid organs and help to maintain peripheral tolerance.

INITIATION OF ADAPTIVE IMMUNE RESPONSES: ROLE OF PRRs

There are a variety of PRRs that play a role in uptake and clearance of pathogenic microbes. Some of them activate the lectin pathway of complement fixation (mannan-binding lectin), some act as opsonins (C-reactive protein) to promote phagocytosis, and some act as receptors for nonopsonic phagocytosis (scavenger receptors) by macrophages and neutrophils (Medzhitov, 2001). A family of PRRs called TLRs plays a critical role in the induction of innate immune responses because of its ability to induce a plethora of antimicrobial and inflammatory genes upon recognition of microbes (Takeda et al., 2003). Some of the TLR-induced signals also have important roles in the initiation of the adaptive immune responses and are involved in many of the regulatory mechanisms discussed earlier in this chapter. In the following subsections, we discuss these mechanisms in greater detail.

TLR Family of PRRs

TLRs represent an ancient system of host defense that is conserved from flies to mammals. There are at least 10 TLR family members in mammals. TLRs have evolved to recognize the conserved molecular products of microorganisms, including bacteria, viruses, fungi, and protozoa (Takeda et al., 2003). Because TLR ligands are unique to microorganisms and not produced by the host, their recognition allows us to distinguish infectious nonself from noninfectious self (Medzhitov and Janeway, 1997). As we will see, the information generated from TLR recognition of microbial infection is used to control many aspects of the ensuing adaptive immune response.

TLRs are type I transmembrane proteins whose extracellular regions contain leucine-rich repeat motifs. All TLRs possess an intracellular region that is homologous to that of the IL-1 receptor and is called the Toll/IL-1R (TIR) domain. The TIR domain is also present in adapters that function downstream of the receptors. All TLRs appear to activate a common signaling pathway that leads to the activation of the transcription factor NF-κB and the expression of a common set of proinflammatory genes (Takeda et al., 2003). In addition to this core set of genes, individual TLRs can induce expression of unique subsets of genes. The molecular basis for this differential gene expression is not yet fully understood. For a more detailed discussion of TLR signal transduction, see chapter 13. Here we focus on the consequences of gene expression induced by TLR activation.

TLRs are expressed on a variety of cell types, including macrophages, dendritic cells (DCs), neutrophils, fibroblasts, epithelial cells, and B cells, and can induce antimicrobial responses in many of these. Many of the genes induced by TLRs are involved in the innate response to infection. As discussed above, the innate immune system must keep infection contained while the adaptive response is initiated. Consequently, many of the genes downstream of TLRs are involved in bacterial killing or preventing viral replication. For example, TLR ligation on macrophages and neutrophils induces production of reactive oxygen and nitrogen intermediates, antimicrobial proteins and peptides, and other effector molecules that help to destroy infectious agents (Huang et al., 2001).

The most important aspect of TLR function in terms of adaptive immune responses is the control of APC activation. TLRs expressed on DCs link microbial recognition with T-cell activation. This complex mechanism plays a central role in the innate control of adaptive immunity and is discussed in more detail in the next subsection.

Control of DC Maturation

A highly specialized APC called a DC is the primary cell involved in priming naive T cells and initiating adaptive immune responses (Steinman et al., 2003). DCs reside in the tissues, where they act as sentinels, constantly scanning for the presence of microbes. When localized in the tissues, before they have encountered pathogens, DCs are highly endocytic and express low levels of MHC and costimulatory molecules. The DC in this state is called "immature" and cannot efficiently prime naive T cells. DCs express TLRs that allow them to recognize pathogens in the tissues. When pathogens enter the host by virtue of a breach in physical barriers or by virtue of their invasive capability, they will be recognized and engulfed by immature DCs. TLRs expressed on DCs initiate intracellular signaling pathways that lead to induction of a differentiation process called DC maturation. The ultimate goal of DC maturation is to present microbial-derived peptides to naive T cells in the proper context to initiate the adaptive response. In this sense, DCs link the recognition of infectious nonself by TLRs to induction of adaptive immunity.

Maturation encompasses a number of coordinated events, all stemming from the initial microbial recognition by TLRs. First, TLR signaling induces the upregulation of genes involved in antigen processing and presentation.

These genes encode proteases involved in degradation of the microbe as well as proteins involved in peptide loading onto MHC molecules. Increasing this activity upon microbial recognition increases the likelihood that pathogen-derived peptides will be bound to MHC molecules and presented to T cells. TLR signals also lead to an upregulation of surface levels of MHC molecules on DCs. Second, TLR ligation leads to the expression of costimulatory molecules on DCs, which greatly enhances their ability to activate naive T cells. Third, DCs that have recognized pathogens via TLRs migrate from the peripheral tissue to the T-cell areas of draining lymph nodes (Fig. 1). This migration is essential for efficient T-cell priming for reasons that were discussed above (Bancherau and Steinman, 1998). To overcome the low precursor frequency of naive T cells for a particular peptide, priming takes place in secondary lymphoid organs. Because of their migration, DCs can present peptides derived from pathogens, which were encountered in peripheral tissues, to naive T cells in the secondary lymphoid organs. Finally, TLR ligation on DCs leads to the production of cytokines. These cytokines have important consequences on the ensuing immune response, in terms of both activating cells of the innate immune system and influencing the nature of the adaptive response. The effect of DC-derived cytokines on the adaptive response is discussed in more detail in later sections.

Over the past several years it has become evident that DCs are actually a heterogeneous population of cells. A number of DC subsets have been defined using different surface markers and functional properties. The interesting aspect of these subsets is that they appear to express different TLR family members. Furthermore, depending on the subset, TLR activation can lead to different responses. For example, a subset of DCs called plasmacytoid DCs expresses TLR7 and TLR9, but not TLR2, TLR4, or TLR5 (Kadowaki et al., 2001). Plasmacytoid DCs produce type I IFNs when stimulated with TLR ligands and are

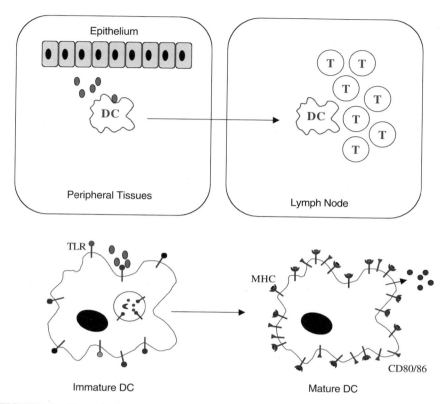

FIGURE 1 Control of DC maturation by TLRs. Microbial infection is recognized by immature DCs in the tissues when TLRs are activated. Signals initiated by TLRs lead to DC maturation, which includes migration to secondary lymphoid organs, upregulation of MHC and costimulatory molecules, and production of cytokines.

involved in responses to viral infections (Asselin-Paturel et al., 2001; Dalod et al., 2002). In contrast, myeloid DCs express TLR2 and TLR4 and do not express the high levels of type I IFNs characteristic of plasmacytoid DCs. Instead, myeloid DCs produce cytokines such as TNF-α and IL-12 in response to TLR2 and TLR4 ligands (Dalod et al., 2002). Many of the functional differences between DC subsets have yet to be clearly defined. Regardless, a general principle is emerging in which certain DC subsets respond to specific types of microbial infections and produce differential responses. These responses, in conjunction with the other more general aspects of DC maturation outlined above, will ultimately

determine the nature of the adaptive immune response.

Control of Induction of Costimulation

As described above, engagement of both TCR and CD28 on naive T cells is a requirement for their activation. Recognition of peptide-MHC complexes on APCs in the absence of costimulatory molecules renders T cells anergic and is one of the mechanisms of maintaining peripheral tolerance to self-antigens. Consequently, expression of costimulatory molecules on DCs is one of the key events controlled by TLRs. TLR activation leads to rapid upregulation of costimulatory molecules, such as CD80 and CD86, and greatly enhances the ability of DCs to activate naive T cells. Importantly, for a T cell to be activated, the peptide-MHC complex and costimulatory molecules must be presented by the same APC. This requirement ensures that the potent ability of DCs to prime naive T cells is physically linked to the recognition, uptake, and presentation of pathogens. Consequently, T-cell priming by DCs is controlled at the level of the recognition of infectious nonself by TLRs.

Regulation of Suppressor T-Cell Function

As discussed above, suppressor T cells can be grouped into two classes on the basis of their function. Treg cells act in an antigen-specific manner and play an important role in inhibiting activation of self-reactive T cells. The TCR beta chain usage by Treg cells is as variable and diverse as that of effector T cells, suggesting a possible antigen recognition repertoire as wide as for effector T cells (Thornton and Shevach, 1998). Although this repertoire includes TCRs capable of recognizing self-antigens, it is likely that Treg cells have specificity toward pathogen-derived antigens as well. Consequently, Treg cells are most likely capable of suppressing protective T-cell responses. Although suppression of self-reactive responses is beneficial to the host, suppression of pathogen-directed responses will render the host susceptible to infections. Therefore, to generate effective T-cell responses against pathogens, it is important for the host to overcome Treg cell-mediated suppression of pathogen-specific T cells. As the primary sensors of microbial infection, TLRs mediate the inhibition of suppressor activity of Treg cells so that pathogen-specific T-cell responses can be initiated. In the absence of infection, TLRs are not engaged and Treg cells suppress self-reactive T-cell responses effectively.

As we have discussed, recognition of microbial infection by TLRs on DCs not only induces upregulation of MHC and costimulatory molecules but also leads to secretion of cytokines such as IL-12, TNF, and IL-6. T-cell recognition of peptide-MHC complexes with high affinity in the presence of costimulation delivers a complete activation signal. Although this signal is sufficient to induce T-cell activation in the absence of Treg cells, it is insufficient to overcome the suppressive signal that is delivered by Treg cells (Pasare and Medzhitov, 2003). Cytokines produced by DCs play a key role in overcoming the suppressive effects of these cells. In particular, IL-6 secreted by DCs makes responding T cells refractory to the suppression mediated by Treg cells (Fig. 2). Importantly, IL-6 does not block the ability of Treg cells to perform their function of suppressing self-reactive responses (Pasare and Medzhitov, 2003). Although the mechanism of suppression is not understood completely, signals delivered through TCR and CD28 are inhibited by Treg cells, leading to cell cycle arrest of responding T cells. However, IL-6 and other cytokines produced by DCs during infection provide additional signals that are not blocked by Treg cells. Consequently, these cytokines enable responding T cells to progress into the cell cycle and mount effective responses. Because IL-6 plays a critical role in overcoming Treg cell function, deregulated induction of this cytokine by TLRs has the potential to lead to development of autoimmunity. In fact, IL-6, TNF-α, and type I IFNs have been implicated in many autoimmune pathologies (Drakesmith et al., 2000). In particular, a role for IL-6 has been demonstrated for such autoimmune diseases as collagen-induced arthritis, pristine-induced lupus, and experimental autoimmune encephalitis (Alonzi et al., 1998; Ohshima et al., 1998; Richards et al., 1998). It is possible that deregulated production of IL-6 during chronic infections can lead to activation of autoreactive T cells, especially when self-peptides are presented along with foreign peptides on DCs. Self-reactive T cells that have escaped thymic deletion and come in contact with DCs presenting self-peptides will become activated because of the ability of IL-6 and other cytokines to render them refractory to suppression. Consistent with this idea, IL-6-deficient mice have been

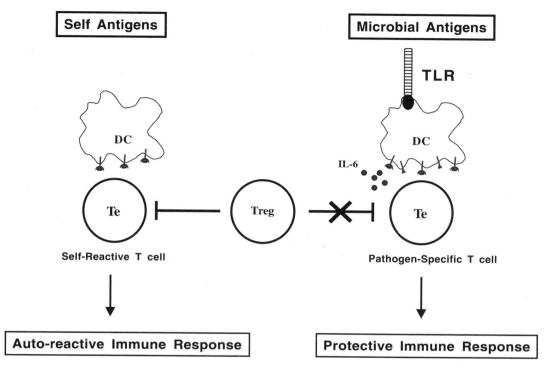

FIGURE 2 Control of T regulatory cell function by TLRs. Treg cells suppress activation of naive T cells and prevent responses to self-antigens. During an infection, TLR ligation on DCs leads to upregulation of MHC and costimulatory molecules as well as production of cytokines such as IL-6. IL-6 provides signals to effector T cells (Te) that render them resistant to the effects of Treg cells, allowing T-cell activation to proceed.

shown to be resistant to several autoimmune diseases (Samoilova et al., 1998; Sasai et al., 1999). This resistance may be due to the role of this cytokine in making effector T cells refractory to Treg cell-mediated suppression.

Cytokines and Their Role in Lymphocyte Differentiation

The wide array of infectious organisms presents a range of challenges to the immune system that must be dealt with using distinct effector responses. After activation, T cells differentiate into distinct subsets of effector cells that influence the nature of the ensuing adaptive immune response. This differentiation can be affected by the type of cytokines produced by DCs during maturation. Within this paradigm, engagement of TLRs on DCs by certain

pathogens will induce expression of cytokines that skew T-cell differentiation. For example, in response to gram-negative bacteria, which activate TLR4, myeloid DCs produce IL-12. IL-12 causes CD4 T cells to differentiate into Th1 cells (Murphy et al., 2000). Th1 cells produce IFN-γ that induces antibody class switching in B cells to produce antibodies of the IgG2 isotype. IgG2 antibodies are effective at eliminating a variety of intracellular and extracellular pathogens because they can fix complement and direct the lysis of infected cells in a process called antibody-dependent cellular cytotoxicity (Janeway et al., 2001). In general, the immune responses that are mounted against pathogens recognized by TLRs (i.e., bacteria, viruses, fungi, and protozoa) are dominated by Th1 cells. This is due to the fact that all TLRs induce the production of IL-12 and other Th1-inducing cytokines by DCs. A more conceptual explanation is that the types of pathogens with the unique features or metabolisms that can be targeted by pattern recognition are generally most effectively combated by Th1 responses.

Interestingly, host defense against multicellular parasites, such as helminthes, appears to follow distinct mechanisms of detection and protection. Worm infection generally leads to differentiation of Th2 cells, which produce IL-4, IL-5, and IL-13 (Maizels and Yazdanbakhsh, 2003). These cytokines induce production of IgE antibodies, which are much better suited for the elimination of large, multicellular pathogens. Cross-linking of IgE bound to FcεR results in degranulation of mast cells, basophils, and eosinophils, creating a microenvironment that is extremely hostile to the invading parasite (Maizels and Yaz-

danbakhsh, 2003). How Th2 effector responses are induced is not well understood and is an area of intense interest. In particular, it is not known how multicellular parasites could be recognized by the innate immune system. Because they are multicellular eukaryotes, it is possible that worms do not possess any unique metabolic products that can be targeted by pattern recognition. Alternatively, some, as yet uncharacterized, PRRs may detect worm-specific glycans (Fig. 3). Another possibility is that multicellular parasites are detected entirely by the missing-self strategy. Whichever is the case, it appears that the strategy of recognition in this case differs considerably from the one mediated by TLRs.

CONCLUSIONS AND PERSPECTIVES

In this chapter we have described the current understanding of how self/nonself discrimination by the innate immune system is linked to

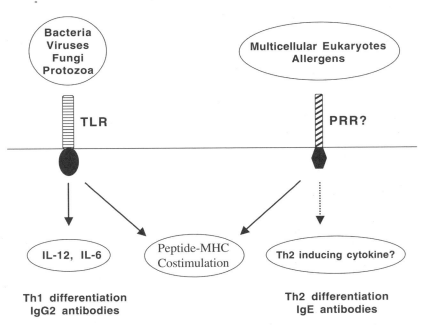

FIGURE 3 Innate immune recognition controls induction of differential immune responses. Microbes that engage TLRs induce a characteristic adaptive immune response leading to Th1 T-cell differentiation and the production of IgG2 antibodies. Large multicellular pathogens, such as worms, induce Th2 T-cell differentiation and the production of IgE antibodies. How innate recognition of worms is achieved and how this recognition leads to induction of Th2 differentiation remain unclear.

induction of adaptive immune responses. As we discussed, the innate immune system has evolved several different mechanisms to distinguish self from nonself. However, pattern recognition by TLRs appears to be the central event by which pathogens are identified as nonself. In this way, recognition of pathogens is linked to the signals necessary for initiation of adaptive immune responses. Most of these signals are delivered through DCs, as these cells recognize pathogens using TLRs, deliver pathogen-derived antigens from the tissues to the secondary lymphoid organs, and prime T cells by providing costimulation and the appropriate cytokines. By linking this series of events to microbial recognition, the system ensures that the responses will not be mounted against self-antigens or innocuous nonself antigens. A number of outstanding questions remain. Most notably, how are responses initiated to pathogens that are not recognized by TLRs, such as helminthes? Further understanding of the innate immune system in general will undoubtedly lead to greater appreciation of the complex mechanisms governing self/nonself discrimination and controlling adaptive immune responses.

REFERENCES

Alonzi, T., E. Fattori, D. Lazzaro, P. Costa, L. Probert, G. Kollias, F. De Benedetti, V. Poli, and G. Ciliberto. 1998. Interleukin 6 is required for the development of collagen-induced arthritis. *J. Exp. Med.* **187:**461–468.

Anderson, M. S., E. S. Venanzi, L. Klein, Z. Chen, S. P. Berzins, S. J. Turley, H. von Boehmer, R. Bronson, A. Dierich, C. Benoist, and D. Mathis. 2002. Projection of an immunological self shadow within the thymus by the aire protein. *Science* **298:**1395–1401.

Asano, M., M. Toda, N. Sakaguchi, and S. Sakaguchi. 1996. Autoimmune disease as a consequence of developmental abnormality of a T cell subpopulation. *J. Exp. Med.* **184:**387–396.

Asselin-Paturel, C., A. Boonstra, M. Dalod, I. Durand, N. Yessaad, C. Dezutter-Dambuyant, A. Vicari, A. O'Garra, C. Biron, F. Briere, and G. Trinchieri. 2001. Mouse type I IFN-producing cells are immature APCs with plasmacytoid morphology. *Nat. Immunol.* **2:**1144–1150.

Banchereau, J., and R. M. Steinman. 1998. Dendritic cells and the control of immunity. *Nature* **392:**245–252.

Borriello, F., M. P. Sethna, S. D. Boyd, A. N. Schweitzer, E. A. Tivol, D. Jacoby, T. B. Strom, E. M. Simpson, G. J. Freeman, and A. H. Sharpe. 1997. B7-1 and B7-2 have overlapping, critical roles in immunoglobulin class switching and germinal center formation. *Immunity* **6:**303–313.

Brunner, T., R. J. Mogil, D. LaFace, N. J. Yoo, A. Mahboubi, F. Echeverri, S. J. Martin, W. R. Force, D. H. Lynch, C. F. Ware, and D. R. Green. 1995. Cell-autonomous Fas (CD95)/Fas-ligand interaction mediates activation-induced apoptosis in T-cell hybridomas. *Nature* **373:**441–444.

Chen, Y., V. K. Kuchroo, J. Inobe, D. A. Hafler, and H. L. Weiner. 1994. Regulatory T cell clones induced by oral tolerance: suppression of autoimmune encephalomyelitis. *Science* **265:**1237–1240.

Cresswell, P., N. Bangia, T. Dick, and G. Diedrich. 1999. The nature of the MHC class I peptide loading complex. *Immunol. Rev.* **172:**21–28.

Cyster, J. G., S. B. Hartley, and C. C. Goodnow. 1994. Competition for follicular niches excludes self-reactive cells from the recirculating B-cell repertoire. *Nature* **371:**389–395.

Dalod, M., T. P. Salazar-Mather, L. Malmgaard, C. Lewis, C. Asselin-Paturel, F. Briere, G. Trinchieri, and C. A. Biron. 2002. Interferon alpha/beta and interleukin 12 responses to viral infections: pathways regulating dendritic cell cytokine expression in vivo. *J. Exp. Med.* **195:**517–528.

Dhein, J., H. Walczak, C. Baumler, K. M. Debatin, and P. H. Krammer. 1995. Autocrine T-cell suicide mediated by APO-1/(Fas/CD95). *Nature* **373:**438–441.

Diefenbach, A., and D. H. Raulet. 2001. Strategies for target cell recognition by natural killer cells. *Immunol. Rev.* **181:**170–184.

Drakesmith, H., B. Chain, and P. Beverley. 2000. How can dendritic cells cause autoimmune disease? *Immunol. Today* **21:**214–217.

Fontenot, J. D., M. A. Gavin, and A. Y. Rudensky. 2003. Foxp3 programs the development and function of CD4+CD25+ regulatory T cells. *Nat. Immunol.* **4:**330–336.

Goodnow, C. C., J. Crosbie, S. Adelstein, T. B. Lavoie, S. J. Smith-Gill, D. Y. Mason, H. Jorgensen, R. A. Brink, H. Pritchard-Briscoe, M. Loughnan, and R. H. Loblay, R. J. Trent, and A. Basten. 1989. Clonal silencing of self-reactive B lymphocytes in a transgenic mouse model. *Cold Spring Harbor Symp. Quant. Biol.* **54**(Pt. 2):907–920.

Gorelik, L., and R. A. Flavell. 2002. Transforming growth factor-beta in T-cell biology. *Nat. Rev. Immunol.* **2:**46–53.

Groux, H., A. O'Garra, M. Bigler, M. Rouleau, S. Antonenko, J. E. de Vries, and M. G. Roncarolo. 1997. A CD4+ T-cell subset inhibits antigen-specific T-cell responses and prevents colitis. *Nature* **389:**737–742.

Hartley, S. B., J. Crosbie, R. Brink, A. B. Kantor, A. Basten, and C. C. Goodnow. 1991. Elimination from peripheral lymphoid tissues of self-reactive B lymphocytes recognizing membrane-bound antigens. *Nature* **353:**765–769.

Hori, S., T. Nomura, and S. Sakaguchi. 2003. Control of regulatory T cell development by the transcription factor Foxp3. *Science* **299:**1057–1061.

Huang, Q., D. Liu, P. Majewski, L. C. Schulte, J. M. Korn, R. A. Young, E. S. Lander, and N. Hacohen. 2001. The plasticity of dendritic cell responses to pathogens and their components. *Science* **294:**870–875.

Janeway, C. A., Jr. 1989. Approaching the asymptote? Evolution and revolution in immunology. *Cold Spring Harb. Symp. Quant. Biol.* **54**(Pt 1):1–13.

Janeway, C. A., Jr., P. Travers, M. Walport, and M. Schlomchik. 2001. *Immunobiology: the Immune System in Health and Disease,* 5th ed. Garland Publishing, New York, N.Y.

Jenkins, M. K., and R. H. Schwartz. 1987. Antigen presentation by chemically modified splenocytes induces antigen-specific T cell unresponsiveness in vitro and in vivo. *J. Exp. Med.* **165:**302–319.

Ju, S. T., D. J. Panka, H. Cui, R. Ettinger, M. el-Khatib, D. H. Sherr, B. Z. Stanger, and A. Marshak-Rothstein. 1995. Fas(CD95)/FasL interactions required for programmed cell death after T-cell activation. *Nature* **373:**444–448.

Kadowaki, N., S. Ho, S. Antonenko, R. W. Malefyt, R. A. Kastelein, F. Bazan, and Y. J. Liu. 2001. Subsets of human dendritic cell precursors express different toll-like receptors and respond to different microbial antigens. *J. Exp. Med.* **194:**863–869.

Kawabe, T., T. Naka, K. Yoshida, T. Tanaka, H. Fujiwara, S. Suematsu, N. Yoshida, T. Kishimoto, and H. Kikutani. 1994. The immune responses in CD40-deficient mice: impaired immunoglobulin class switching and germinal center formation. *Immunity* **1:**167–178.

Khattri, R., T. Cox, S. A. Yasayko, and F. Ramsdell. 2003. An essential role for Scurfin in CD4+CD25+ T regulatory cells. *Nat. Immunol.* **4:**337–342.

Kuhn, R., J. Lohler, D. Rennick, K. Rajewsky, and W. Muller. 1993. Interleukin-10-deficient mice develop chronic enterocolitis. *Cell* **75:**263–274.

Lantz, O., I. Grandjean, P. Matzinger, and J. P. Di Santo. 2000. Gamma chain required for naive CD4+ T cell survival but not for antigen proliferation. *Nat. Immunol.* **1:**54–58.

Liston, A., S. Lesage, J. Wilson, L. Peltonen, and C. C. Goodnow. 2003. Aire regulates negative selection of organ-specific T cells. *Nat. Immunol.* **4:**350–354.

Liu, Y., and C. A. Janeway, Jr. 1992. Cells that present both specific ligand and costimulatory activity are the most efficient inducers of clonal expansion of normal CD4 T cells. *Proc. Natl. Acad. Sci. USA* **89:**3845–3849.

Maizels, R. M., and M. Yazdanbakhsh. 2003. Immune regulation by helminth parasites: cellular and molecular mechanisms. *Nat. Rev. Immunol.* **3:**733–744.

Medzhitov, R. 2001. Toll-like receptors and innate immunity. *Nat. Rev. Immunol.* **1:**135–145.

Medzhitov, R., and C. A. Janeway, Jr. 1997. Innate immunity: the virtues of a nonclonal system of recognition. *Cell* **91:**295–298.

Mellman, I., S. J. Turley, and R. M. Steinman. 1998. Antigen processing for amateurs and professionals. *Trends Cell. Biol.* **8:**231–237.

Murphy, K. M., W. Ouyang, J. D. Farrar, J. Yang, S. Ranganath, H. Asnagli, M. Afkarian, and T. L. Murphy. 2000. Signaling and transcription in T helper development. *Annu. Rev. Immunol.* **18:**451–494.

Nakagawa, T. Y., and A. Y. Rudensky. 1999. The role of lysosomal proteinases in MHC class II-mediated antigen processing and presentation. *Immunol. Rev.* **172:**121–129.

Ohshima, S., Y. Saeki, T. Mima, M. Sasai, K. Nishioka, S. Nomura, M. Kopf, Y. Katada, T. Tanaka, M. Suemura, and T. Kishimoto. 1998. Interleukin 6 plays a key role in the development of antigen-induced arthritis. *Proc. Natl. Acad. Sci. USA* **95:**8222–8226.

Pasare, C., and R. Medzhitov. 2003. Toll pathway-dependent blockade of CD4+CD25+ T cell-mediated suppression by dendritic cells. *Science* **299:**1033–1036.

Raulet, D. H., R. E. Vance, and C. W. McMahon. 2001. Regulation of the natural killer cell receptor repertoire. *Annu. Rev. Immunol.* **19:**291–330.

Ravetch, J. V., and L. L. Lanier. 2000. Immune inhibitory receptors. *Science* **290:**84–89.

Richards, H. B., M. Satoh, M. Shaw, C. Libert, V. Poli, and W. H. Reeves. 1998. Interleukin 6 dependence of anti-DNA antibody production: evidence for two pathways of autoantibody formation in pristane-induced lupus. *J. Exp. Med.* **188:**985–990.

Rose, N. R. 1998. The role of infection in the pathogenesis of autoimmune disease. *Semin. Immunol.* **10:**5–13.

Sadlack, B., H. Merz, H. Schorle, A. Schimpl, A. C. Feller, and I. Horak. 1993. Ulcerative colitis-like disease in mice with a disrupted interleukin-2 gene. *Cell* **75:**253–261.

Sadlack, B., J. Lohler, H. Schorle, G. Klebb, H. Haber, E. Sickel, R. J. Noelle, and I. Horak. 1995. Generalized autoimmune disease in interleukin-2-deficient mice is triggered by an uncontrolled activation and proliferation of CD4+ T cells. *Eur. J. Immunol.* **25:**3053–3059.

Sakaguchi, S., N. Sakaguchi, M. Asano, M. Itoh, and M. Toda. 1995. Immunologic self-tolerance maintained by activated T cells expressing IL-2 receptor alpha-chains (CD25). Breakdown of a single mechanism of self-tolerance causes various autoimmune diseases. *J. Immunol.* **155:**1151–1164.

Samoilova, E. B., J. L. Horton, B. Hilliard, T. S. Liu, and Y. Chen. 1998. IL-6-deficient mice are resistant to experimental autoimmune encephalomyelitis: roles of IL-6 in the activation and differentiation of autoreactive T cells. *J. Immunol.* **161:**6480–6486.

Sasai, M., Y. Saeki, S. Ohshima, K. Nishioka, T. Mima, T. Tanaka, Y. Katada, K. Yoshizaki, M. Suemura, and T. Kishimoto. 1999. Delayed onset and reduced severity of collagen-induced arthritis in interleukin-6-deficient mice. *Arthritis Rheum.* **42:**1635–1643.

Schwartz, R. H. 2003. T cell anergy. *Annu. Rev. Immunol.* **21:**305–334.

Seder, R. A., and R. Ahmed. 2003. Similarities and differences in CD4+ and CD8+ effector and memory T cell generation. *Nat. Immunol.* **4:**835–842.

Shahinian, A., K. Pfeffer, K. P. Lee, T. M. Kundig, K. Kishihara, A. Wakeham, K. Kawai, P. S. Ohashi, C. B. Thompson, and T. W. Mak. 1993. Differential T cell costimulatory requirements in CD28-deficient mice. *Science* **261:**609–612.

Shull, M. M., I. Ormsby, A. B. Kier, S. Pawlowski, R. J. Diebold, M. Yin, R. Allen, C. Sidman, G. Proetzel, D. Calvin, N. Annunziata, and T. Doetschman. 1992. Targeted disruption of the mouse transforming growth factor-beta 1 gene results in multifocal inflammatory disease. *Nature* **359:**693–699.

Starr, T. K., S. C. Jameson, and K. A. Hogquist. 2003. Positive and negative selection of T cells. *Annu. Rev. Immunol.* **21:**139–176.

Steinman, R. M., D. Hawiger, and M. C. Nussenzweig. 2003. Tolerogenic dendritic cells. *Annu. Rev. Immunol.* **21:**685–711.

Takeda, K., T. Kaisho, and S. Akira. 2003. Toll-like receptors. *Annu. Rev. Immunol.* **21:**335–376.

Teague, T. K., P. Marrack, J. W. Kappler, and A. T. Vella. 1997. IL-6 rescues resting mouse T cells from apoptosis. *J. Immunol.* **158:**5791–5796.

Thornton, A. M., and E. M. Shevach. 1998. CD4+CD25+ immunoregulatory T cells suppress polyclonal T cell activation in vitro by inhibiting interleukin 2 production. *J. Exp. Med.* **188:**287–296.

Tonegawa, S. 1983. Somatic generation of antibody diversity. *Nature* **302:**575–581.

Tough, D. F., P. Borrow, and J. Sprent. 1996. Induction of bystander T cell proliferation by viruses and type I interferon in vivo. *Science* **272:**1947–1950.

Zheng, L., G. Fisher, R. E. Miller, J. Peschon, D. H. Lynch, and M. J. Lenardo. 1995. Induction of apoptosis in mature T cells by tumour necrosis factor. *Nature* **377:**348–351.

ANTIGEN-PRESENTING CELL RECEPTORS AND INNATE IMMUNITY: DIVERSITY, RECOGNITION, AND RESPONSES

Siamon Gordon

15

Macrophages (MΦs) and their specialized antigen-presenting derivatives, myeloid dendritic cells (DCs), are widely distributed throughout lympho-hematopoietic and other tissues. (For general reviews, see Gordon [2001, 2003b].) They maintain tissue homeostasis and are able to respond to local infection and injury by cell activation and destruction of invading microorganisms or by induced migration and presentation of antigens to T and B lymphocytes. Antigen-presenting cells (APCs) play an important role in innate immunity as well as in the regulation of an adaptive immune response. Their ability to recognize foreign and modified self, mediating clearance with or without inflammation, is central to these cellular responses. The nature of the APC receptors utilized and their complex functions have received a great deal of attention in the past decade. The emphasis in studies of immune recognition has to some extent shifted from lymphoid to myeloid cells, and in the latter case from classic receptors for opsonins such as antibody and complement to opsonin-independent receptors. Work on Toll-like receptors

(TLRs) revealed evolutionarily conserved pathways of mammals and flies and links between developmental and host defense mechanisms. However, the variety of nonopsonic, TLR-independent receptors and their role in immune recognition have not been integrated sufficiently into current concepts. In this chapter I consider selected scavenger and lectinlike APC receptors in relation to innate immunity to illustrate principles and provide questions for further study.

A BRIEF HISTORY

The modern era of MΦ receptor knowledge dates from the studies of Nussenzweig, Bianco, Silverstein, Rabinovitch, and their colleagues in the 1960s and 1970s. (For reviews, see Rabinovitch, 1995; Silverstein et al., 1977; Steinman and Moberg, 1994). The investigation of antibody- and complement-mediated phagocytosis of opsonized particles yielded insights into receptor delineation, functional activation, and the mechanism of uptake by zipperlike interactions between ligands and receptors, then still poorly defined. The generation of monoclonal antibodies (MAbs) for FcR by Unkeless (1979) and for the type 3 complement receptor (CR3) by Springer (Beller et al., 1982; Springer et al., 1978), Wright and

Siamon Gordon, Sir William Dunn School of Pathology, University of Oxford, South Parks Rd., Oxford OX1 3RE, United Kingdom

The Innate Immune Response to Infection
Ed. by S. H. E. Kaufmann, R. Medzhitov, and S. Gordon
©2004 ASM Press, Washington, D.C.

Detmers (1988), and other workers provided specific tools for further cellular studies (late 1970s). Subsequent cloning and molecular definition by Mellman et al. (1988), Law (1988), and others (1980s) and genetic ablation by Ravetch and Bolland (2001), Hogarth (FcR) (2002), Norton-Mayadas (Coxon et al., 1996), Beaudet (Lu et al., 1997), and others (CR3) (1990s) defined the roles of distinct receptors in effector and inhibitory functions. Concurrently, Aderem (Allen and Aderem, 1995), Cohn (Steinman and Moberg, 1994), and their colleagues contributed to improved understanding of the mechanisms of particle uptake, the role of the cytoskeleton in this process, and the link between phagocytosis and secretion of arachidonates and other metabolic products.

It became apparent that CR3 could mediate a range of functions, interacting with a cleaved complement-derived protein (iC3b), as well as poorly defined ligands on pathogens and host components, even in the absence of an exogenous source of complement (Ezekowitz et al., 1985). Another apparently promiscuous scavenger receptor (SR) for artificially modified low-density lipoproteins (acetylated LDLs) was discovered by Brown and Goldstein (1983) and later cloned by Krieger, Kodama, and colleagues (Rohrer et al., 1990). From initial emphasis on foam cell formation and atherogenesis, studies of the role of this and other SRs in apoptotic cell clearance (Platt et al., 1996) and host defense (Dunne et al., 1994) gathered pace. At the same time, an endocytosis receptor for mannosyl glycoconjugates and lysosomal hydrolases (mannose receptor [MR]) was discovered by Stahl (reviewed by East and Isacke, 2002). The MR was cloned by Taylor et al. (1992) and by Ezekowitz and colleagues (1990). These prototype receptors set the stage for, but were rapidly overtaken by, the explosive interest that followed the discovery of TLRs in mammalian cells and of their role in lipopolysaccharide (LPS)-induced activation of NF-κB pathways and proinflammatory cytokine secretion (Poltorak et al., 1998). This work meshed with the earlier discovery of CD14 and the LPS-binding protein (LBP) as transducers of LPS responses (reviewed by Triantafilou and Triantafilou, 2002).

Many groups have contributed to the molecular, genetic, and functional characterization of the TLR, as described elsewhere in this volume. Perhaps most intriguing is the apparent ability of *Drosophila* (Imler and Hoffmann, 2001), as well as mammalian phagocytes, to respond differentially to different classes of organism (gram-positive and -negative bacteria and fungi), utilizing TLRs and other microbial recognition molecules, including receptors for peptidoglycans (Liu et al., 2001).

SOME GENERAL FEATURES

APC Heterogeneity

Tissue MΦs display considerable heterogeneity, including their expression of differentiation antigens such as F4/80, macrosialin (FA.11), and sialoadhesin (see Gordon et al. [1992] for a review). It is useful to distinguish resident MΦs, constitutively distributed during development and throughout adult life in the absence of inflammation, from elicited and activated MΦs recruited in response to sterile and immune inflammatory stimuli, respectively (Fig. 1). Resident MΦs differ from monocytes and vary in different microenvironments such as brain, liver, and gut. Inflammatory MΦs resemble monocytes more closely and express different properties depending on their cytokine milieu and local interactions with microorganisms. Innate activation is characterized by induction of APC costimulatory antigens and secretion of proinflammatory cytokines; classical immune activation is a feature of gamma interferon-induced gene expression, upregulated major histocompatibility complex (MHC) class II antigens and priming to secrete reactive oxygen and nitrogen metabolites and proinflammatory cytokines; alternative immune activation, on the other hand, is associated with interleukin-4 (IL-4)- and IL-13-induced upregulation of MHC class II antigens, enhanced MR expression, and promotion of antibody production and tissue repair

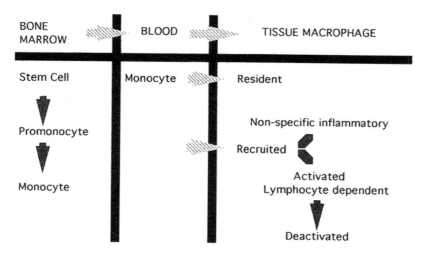

FIGURE 1 Heterogeneity of MΦs, including activation.

(Gordon, 2003a). Classical activation is mainly directed at intracellular pathogens, for example, *Mycobacterium tuberculosis,* and alternate activation is mainly directed at extracellular parasites such as schistosomes. Innate and immune deactivation are brought about by cytokines such as IL-10 and transforming growth factor β (TGF-β), which downregulate MHC class II expression and production of inflammatory mediators.

Myeloid DCs can be generated from bone marrow or blood mononuclear cells in vitro and are distinguished as immature cells, able to capture antigen, or as mature APCs, after exposure to various signals including LPS, that act through TLRs to induce cell activation (Banchereau et al., 2000). Maturation is accompanied by surface expression of MHC class II and costimulatory molecules, and the cells acquire the ability to present processed antigens efficiently to naive as well as primed T lymphocytes. In vivo DCs are markedly heterogeneous and do not necessarily correspond to in vitro-generated DCs; immature precursors, such as Langerhans cells, are present in epithelia and can be induced to migrate to draining lymph nodes and to T- and B-cell areas in the spleen by antigenic stimuli. Recently a distinct form of differentiation into

plasmacytoid DCs has been identified, with different functions (Shortman and Liu, 2002). Differentiation of DCs as well as extrinsic factors determines their ability to modulate the adaptive immune response to enhance or suppress immunity. MΦs are also able to present antigens to primed T lymphocytes, but additionally contribute potently to immune suppression and even tolerance.

Pattern Recognition and APC Repertoire

The concept of pattern recognition receptors (PRRs) interacting with pathogen-associated molecular patterns has received widespread attention following the work of Janeway (1989) and Medzhitov et al. (1997). Genes for the PRRs of the innate immune system have become fixed in the germ line during evolution, unlike the recombinant genes generated in somatic cells, which determine clonotypic recognition by T and B lymphocytes in the acquired immune response. The diversity of the repertoire generated in lymphoid cells by gene rearrangement is responsible for improved specificity and for immunological memory. However, it is now apparent that the recognition repertoire of APCs is also broad; preformed receptors exist not mainly for

MHC-associated peptides, as in the adaptive response, but for a broad spectrum of ligands including proteins, saccharides, lipids, and nucleic acids. These receptors, examples of which are shown in Fig. 2 and 3 and discussed below, often work in combination with one another. Their expression on APCs is regulated by diverse endogenous and exogenous stimuli, and individual receptors themselves often bind a range of ligands, including foreign structures (e.g., microbial) and altered self-structures (e.g., apoptotic cells, protein complexes, or modified proteins) (Gordon, 2002). In addition, other plasma membrane molecules such as SIRPα and C1q receptor-related proteins (Brown and Frazier, 2001), several members of the epidermal growth factor–TM7 family of adhesion receptors (Stacey et al., 2000), and CD200R (Barclay et al., 2002) are able to regulate the functions of primary endocytic and phagocytic receptors and to modulate recognition and cell activation.

APC Responses

Recognition can result in efficient uptake of ligands or particles by receptor-mediated endocytosis or phagocytosis. Involvement of the cytoskeleton depends on the size of the captured ligand and the requirement for bulk membrane engagement. The recruitment and assembly of cytosolic and membrane-associated signal transduction molecules by nonopsonic receptors is poorly defined, compared with knowledge of opsonic CR3 and FcR and TLR-dependent pathways (Aderem and Underhill, 1991; Greenberg and Grinstein, 2002). Examples of possible cooperation between nonopsonic receptors and TLRs have been reported and are considered below. Gene expression programs induced by different agents and cytokines are under investigation in an ever-growing number of microarray studies (Boldrick et al., 2002; Ehrt et al., 2001; Nau et al., 2002). Responses by receptors to distinct ligand stimuli can overlap or be largely independent. The generation of MHC-associated peptide complexes for antigen presentation and induction of cell migration and altered adhesion is a characteristic property of APC that cannot yet be ascribed to the engagement of particular recognition receptors.

SELECTED RECEPTORS

TLR and CD14

The role of TLR and CD14 in the innate immune response is described in detail elsewhere in this volume and has been reviewed extensively elsewhere (Imler and Hoffmann, 2001). Here, I briefly note some features pertinent to the present discussion. CD14 is a GPI-linked receptor for LBP and plays a central role in LPS responses, but other functions (for example, apoptotic cell clearance [Devitt et al., 1998], lipoprotein homeostasis) have also been described. Because CD14 lacks a cytoplasmic tail, the TLRs have been implicated in CD14-dependent signal transduction, together with other peripheral and cytosolic proteins. The TLRs are a family of transmembrane molecules, related to the IL-1 receptor (IL-1R), and achieve the ability to transduce signals from a range of microbial ligands through combinatorial homo- and heterodimerization (Ozinsky et al., 2000). Because the TLRs probably do not bind directly to ligands such as LPS, they may associate with more proximal ligand-binding receptors such as CD14 or dectin-1 (see below) in a signal relay process. It is likely that multiple APC receptors interact simultaneously with the complex arrays of ligands on the surface of a bacterium, influencing their avidity, selectivity, and signaling capacity. Although the majority of known ligands upstream of TLR are exogenous, it is possible that endogenous ligands, generated extra- as well as intracellularly, can signal through TLRs.

CR3

As alluded to above, the myeloid cell receptor CR3 exemplifies many of the issues relating to nonopsonic as well as opsonic recognition. Opsonization by classical, alternative, or lectin pathways can result in the deposition, and thiolester-dependent covalent attachment, of cleaved iC3b on the surface of a particle. The

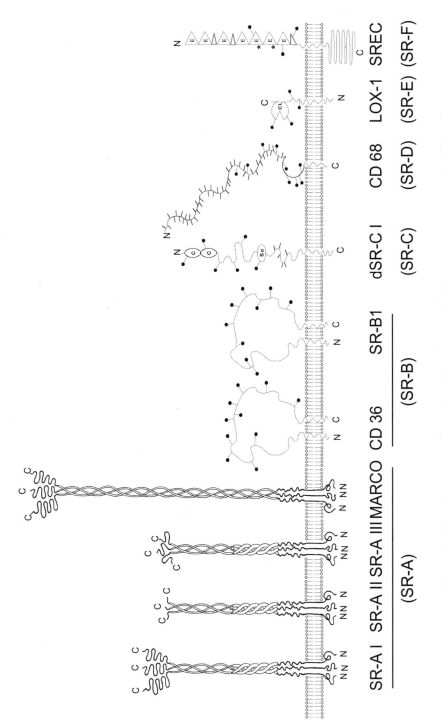

FIGURE 2   SRs. LOX-1, lectin–like oxidized LDL receptor; SREC, scavenger receptor, endothelial cells.

phagocytic mechanism of complement versus antibody-opsonized targets can be distinguished morphologically (Aderem and Underhill, 1999) and by its dependence on different small GTPases (Caron and Hall, 1998). In the absence of an exogenous source of complement, CR3 can bind directly to selected targets (e.g., saccharides of zymosan) or to other protein ligands derived from the coagulation cascade or activated adhesion molecules, such as intercellular adhesion molecule 1. It is also possible that MΦs themselves are able to opsonize zymosan, an extremely efficient trap for complement activation, by local secretion of alternative pathway components in their local in vitro microenvironment (Ezekowitz et al., 1985). Apart from its role in phagocytosis, CR3 contributes to adhesion to inflamed endothelium, together with other β_2 integrins, as shown by genetic absence (Anderson and Springer, 1987), ablation (Coxon et al., 1996; Lu et al., 1997), or monoclonal antibody blockade (Rosen and Gordon, 1987). This is an important step in diapedesis of myelomonocytic cells. The ligands critical for CR3 binding to endothelium in vivo, or to serum-coated bacteriologic plastic substrates in vivo, are not defined. CR3 ligation does not result in secretory responses by MΦs, although it has been reported to upregulate MHC class II expression (Ding et al., 1987). Thus there is no triggered release of arachidonate (Steinman and Moberg, 1994) or respiratory burst metabolites (Wright and Silverstein, 1983; Yamamoto and Johnston, 1984), unlike that mediated by ligation of selected FcRs. This property may be physiologically important in the "silent" uptake of apoptotic cells (Mevorach et al., 1998), but is also inviting to pathogens such as *M. tuberculosis,* providing a potentially safe entry mechanism into MΦs (Ehlers, 1999).

There are many puzzles regarding CR3 expression and functions that remain unanswered. What is the molecular basis for the "activation" of CR3 as an ingestion receptor by inflammatory stimuli such as thioglycolate broth, widely used as an inflammation-eliciting stimulus (Bianco et al., 1975)? What is the significance of abundant constitutive CR3 expression on microglia (Reid et al., 1994) given that many other resident tissue MΦs at portals of entry (lung) or in contact with blood (Kupffer cells) fail to express CR3? Inflammatory stimuli, on the other hand, induce newly recruited CR3[+] monocytes to enter these sites while upregulating CR3 expression in circulating myeloid cells. Further issues are the possible interactions between CR3 and other receptors, e.g., lectins or FcR, in the uptake of complex ligands such as *Leishmania* promastigotes (Blackwell et al., 1985) and the distinctive functions of CR3 on polymorphonuclear leukocytes and NK cells.

SR, Class A

The SR-A molecule has two functional (I and II) and one nonfunctional (III) isoforms (Fig. 2), depending on differential exon splicing (Peiser et al., 2002a). It is a distinct gene product from MARCO (macrophage collagenous receptor), a similar collagenlike type 2 transmembrane glycoprotein (Elomaa et al., 1995). Other so-called SRs have completely different structures, but may share functional properties, for example, the uptake of polyanionic ligands such as DII–acetylated LDL, apoptotic cells, and, where examined, bacteria. Here we restrict discussion to SR-A I/II and MARCO, best studied in relation to innate immunity.

Murine SR-A I/II can be defined antigenically by means of a rat MAb, 2F8 (Fraser et al., 1993), and its function has been analyzed in knockout mice (Suzuki et al., 1997). SR-A is expressed by many tissue MΦs and selected endothelia (Hughes et al., 1995). Early reports indicated that SR-A is host protective following in vivo challenge by *Listeria monocytogenes* and *Staphylococcus aureus,* as well as herpesvirus (Suzuki et al., 1997). After priming of MΦs by *Mycobacterium bovis* BCG infection followed by challenge with LPS, the presence of SR-A limits tumor necrosis factor alpha (TNF-α) release into the blood and results in septic shock (Haworth et al., 1997). SR-A function in innate immunity has not been fully analyzed in vivo, but in vitro model systems have contributed to our understanding of its role in uptake of bacteria (Peiser et al., 2000, 2002b).

SR-A I/II plays a variable role in the binding and uptake of unopsonized live and ethanol-killed bacteria. Phagocytosis of *Neisseria meningitidis* shows a strong dependence (>90%) on SR-A I/II when bone marrow culture-derived MΦs from wild-type and SR-A knockout mice are challenged with fluorescein isothiocyanate-labeled organisms. In the case of *Escherichia coli* and *S. aureus*, SR-A-specific polyanion-sensitive receptors contribute one half or more to the uptake, whereas organisms such as *Haemophilus influenzae* can be essentially independent of SR-A I/II. Other variables include the expression of SR-A I/II, depending on culture conditions (e.g., the presence of MΦ colony-stimulating factor, an upregulator of SR-A I/II, or of a serum ligand that serves to downregulate SR-A I/II on adherent cells) and the source of the MΦs. Freshly isolated peritoneal MΦs elicited by Bio-Gel polyacrylamide bead injection 4 days prior to harvest utilize SR-A I/II (about one third to one half), but also other still undefined SRs. Binding of *N. meningitidis* via SR-A I/II in MΦs is followed by rapid ingestion, cytokine release (TNF-α, IL-12, IL-6, IL-10), and killing. In the bone marrow–cultured MΦ model and depending on the multiplicity of infection, some organisms survive and may eventually escape into the extracellular medium. Although lipid A is a known ligand for SR-A I/II, uptake of LPS-deficient mutant *Neisseria* shows an SR-A dependence similar to that of wild-type bacteria, indicating that other ligands are also present on the bacteria. Study of the in vitro model has shown that phagocytosis via SR-A can be dissociated from TNF-α production, which depends on LPS and TLR4, as shown with MΦ from C3H/HeJ strain mice.

N. meningitidis is a potent immune adjuvant, inducing the expression of costimulatory molecules, but not MHC class II, as well as that of MARCO. Many interesting questions remain regarding the nature of the SR-A ligands and the role of uptake of the organism by MΦs in pathogenesis of infection and its sequelae. The further analysis of innate activation and of its regulation in MΦs should benefit from studies with this and related organisms.

MARCO is constitutively expressed by few MΦs (strongly on marginal zone, weakly on resident peritoneal MΦs), but is rapidly upregulated by microbial challenge, or LPS, in vivo or in vitro; its natural ligands and functions remain undefined (Van der Laan et al., 1999).

LECTINS AND LECTINLIKE RECEPTORS

MΦs and other myeloid cells express a range of lectins and lectinlike molecules that contribute to interactions with organisms as well as host ligands. Perhaps best characterized are the receptor for β-glucans, dectin-1, and the multilectin MΦ MR (Fig. 3).

Dectin-1

Dectin-1 was originally described as a DC-restricted molecule of unknown function, but retrovirus-based expression cloning by Brown and Gordon (2001) identified it as a β-glucan receptor of MΦs and other myeloid cells, which efficiently bound and ingested zymosan particles and various fungi when expressed at high levels on 3T3 fibroblast-like cells. Dectin-1 is a type II transmembrane molecule with a C-type lectin-like extracellular domain and contains an immunoreceptor tyrosine-based activation (ITAM) motif in its cytoplasmic tail, which has been implicated in phagocytic uptake. Dectin-1-transfected fibroblasts bind and ingest zymosan with the appropriate sugar specificity (linear and branched β-1,3- and β-1,6-glucans, competed for by laminarin and glucan phosphate). Live *Saccharomyces cerevisiae*, *Pneumocystis carinii*, and heat-killed *Candida albicans* express ligands readily, unlike live *Candida* and other fungi such as *Histoplasma capsulatum* (although their walls are rich in β-glucans), consistent with masking of surface expression of β-glucan structures by pathogenic fungi.

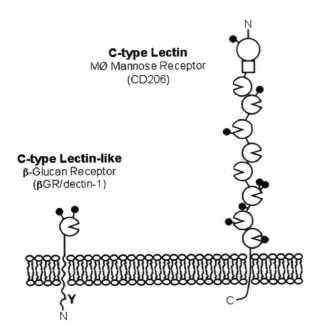

C-type Lectin
MØ Mannose Receptor
(CD206)

C-type Lectin-like
β-Glucan Receptor
(βGR/dectin-1)

FIGURE 3 Lectin and lectinlike receptors.

CR3, another candidate receptor for binding of yeast, is not essential for yeast uptake, as shown with MΦs from CR3 knockout mice (Brown et al., 2002). However, CR3 and other receptors such as the MR may cooperate with dectin-1 in yeast uptake in vivo. Similarly, dectin-1 contributes to uptake of zymosan even in the presence of complement. Apart from phagocytosis, the dectin-1 receptor mediates signalling of TNF-α secretion following initial binding (Brown et al., 2003). Signal transduction is also dependent on TLR2 for several secretory responses, but not for particle ingestion. Recent studies by two groups of investigators have explored the cooperation of dectin-1 and TLR in zymosan and fungal uptake and induced secretion (Brown et al., 2003; Gantner et al., 2003). This may prove to be a paradigm for a more general requirement of proximal recognition by a PRR, coupled to selective signal transduction involving TLR, adaptor molecules such as myeloid differentiation primary response protein 88, and NF-κB activation. Distinct receptors, which can be coexpressed on the cell surface or be recruited to phagosomes, can function synergistically or

independently of each other. This reinforces the notion that important cellular responses such as phagocytosis and secretion of inflammatory mediators can be dissociated.

MR

It is now clear that there are several distinct mannose recognition molecules expressed by mature MΦs and selected endothelia, including the classic multilectin MR (East and Isacke, 2002), DC-SIGN and DC-SIGN-related molecules (Geijtenbeek et al., 2002), and Langerin (Valladeau et al., 2000). Here we summarize studies on the MR, for which a range of exogenous and endogenous ligands has been defined.

The MR (Fig. 3) has eight calcium-dependent carbohydrate recognition domains (CRDs) and a cysteine-rich (CR) domain for which a role has been proposed in antigen transport (Martinez-Pomares and Gordon, 1999). Microbial ligands for the CRD include bacteria, viruses, fungi, and parasites. Microbial constituents thought to bind to the MR and related molecules include capsular polysaccharides, mannans, lipoarabinomannan, and selected

LPSs. Binding results in endocytic or phagocytic uptake of particulate or soluble ligands. Secretory responses and signaling pathways are still poorly understood.

Endogenous ligands for CRD include a group of lysosomal hydrolases, as confirmed by studies with MR knockout mice (Lee et al., 2002). In addition, CRD4-7 has been utilized as an Fc-chimeric fusion protein to identify ligands in endocrine and exocrine organs, such as thyroglobulin (Linehan et al., 2001). Other naturally occurring ligands include myeloperoxidase and tissue plasminogen activator.

The CR domain was also used as an Fc fusion protein to identify sulfated saccharide ligands in peripheral lymphoid organs (marginal metallophilic MΦs in spleen and subcapsular sinus MΦs in lymph nodes) (Martinez-Pomares et al., 1996). Similar ligands for the CR domain were implicated in clearance of anterior pituitary hormones by Fiete and colleagues (1998). No exogenous ligands have been described for the MR CR domain.

A soluble form of the MR has been detected in MΦ culture fluids and in plasma (Martinez-Pomares et al., 1998). This seems to be constitutively present, in contrast with the acute-phase mannose-binding lectin with similar specificity produced by hepatocytes.

The role of the MR in innate immunity and responses requires further study in vivo with defined reagents, e.g., MAb and knockout mice. Microbial products such as LPS induce changes in the distribution of CR ligand-bearing cells and may influence their uptake and processing of potential antigens. Thus, the MR plays a complex role in targeting and clearance of glycoconjugates, including microbial constituents. Early studies indicate that such targeting could serve to limit humoral responses.

Role of MΦ PRRs in the Induction of Acquired Immunity

Several in vitro models have shown that antigens captured by APCs via PRRs can be presented to T lymphocytes. These include modification epitopes reacting with SRs (unspecified) (Abraham et al., 1995) and mannosylated ligands recognized by MR (Engering et al., 1997; Prigozy et al., 1997). There is still limited knowledge of expression of SR-A by immature and mature DCs in vitro and expression of MR or SR-A by DCs in vivo. The competing fates (clearance, failure to elicit humoral or cellular immune responses versus enhanced immunogenicity) and effects of concurrent presence of microbial adjuvants should be borne in mind. Uptake of apoptotic cells by APC PRRs can bring about cross-presentation, but is more likely to result in immunosuppression. In vitro uptake of apoptotic cells via receptors, such as vitronectin receptors and CD36, CR3, and several other receptors, results in release of IL-10, TGF-β, and prostaglandin E_2, rather than of proinflammatory cytokines (Henson et al., 2001).

The TLR and other elements of the TLR signaling pathway play a critical role in the induction of a Th1-type acquired immune response, as shown with myeloid differentiation primary response protein 88 and Toll-IL-1 adaptor protein knockout mice (Barton and Medzhitov, 2003; Yamamoto et al., 2002). Innate microbial stimuli can also upregulate various TLRs. The role, if any, of non-TLR PRRs in induction of acquired immunity is less well understood.

The MR is a useful marker of alternative MΦ activation in vitro and may be induced by Schistosomal antigens on Th2 granulomata in vivo (Linehan et al., 2003). There is still no indication whether or how APCs discriminate between Th2- and Th1-inducing ligands.

CONCLUSION

Our knowledge of innate immune recognition by APC receptors and of the pathways leading to distinct responses is limited. This subject has become topical and will have considerable theoretical and practical implications in therapeutic modulation of host resistance to infection and vaccine development. In addition, improved understanding will bring insights into the pathogenesis of autoimmunity and of a range of inflammatory disease syndromes.

With the advent of powerful new tools for in situ as well as in vitro analysis, we can expect rapid progress in this field.

ACKNOWLEDGMENTS

Work in the author's laboratory has been supported by the Medical Research Council UK, The Wellcome Trust, the Arthritis Research Campaign, the Jenner Institute, and British Heart Foundation. I appreciate the stimulating discussions of my colleagues and collaborators and thank Christine Holt for her help in preparing this manuscript.

REFERENCES

Abraham, R., N. Singh, A. Mukhopadhyay, S. K. Basu, V. Bal, and S. Rath. 1995. Modulation of immunogenicity and antigenicity of proteins by maleylation to target scavenger receptors on macrophages. *J. Immunol.* **154:**1–8.

Aderem, A., and D. M. Underhill. 1999. Mechanisms of phagocytosis in macrophages. *Annu. Rev. Immunol.* **17:**593–623.

Allen, L. A. H., and A. Aderem. 1995. A role for MARCKS, the α isozyme of protein kinase C and a myosin I in zymosan phagocytosis by macrophages. *J. Exp. Med.* **182:**829–840.

Anderson, D. C., and T. A. Springer. 1987. Leukocyte adhesion deficiency: an inherited defect in Mac-1, LFA-1 and p150,95 glycoproteins. *Annu. Rev. Med.* **38:**175–194.

Banchereau, J., F. Briere, C. Caux, J. Davoust, S. Lebecque, Y. J. Liu, B. Pulendran, and K. Palucka. 2000. Immunobiology of dendritic cells. *Annu. Rev. Immunol.* **18:**767–811.

Barclay, A. N., G. J. Wright, G. Brooke, and M. H. Brown. 2002. CD200 and membrane protein interactions in the control of myeloid cells. *Trends Immunol.* **213:**285–290.

Barton, G. M., and R. Medzhitov. 2003. Toll-like receptor signaling pathways. *Science* **300:**1524–1525.

Beller, D. I., T. A. Springer, and R. D. Schreiber. 1982. Anti Mac-1 selectively inhibits the mouse and human type three complement receptor. *J. Exp. Med.* **156:**1000–1009.

Bianco, C., F. M. Griffin, Jr., and S. C. Silverstein. 1975. The macrophage complement receptor. Alteration of receptor function upon macrophage activation. *J. Exp. Med.* **141:**1278–1290.

Blackwell, J. M., R. A. B. Ezekowitz, M. B. Roberts, J. Y. Channon, R. B. Sim, and S. Gordon. 1985. Macrophage complement and lectin-like receptors bind Leishmania in the absence of serum. *J. Exp. Med.* **162:**324–331.

Boldrick, J. C., A. A. Alizadeh, M. Diehn, S. Dudoit, C. L. Liu, C. E. Belcher, D. Botstein, L. M. Staudt, P. O. Brown, and D. A. Relman. 2002. Stereotyped and specific gene-expression programs in human innate immune responses to bacteria. *Proc. Natl. Acad. Sci. USA* **99:**972–977.

Brown, E. J., and W. A. Frazier. 2001. Integrin-associated protein (CD47) and its ligands. *Trends Cell Biol.* **11:**130–135.

Brown, G. D., and S. Gordon. 2001. A new receptor for β-glucans. *Nature* **413:**36–37.

Brown, G. D., P. R. Taylor, D. M. Reid, D. L. Williams, J. A. Willment, L. Martinez-Pomares, S. Y. C. Wong, and S. Gordon. 2002. Dectin-1 is a major β-glucan receptor on macrophages. *J. Exp. Med.* **196:**407–412.

Brown, G. D., J. Herre, D. L. Williams, J. A. Willment, A. S. J. Marshall, and S. Gordon. 2003. Dectin-1 mediates the biological effects of β-glucans. *J. Exp. Med.* **197:**1119–1124.

Brown, M. S., and J. L. Goldstein. 1983. Lipoprotein metabolism in the macrophage: implications for cholestrol deposition in atherosclerosis. *Annu. Rev. Biochem.* **52:**223–261.

Caron, E., and A. Hall. 1998. Identification of two distinct mechanisms of phagocytosis controlled by different Rho GTPases. *Science* **282:**1717–1721.

Coxon, A., P. Rieu, F. J. Barkalow, S. Askari, A. H. Sharpe, U. H. von Andrian, M. A. Arnaout, and T. Norton-Mayadas. 1996. A novel role for the β2 integrin CD11b/CD18 in neutrophil apoptosis: a homeostatic mechanism in inflammation. *Immunity* **5:**653–666.

Devitt, A., O. D. Moffatt, C. Raykundalia, J. D. Capra, D. J. Simmons, and C. D. Gregory. 1998. Human CD14 mediates recognition and phagocytosis of apoptotic cells. *Nature* **392:**505–509.

Ding, A., S. D. Wright, and C. Nathan. 1987. Activation of mouse peritoneal macrophages by monoclonal antibody to Mac-1 (complement receptor three). *J. Exp. Med.* **165:**733–749.

Dunne, D. W., D. Resnick, J. Greenberg, M. Krieger, and K. A. Joiner. 1994. The type I macrophage scavenger receptor binds to gram-positive bacteria and recognizes lipoteichoic acid. *Proc. Natl. Acad. Sci. USA* **91:**1863–1867.

East, L., and C. M. Isacke. 2002. The mannose-receptor family. *Biochim. Biophys. Acta* **1572:**364–386.

Ehlers, M. R. W. 1999. The role of complement receptor type 3 in the invasion strategies of *Mycobacterium tuberculosis*, p. 81–105. *In* S. Gordon (ed.), *Phagocytosis: Microbial Invasion,* vol. 6. JAI Press Inc., Stamford, Conn.

Ehrt, S., D. Schnappinger, S. Bekiranov, J. Drenkow, S. Shi, T. R. Gingeras, T. Gaasterland, G. Schoolnik, and C. Nathan. 2001. Reprogramming of the macrophage transcriptome in response to Interferonγ and *Mycobacterium tuberculosis.* Signalling roles of nitric oxide synthase-2 and phagocyte oxidase. *J. Exp. Med.* **194:**1123–1140.

Elomaa, O., M. Kangas, C. Sahlberg, J. Tuukkanen, R. Sormunen, A. Liakka, I. Thesleff, G. Kraal, and K. Tryggvason. 1995. Cloning of a novel bacteria-binding receptor structurally related to scavenger receptors and expressed in a subset of macrophages. *Cell* **80:**603–609.

Engering, A. J., M. Cella, D. Fluitsma, M. Brockhaus, E. C. Hoefsmit, A. Lanzavecchia, and J. Pieters. 1997. The mannose receptor functions as a high capacity and broad specificity antigen receptor in human dendritic cells. *Eur. J. Immunol.* **27:**2417–2425.

Ezekowitz, R. A. B., R. B. Sim, G. G. MacPherson, and S. Gordon. 1985. Interaction of human monocytes, macrophages and polymorphonuclear leukocytes with zymosan in vitro. Role of type 3 complement receptors and macrophage-derived complement. *J. Clin. Invest.* **76:**2368–2376.

Ezekowitz, R. A. B., K. Sastry, P. Bailly, and A. Warner. 1990. Molecular characterization of the human macrophage mannose receptor: demonstration of multiple carbohydrate recognition-like domains and phagocytosis of yeasts in Cos-1 cells. *J. Exp. Med.* **172:**1785–1794.

Fiete, D. J., M. C. Beranek, and J. U. Baenziger. 1998. A cysteine-rich domain of the "mannose" receptor mediates Ga1NAc-4-SO4 binding. *Proc. Natl. Acad. Sci. USA* **95:**2089–2093.

Fraser, I., D. Hughes, and S. Gordon. 1993. Divalent cation-independent macrophage adhesion inhibited by monoclonal antibody to murine scavenger receptor. *Nature* **364:**343–346.

Gantner, B. N., R. M. Simmons, S. J. Canavera, S. Akira, and D. M. Underhill. 2003. Collaborative induction of inflammatory responses by Dectin-1 and Toll-like receptor 2. *J. Exp. Med.* **197:**1107–1117.

Geijtenbeek, T. B. H., A. Engering, and Y. van Kook. 2002. DC-SIGN, a C-type lectin on dendritic cells that unveils many aspects of dendritic cell biology. *J. Leukoc. Biol.* **71:**921–931.

Gordon, S. 2001. Mononuclear phagocytes in immune defence, p. 147–162. *In* I. Roitt, B. Brostoff, and D. Male (ed.), *Immunology*, 6th ed. Mosby, Edinburgh, United Kingdom.

Gordon, S. 2002. Pattern recognition receptors: doubling up for the innate immune response. *Cell* **11:**1–4.

Gordon, S. 2003a. Alternative activation of macrophages. *Nat. Rev. Immunol.* **3:**23–35.

Gordon, S. 2003b. Macrophages and the immune response, p. 481–495. *In* W. Paul (ed.), *Fundamental Immunology*, 5th ed. Lippincott Raven, Philadelphia, Pa.

Gordon, S., L. Lawson, S. Rabinowitz, P. R. Crocker, L. Morris, and V. H. Perry. 1992. Antigen markers of macrophage differentiation in murine tissues. *Curr. Top. Microbiol. Immunol.* **181:**1–37.

Greenberg, S., and S. Grinstein. 2002. Phagocytosis and innate immunity. *Curr. Opin. Immunol.* **14:**136–145.

Haworth, R., N. Platt, S. Keshav, D. Hughes, E. Darley, H. Suzuki, Y. Kurihara, T. Kodama, and S. Gordon. 1997. The Macrophage Scavenger Receptor Type A (SR-A) is expressed by activated macrophages and protects the host against lethal endotoxic shock. *J. Exp. Med.* **186:**1431–1439.

Henson, P. M., D. L. Bratton, and V. A. Fadok. 2001. Apoptotic cell removal. *Curr. Biol.* **11:**R795–R805.

Hogarth, P. M. 2002. Fc receptors are major mediators of antibody based inflammation in autoimmunity. *Curr. Opin. Immunol.* **14:**798–802.

Hughes, D. A., I. P. Fraser, and S. Gordon. 1995. Murine Macrophage Scavenger Receptor: in vivo expression and function as receptor for macrophage adhesion in lymphoid and non-lymphoid organs. *Eur. J. Immunol.* **25:**466–473.

Imler, J. L., and J. A. Hoffmann. 2001. Toll receptors in innate immunity. *Trends Cell Biol.* **11:**304–311.

Janeway, C. A., Jr. 1989. Approaching the asymptote? Evolution and revolution in immunology. *Cold Spring Harbor Symp. Quant. Biol.* **54:**1–13.

Law, S. K. A. 1988. C3 receptors on macrophages. *J. Cell Sci.* **9**(Suppl.)**:**67–97.

Lee, S. J., S. Evers, D. Roeder, A. F. Parlow, J. Risteli, L. Risteli, Y. C. Lee, T. Feizi, H. Langen, and M. C. Nussenzweig. 2002. Mannose receptor-mediated regulation of serum glycoprotein homeostasis. *Science* **295:**1898–1901.

Linehan, S. A., L. Martinez-Pomares, R. Da Silva, and S. Gordon. 2001. Endogenous ligands of carbohydrate recognition domains of the mannose receptor in murine macrophages, endothelial cells and secretory cells; potential relevance to inflammation and immunity. *Eur. J. Immunol.* **31:**1857–1866.

Linehan, S. A., P. A. Coulson, R. A. Wilson, A. P. Mountford, F. Brombacher, L. Martinez-Pomares, and S. Gordon. 2003. IL-4 receptor signalling is required for mannose receptor expression by macrophages recruited to granulomata but not resident cells in mice infected with *Schistosoma mansoni*. *Lab. Invest.* **83:**1223–1231.

Liu, C., Z. Xu, D. Gupta, and R. Dziarski. 2001. Peptidoglycan recognition proteins: a novel family of four human innate immunity pattern recognition molecules. *J. Biol. Chem.* **276:**34686–34694.

Lu, H., C. W. Smith, J. Perrard, D. Bullard, L. Tang, S. B. Shappell, M. L. Entman, A. L. Beaudet, and C. M. Ballantyne. 1997. LFA-1 is sufficient in mediating neutrophil emigration in Mac-1-deficient mice. *J. Clin. Invest.* **99:**1340–1350.

Martinez-Pomares, L., and S. Gordon. 1999. The Mannose receptor and its role in antigen presentation. *Immunologist* **7:**119–123.

Martinez-Pomares, L., M. Kosco-Vilbois, E. Darley, P. Tree, S. Herren, J. Y. Bonnefoy, and S. Gordon. 1996. Fc chimeric protein containing the cysteine-rich domain of the murine mannose receptor binds to macrophages from splenic marginal zone and lymph node subcapsular sinus, and to germinal centres. *J. Exp. Med.* **184:**1927–1937.

Martinez-Pomares, L., J. A. Mahoney, R. Kaposzta, S. A. Linehan, P. D. Stahl, and S. Gordon. 1998. A functional soluble form of the murine mannose receptor is produced by macrophages in vitro and is present in mouse serum. *J. Biol. Chem.* **273:**23376–23380.

Medzhitov, R., P. Preston-Hurlburt, and C. A. Janeway, Jr. 1997. A human homologue of the *Drosophila* Toll protein signals activation of adaptive immunity. *Nature* **388:**394–397.

Mellman, I., T. Koch, G. Healey, W. Hunziker, V. Lewis, H. Plutner, H. Mettinen, D. J. Vaux, K. Moore, and S. Stuart. 1988. Structure and function of Fc receptors on macrophages and lymphocytes. *J. Cell Sci.* **9**(Suppl.):45–65.

Mevorach, D., J. O. Mascarenhas, D. Gershov, and K. B. Elkon. 1998. Complement-dependent clearance of apoptotic cells by human macrophages. *J. Exp. Med.* **188:**2313–2320.

Nau, G. J., J. F. L. Richmond, A. Schlesinger, E. G. Jennings, E. S. Lander, and R. A. Young. 2002. Human macrophage activation programs induced by bacterial pathogens. *Proc. Natl. Acad. Sci. USA* **99:**1503–1508.

Ozinsky, A., D. M. Underhill, J. D. Fontenot, A. M. Hajjar, K. D. Smith, C. B. Wilson, L. Schroeder, and A. Aderem. 2000. The repertoire for pattern recognition of pathogens by the innate immune system is defined by co-operation between Toll-like receptors. *Proc. Natl. Acad. Sci. USA* **97:**13766–13771.

Peiser, L., P. J. Gough, T. Kodama, and S. Gordon. 2000. Macrophage class A scavenger receptor-mediated phagocytosis of *Escherichia coli:* role of cell heterogeneity, microbial strain and culture conditions in vitro. *Infect. Immun.* **68:**1953–1963.

Peiser, L., S. Mukhopadhyay, and S. Gordon. 2002a. Scavenger receptors in innate immunity. *Curr. Opin. Immunol.* **14:**123–128.

Peiser, L., M. P. J. de Winther, K. Makepeace, M. Hollinshead, P. Coull, J. Plested, T. Kodama, E. R. Moxon, and S. Gordon. 2002b. The class A macrophage scavenger receptor is a major pattern-recognition receptor for *Neisseria meningitidis*, which is independent of lipopolysaccharide and not required for secretory responses. *Infect. Immun.* **70:**5346–5354.

Platt, N., H. Suzuki, Y. Kurihara, T. Kodama, and S. Gordon. 1996. Role for the Class A macrophage scavenger receptor in the phagocytosis of apoptotic thymocytes in vitro. *Proc. Natl. Acad. Sci. USA* **93:**12456–12460.

Poltorak, A., X. He, I. Smirnova, M. Y. Liu, C. V. Huffel, X. Du, D. Birdwell, E. Alejos, M. Silva, C.

Galanos, M. Freudenberg, P. Ricciardi-Castagnoli, B. Layton, and B. Beutler. 1998. Defective LPS signalling in C3H/HeJ and C57BL/10ScCr mice: mutations in TLR4 gene. *Science* **282:**2085–2088.

Pontow, S. E., V. Kery, and P. D. Stahl. 1992. Mannose receptor. *Int. Rev. Cytol.* **137B:**221–244.

Prigozy, T. I., P. A. Sieling, D. Clemens, P. L. Stewart, S. M. Behar, S. A. Porcelli, M. B. Brenner, R. L. Modlin, and M. Kronenberg. 1997. The mannose receptor delivers lipoglycan antigens to endosomes for presentation to T cells by CD1b molecules. *Immunity* **6:**187–197.

Rabinovitch, M. 1995. Professional and non-professional phagocytes: an introduction. *Trends Cell Biol.* **5:**85–87.

Ravetch, J. V., and S. Bolland. 2001. IgG Fc receptors. *Annu. Rev. Immunol.* **19:**275–290.

Reid, D. M., V. H. Perry, P. B. Andersson, and S. Gordon. 1994. Mitosis and apoptosis of microglia in vivo induced by an anti-CR3 antibody which crossed the blood-brain barrier. *Neuroscience* **56:**529–533.

Rohrer, L., M. Freeman, T. Kodama, M. Penman, and M. Krieger. 1990. Coiled-coil fibrous domains mediate ligand binding by macrophage scavenger receptor type III. *Nature* **343:**570–572.

Rosen, H., and S. Gordon. 1987. Monoclonal antibody to the murine type 3 complement receptor inhibits adhesion of myelomonocytic cells in vitro and inflammatory cell recruitment in vivo. *J. Exp. Med.* **166:**1685–1701.

Shortman, K., and Y. J. Liu. 2002. Mouse and human dendritic cell sub-types. *Nat. Immunol.* **2:**151–161.

Silverstein, S. C., R. M. Steinman, and Z. A. Cohn. 1977. Endocytosis. *Annu. Rev. Biochem.* **46:**669–722.

Springer, T., G. Galfré, D. S. Secher, and C. Milstein. 1978. Monoclonal xenogeneic antibodies to murine cell surface antigens: identification of novel leukocyte differentiation antigens. *Eur. J. Immunol.* **8:**539–551.

Stacey, M., H. H. Lin, S. Gordon, and A. J. McKnight. 2000. LNB-TM7, a novel group of seven-transmembrane proteins related to family-B G-protein-coupled receptors. *Trends Biochem. Sci.* **25:**284–289.

Steinman, R. M., and C. L. Moberg. 1994. Zanvil Alexander Cohn—1926–1993. *J. Exp. Med.* **179:**1–30.

Suzuki, H., Y. Kurihara, M. Takeya, N. Kamada, M. Kataoka, K. Jishage, O. Ueda, H. Sakaguchi, T. Higashi, T. Suzuki, Y. Takashima, Y. Kawabe, O. Cynshi, Y. Wada, M. Honda, H. Kirihara, H. Aburatani, T. Doi, A. Matsumoto, S. Azuma, T. Noda, Y. Toyoda, H. Itakura, Y. Yazaki, S. Horiuchi, K. Takashi, J. Kar Kruijt, T. J.C. van

Berkel, U. P. Steinbrecher, S. Ishibashi, N. Maeda, S. Gordon, and T. Kodama. 1997. A role for macrophage scavenger receptors in atherosclerosis and susceptibility to infection. *Nature* **386:**292–296.

Taylor, M. E., K. Bezouska, and K. Drickamer. 1992. Contribution to ligand binding by multiple carbohydrate-recognition domains in the macrophage mannose receptor. *J. Biol. Chem.* **267:**1719–1726.

Triantafilou, M., and K. Triantafilou. 2002. Lipopolysaccharide recognition: CD14, TLRs and the LPS-activation cluster. *Trends Immunol.* **23:**301–304.

Unkeless, J.C. 1979. Characterization of a monoclonal antibody directed against mouse macrophage and lymphocyte Fc receptors. *J. Exp. Med.* **150:**580–596.

Valladeau, J., O. Ravel, C. Dezutter-Dambuyant, K. Moore, M. Kleijmeer, Y. Liu, Y. Duvert-Frances, C. Vincent, D. Schmitt, J. Davoust, C. Caux, S. Lebeque, and S. Saeland. 2000. Langerin, a novel C-type lectin specific to Langerhans cells, is an endocytic receptor that induces the formation of Birbeck granules. *Immunity* **12:**71–81.

Van der Laan, L. J. W., E. A. Döpp, R. Haworth, T. Pikkarainen, M. Kangas, O. Elomaa, C. D. Dijkstra, S. Gordon, K. Tryggvason, and G. Kraal. 1999. Regulation and functional involvement of macrophage scavenger receptor MARCO in clearance of bacteria *in vivo. J. Immunol.* **2:**939–947.

Wright, S. D., and P. Detmers. 1988. Adhesion-promoting receptors in phagocytes. *J. Cell Sci.* **9**(Suppl.):99–120.

Wright, S. D., and S. C. Silverstein. 1983. Receptors for C3b and C3bi promote phagocytosis but not the release of toxic oxygen from human phagocytes. *J. Exp. Med.* **158:**2016–2023.

Yamamoto, K., and R. B. Johnston, Jr. 1984. Dissociation of phagocytosis from stimulation of the oxidative metabolic burst in macrophages. *J. Exp. Med.* **159:**405–416.

Yamamoto, M., S. Sato, H. Hemmi, H. Sanjo, S. Uematsu, T. Kaisho, K. Hoshino, O. Takeuchi, M. Kobayashi, T. Fujita, K. Takeda, and S. Akira. 2002. Essential role for TIRAP in activation of the signaling cascade shared by TLR2 and TLR4. *Nature* **420:**324–329.

THE FUNCTION OF LEUKOCYTE IMMUNOGLOBULIN-LIKE RECEPTORS IN SELF-TOLERANCE, VIRAL RECOGNITION, AND REGULATION OF ADAPTIVE RESPONSES

Marco Colonna and Winfried Barchet

16

INHIBITORY RECEPTORS: A MECHANISM FOR SELF-TOLERANCE

Immune cells have evolved multiple mechanisms to avoid immune responses against "self" (Goodnow, 1996; Miller and Morahan, 1992; Sprent and Kishimoto, 2000). One relatively straightforward way for immune cells to maintain tolerance is the expression of inhibitory receptors that recognize self. These receptors are quite diverse as they recognize a variety of ligands on different cell types (Ravetch and Lanier, 2000). Despite their diversity, all inhibitory receptors share tyrosine-based motifs in their cytoplasmic domains, called immunoreceptor tyrosine-based inhibitory motifs (ITIMs), which recruit protein tyrosine phosphatases and inositol phosphatases (Ravetch and Lanier, 2000). These phosphatases, including SHP-1, SHP-2, and SHIP, dephosphorylate and deactivate multiple intracellular-activating mediators (Bolland and Ravetch, 1999; Brauweiler et al., 2000). Thus, all inhibitory receptors, upon engagement with their cognate ligands, deliver intracellular

signals that prevent immune cell activation in the absence of an infection. This mechanism of maintaining tolerance is particularly important for cells involved in innate responses, such as monocytes and macrophages, natural killer (NK) cells, and other innate effector cells capable of recognizing self that are not subject to selection during maturation. Furthermore, when pathogens trigger an immune response, inhibitory receptors are required to prevent excessive activation of the immune system and facilitate the termination of immune responses.

THE HUMAN INHIBITORY RECEPTORS FOR MHC-I MOLECULES

To achieve self-tolerance, many inhibitory receptors recognize major histocompatibility complex class I (MHC-I) molecules, which are normally expressed on healthy cells. Additional inhibitory ligands include CD47, CD200, and sialic acids (Barclay et al., 2002; Crocker, 2002). In humans, inhibitory MHC-I receptors include the killer cell immunoglobulin (Ig)-like receptors (KIRs), the leukocyte Ig-like receptors (LILRs), and the CD94/NKG2A heterodimer. KIRs and LILRs consist of multiple Ig-like molecules encoded by two

Marco Colonna and Winfried Barchet, Department of Pathology and Immunology, Washington University School of Medicine, Box 8118, 660 South Euclid Ave., St. Louis, MO 63110.

The Innate Immune Response to Infection
Ed. by S. H. E. Kaufmann, R. Medzhitov, and S. Gordon
©2004 ASM Press, Washington, D.C.

adjacent gene clusters on human chromosome 19q13.4 (Trowsdale, 2001). Two LILRs recognize all HLA molecules (Borges and Cosman, 2000; Dietrich et al., 2000), whereas inhibitory KIR isoforms recognize either HLA-C, -B, or -A (Lanier, 1998; Long et al., 2001; Vilches and Parham, 2002). In contrast, the CD94/NKG2A heterodimer is composed of two lectin-like subunits and recognizes HLA-E, a unique MHC-I molecule that presents peptides derived from the leader sequence of other MHC-I molecules (Braud and McMichael, 1999). Therefore, HLA-E levels reflect the global MHC-I expression.

Inhibitory MHC-I receptors have different but overlapping cellular distribution patterns. One LILR is broadly expressed on T, B, NK, and myeloid cells, whereas other LILRs are preferentially expressed on myeloid cells, including monocytes and macrophages, dendritic cells (DCs), and granulocytes. KIRs and CD94/NKG2A are selectively expressed on NK cells, subsets of cytotoxic T lymphocytes (CTLs), and γδ T cells. Together, KIRs, LILRs, and CD94/NKG2A provide a comprehensive system of inhibitory MHC-I receptors that ensure self-tolerance in a variety of innate immune cells. The importance of KIRs and CD94/NKG2A in regulating NK and CTL functions has been reviewed extensively (Braud and McMichael, 1999; Lanier, 1998; Long et al., 2001; Vilches and Parham, 2002). Here, we focus on LILRs and, in particular, on their function during cytomegalovirus (CMV) infection and their ability to regulate adaptive responses during bacterial infection and following organ transplantation.

DIVERSITY OF LILRs: IMPACT ON SPECIFICITY AND SIGNALING

The members of the LILR family—also known as immunoglobulin-like transcript (ILT), leukocyte Ig-like receptor (LIR), monocyte and macrophage Ig-like receptor (MIR), or CD85—include at least 11 distinct molecules, which have either two or four homologous extracellular Ig-like domains of the C2 type (Fig. 1) (Arm et al., 1997; Borges

and Cosman, 2000; Dietrich et al., 2000; Liu et al., 2000; Trowsdale, 2001; Volz et al., 2001; Young et al., 2001a). Inhibitory LILRs (LILRB1, LILRB2, LILRB3, LILRB4, and LILRB5) contain long cytoplasmic domains with two to four ITIMs (Fig. 1). Another group of LILRs (LILRA1, LILRA2, ILT7, ILT8, and ILT11) have short cytoplasmic domains that lack ITIMs or recognizable docking motifs for signaling mediators (Fig. 1). Instead, they are characterized by the presence of a single basic arginine residue within the hydrophobic transmembrane domain. These LILRs do not mediate inhibition but rather associate with the gamma chain of Fc receptors (FcRγ), which contains an immunoreceptor tyrosine-based activation motif (ITAM) (Nakajima et al., 1999). Upon phosphorylation, FcRγ recruits p70Syk protein tyrosine kinase, which promotes tyrosine phosphorylation and activation of multiple intracellular signaling mediators (Ravetch and Kinet, 1991). A third type of LILR (LILRA3) has no transmembrane or cytoplasmic domains and may be secreted as soluble receptor (Fig. 1).

The inhibitory LILRB1 and LILRB2 recognize all MHC-I molecules (Borges et al., 1997; Colonna et al., 1997, 1998; Cosman et al., 1997). The molecular details of this interaction have recently been revealed by structural analysis of the LILRB1/HLA-A2 complex (Willcox et al., 2003). The two LILRB1 N-terminal domains primarily interact with amino acid side chains of the HLA-A2 α3 domain and β$_2$ microglobulin. The MHC-I contact residues are highly conserved in HLA-A, -B, -C, -E, and -F, which accounts for the broad recognition spectrum of LILRB1.

HLA-G differs in two contact residues, which may explain its recently observed threefold to fourfold higher affinity for LILRB1 (Shiroishi et al., 2003). Moreover, an alignment of LILRB1 amino acid contacts with putative contact residues on other LILRs divides these receptors into two distinct groups (Willcox et al., 2003). Contact amino acids within group 1, which includes the MHC-I receptors LILRB1 and LILRB2, are highly conserved,

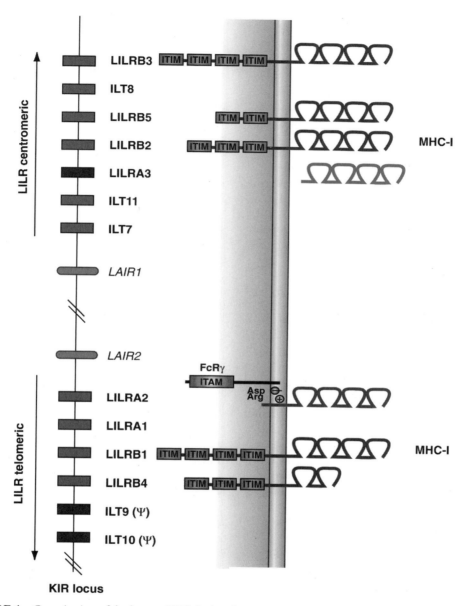

FIGURE 1 Organization of the human LILR loci on human chromosome 19q13.4. LILR genes are organized in a centromeric and a telomeric gene cluster encoding inhibitory (LILRB3, LILRB5, LILRB2, LILRB1, and LILRB4), activating (ILT8, ILT11, ILT7, LILRA2, LILRA1), and soluble (LILRA3) isoforms. Two further LILR genes are pseudogenes (ILT9, ILT10, ψ). Schematic models of the encoded molecules are also shown. The five inhibitory LILRs comprise two to four extracellular Ig-like domains and signal through two to four ITIMs in the cytoplasmic domain. LILRB1 and LILRB2 recognize all MHC-I molecules but ligands for other inhibitory LILRs remain unknown. LILRA1 is shown as an example for activating LILRs that lack a cytoplasmic signaling domain but associate with the FcRγ adaptor via charged residues in the transmembrane region. FcRγ signals through an ITAM. LILRA3 is lacking cytoplasmic as well as transmembrane domains and is probably secreted as a soluble molecule. LILRs are also known as ILTs, LILRs, MIRs, or CD85. See the official HUGO nomenclature at http://www.gene.ucl.ac.uk/ nomenclature.

whereas group 2 members display a significant degree of nonconservative substitutions. Thus, group 2 members are unlikely to bind MHC-I molecules in a similar fashion, and hence probably engage a different set of ligands. Indeed, all attempts to demonstrate that group 2 LILRs bind MHC-I have failed (Borges et al., 1997). MHC-I-like molecules may be more likely ligands.

In conclusion, LILRs are characterized by significant variability that involves both extracellular and intracellular domains. The functional significance of extracellular variability is still poorly understood, as only two LILRs have definite MHC-I ligands. Intracellular variability allows LILRs to mediate either inhibitory or activating functions.

INHIBITORY AND ACTIVATING LILRs IN HERPESVIRUS INFECTIONS

Many in vitro experiments have demonstrated that inhibitory LILRs mediate tolerance to self. Engagement of LILRB1 and LILRB2 with MHC-I or agonistic antibodies inhibits NK cell-mediated cytotoxicity (Colonna et al., 1997; Cosman et al., 1997), CTL activation and proliferation, and cytokine secretion (Colonna et al., 1997; Dietrich et al., 2001; Saverino et al., 2000, 2002; Young et al., 2001b) as well as monocyte and macrophage and DC activation and secretion of proinflammatory cytokines (Cella et al., 1997; Colonna et al., 1999; Fanger et al., 1998). However, the inhibitory function of LILRB1 may be exploited by the human CMV (HCMV) to facilitate host infection. HCMV is a β-herpesvirus that is commonly acquired during childhood with minor or no symptoms and persists for the lifetime of the host in a latent state (Mocarski, 1996). However, in immunosuppressed individuals, such as transplant recipients, the virus can reactivate and cause life-threatening infections (Britt and Alford, 1996). In order to coexist with the immune system of a healthy individual, the HCMV genome has incorporated a number of host genes encoding proteins that interfere with immune responses in various ways. Several

HCMV proteins interfere with the expression and assembly of MHC-I molecules, allowing HCMV-infected cells to downmodulate MHC-I expression and thus avoid CD8[+] T-cell surveillance (Tortorella et al., 2000). In addition, one HCMV protein, UL18, mimics MHC-I molecules and interacts with the inhibitory receptor LILRB1 with a 1,000-fold higher affinity than endogenous MHC-I (Chapman et al., 1999; Cosman et al., 1997). This interaction may allow the virus to directly inhibit host leukocyte responses against HCMV-infected cells (Lopez-Botet et al., 2001).

In an intriguing parallel, it has recently been shown that mouse strains susceptible to murine CMV (MCMV) recognize an MCMV-encoded MHC-I antigen, called m157, through Ly-49I, an inhibitory isoform of the Ly-49 receptor family (Arase and Lanier, 2002; Arase et al., 2002). Importantly, resistant strains lack Ly-49I and recognize m157 through the Ly-49H activating isoform, which presumably evolved as a pathogen-specific activating receptor (Arase and Lanier, 2002; Arase et al., 2002; Smith et al., 2002). Thus, the ability of HMCV to encode MHC-I homologs may have provided the selective pressure that led to the evolution of the LILR locus as a cluster of genes encoding diverse inhibitory, activating, and soluble receptors. To avoid blockade by UL18, an originally inhibitory LILR gene could plausibly have been duplicated and converted into an activating version capable of recruiting FcRγ (Fig. 2). This transition would require only minor variation, introducing a charged residue in the transmembrane region and a stop codon in the cytoplasmic domain. This evolutionary mechanism would provide the host with UL18-specific activating LILRs. Conversion of an inhibitory LILR into a soluble isoform would be equally effective in counteracting UL18-mediated inhibition of immune responses.

Demonstrating this hypothesis in the human is obviously a challenge. Are inhibitory LILRs associated with susceptibility to HCMV infections? Berg and colleagues (2003) recently reported that several lung transplant patients

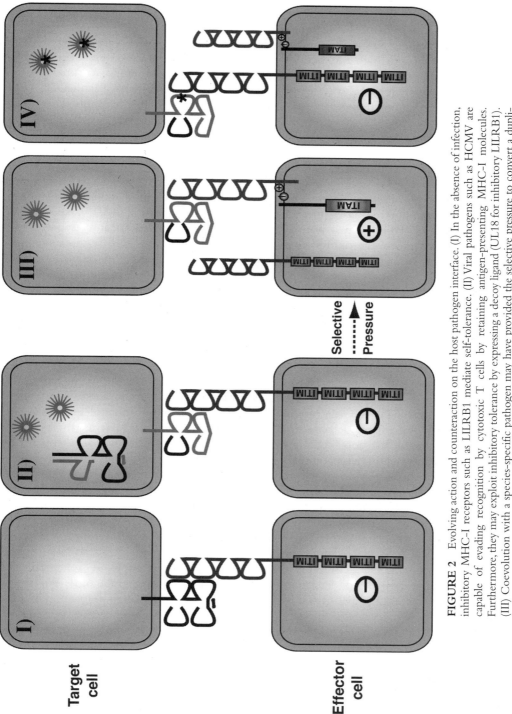

FIGURE 2 Evolving action and counteraction on the host pathogen interface. (I) In the absence of infection, inhibitory MHC–I receptors such as LILRB1 mediate self-tolerance. (II) Viral pathogens such as HCMV are capable of evading recognition by cytotoxic T cells by retaining antigen-presenting MHC–I molecules. Furthermore, they may exploit inhibitory tolerance by expressing a decoy ligand (UL18 for inhibitory LILRB1). (III) Coevolution with a species-specific pathogen may have provided the selective pressure to convert a duplicated receptor gene into a pathogen-specific activating isoform. (IV) Mutations that were identified in the contact residues of the viral decoy indicate a viral strategy to evade specific detection of infected cells by innate effectors. Endogenous molecules in the target cells are shown in black and viral proteins are depicted in gray.

have increased numbers of cytotoxic lymphocytes (i.e., NK and CD8$^+$ T cells) that express the inhibitory receptor LILRB1 in their blood. Remarkably, among all lung transplant patients studied, those with high numbers of LILRB1$^+$ lymphocytes subsequently developed a pneumonitis caused by HCMV. Thus, expression of LILRB1 on lymphocytes may actively contribute to HCMV infection in lung transplant patients. Two scenarios can be proposed. (i) Patients with constitutively high numbers of LILRB1$^+$ lymphocytes may be highly susceptible to HCMV reactivation, as expression of LILRB1 can be exploited by HCMV to inhibit immune responses through UL18. Or, (ii) upon HCMV reactivation, infected cells may release cytokines that induce de novo expression of LILRB1 on cytotoxic lymphocytes. Transforming growth factor β is an obvious candidate, as it induces expression of CD94/NKG2A on T cells (Bertone et al., 1999).

If LILRs have evolved under the selective pressure of UL18, one would also expect that UL18 mutates to neutralize this strategy of the host immune system. In support of this hypothesis, we have recently identified two variants of UL18 from the HCMV strain AD169, UL18A, and UL18B, which are significantly mutated in the α3 domain in the putative region of interaction with LILRB1 (M. Colonna, unpublished observation). Given this, UL18 is likely to vary considerably in clinical isolates of HCMV. To understand the physiological significance of this variability, it will be necessary to determine whether UL18 is on the surface of HCMV-infected cells and inhibits LILRB1$^+$ immune cell activation. In addition, it will be important to determine whether UL18 variants engage any of the ligand-orphan LILRs. Whatever the answers, LILRB1 expression may provide an important clinical marker for HCMV infection following lung transplantation as well as in other medically relevant conditions, including patients on immunosuppressive regimens or with intrinsic immune deficiencies.

ACTIVATING LILRs THAT REGULATE THE TYPE OF HOST RESPONSES TO BACTERIAL INFECTIONS

Host responses to bacteria are triggered by the Toll-like receptors (TLRs) expressed on cells involved in innate responses, particularly monocytes and macrophages and DCs. TLRs recognize microbial structures shared by pathogens, such as lipopolysaccharide, lipoproteins, double-stranded RNA, and bacterial DNA, and initiate a cascade of signaling events leading to activation of NF-κB and secretion of proinflammatory cytokines, such as tumor necrosis factor α, interleukin-1 (IL-1), IL-6, and IL-12 (Medzhitov, 2001; Takeda et al., 2003). TLR-mediated innate responses promote inflammation as well as the subsequent development of type 1 T-cell responses, activation of cell-mediated immunity, and, ultimately, clearance of pathogens (Medzhitov, 2001; Takeda et al., 2003). Recent studies indicate that LILRs, in contrast to TLRs, may promote susceptibility versus resistance to infections by microbial pathogens. Modlin and colleagues (Bleharski et al., 2003) analyzed human immune responses to the pathogen *Mycobacterium leprae*, which can lead to two types of leprosy with opposite clinical manifestations: (i) tuberculoid leprosy (T-lep), which exhibit limited lesions with few bacteria and is associated with expression of type 1 cytokines characteristic of cell-mediated immunity, or (ii) lepromatous leprosy (L-lep), which displays disseminated lesions and high bacterial loads and is associated with the expression of type 2 cytokines, activation of humoral immunity, and suppression of cell-mediated responses.

Analysis of the gene expression profiles of T-lep and L-lep skin granulomas confirmed the type 1/type 2 paradigm. Most importantly, L-lep granulomas revealed a preferential expression of LILR transcripts, including LILRA2 and LILRA3 (Bleharski et al., 2003). This observation raises the question of whether LILRs are simply associated with type 2 lesions or if they can actually induce susceptibility to progressive infection. To address this question, Modlin and colleagues (Bleharski et al., 2003) examined the effect of the activating LILRA2 on TLR-dependent production of IL-12 and IL-10, which potentiate type 1 and type 2 immune responses, respectively. LILRA2 engagement with activating anti-LILRA2 antibodies enhanced TLR-dependent secretion of IL-10. This resulted in almost complete abrogation of IL-12 production in response to two different TLR ligands. Thus, LILRA2 on macrophages and DCs may influence the balance of cytokines produced during the innate response, diverting it away from the proinflammatory program required for the development of type 1 T-cell responses and cell-mediated immunity (Fig. 3). Interestingly, although LILRA2 is an activating receptor because of its association with the adaptor FcRγ, its engagement inhibits type 1 cytokines and deflects T cells to the type 2 cytokine pattern, resulting in immune unresponsiveness to intracellular pathogens.

Bronchial asthma and atopy are further examples of type 2 T-cell immune deviation. Recently, genome-wide screens for the identification of susceptibility loci for bronchial asthma and atopy identified the KIR–LILR locus as one of the candidates, corroborating the hypothesis that LILR may promote type 2 adaptive responses (Collaborative Study on the Genetics of Asthma, 1997; Ober et al., 1998; Venanzi et al., 2001). Finally, a role for activating LILRs in the regulation of type 2 versus type 1 responses is also supported by studies in the mouse. The murine counterparts of LILRs are called paired Ig-like receptors (PIRs) (Hayami et al., 1997; Kubagawa et al., 1997). These molecules are characterized by six extracellular Ig-like domains and include one inhibitory (PIR-B) and several activating (PIR-A) isoforms. All receptors are encoded by a gene cluster on mouse chromosome 7 that is syntenic to the KIR and LILR locus (Hayami et al., 1997; Kubagawa et al., 1997). PIR interaction with MHC-I molecules has been suggested by the lack of PIR phosphorylation in MHC-I-deficient mice (Ho et al., 1999). Direct evidence of PIR–MHC-I binding, however, has not yet been obtained. Takai and colleagues have recently generated PIR-B-deficient (PIR-B$^{-/-}$) mice (Ujike et al., 2002). Upon immunization of mice with T-dependent antigens, they observed a diversion of T-cell responses in PIR-B$^{-/-}$ mice toward a type 2 pattern, which was characterized by increased IL-4 and decreased gamma interferon responses, as well as enhanced IgG1 and IgE production. Skewed responses were caused by impaired activation of DCs and, in particular, reduced IL-12 secretion. These results are consistent with a model in which, in the absence of the inhibitory PIR-B, DC function is dominated by activating PIR-As, diverging T-cell differentiation toward type 2 immune responses (Fig. 3).

INHIBITORY LILRs AND TOLERANCE TO ALLOGENEIC GRAFT AND MATERNAL FETAL TOLERANCE

A recent study suggests that the ability of inhibitory LILRs to regulate the function of antigen-presenting cells (APCs) may be an important mechanism utilized by suppressor T (Ts) cells to induce immunological tolerance. Several subsets of Ts and T regulatory cells with distinct phenotypes and mechanisms to induce tolerance have been identified (Bluestone and Abbas, 2003; Sakaguchi, 2000). One of these, known as CD8$^+$CD28$^-$ Ts, can be generated in vitro by repeated stimulation of CD8$^+$ Ts cells with allogeneic APCs (Chang et al., 2002). Recently, Suciu-Foca and colleagues demonstrated that incubation of CD8$^+$CD28$^-$ Ts cells with DCs induced upregulation of the inhibitory LILRB2 and LILRB4 on DCs (Chang et al., 2002) (Fig. 3). Engagement of LILRs inhibited CD40-mediated activation of DCs and, in particular, prevented the expression of T-cell costimulatory molecules B7.1 and B7.2. In vivo, LILRB2 and LILRB4 may inhibit additional DC functions, including migration to lymph nodes in response to chemokines, adhesion to T cells,

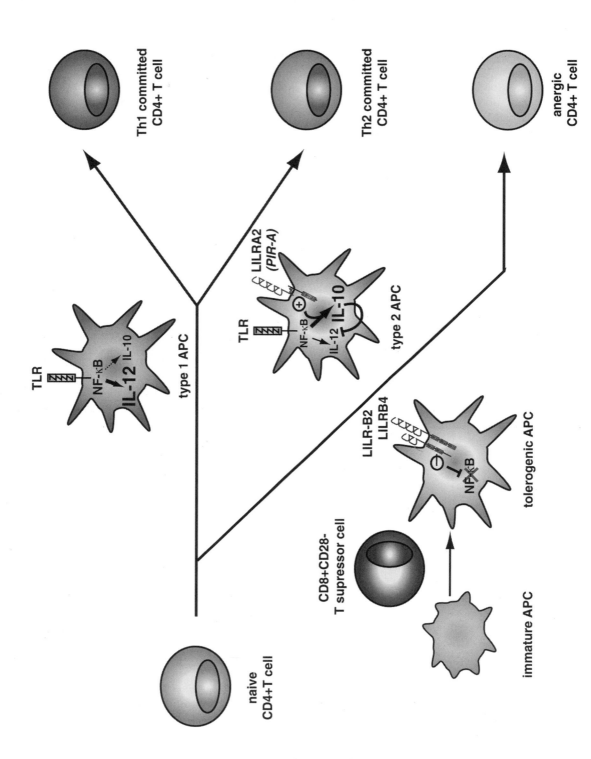

expression of T-cell costimulatory molecules, and secretion of cytokines. Thus, inhibitory LILRs may steer DCs from an immunogenic to a tolerogenic phenotype. This mechanism of tolerance may be particularly important in recipients of organ allografts, as CD8$^+$CD28$^-$ Ts cells are generated by allogeneic stimulation.

Inhibitory LILR may also contribute to tolerance during pregnancy, in which the maternal immune system tolerates the fetus semiallograft. LILRB1 and LILRB2 are among the few MHC-I receptors capable of interacting with HLA-G (Allan et al., 1999; Colonna et al., 1997; Lopez-Botet et al., 2000; Ponte et al., 1999). HLA-G is selectively expressed in the trophoblast, a tissue of fetal origin devoid of HLA-A, -B, and -C molecules that separates the developing embryo from the mother (Le Bouteiller and Blaschitz, 1999). Thus, the interaction of HLA-G with LILRB1 and LILRB2 may inhibit DCs and other immune cells that are present within the decidua, contributing to maternal–fetal tolerance. Expression and engagement of inhibitory LILRs on antigen-presenting cells block their function in vitro and may represent an important mechanism of tolerance to allografts and fetal semiallografts in vivo.

THE FUTURE OF LILRs

Since the discovery of LILRs, a number of sensitive assays have been developed for identifying their ligands. Thus, rapid progress can be foreseen in the characterization of LILR ligand specificities and their relationship with MHC-I, MHC-I-like, and HCMV-encoded molecules. It is noteworthy that LILR sequence analysis in a random population has revealed the presence of ~15 different LILRB3 alleles (Colonna et al., 1997). This polymorphism indicates that the LILR locus is undergoing rapid evolution, possibly under the selective pressure of pathogens. Thus, LILR ligand identification will elucidate why humans have developed such a large number of LILR genes and whether any of them is responsible for susceptibility and/or resistance to infections by HCMV or other herpesviruses encoding MHC-I-like molecules.

Although initial studies focused on the ability of LILRs to control effector responses by cells of the innate immune system, more recent studies have pointed out the importance of LILRs in regulating antigen-presenting cells and thereby instructing adaptive T-cell responses. Both lines of research indicate a role for LILRs in preventing type 1 T-cell responses characteristic of cell-mediated immunity. Activating LILRs promote type 2 responses, whereas inhibitory LILRs induce tolerogenic responses, at least in vitro. It will be important to substantiate these models in vivo by analyzing immunopathological conditions characterized by type 2 T-cell responses, such as allergies. Moreover, comparing LILR functions in graft acceptance and graft rejection is essential to corroborate their potential tolerogenic function. As more immune cell subsets with tolerogenic functions are identified, it will be important to verify a preferential expression or function of individual LILRs on these subsets.

FIGURE 3 Differential expression of LILR on APCs regulates CD4$^+$ T-cell responses and a pattern emerges. TLR signaling in maturing APCs activates NF-κB, leading to the production of IL-12 and to a lesser degree IL-10. APCs activated in this fashion promote a Th1 response. Modlin and colleagues (Bleharski et al., 2003) have shown that coengagement of activating LILRA2 can shift the balance toward enhanced production of IL-10 and a significant reduction in IL-12. CD4$^+$ T cells polarized by IL-10-producing APCs may deviate toward a Th2 phenotype. Strong Th2 bias has also been observed in mice deficient for the inhibitory LILR homolog PIR-B, presumably due to the dominance of activating PIRs (PIR-As). Chang and colleagues (2002) report that the presence of CD8$^+$CD28$^-$ Ts cells induces the expression of inhibitory LILRB2 and LILRB4 on maturing APCs. Inhibitory LILR signals downmodulate NF-κB activity, APCs become tolerogenic, and CD4 T cells cocultured with tolerogenic APCs become unresponsive to further antigenic stimuli.

ACKNOWLEDGMENTS
We thank Susan Gilfillan for reading the manuscript.

REFERENCES

Allan, D. S., M. Colonna, L. L. Lanier, T. D. Churakova, J. S. Abrams, S. A. Ellis, A. J. McMichael, and V. M. Braud. 1999. Tetrameric complexes of human histocompatibility leukocyte antigen (HLA)-G bind to peripheral blood myelo-monocytic cells. *J. Exp. Med.* **189:**1149–1156.

Arase, H., and L. L. Lanier. 2002. Virus-driven evolution of natural killer cell receptors. *Microbes Infect.* **4:**1505–1512.

Arase, H., E. S. Mocarski, A. E. Campbell, A. B. Hill, and L. L. Lanier. 2002. Direct recognition of cytomegalovirus by activating and inhibitory NK cell receptors. *Science* **296:**1323–1326.

Arm, J. P., C. Nwankwo, and K. F. Austen. 1997. Molecular identification of a novel family of human Ig superfamily members that possess immunoreceptor tyrosine-based inhibition motifs and homology to the mouse gp49B1 inhibitory receptor. *J. Immunol.* **159:**2342–2349.

Barclay, A. N., G. J. Wright, G. Brooke, and M. H. Brown. 2002. CD200 and membrane protein interactions in the control of myeloid cells. *Trends Immunol.* **23:**285–290.

Berg, L., G. C. Riise, D. Cosman, T. Bergstrom, S. Olofsson, K. Karre, and E. Carbone. 2003. LIR-1 expression on lymphocytes, and cytomegalovirus disease in lung-transplant recipients. *Lancet* **361:**1099–1101.

Bertone, S., F. Schiavetti, R. Bellomo, C. Vitale, M. Ponte, L. Moretta, and M. C. Mingari. 1999. Transforming growth factor-beta-induced expression of CD94/NKG2A inhibitory receptors in human T lymphocytes. *Eur. J. Immunol.* **29:**23–29.

Bleharski, J. R., H. Li, C. Meinken, T. G. Graeber, M.-T. Ochoa, M. Yamamura, A. Burdick, E. N. Sarno, M. Wagner, M. Rollinghoff, T. H. Rea, M. Colonna, S. Stenger, B. R. Bloom, D. Eisenberg, and R. L. Modlin. 2003. Use of genetic profiling in leprosy to discriminate clinical forms of the disease. *Science* **301:**1527–1530.

Bluestone, J. A., and A. K. Abbas. 2003. Natural versus adaptive regulatory T cells. *Nat. Rev. Immunol.* **3:**253–257.

Bolland, S., and J. V. Ravetch. 1999. Inhibitory pathways triggered by ITIM-containing receptors. *Adv. Immunol.* **72:**149–177.

Borges, L., and D. Cosman. 2000. LIRs/ILTs/MIRs, inhibitory and stimulatory Ig-superfamily receptors expressed in myeloid and lymphoid cells. *Cytokine Growth Factor Rev.* **11:**209–217.

Borges, L., M. L. Hsu, N. Fanger, M. Kubin, and D. Cosman. 1997. A family of human lymphoid and myeloid Ig-like receptors, some of which bind to MHC class I molecules. *J. Immunol.* **159:**5192–5196.

Braud, V. M., and A. J. McMichael. 1999. Regulation of NK cell functions through interaction of the CD94/NKG2 receptors with the nonclassical class I molecule HLA-E. *Curr. Top. Microbiol. Immunol.* **244:**85–95.

Brauweiler, A. M., I. Tamir, and J. C. Cambier. 2000. Bilevel control of B-cell activation by the inositol 5-phosphatase SHIP. *Immunol. Rev.* **176:**69–74.

Britt, W. J., and C. A. Alford. 1996. Cytomegalovirus, p. 2493–2524. *In* B. N. Fields (ed.), *Virology*, vol. 2. Lippincott-Raven, Philadelphia, Pa.

Cella, M., C. Dohring, J. Samaridis, M. Dessing, M. Brockhaus, A. Lanzavecchia, and M. Colonna. 1997. A novel inhibitory receptor (ILT3) expressed on monocytes, macrophages, and dendritic cells involved in antigen processing. *J. Exp. Med.* **185:**1743–1751.

Chang, C. C., R. Ciubotariu, J. S. Manavalan, J. Yuan, A. I. Colovai, F. Piazza, S. Lederman, M. Colonna, R. Cortesini, R. Dalla-Favera, and N. Suciu-Foca. 2002. Tolerization of dendritic cells by T(S) cells: the crucial role of inhibitory receptors ILT3 and ILT4. *Nat. Immunol.* **3:**237–243.

Chapman, T. L., A. P. Heikeman, and P. J. Bjorkman. 1999. The inhibitory receptor LIR-1 uses a common binding interaction to recognize class I MHC molecules and the viral homolog UL18. *Immunity* **11:**603–613.

Collaborative Study on the Genetics of Asthma (CSGA). 1997. A genome-wide search for asthma susceptibility loci in ethnically diverse populations. *Nat. Genet.* **15:**389–392.

Colonna, M., F. Navarro, T. Bellon, M. Llano, P. Garcia, J. Samaridis, L. Angman, M. Cella, and M. Lopez-Botet. 1997. A common inhibitory receptor for major histocompatibility complex class I molecules on human lymphoid and myelomonocytic cells. *J. Exp. Med.* **186:**1809–1818.

Colonna, M., J. Samaridis, M. Cella, L. Angman, R. L. Allen, C. A. O'Callaghan, R. Dunbar, G. S. Ogg, V. Cerundolo, and A. Rolink. 1998. Human myelomonocytic cells express an inhibitory receptor for classical and nonclassical MHC class I molecules. *J. Immunol.* **160:**3096–3100.

Colonna, M., H. Nakajima, F. Navarro, and M. Lopez-Botet. 1999. A novel family of Ig-like receptors for HLA class I molecules that modulate function of lymphoid and myeloid cells. *J. Leukoc. Biol.* **66:**375–381.

Cosman, D., N. Fanger, L. Borges, M. Kubin, W. Chin, L. Peterson, and M. L. Hsu. 1997. A novel immunoglobulin superfamily receptor for cellular and viral MHC class I molecules. *Immunity* **7:**273–282.

Crocker, P. R. 2002. Siglecs: sialic-acid-binding immunoglobulin-like lectins in cell-cell interactions and signalling. *Curr. Opin. Struct. Biol.* **12:**609–615.

Dietrich, J., H. Nakajima, and M. Colonna. 2000. Human inhibitory and activating Ig-like receptors which modulate the function of myeloid cells. *Microbes Infect.* **2**:323–329.

Dietrich, J., M. Cella, and M. Colonna. 2001. Ig-like transcript 2 (ILT2)/leukocyte Ig-like receptor 1 (LIR1) inhibits TCR signaling and actin cytoskeleton reorganization. *J. Immunol.* **166**:2514–2521.

Fanger, N. A., D. Cosman, L. Peterson, S. C. Braddy, C. R. Maliszewski, and L. Borges. 1998. The MHC class I binding proteins LIR-1 and LIR-2 inhibit Fc receptor-mediated signaling in monocytes. *Eur. J. Immunol.* **28**:3423–3434.

Goodnow, C. C. 1996. Balancing immunity and tolerance: deleting and tuning lymphocyte repertoires. *Proc. Natl. Acad. Sci. USA* **93**:2264–2271.

Hayami, K., D. Fukuta, Y. Nishikawa, Y. Yamashita, M. Inui, Y. Ohyama, M. Hikida, H. Ohmori, and T. Takai. 1997. Molecular cloning of a novel murine cell-surface glycoprotein homologous to killer cell inhibitory receptors. *J. Biol. Chem.* **272**:7320–7327.

Ho, L. H., T. Uehara, C. C. Chen, H. Kubagawa, and M. D. Cooper. 1999. Constitutive tyrosine phosphorylation of the inhibitory paired Ig-like receptor PIR-B. *Proc. Natl. Acad. Sci. USA* **96**:15086–15090.

Kubagawa, H., P. D. Burrows, and M. D. Cooper. 1997. A novel pair of immunoglobulin-like receptors expressed by B cells and myeloid cells. *Proc. Natl. Acad. Sci. USA* **94**:5261–5266.

Lanier, L. L. 1998. NK cell receptors. *Annu. Rev. Immunol.* **16**:359–393.

Le Bouteiller, P., and A. Blaschitz. 1999. The functionality of HLA-G is emerging. *Immunol. Rev.* **167**:233–244.

Liu, W. R., J. Kim, C. Nwankwo, L. K. Ashworth, and J. P. Arm. 2000. Genomic organization of the human leukocyte immunoglobulin-like receptors within the leukocyte receptor complex on chromosome 19q13.4. *Immunogenetics* **51**:659–669.

Long, E. O., D. F. Barber, D. N. Burshtyn, M. Faure, M. Peterson, S. Rajagopalan, V. Renard, M. Sandusky, C. C. Stebbins, N. Wagtmann, and C. Watzl. 2001. Inhibition of natural killer cell activation signals by killer cell immunoglobulin-like receptors (CD158). *Immunol. Rev.* **181**:223–233.

Lopez-Botet, M., M. Llano, F. Navarro, and T. Bellon. 2000. NK cell recognition of non-classical HLA class I molecules. *Semin. Immunol.* **12**:109–119.

Lopez-Botet, M., M. Llano, and M. Ortega. 2001. Human cytomegalovirus and natural killer-mediated surveillance of HLA class I expression: a paradigm of host-pathogen adaptation. *Immunol. Rev.* **181**:193–202.

Medzhitov, R. 2001. Toll-like receptors and innate immunity. *Nat. Rev. Immunol.* **1**:135–145.

Miller, J. F., and G. Morahan. 1992. Peripheral T cell tolerance. *Annu. Rev. Immunol.* **10**:51–69.

Mocarski, E. S. 1996. Cytomegaloviruses and their replication, p. 2447–2492. *In* B. N. Fields (ed.), *Virology,* 3rd ed., vol. 2. Lippincott-Raven, Philadelphia, Pa.

Nakajima, H., J. Samaridis, L. Angman, and M. Colonna. 1999. Human myeloid cells express an activating ILT receptor (ILT1) that associates with Fc receptor gamma-chain. *J. Immunol.* **162**:5–8.

Ober, C., N. J. Cox, M. Abney, A. Di Rienzo, E. S. Lander, B. Changyaleket, H. Gidley, B. Kurtz, J. Lee, M. Nance, A. Pettersson, J. Prescott, A. Richardson, E. Schlenker, E. Summerhill, S. Willadsen, and R. Parry. 1998. Genome-wide search for asthma susceptibility loci in a founder population. The Collaborative Study on the Genetics of Asthma. *Hum. Mol. Genet.* **7**:1393–1398.

Ponte, M., C. Cantoni, R. Biassoni, A. Tradori-Cappai, G. Bentivoglio, C. Vitale, S. Bertone, A. Moretta, L. Moretta, and M. C. Mingari. 1999. Inhibitory receptors sensing HLA-G1 molecules in pregnancy: decidua-associated natural killer cells express LIR-1 and CD94/NKG2A and acquire p49, an HLA-G1-specific receptor. *Proc. Natl. Acad. Sci. USA* **96**:5674–5679.

Ravetch, J. V., and J. P. Kinet. 1991. Fc receptors. *Annu. Rev. Immunol.* **9**:457–492.

Ravetch, J. V., and L. L. Lanier. 2000. Immune inhibitory receptors. *Science* **290**:84–89.

Sakaguchi, S. 2000. Regulatory T cells: key controllers of immunologic self-tolerance. *Cell* **101**:455–458.

Saverino, D., M. Fabbi, F. Ghiotto, A. Merlo, S. Bruno, D. Zarcone, C. Tenca, M. Tiso, G. Santoro, G. Anastasi, D. Cosman, C. E. Grossi, and E. Ciccone. 2000. The CD85/LIR-1/ILT2 inhibitory receptor is expressed by all human T lymphocytes and down-regulates their functions. *J. Immunol.* **165**:3742–3755.

Saverino, D., A. Merlo, S. Bruno, V. Pistoia, C. E. Grossi, and E. Ciccone. 2002. Dual effect of CD85/leukocyte Ig-like receptor-1/Ig-like transcript 2 and CD152 (CTLA-4) on cytokine production by antigen-stimulated human T cells. *J Immunol.* **168**:207–215.

Shiroishi, M., K. Tsumoto, K. Amano, Y. Shirakihara, M. Colonna, V. M. Braud, D. S. Allan, A. Makadzange, S. Rowland-Jones, B. Willcox, E. Y. Jones, P. A. van der Merwe, I. Kumagai, and K. Maenaka. 2003. Human inhibitory receptors Ig-like transcript 2 (ILT2) and ILT4 compete with CD8 for MHC class I binding and bind preferentially to HLA-G. *Proc. Natl. Acad. Sci. USA* **100**:8856–8861.

Smith, H. R., J. W. Heusel, I. K. Mehta, S. Kim, B. G. Dorner, O. V. Naidenko, K. Iizuka, H. Furukawa, D. L. Beckman, J. T. Pingel, A. A. Scalzo, D. H. Fremont, and W. M. Yokoyama. 2002. Recognition of a virus-encoded ligand by a natural killer cell activation receptor. *Proc. Natl. Acad. Sci. USA* **99**:8826–8831.

Sprent, J., and H. Kishimoto. 2002. The thymus and negative selection. *Immunol. Rev.* **185**:126–135.

Takeda, K., T. Kaisho, and S. Akira. 2003. Toll-like receptors. *Annu. Rev. Immunol.* **21**:335–376.

Tortorella, D., B. E. Gewurz, M. H. Furman, D. J. Schust, and H. L. Ploegh. 2000. Viral subversion of the immune system. *Annu. Rev. Immunol.* **18**:861–926.

Trowsdale, J. 2001. Genetic and functional relationships between MHC and NK receptor genes. *Immunity* **15**:363–374.

Ujike, A., K. Takeda, A. Nakamura, S. Ebihara, K. Akiyama, and T. Takai. 2002. Impaired dendritic cell maturation and increased T(H)2 responses in PIR-B(−/−) mice. *Nat. Immunol.* **3**:542–548.

Venanzi, S., G. Malerba, R. Galavotti, M. C. Lauciello, E. Trabetti, G. Zanoni, L. Pescoll-derungg, L. C. Martinati, A. L. Boner, and P. F. Pignatti. 2001. Linkage to atopy on chromosome 19 in north-eastern Italian families with allergic asthma. *Clin. Exp. Allergy* **31**:1220–1224.

Vilches, C., and P. Parham. 2002. KIR: diverse, rapidly evolving receptors of innate and adaptive immunity. *Annu. Rev. Immunol.* **20**:217–251.

Volz, A., H. Wende, K. Laun, and A. Ziegler. 2001. Genesis of the ILT/LIR/MIR clusters within the human leukocyte receptor complex. *Immunol. Rev.* **181**:39–51.

Willcox, B. E., L. M. Thomas, and P. J. Bjorkman. 2003. Crystal structure of HLA-A2 bound to LIR-1, a host and viral major histocompatibility complex receptor. *Nat. Immunol.* **4**:913–919.

Young, N. T., F. Canavez, M. Uhrberg, B. P. Shum, and P. Parham. 2001a. Conserved organization of the ILT/LIR gene family within the polymorphic human leukocyte receptor complex. *Immunogenetics* **53**:270–278.

Young, N. T., M. Uhrberg, J. H. Phillips, L. L. Lanier, and P. Parham. 2001b. Differential expression of leukocyte receptor complex-encoded Ig-like receptors correlates with the transition from effector to memory CTL. *J. Immunol.* **166**:3933–3941.

EFFECTOR RESPONSES

ANTIMICROBIAL PEPTIDES: EFFECTORS OF INNATE IMMUNITY

Michael Zasloff

17

As you walk through a field, appreciate that plants, and animals including yourself, rely on antimicrobial peptides to defend themselves against environmental microbes. Consider a radish seed. Packaged within the seed are preformed potent antimicrobial peptides; they leak out from the seed when the sprouting embryo tears through the coat, creating in the surrounding soil a powerful antimicrobial shield (Terras et al., 1992). What sorts of molecules are invested with this degree of responsibility, considering the complexity and uncertainty of the microbial challenge? Antimicrobial peptides are evolutionarily ancient weapons, which along with regulatory proteins such as the Toll receptor families have provided complex multicellular organisms with the defenses needed to effectively compete in a world dominated by microbes. Indeed, their widespread distribution suggests that antimicrobial peptides have served a fundamental role in the successful evolution of complex multicellular organisms. Despite their ancient lineage, antimicrobial peptides have remained effective defensive weapons, confounding the general belief that bacteria, fungi, and viruses can and

will develop resistance to any conceivable substance. The insights provided by this large body of research have spawned considerable commercial effort to create new classes of anti-infective therapeutics.

NATURAL PEPTIDES

Antibiotic peptides have been isolated from single-celled protozoans (Andra et al., 2003); from the blood cells of invertebrates, such as shrimp (Munoz et al., 2003), and all vertebrates; from the epithelia of all animals studied; from the hemolymph of insects; from various tissues of plants; and in specialized settings such as the venom used by ants and spiders (Kuhn-Nentwig et al., 2002; Corzo et al., 2002) to sterilize prey or by bees, in secretions they infuse into royal jelly as preservatives.

The diversity of antibiotics discovered to date is so great that it is difficult to categorize them except in broad generalities based on their secondary structure. (An up-to-date online catalog of all such reported molecules, now over 800, can be found at www.bbcm. univ.trieste.it/~tossi/antimic.html.) The fundamental structural principle underlying all classes is the ability of the molecule to adopt a shape in which the hydrophobic amino acids are organized on one side of the molecule

Michael Zasloff, Georgetown University Medical Center, 3900 Reservoir Rd., Washington, D.C. 20057.

The Innate Immune Response to Infection
Ed. by S. H. E. Kaufmann, R. Medzhitov, and S. Gordon
©2004 ASM Press, Washington, D.C.

while cationic hydrophilic amino acids are located on the other ("amphipathic design"). Linear peptides like the silk moth's cecropin (Steiner et al., 1981), the African clawed frog's magainin (Zasloff, 1987), and the cathelicidin-derived antimicrobial peptide (CRAMP) (Yu et al., 2002) adopt this organization only when they enter a membrane, whereupon they assume an amphipathic α-helical secondary structure (Bechinger et al., 1993). Peptides, such as bactenecins (Romeo et al., 1988) and defensins (Selsted et al., 1985), utilize a relatively rigid antiparallel β-sheet constrained by disulfide bonds as the framework (Schibili et al., 2002a). Tachyplesin, the 17-residue peptide from the horseshoe crab, adopts a β-hairpin conformation in solution stabilized by two cross-strand disulfide bonds; upon insertion into a membrane, several of the hydrophobic side chains exhibit significant conformational rearrangement compared with their structure in aqueous solution (Laederbach et al., 2002). The extremely large and diverse family of peptides found in the skin of frogs of the *Rana* species has a single loop imposed by a single disulfide bond, in which the cationic groups are segregated, with an α-helical stem containing hydrophobic amino acids (reviewed by Simmaco et al., 1998; Rinaldi, 2002; Isaacson et al., 2002). A large family of linear peptides characterized by a predominance of one or two amino acids, such as the tryptophan-rich indolicidin of the cow neutrophil (Selsted et al., 1992) or the proline-arginine-rich PR39 (Agerberth et al., 1991) of the pig neutrophil (Table 1 and Color Plate 4), segregate hydrophobic and hydrophilic side chains around an extended peptide scaffold in the setting of the membrane. Model studies of the interaction between indolicidin and bacterial endotoxin have highlighted the importance of both hydrophobic and electrostatic interactions, along with conformational plasticity of the peptide, for effective binding (Nagpal et al., 2002).

The amphipathic property of antimicrobial peptides permits them to achieve high concentrations both in the aqueous solution

TABLE 1 Overview of antimicrobial peptides from plants and animals[a]

Peptide	Sequence	Origin	Tissue
α-Helix			
Cecropin A	KWKLFKKIEKVGQNIRDGIIKAGPAVAVVGQATQIAK*a*	Silk moth	E, BC, H
Magainin 2	GIGKFLHSAKKFGKAFVGEIMNS	Frog	E
Pexiganan	GIGKFLKKAKKFGKAFVKILKK*a*	Synthetic	E
Dermaseptin 1	ALWKTMLKKLGTMALHAGKAALGAAADTISQGTQ	Frog	E, BC, ES
LL-37	LLGDFFRKSKEKIGKEFKRIVQRIKDFLRNLVPRTES	Human	E
Buforin II	TRSSRAGLQFPVGRVHRLLRK	Vertebrate	
1 Disulfide bond			
Bactenecin 1	RLCRIVIRVCR	Cow	BC
Thanatin	GSKKPVPIIYCNRRTGKCQRM	Insect	BC
Brevinin 1T	VNPIILGVLPKVCLITKKC	Frogs of the *Rana* genus	E
Ranalexin	FLGGLIKIVPAMICAVTKKC		
Ranateurin 1	SMLSVLKNLGKVGLGFVACKINKQC		
Esculentin 1	GIFSKLGRKKIKNLLISGLKNVGKEVGMDVVRTGIDIAGCKIKGEC		

	Sequence	Source	Tissue
2 Disulfide bonds			
Tachyplesin	$RWC_1FRVC_2YRGIC_2YRKC_1R$a	Horseshoe crab	BC
Androctonin	$RSVC_1RQIKIC_2RRRGGC_2YYKC_1TNRPY$	Scorpion	H
Protegrin 1	$RGGRLC_1YC_2RRRFC_2VC_1VGR$a	Pig	BC
3 Disulfide bonds			
α-Defensin (human neutrophil protein 3)	$DC_1YC_2RIPAC_3IAGERRYGTC_2IYQGRLWAFC_3C_1$	Human	BC, E
β-Defensin (tracheal antimicrobial peptide)	$NPVSC_1VRNKGIC_2VPIRC_3PGSMKQIGTC_2VGRAVKC_1C_3RKK$	Cow	E, BC
θ-Defensin	$GFC_1RC_2LC_3RRGVC_3RC_2IC_1TR$	Monkey	BC
Kalata B5 (cyclotide)	$GTPC_1GSSC_2VYIPC_3ISGVIGC_1SC_2TDKYC_3YLN$	Plant	E
Defensin (sapecin A)	$ATC_1DLLSGTGINHSAC_2AAHC_3LLRGNRGGYC_2NGKAVC_3VC_1RN$	Insect	E, BC, H
Thionin (crambin)	$TTC_1C_2PSIVARSNFNVC_3RIPGTPEAIC_3ATYTGC_2IIIPGATC_1PGDYAN$	Plant	E
4 Disulfide bonds			
Defensin	$QKLC_1QRPSGTWSGVC_2GNNNAC_3KNQC_4IRLEKARHGSC_2NYVFPAHC_3IC_4YFPC_1$	Radish	Seeds, E
Drosomycin	$DC_1LSGRYKGPC_2AVWDNETC_3RRVC_4KEEGRSSGHC_2SPSLKC_3WC_4EGC_1$	*Drosophila*	H
Hepcidin	$DTHFPIC_1IFC_2C_3GC_4C_1HRSKC_2GMC_3C_4KT$	Human	Liver
Linear, not α-helical			
Bac 5	$RFRPPIRRPPIRPPFYPPFRPPIRPPIFPPIRPPFRPPLGRPFP$a	Cow	BC
PR39	$RRRPRPPYLPRPRPPPFFPPRLPPRIPPGFPPRFPPRFP$a	Pig	BC
Indolicidin	$ILPWKWPWWPWRR$a	Cow	H
Apidaecin	GNNRPVYIPQPRPPHPRI	Honeybee	H
Pyrrhocoricin	VDKGSYLPRPTPPRIPYNRN	Insect	H
Histatin 5	DSHAKRHHGYKRKFHEKHHSHRGY	Human	Saliva
Lactoferricin	FKCRRWQWRM KKLGAPSITC VRRAF	Cow	ES, BC

[a]BC, blood cell; H, hemolymph; E, epithelial tissue; ES, exocrine gland secretions. Cysteines paired in disulfide linkages are noted by common numerical subscripts. Carboxyl–terminal amides are noted by lowercase a. In θ-defensin the first and last residues are joined in a peptide bond. Kalata B5 forms a "cystine knot."

through which they must travel to reach their targets and in the fatty membranes of microbes into which they must penetrate.

Most organisms secrete a cocktail of peptides of several classes from their immune tissues. In addition, the antimicrobial peptides act synergistically with secreted proteins with antimicrobial activity such as lysozyme, lactoferrin, and phospholipase A2 (Cole et al., 2002; Zhao and Kinnunen, 2003).

All peptides are derived from larger precursors. Posttranslational modifications include proteolytic processing and, in some cases, glycosylation (Bulet et al., 1993), carboxyl-terminal amidation and amino acid isomerization (reviewed by Simmaco et al. [1998]), and halogenation (Shinnar et al., 1996). Plictamide, an antimicrobial octapeptide from the blood cells of a tunicate, carries a highly modified amino acid, decarboxy-α,β-dehydro-3,4-dihydroxyphenylalanine (Tincu et al., 2003). A rather complex modification involves the cyclization of two short peptides leading to the fully circular θ-defensin isolated from rhesus neutrophils (Tang et al., 1999).

Some peptides are derived by proteolysis from larger proteins, such as buforin II from histone 2A (Kim et al., 2000) in the stomachs of frogs and mammals; the 19-residue parasin I from histone 2a in the skin mucus of wounded catfish (Cho et al., 2002); and lactoferricin from lactoferrin (Ulvatne and Vorland, 2001; Vogel et al., 2002; Strom et al., 2002) as well as from fragments of ubiquitin (Kieffer et al., 2003) and hemoglobin (Nakajima et al., 2003). Fragments of eukaryotic viral coat proteins involved in membrane fusion have also been shown to have antimicrobial properties, which is of interest in terms of peptide design but of uncertain biological significance (Phadke et al., 2002).

The availability of large bodies of genomic sequence data has permitted an estimate of the number of antimicrobial peptide genes represented in various species. In humans, only one cathelicidin gene has been identified (Termen et al., 2003). In one study, a genome-wide search of β-defensins identified six new genes beyond the four that are currently known; two of the novel sequences are expressed in lung (Kao et al., 2003). Another study that used a different searching algorithm suggested that there are as many as 28 new human and 43 new mouse β-defensins in the respective genomic databases (Scheetz et al., 2002). A detailed analysis of the murine β-defensin cluster on chromosome 8 identified six novel exon 2-like β-defensin sequences, expressed in brain and reproductive tissues (Morrison et al., 2003).

Single-nucleotide polymorphisms in both noncoding and coding regions of human β-defensin 1 (HBD1) and human β-defensin 2 (HBD2) have been identified within human ethnic populations (Jurevic et al., 2002); in the case of HBD1, they were associated with differences in carriage of *Candida albicans* in the oral cavity (Jurevic et al., 2003). A polymorphism identified in HBD1 (Ile 38) was seen in 15% of patients with chronic obstructive pulmonary disease versus 2.8% of healthy individuals, suggesting association with pulmonary infection (Matsushita et al., 2002). A coding single-nucleotide polymorphism in HBD1 (Ser 35) eliminates a cysteine, thus profoundly altering the peptide's structure; despite this, the synthetic peptide is as active as HBD1 (Circo et al., 2002). A β-defensin from mouse, DEFr1, lacking one of the conserved cysteines, was recently cloned; it was found to be expressed most abundantly in testes and heart, and shown to retain antimicrobial activity (Morrison et al., 2002b). Analysis of HBD1 variation among nonhuman primates suggested that mutation in this gene between these species was driven by random events rather than through selective pressure or positive selection (Del Pero et al., 2002).

The diversity of sequences is such that the same peptide sequence is rarely recovered from two different species of animal, even those that are closely related, be they insect, frog, or mammal (exceptions include peptides cleaved from highly conserved proteins, such as those from histones or hemoglobin). However, within the antimicrobial peptides from a single species and even between certain classes of different peptides from diverse species (reviewed by Simmaco et al. [1998] and Cuthbertson et al. [2002]), significant conservation of amino acid sequences can be recognized in the pre-pro-region of the precursor molecules. The design suggests that constraints exist on the sequences involved in the translation, secretion, or intracellular trafficking of this class of membrane-disruptive peptide. This feature is dramatically illustrated by the cathelicidins (reviewed by Zanetti et al., 2000).

Because single mutations can dramatically alter the biological activity of each peptide (e.g., Sawai et al., 2002), the diversity likely reflects the species' adaptation to the unique microbial environments that characterize the niche occupied, including the microbes associated with acceptable food sources (reviewed by Simmaco et al. [1998], Boman [2000], and Duda et al. [2002]). The worldwide decline of amphibian populations, which has been linked to microbial infections (Rollins-Smith et al., 2002a, 2002b, 2002c), might represent a visible demonstration of the type of selection pressure that leads to antimicrobial peptide diversity.

SYNTHETIC PEPTIDES

With respect to the diversity created in the synthetic laboratory, almost all active molecules are composed of hydrophilic, hydrophobic, and cationic amino acids arranged in a molecule that can organize into an amphipathic structure (reviewed by Maloy and Kari, 1995; Muhle and Tam, 2001; Tossi et al., 2000). Straightforward chemical synthesis of analogues of naturally occurring disulfide cross-linked peptides such as the α-defensins has been achieved through solid-phase synthesis and controlled cysteine cross-linking (Mandal and Nagaraj, 2002). Natural peptides composed of all D-amino acids, in place of L-amino acids, retain full antibiotic potency while exhibiting expected resistance to enzymatic proteolysis (Maloy and Kari, 1995). Analogues of protegrins, lacking the cross-chain disulfide bridges but designed with sequences that create stable β-hairpin secondary structures, have been created (Lai et al., 2002). Short linear or cyclic amphiphilic peptides containing both L- and D-amino acids can be generated with various degrees of selectivity, antimicrobial potency (Fernandez-Lopez et al., 2001; Oren and Shai, 2000; Papo et al., 2002), and resistance to proteolytic degradation (Hamamoto et al., 2002). Cyclic peptides containing L- and D-amino acids have been synthesized which form highly organized "nanotubes," created through the self-organizing stacking of the peptide rings which possibly form on the surfaces of microbial membranes (Fernandez-Lopez et al., 2001). Dendrimeric peptides, consisting of a lysine core with several tetrapeptides or octapeptides decorating the root, show surprising potency and selectivity (Tam et al., 2002). Fatty acid-modified peptides with impressive antifungal properties (Avrahami and Shai, 2002; Mak et al., 2003) and systemic antibacterial activity (Zasloff, 2003) have been created. Reversible masking of the cationic charges on synthetic antimicrobial peptides with methane sulfonate, previously used in the case of polymyxin, can extend the therapeutic window for certain peptides designed for systemic use (Zasloff, 2003). Protease-resistant antimicrobial peptides composed of β-amino acids have been constructed (Porter et al., 2000; Hamuro et al., 1999; Epand et al., 2003). Antimicrobial polymers created off an acrylamide backbone have been designed with amphiphilic properties that mimic the physical and biological activities of antimicrobial peptides (Tew et al., 2002). The principal issues, beyond efficacy and toxicity, that will determine whether these polymeric substances or synthetic peptides containing unnatural amino acids can be commercially developed will depend on the cost of synthesis, since such molecules cannot be prepared by recombinant methodologies.

MECHANISM OF ACTION

Antimicrobial peptides have targeted a surprising but clearly fundamental difference in the design of the membranes of microbes and multicellular animals. Bacterial membranes, for example, are organized in such a way that the outermost leaflet of the bilayer, the surface exposed to the outer world, is heavily populated by lipids with negatively charged phospholipid head groups. In contrast, the outer leaflet of the membranes of plants and animals is composed principally of lipids with no net charge; most of the lipids with negatively charged head groups are segregated into the inner leaflet, facing the cytoplasm (Color Plate 5) (reviewed by Matsuzaki [1999]). A basic model that explains the activity of most antimicrobial peptides is the Shai–Matsuzaki–Huang (SMH) model (Matsuzaki, 1999; Yang et al., 2000b; Shai, 1999) (Color Plate 6). Random collisions result in electrostatic interaction between the negatively charged phospholipid head groups of the lipids on the outer leaflet of the target cell's membrane and the positively charged amino acids of the peptide. We visualize the membrane as initially "carpeted" by a layer of peptides, attracted by electrostatic forces (Shai, 1999) (Color Plate 6A and B). As the peptides accumulate within the outer leaflet of the bilayer, they spread the head groups, displacing lipids by their presence (Color Plate 6C). The surface area of the outer leaflet expands relative to the inner leaflet, causing the bilayer to assume a convex shape, or positive curvature (Matsuzaki, 1999; Yang et al., 2000b), and at the same time the membrane weakens due to the dilution of lipids by peptides. Strain is relieved by a phase transition in which peptides along with associated lipids collapse down a torus-shaped "wormhole" (Color Plate 6C), representing a transient pore. In some cases highly organized arrays of lipids and peptides can be detected within these wormholes (Yang et al., 2000b). Peptides begin to accumulate within the inner leaflet of the bilayer (Color Plate 6D), and some fraction escape and diffuse into the interior of the cell (Color Plate 6E). As peptides continue to invade the upper face of the bilayer, the membrane, heavily contaminated by peptides, disintegrates into fragments carpeted with peptides (Shai, 1999) (Color Plate 6F).

The precise orientation of particular peptides within artificial phospholipid membranes and their interactions with component phospholipids have been studied in detail by various methods (Konovalov et al., 2002; Schibili et al., 2002b). Interactions between lipid bilayers and specific peptides, as depicted by computer simulation, appear to reasonably predict properties discovered by biophysical methods (Shepherd et al., 2003). The presence of cholesterol in the target membrane in general reduces the activity of antimicrobial peptides due to either stabilization of the lipid bilayer or interactions between cholesterol and the peptide (Matsuzaki, 1999). Phospholipids with relatively small head groups, such as phosphatidylserine and phosphatidylethanolamine, decrease the activity of most peptides because more peptide is required to be adsorbed per unit area to achieve the same degree of lateral expansion compared to a leaflet composed of lipids with larger-volume head groups, such as phosphatidylglycerol (Yang et al., 2000b). Similarly, it is believed that increasing ionic strength, which in general reduces the activity of most antimicrobial peptides, does so, in part, by weakening the electrostatic charge interactions required for the initial interaction.

In general, peptides operating by the SMH mechanism kill microbes at micromolar concentrations. In contrast, the peptide nisin, a 14-amino-acid amphipathic molecule produced by lactobacilli, operates at nanomolar concentrations. Nisin binds with high affinity to lipid II, the fatty acyl proteoglycan anchor in the bacterial membrane, and thereupon adopts a transmembrane orientation leading to pore formation and membrane permeabilization (Brotz et al., 1998; Van Heusden et al., 2002). Certain plant defensins use a similar strategy. The *Dahlia merckii* defensin binds to the major membrane lipid mannosyl innositol diphosphate ceramide in the membrane of the yeast *Saccharomyces cerevisiae*, subsequently disrupting membrane permeability (Thevissen et al., 2000).

How do antimicrobial peptides actually kill microbes? Many hypotheses have been presented, including fatal depolarization of the normally energized bacterial membrane (Westerhoff et al., 1989); membrane damage resulting in leakage of ions such as potassium, leading to loss of internal osmotic pressure, with subsequent water influx and fatal cellular swelling (Orlov et al., 2002); the creation of physical holes that cause macromolecular cellular contents to leak out (Yang et al., 2000b); the activation of deadly processes such as induction of cell wall-degrading hydrolases (Bierbaum and Sahl, 1985); the scrambling of the usual distribution of lipids between the leaflets of the bilayer, resulting in disturbance of membrane functions (Matsuzaki, 1999); and the damaging of critical intracellular targets following internalization of the peptide (Kragol et al., 2001, 2002; Patrzykat et al., 2002; Cudic and Otvos, 2002). A recent study using microarray analysis of *Escherichia coli* treated with cecropin suggests that specific gene sets are induced by exposure, which differs from responses to nutritional, thermal, osmotic, or oxidative stress (Hong et al., 2003). In my opinion, it is likely each of these mechanisms contributes to the activity of most peptides, with certain mechanisms more critical than others depending on the peptide and the microbe.

Although most studies of mechanism have focused on the antimicrobial activity of these molecules, activity of various antimicrobial peptides against protozoans such as plasmodia (Ghosh et al., 1997), *Leishmania* spp. (Bera et al., 2003), and *Trypanosoma* spp. (Vizioli and Salzet, 2002; Jacobs et al., 2003) has been reported. Limited studies of mechanism suggest that membrane damage to the outmost limiting membrane of the protozoan is involved in the killing activity, but details of this mechanism are incompletely understood. Studies reported from this laboratory on the effects of magainin on the freshwater protozoan *Paramecium caudatum* described a complex effect of the peptide on the organism's handling of water flux, as evident initially by the progressive swelling of the contractile vacuole, resulting in swelling of the organism, followed by rupture (Zasloff et al., 1988). Molecules

optimized for certain strains of *Plasmodium* in the sporogonic stage have been recently developed, likely with the intent of engineering insects that can effectively destroy the parasite (Arrighi et al., 2002). Curiously, insects respond with antimicrobial defense reactions as they become infected with certain parasites, such as seen in the case of the tsetse fly and the trypanosome (Boulanger et al., 2002). These innate defensive responses likely control the systemic spread of the protozoan and permit the insect to survive as a "vector," suggesting a novel mode of controlling the spread of insect-borne diseases.

HEPCIDIN AND IRON METABOLISM

An interesting class of newly described antimicrobial peptides is represented by the hepcidins. The peptide was isolated from human urine and subsequently shown to be expressed in the liver (Park et al., 2001). Hepcidin was found to be identical to a liver-encoded protein linked genetically to iron storage in mammals (Nicolas et al., 2001; Roetto et al., 2003). Levels of hepcidin fall in the setting of iron excess and rise in the setting of total body iron deficiency; iron uptake from the gastrointestinal tract appears to correlate inversely with serum hepcidin levels; inactivating mutations in humans result in a state of pathological iron overload, suggesting that hepcidin in some fashion restricts iron absorption (Roetto et al., 2003). Because hepcidin levels rise in the setting of infection, which in turn results in decreased plasma iron, a nutrient required for bacterial growth, it is believed that hepcidin plays a role in host defense as a "physiological" mediator. The precise role of hepcidin's antimicrobial properties in this setting remains unclear. Hepcidins have recently been isolated from other vertebrates, including fish. Bass hepcidin is a 21-amino-acid antimicrobial peptide with four disulfide bonds; it was isolated initially from gills and dramatically induced in liver following a challenge with a fish pathogen; the gene has regulatory elements that include NF-κB (Shike et al., 2002).

INTERNALIZATION OF ANTIMICROBIAL PEPTIDES INTO EUKARYOTIC CELLS

Although antimicrobial peptides display selectivity for microbes over the cells of metazoan organisms, numerous studies have reported the activity of antimicrobial peptides against cancer cells (Jacob and Zasloff, 1994; Hui et al., 2002). Earlier reports suggested that susceptibility of transformed cells over their normal counterparts was due, in part, to the anionic lipid composition of the outer resulting leaflet of the transformed cell, leading to electrostatic interaction and subsequent lysis, not unlike the mechanism proposed for antibacterial action. However, recent studies suggest that in some cases, peptides are internalized and cause cellular damage through perturbation of intracellular events. Structural studies on the Bac 7 peptide demonstrate that internalization is promoted by the presence of proline residues, in addition to cationic charges (Sadler et al., 2002). A detailed study of analogues of magainin and buforin, in their capacity to translocate across the membranes of HeLa cells and a fibroblast line, suggested that various translocation mechanisms are utilized by different peptides (Takeshima et al., 2003). Studies with BMAP-28 (bone marrow antimicrobial peptide), a bovine cathelicidin, causes cell death in human tumor lines and activated lymphocytes, likely through translocation across the cell membrane and subsequent damage to mitochondrial permeability (Risso et al., 2002). A similar mechanism has been proposed for the anticandidal activity of the salivary peptide histatin 5 (Helmerhorst et al., 2001). Indeed, derivatives of dermaseptin were shown to kill intraerythrocyte malarial parasites without erythrocyte lysis (Efron et al., 2002). Derivatives based on dermaseptin S4 with various fatty acids have been created with increased selectivity (Dagan et al., 2002).

RESISTANCE

Unlike conventional antibiotics such as penicillin, which microbes readily circumvent, acquisition of resistance by a sensitive microbial strain against antimicrobial peptides is surprisingly improbable. Certain bacterial species are intrinsically resistant to antimicrobial peptides, in the sense that they survive killing at concentrations in excess of what they might be expected to encounter in vivo. Resistant species of genera such as *Morganella* and *Serratia* express an outer membrane that lacks the appropriate density of acidic lipids to provide peptide binding sites. Indeed, measurement of binding sites of protegrin on the lipopolysaccharide (LPS) from sensitive *Pseudomonas aeruginosa* versus resistant *Burkholderia* species suggests that resistance correlates with reduced peptide binding sites to critical membranes (Albrect et al., 2002). Other resistant species, such as *Porphyromonas gingivalis*, secrete digestive proteases that destroy peptides. Proteinases secreted by organisms such as *Enterococcus faecalis* and *P. aeruginosa* have been shown to degrade natural peptides such as LL-37 in vitro, but their role as virulence factors in vivo has not been determined (Schmidtchen et al., 2002). No published data exist documenting the transfer of a resistant phenotype from a resistant to a sensitive species via either a plasmid or chromosomal DNA. Published studies of "acquired resistance" against antimicrobial peptides, by and large, have identified genes that, when disrupted, make sensitive organisms more susceptible to a particular antimicrobial peptide; indeed, these genes usually appear to play a role in virulence: compelling evidence that harmless bacteria become pathogenic in part by evolving defenses against antimicrobial peptides they encounter on invasion of the host.

A recent report of a survey of thousands of clinical isolates against the synthetic magainin analogue pexiganan illustrates the general picture that has emerged over the past decade regarding the issues of resistance (Ge et al., 1999). Bacterial species exhibit a wide range of susceptibilities, with some, such as anaerobes in the case of pexiganan, among the most sensitive. The basis for the different susceptibilities of bacterial and fungal species to particular peptides remains unexplained. Attempts at inducing pexiganan resistance in *E. coli* and *Staphylococcus aureus* by chemical mutagenesis have been unsuccessful to date. Repeated passage of bacteria such as *S. aureus, Staphylococcus epidermidis, Enterobacter cloacae, Klebsiella pneumoniae, P. aeruginosa, Acinetobacter baumannii,* and *Stenotrophomonas maltophilia* at sublethal concentrations of pexiganan failed to select resistant isolates, under conditions at which isolates resistant to conventional agents such as quinolones and β-lactams could readily be selected. As expected, no evidence of cross-resistance between pexiganan and any antibiotic in clinical use has been documented.

To kill a microbe, the antimicrobial peptide must initially dock onto negatively charged moieties exposed on the membrane surface, and high-affinity interactions between certain antimicrobial peptides and LPS have been described (Hancock et al., 1995; Hirakura et al., 2002). The best-characterized resistance strategies involve modifications that make the overall charge of the barrier more positive, reducing electrostatic interaction.

Gram-negative bacteria possess an outer membrane composed of LPS, which is held together by magnesium and calcium ions that bridge negatively charged phosphosugars. The addition of cationic peptides results in displacement of metal, damaging the outer membrane, and facilitates entry of additional molecules from the exterior (as reviewed by Hancock et al. [1995]). Peptides, having gained access to the periplasmic space, can now integrate into the cytoplasmic membrane.

In many species of gram-negative bacteria the charge on the outer membrane is modulated by the PhoPQ regulon, a two-component system that utilizes a sensor (PhoQ) and an intracellular effector, PhoP (Groisman, 1998). The PhoP/PhoQ regulon affects antimicrobial peptide sensitivity through modulation of the polymyxin resistance A regulon, which controls a bank of genes that mediate decoration of the outer membrane with the positively charged moieties ethanolamine and 4-aminoarabinose (Tamayo et al., 2002; Gunn et al., 2000). The crystal structure of a

Salmonella 4-aminoarabinose LPS transferase has recently been published, opening the possibility of designing classes of agents that might lessen the virulence of certain pathogens by blocking modifications directed at antimicrobial peptides (Noland et al., 2002). In the case of *Haemophilus influenzae,* an organism that causes meningitis in young children, LPS is made more cationic by decoration with phosphorylcholine (PC). This modification requires the enzyme phosphorylcholine kinase (PCK). The PCK gene exhibits phase variation, a random activation or inactivation due to variability in the inheritance of a repetitive sequence within the translation frame of PCK. Analysis of isolates from the airway show high PC decoration (selection for gene turned on), suggesting that variants more resistant to antimicrobial peptide assault are selected (Lysenko et al., 2000).

S. aureus, a common human pathogen, has two normally expressed loci that, when disrupted, increase the sensitivity of this species to antimicrobial peptides. *dlt* effects the addition of alanine, via its carboxyl group, onto the sugar hydroxyls of the proteoglycan coat, adding a positive charge to the coat; *mprF* encodes a protein that is involved in the coupling of lysine onto the glycerol of phosphatidylglycerol, yielding the strongly cationic phospholipid lysyl phosphatidylglycerol (Peschel et al., 2001; Peschel, 2002).

Other bacterial genes that influence the activity of specific antimicrobial peptides and are associated with the virulence of certain bacterial species include modifications that affect the chain length of the LPS lipid moieties, leading to a more intrinsically stable outer membrane (Ernst et al., 1999), and several involved in maintaining ionic homeostasis after initial damage, peptide transporters that can eliminate internalized molecules, and highly selective proteases (as reviewed by Peschel [2002] and Groisman [1995]).

Why have microbes not been more successful in resisting the activity of antimicrobial peptides, considering the span of time over which such mechanisms could have evolved?

The usual strategies of resistance include altering the microbial target or destroying the antibiotic, via a mechanism that does not impair the growth or viability of the microbe. Since the target of antimicrobial peptides is the bacterial membrane, a microbe would have to redesign its membrane, changing the composition and/or organization of its lipids, most likely a very "costly" solution for most microbial species. Destruction of the antimicrobial peptide poses several problems. Most peptides are created from nondescript sequences of amino acids lacking unique epitopes that could serve as the recognition site of a protease required for selective destruction of the antibiotic in the presence of cellular protein constituents. In addition, multicellular organisms attack microbes with multiple peptides of different structural classes, and hence destruction of one peptide might not suffice to ward off the lethal assault. Perhaps the virulence genes that bacteria now express which affect susceptibility toward antimicrobial peptides represent the best defenses that most microbes can mount without suffering a loss of viability, the selection having already taken place over the period of time microbes and multicellular organisms have coexisted.

REGULATION

We have come to realize that plants and animals not only share a dependence on antimicrobial peptides, but also utilize common intracellular circuits to regulate the activity of their corresponding genes.

Insects

Following the discovery of inducible antimicrobial peptides in silk moths and *Drosophila* by Boman's laboratory (Kylsten et al., 1990), the corresponding genes were cloned and sequenced. The genes are expressed in blood cells, epithelia, and the insects' fat body, an organ resembling the vertebrate liver that secretes proteins and peptides directly into the animals' hemolymph. The 5′ flanking regions harbored sequences that bound Rel transcription factors, analogues of the NF-κB-binding motifs of mammals (Engström et al., 1993; Kappler et al., 1993). These putative regulatory regions had previously been implicated in *Drosophila* in early embryonic development (as reviewed by Imler and Hoffmann [2000]). Examination of the intracellular pathway involved in the regulation of antimicrobial peptides revealed that much of the early embryonic circuit was co-opted for a defensive function. A recent view of this pathway shows it to involve initiation of the signal through proteolytic generation of the protein Spaetzle from its precursor; the presumed interaction of Spaetzle with a receptor called Toll; subsequent communication through a series of intracellular proteins resulting in the chemical modification of Cactus, which is then released from its physical union with the Dorsal-related protein called Dif; Dif then moves into the nucleus, where it binds to a DNA sequence in the vicinity of the antimicrobial gene, activating transcription. Drosomycin, an important antifungal peptide in *Drosophila*, appears to be regulated by this circuit (Imler and Hoffmann, 2000; Lemaitre et al., 1996).

As predicted, mutant flies that have lost the function of certain genes within this pathway can no longer express Drosomycin following a fungal challenge and succumb to overwhelming fungal infection (Lemaitre et al., 1996). Conversely, mutants that are created to overexpress Spaetzle, the Toll ligand, produce Drosomycin in the absence of fungal challenge (Levashina et al., 1999). Mutants defective in the Toll-Drosomycin circuit can still express antibacterial peptides such as cecropin and defensins (Lemaitre et al., 1996). The residual circuit is called the *imd* pathway, regulated by a pathway that is activated by a Dif-related protein called relish (Hendengren et al., 1999). Like Dif, relish resides in the cytoplasm in union with a partner from which it must be liberated by upstream events (Stoven et al., 2000). *imd* appears to encode a protein with a sequence similarity to that of mammalian RIP and associates with the *Drosophila* death protein dFADD (Naitza et al., 2002). The actual receptor that turns on the *imd* intracellular pathway may be the proteoglycan recognition protein (PGRP)-LC receptor (Choe et al., 2002), a membrane-associated protein of the proteoglycan recognition family.

Deletion of both *imd* and Toll pathways creates *Drosophila* insects which fail to produce any known antimicrobial peptide; constitutive expression of a single peptide, introduced genetically into these double-null mutants, can rescue these insects from susceptibility to certain microbial infections, highlighting the importance of antimicrobial peptides in immune defense in *Drosophila* (Tzou et al., 2002). Deletion of the Rel locus in mosquitoes is associated with depressed defensin and cecropin synthesis and susceptibility to gram-negative infections (Shin et al., 2003), demonstrating the conservation of intracellular circuitry between widely separated insect species.

The *Drosophila* story also demonstrates the role of proteins in the defense circuitry that recognize distinct proteoglycan "patterns" in the initiation of the defensive cascade (Hoffmann and Reichhart, 2002). Pro-Spaetzle is converted to Spaetzle when a PGRP, PGRP-SA, binds to the proteoglycan from gram-positive bacteria (Michel et al., 2001). This complex, in turn, activates an as yet uncharacterized protease that cleaves pro-Spaetzle (Michel et al., 2001). Gram-negative bacteria interact with the putative transmembrane protein, PGRP-LC, which functions, in some undefined fashion, upstream of the *imd* pathway (Gottar et al., 2002). Fungal organisms activate, via binding to an uncharacterized PGRP, the serine protease Persephone, which processes Spaetzle (Ligoxygakis et al., 2002).

Vertebrates

Expression of the antimicrobial β-defensins TAP (Diamond et al., 1991) in epithelial cells of the bovine respiratory tract and LAP in the tongue (Schonwetter et al., 1995) were shown to be stimulated by LPS, interleukin-1β (IL-1β), and tumor necrosis factor (TNF) (Russell et al., 1996) and were upregulated in vivo in the setting of inflammation and following acute bacterial challenge. Reports followed that described the induction of β-defensins in various epithelia including the human gastrointestinal (O'Neil et al., 1999) and respiratory (Singh et al., 1998; Harder et al., 2000) tracts and skin (Harder et al., 1997). Analysis of the 5′ flanking regions of several inducible epithelial antimicrobial peptide genes from mammals (Tarver et al., 1998; Liu et al., 1998) and frogs (reviewed by Simmaco et al., 1998), like insects, revealed NF-κB binding sites. Exposure to the appropriate stimulus resulted in an increase in intracellular levels of NF-κB, its translocation into the nucleus, and activation of the corresponding antimicrobial gene.

The inducing activity of IL-1β implicated a role for the IL-1 receptor (IL-1R) in the regulation of epithelial defensin production. The IL-1R is a close structural relative of Toll, and both respond to a protein ligand which must be proteolytically processed. Furthermore, the intracellular pathways involved in IL-1 signaling converge on NF-κB like the corresponding Toll pathway in insects. In mammals, IL-1 can be liberated from monocytes, macrophages, dendritic cells, or injured epithelial cells (Murphy et al., 2000). LPS-stimulated monocytes produce large quantities of pro-IL-1β, requiring processing to the mature species for secretion. Several antimicrobial peptides, such as protegrin 1 and magainin, but not the natural peptides PR26 or PR39, stimulate coupled processing and secretion of the mature active form of IL-1β, suggesting that the expression of certain antimicrobial peptides can be governed by positive autoregulatory loops (Perregaux et al., 2002).

The discovery that Toll and Toll-like receptors (TLRs) played a role in antimicrobial peptide gene expression in insects and mammals led to a search for additional human homologues, driven by the hypothesis that the innate immune system utilizes specially tuned receptors to recognize specific and unique microbial chemical constituent patterns presented when microbes attack a multicellular organism (reviewed by Perregaux et al. [2002] and Kimbrell and Beutler [2001]).

Subsequent studies have demonstrated that at least 10 TLR genes exist in humans (Kimbrell and Beutler, 2001; Imler and Hoffmann, 2002). TLRs are located in just the right places one would imagine them to be were they serving as the sentinels of attack to activate antimicrobial peptides; they are expressed, for example, on the epithelial cells of the lungs (Becker et al., 2000; Droemann et al., 2003), the oral cavity (A. Weinberg, personal communication), and the bowel (Melmed et al., 2003). Studies linking TLRs with antimicrobial gene expression with the strong experimental support that has been gathered in *Drosophila* have emerged from several laboratories (Birchler et al, 2001; Wang et al., 2002). For example, in the human gingival epithelium, TLR4 has been implicated in the activation by bacteria of the inducible β-defensin HBD2 (Weinberg, personal communication). The current model suggests that microbial products, such as LPS, bind directly to these TLRs, in some cases in association with specific binding proteins that might enhance specificity (such as the LPS-binding protein CD14), but the full story regarding ligand–receptor interactions as well the intracellular circuitry utilized to modulate antimicrobial peptide gene expression is still very incomplete. Since specific TLR receptors recognize particular microbial products (Kimbrell and Beutler, 2001; Imler and Hoffmann, 2002), it will be interesting to see which microbial products these sentinels are designed to detect in their specific microenvironments.

Plants

Like animals, plants express antimicrobial peptides such as defensins (Thomma et al., 2003; Park et al., 2002), thionins (Vila-Perelló et al., 2003), "cyclotides" (Jennings et al., 2001; Tam et al., 1999), and potato "snakins" (Berrocal-Lobo et al., 2002), both constitutively and in response to microbial assault. The initial insult is transmitted by highly specific pattern recognition receptors called Toll–interleukin-related–nucleotide domain (ND)–leucine-rich repeat (TIR–ND–LRR) receptors, analogues of the mammalian TLRs; they in turn activate a relatively specific hard-wired response against the specific organism to which it is tuned, a concept termed the "gene-for-gene" defensive strategy in the plant literature (Dangl and Jones, 2001). Although the precise ligands and intracellular circuits involved are largely unknown, even at this rudimentary stage of knowledge, the similarities between the plant and vertebrate innate systems seem to be remarkable.

ROLES IN HEALTH AND DISEASE

Antimicrobial peptides provide epithelial surfaces with protective agents that permit an animal to construct a physical barrier out of materials that could otherwise serve as a source of nutrients for microbes.

Epithelial Surfaces

Antimicrobial peptides are both expressed by the epithelial cells within the barrier and delivered to the site by circulating white blood cells. This generalization is valid for both all vertebrates studied to date (e.g., fish gills [Iijima et al., 2003]) and very likely every invertebrate, including insects (Brey et al., 1993). The particular peptides contained in the circulating cells and expressed in the epithelium differ between species, presumably creating an antimicrobial shield "tuned" for that organism, and act in synergy with proteins such as lysozyme, granulysin, and lactoferrin (Cole et al., 2002). In humans and other mammals, fully processed active peptides can be isolated from keratinized epithelial sheets of both dry skin and tongue, where they likely act as epithelial "preservatives." HBD2 can be found within the keratinocytes at the lower layer and surrounding the keratinocytes in the more superficial layers, suggesting a complex transport pathway, observed both in vivo (Huh et al., 2002) and in vitro (Liu et al., 2002). A microarray analysis of human epidermis following exposure to IL-1 demonstrated that the HBD2 gene was among the most inducible of the genes expressed (Liu et al., 2003). LL-37 is secreted onto the ductal epithelium of exocrine glands, such as the salivary (Murakami et al., 2002a) and sweat (Murakami et al., 2002b) glands, both protecting the gland itself from microbial invasion (an otherwise acceptable bacterial niche) and providing protection to the epithelial surface via the secretion (Murakami et al., 2002b). In the human upper respiratory tract (nasal mucosa [Lee et al., 2002; Kim et al., 2003] and larynx [Kutta et al., 2002]) and lower respiratory tract (Schaller-Bals et al., 2002), expression of the inducible defensin HBD2 and the cathelicidin LL-37 appears to be consistently elevated in states of infection, suggesting a defensive function. In one report, mice in which the mouse β-defensin MBD1 was knocked out exhibited delayed clearance of *H. influenzae* from the lung (Moser et al., 2002); in another study of a similar knockout, carriage of *Staphylococcus* species in the bladder was higher than in controls (Morrison et al., 2002b).

In other sites in humans, such as the columnar epithelium of the airway, antimicrobial peptides are secreted into a micrometer-thick biofilm directly overlying the epithelium. The concentration and composition of electrolytes within this antimicrobial-rich unstirred layer are regulated by a variety of pumps and channels, which maintain conditions that maximize the antimicrobial activity of these defenses. In cystic fibrosis, this homeostasis is disturbed due to the genetic defect in cystic fibrosis transmembrane regulator; antimicrobial peptide defenses fail to provide an effective barrier, resulting in bacterial overgrowth and chronic tissue-destructive inflammation (Smith et al., 1996; Goldman et al., 1997). In addition, anionic polyelectrolytes within the sputum of the cystic fibrosis patient, such as DNA and F actin, further sequester these peptides (Weiner et al., 2003).

The skin of an animal is under constant microbial assault, and a recent study highlights the defensive contribution to this barrier provided by antimicrobial peptides. The mouse has only a single member of the cathelicidin gene family, called MCRAMP, which it expresses in both leukocytes and epithelial tissues. Knockout mutants of MCRAMP exhibit hypersusceptibility to group A *Streptococcus* and succumb to destructive necrotic ulceration following inoculation of a dose of bacteria that causes only a mild self-limited reaction in wild-type mice (Nizet et al., 2001). Similarly, mutants of group A streptococci selected for reduced susceptibility to MCRAMP (which, curiously, seem to grow more slowly than the wild type) exhibit an enhanced virulence when introduced into the dermis of wild-type mice. In this model, although neutrophils appear to be functionally intact in killing, the mast cells, which also express MCRAMP, appear to be somewhat impaired in activity against *Streptococcus* spp., making it somewhat difficult to ascribe a defect in this knockout to the epithelium alone (Di Nardo et al., 2003). Does a comparable balance between pathogen and antimicrobial peptide exist for the human, who like the mouse expresses a sole cathelicidin?

Perhaps. Although both psoriasis and atopic dermatitis are inflammatory skin conditions, associated with physical disruption of the normal structure of the epidermis, infection is rarely associated with psoriasis, whereas *S. aureus* infections commonly complicate eczematous lesions. A recent report demonstrates that, whereas HBD2 and LL-37 are robustly expressed in psoriasis, they are not significantly expressed in eczematous lesions. Apparently, the cytokines associated with the atopic state, such as IL-13, suppress the induction of these antimicrobial peptides, leading to colonization and infection by *S. aureus* (Ong et al., 2002).

A deficiency state in neutrophil-associated antimicrobial peptides, defensins, and LL-37 has recently been described. Morbus Kostmann is a rare, genetically transmitted neutropenic condition, identified in a Swedish cohort, associated with fatal infections, usually arising during childhood. Treatment with the granulocyte-monocyte colony-stimulating factor restores neutrophil populations, but neutrophils appear to be selectively deficient in LL-37 and α-defensins. Severe periodontal disease suggests a role for neutrophil cathelicidins in gingival health (Putsep et al., 2002). Neutrophils populate the gingival sulcus and appear to secrete the cathelicidin LL-37 into the oral cavity, since LL-37 can be found in saliva. In patients suffering from Morbus Kostmann, salivary LL-37 is absent (Putsep et al., 2002).

Although we tend to regard circulating mature polymorphonuclear white cells as end-stage transcriptionally inactive cells, it appears that in some settings this is not the case. Bovine neutrophils, exposed to LPS in vitro, respond in the transcription of Bac 5, a cathelicidin which like LL-37 is released extracellularly. This study suggests that, in some physiological settings where collections of neutrophils are normally resident, such as the oral cavity, induction of antimicrobial peptide synthesis and subsequent secretion into the oral cavity by "secretory" neutrophils resident in the gingival sulcus might occur physiologically (Tomasinsig et al., 2002).

The gastrointestinal tract of mammals is covered by a continuous sheet of epithelial cells that is folded into villous projections and crypts. Within the base of the crypts, where the stem cells of the gastrointestinal tract can be found, we find specialized granular cells called Paneth cells in both humans and mice. Both the enterocytes and the Paneth cells produce antimicrobial peptides (as reviewed by Oulette and Bevins [2001]). The enterocytes synthesize and secrete antimicrobial peptides both constitutively and upon induction and either secrete them onto their surface as in the respiratory tract or, as in the rectum, retain them in a cell-associated fashion in the superficial nonviable sheets of epithelium. The Paneth cells at the base of the intestinal crypts, in contrast, secrete α-defensins into the cryptal well, following a microbial stimulus resulting in concentrations estimated at milligram-per-milliliter level, which eventually flush into the gut lumen (Ayabe et al., 2000). In humans, the precursors of α-defensins (HD5 and HD6) are stored in intracellular granules along with trypsinogen, with processing occurring following secretion (Ghosh et al., 2002). Although both precursor and mature forms have antimicrobial activity, their spectra differ (Ghosh et al., 2002).

The defensins released by Paneth cells influence the virulence of orally ingested bacteria.

Transgenic mice expressing human α-defensins, which are more active against *Salmonella typhimurium* than respective mouse defensins, are relatively resistant to oral inoculation of this normally pathogenic bacterial species compared to wild-type mice (Salzman et al., 2003a). In this chapter I strongly support the hypothesis that organisms that cause disease through entry of the gastrointestinal tract must survive the innate antimicrobial defenses provided by Paneth cell defensins if they are to cause infection.

In children and adults suffering from diarrhea caused by *Shigella* spp., synthesis of the colonic enterocyte β-defensin HBD1 and the cathelicidin LL-37 is markedly depressed; expression recovers in time during resolution of the illness (Islam et al., 2001). Similarly, mice lacking the proteolytic enzyme required for processing cryptdins, the murine Paneth cell α-defensins, and consequently lacking functional cryptdins, exhibit increased susceptibility to orally administered *Salmonella* spp. (Wilson et al., 1999). Virulent salmonellae have been shown to depress Paneth cell secretion, with the SPI1 type III secretion system implicated as the determinant (Salzman et al., 2003b).

Crohn's disease is a chronic inflammatory condition involving the mucosa of the distal small bowel and portions of the ascending colon. The cause of this disease is unknown, but there is general agreement that inflammation occurs as an abnormal response to commensal flora (Shanahan, 2002). Consistent with this view is the observation that inactivating mutations in NOD2, a membrane-associated protein similar in structure to an LPS sensor in plants, have been linked to certain cohorts of patients with Crohn's disease (Hampe et al., 2002). A recent report demonstrates that HBD2 expression is markedly depressed in the enterocytes of the ileum and colon of individuals with Crohn's disease, compared with comparable studies in patients with ulcerative colitis and nonspecific colitis (Wehkamp et al., 2002). The precise mechanism underlying the depressed expression of HBD2 is not yet clear, but one might imagine that the inflammatory process, sustained by the adaptive immune system, has responded to a failure of the innate system to properly defend the mucosal barrier.

Curiously, in both Crohn's disease and ulcerative colitis, neutrophil human neutrophil defensins proteins 1 to 3 (HNP1–3) are expressed in enterocytes in inflamed mucosa (Fahlgren et al., 2003; Cunliffe et al., 2002). The basis for ectopic expression of these defensins is unknown.

A rather surprising scenario has been discovered to operate in the gastric mucosa of humans, mice, and other vertebrates. It appears that histone 2A is synthesized in excess of the amount required for DNA packaging in the gastric mucosal cell and accumulates within cytoplasmic secretory granules. Upon secretion, the histone is processed by pepsin to the potent antimicrobial peptide buforin II, which remains adherent to the mucous biofilm coating the stomach surface, thus providing the stomach with a protective antimicrobial coat (Kim et al., 2000). A similar process involving proteolytic cleavage of histone 2A also occurs in the mucous layer of catfish. However, as in other parts of the gastrointestinal tract, the enterocytes of the gastric mucosa also produce β-defensins in inflammatory conditions such as *Helicobacter pylori*-associated gastritis; this microbe is susceptible to HBD2 (Uehara et al., 2003). In vitro, both *H. pylori* and IL-1β have been shown to be effective inducers of HBD2 (Bajaj-Elliot et al., 2002).

The healthy human is inhabited by a population of bacteria called "commensals," which include organisms such as *Fusobacterium nucleatum* in the mouth or *Lactobacillus acidophilus* in the gut. These bacteria both are relatively resistant to the action of endogenous antimicrobial peptides and, at the same time, induce epithelial defensins. In the gingival epithelium, *F. nucleatum* stimulates the inducible defensin HBD2, while *P. gingivalis*, the anaerobe that destroys gum tissue, does not, behaving as a silent invader (Krisanaprakornkit et al., 2000). Hence, commensals can provide a chronic inducing stimulus to maintain "protective" levels of certain antimicrobial peptides in and

on epithelial surfaces, protecting by stimulating the underlying epithelium to synthesize a suite of molecules that suppresses potential pathogens. In addition, antimicrobial substances secreted by lactobacilli (bacteriocins) have been shown to synergize with certain epithelial antimicrobial peptides, extending the antimicrobial spectrum of both classes of agent (Luders et al., 2003). Frogs that have been pharmacologically depleted of skin antimicrobial peptides will not reaccumulate skin antimicrobial peptides unless the animals are exposed to bacteria in their environment, and they will succumb to overwhelming infection if suddenly exposed (Mangoni et al., 2001).

Urogenital and Reproductive Tract

Antimicrobial peptides, including both α- and β-defensins, are widely expressed in the male reproductive tracts of rats, mice, and humans. They are distributed not only in the epithelial linings of the epididymis and seminiferous tubules but also in the germ cells, Leydig cells, Sertoli cells, and various interstitial cells, suggesting an as yet not fully appreciated function (Yamaguchi et al., 2002; Com et al., 2003). Human antibacterial cathelicidin-18 (HCAP-18), the precursor of LL-37, can be found in high concentrations in human seminal plasma, associated with both sperm and high-molecular-weight complexes called prostasomes (Andersson et al., 2002). In the rat, expression of β-defensin 1 in the epididymis appears to be regulated by androgens (Palladino et al., 2003). Several novel antimicrobial peptides, specifically expressed in human epididymis (HE2 peptides), encoded by genes that lie within the defensin gene cluster, have been described (VonHorsten et al., 2002).

The fetal-placental unit is poised in a very fragile environment. The mechanisms that operate to maintain control over infection of the fetus are still poorly understood. Recent studies suggest that placental tissues, including amniotic fluid, are protected by intact H2A and H2B secreted into the fluid and expressed in the cytoplasm of synciotrophoblasts and amnion cells (Kim et al., 2002). Proinflammatory mediators such as IL-1β have been shown to stimulate induction of HBD2 in endometrial cells in vitro (King et al., 2002). The cervical mucous plug, which provides a physical barrier between the cervix and the bacteria-laden perineal area of the woman, exhibits antimicrobial activity resulting from a cocktail of antimicrobial peptides including lysozyme, lactoferrin, and neutrophil defensins (Hein et al., 2002). The fetus itself, during the third trimester in utero, becomes covered by a greasy, creamy substance, vernix caseosa, which has also been shown recently to contain a collection of antimicrobial peptides that are especially active against gram-negative bacteria (Yoshio et al., 2003).

The kidney is known to be surprisingly free from infection, both from organisms ascending from the urethra and from blood-borne microbes entering the parenchyma. In the normal uninfected kidney, HBD1 is widely expressed and can be found in urine. In states of infection, such as pyelonephritis, HBD2 is induced throughout the kidney epithelia, such as distal tubules, loops of Henle, and the collecting ducts. In vitro studies with renal cell lines demonstrate the inducing activity of IL-1β, TNF-α, and LPS (Lehmann et al., 2002).

Platelets

In many invertebrates, such as the horseshoe crab, a specific blood cell collects at a site of injury, degranulates, and discharges its contents into the vicinity of the wound, releasing proteins required for coagulation, growth factors to stimulate tissue repair, and large quantities of antimicrobial peptides (Iwanaga, 2002; Iwanaga and Kawabata, 1998). Similarly, the platelets of humans and several other mammals contain a collection of multifunctional antimicrobial peptides (Tang et al., 2002; Krijgsveld et al., 2000) which they release at the site of a thrombus, such as those that form continuously on native and prosthetic heart valves, making them less hospitable to circulating bacteria of the species of *Streptococcus* and *Staphy-*

lococcus (Wu et al., 1994). Failure of this system is linked to infectious endocarditis in humans (Wu et al., 1994).

ANTIMICROBIAL PEPTIDES AND ADAPTIVE IMMUNITY

Antimicrobial peptides, released from circulating cells or induced in epithelia, can alert the adaptive immune system to trouble brewing. The α-defensins of the human neutrophil directly attract CD4$^+$/CD45RA$^+$ (naive) and CD8$^+$ human peripheral blood T cells and immature dendritic cells both in vitro and following injection under the skin of mammals (as reviewed by Chertov et al., 2000). When administered simultaneously with antigens, these neutrophil defensins enhance antigen-specific immune responses. Fusion of antigenic peptides with β-defensin was shown to interact with the TLR4 receptor on dendritic cells, markedly increasing the immunogenicity of the antigen for TH1 polarized responses (Biragyn et al., 2002). The cathelicidin LL-37 attracts neutrophils along with monocytes and certain peripheral T cells. LL-37 appears to act via a formyl peptide receptor-like-1 (FPRL1) receptor, a G-protein-coupled receptor that also recognizes ligands such as the bacterial formyl peptides (Yang et al., 2000a). The mast cell also responds to LL-37 as a chemokine and, in addition, degranulates in its presence; the receptor utilized in this case, however, appears not to be FPRL1 (Niyonsaba et al., 2002).

LL-37 is induced within epithelial cells of skin and lung in states of inflammation by some 10- to 50-fold and would be expected to attract neutrophils, monocytes, and T cells to the site of damage. In a recent study, using expression profiling, exposure of macrophages to LL-37 was shown to stimulate expression of 29 genes including those for several chemokine receptors such as CXCR4, CCR2, and IL-8R, suggesting that antimicrobial peptides can profoundly modulate the chemokine response characteristics of certain defensive cells (Scott et al., 2002). The epithelial β-defensins, constitutively expressed HBD1, and the inducible

HBD2 and HBD3 are also chemoattractants. HBD2 selectively attracts the memory subset of peripheral T cells (CD4$^+$/CD45RO$^+$). The receptor utilized in this case has been identified to be CCR6, which also recognizes the selective dendritic cell attractant MIP-3α (Chertov et al., 2000). Curiously, CCR6 expression is restricted to the cells comprising the mantle and marginal zones of secondary lymphoid tissue within the submucosa (Rodig et al., 2002). The recent observation that HNP1 can be ADP-ribosylated by ADP ribosyltransferases on airway epithelial cells, resulting in a defensin modified at Arg 14 (inactive as an antimicrobial but retaining chemokine activity), suggests that regulatory loops exist (Paone et al., 2002).

What is striking about the chemokine role ascribed to antimicrobial peptides is their relatively low affinity (10^{-6} to 10^{-5} M) compared with optimal concentrations observed for classical chemotactic factors (10^{-8} to 10^{-7} M). High-affinity receptors generally reach maximal stimulation at a certain concentration of ligand, and in many cases they experience inactivation as the concentration of ligand exceeds optimal concentrations. A cell relying solely on high-affinity ligands for directing movement might experience a "stunning" as it approaches the source of the chemokine. However, low-affinity interactions will still operate, and as a consequence of the presence of a large concentration gradient, perhaps stabilized by the semisolid matrix of the epithelium, cellular traffic will be directed with greater precision to specific sites of injury.

CYTOKINES, PEPTIDE HORMONES, GROWTH FACTORS, AND ANTIMICROBIAL PEPTIDES

Over the past several years the functional categorization of antimicrobial peptides has been blurred somewhat by the discovery that numerous peptide hormones and cytokines exhibit potent antimicrobial activity in vitro. Whether these substances, in vivo, actually function in host defense remains controversial. α-Melanocyte-stimulating hormone has anti-inflammatory properties and is also antimicrobial (Grieco et al., 2003). Substance P exhibits antimicrobial activity against *S. aureus* (Kowalska et al., 2002). Neuropeptide Y, present in Langerhans cells in the skin, might serve a protective function in the skin (Lambert et al., 2002). Chromogranin A and B are processed to the antimicrobial fragments vasostatin and secretolytin, which appear in plasma following surgical procedures, suggesting either a direct antimicrobial role for this system or its presence as a sentinel for injury (Tasiemki et al., 2002). Several cytokines, such as CCL28, are secreted from human and mouse salivary and acinar cells and CC chemokines and appear in the saliva. The likely responding cells are plasma cells. CCL28 exhibits antibacterial and antifungal activity, suggesting a possible role as both a signaling molecule and an antimicrobial activity (Hieshima et al., 2003).

MIP-3α or CCL20 is a chemokine that activates the CCR6 receptor, a receptor it shares with no other chemokines. HBD1 and HBD2 were previously shown to bind to CCR6 and activate it. Surprisingly, MIP-3α exhibits greater potency towards *E. coli* and *S. aureus* than the defensins. Little sequence similarity exists between these molecules, but several structural features are shared, demonstrated by a comparison of crystal structures (Hoover et al., 2002).

Neutrophil defensins have been shown to enhance proliferation of epithelial cells, likely through a pathway that involves, indirectly, the epidermal growth factor receptor, including the MAP kinase signaling pathway; the study suggests that these defensins play a role in epithelial repair in the airway (Aarbiou et al., 2002).

APPLICATIONS

The growing problem of resistance to conventional antibiotics and the need for new antibiotics has stimulated interest in the development of antimicrobial peptides as human therapeutics. Most pharmaceutical effort to date has been devoted to the development of topically applied agents, such as the magainin analogue pexiganan (Zasloff, 2001) and the orally applied protegrin analogue (Chen et al., 2000), in large part because of the relative safety of topical therapy and the uncertainty surrounding the long-term toxicology of any new class of drug administered systemically. Furthermore, many of the naturally occurring peptides, such as magainin, although active in vitro, are effective in animal models of infection only at very high doses, often close to the 50% lethal dose of the peptide (Darveau et al., 1991; Pacor et al., 2002). Considerable effort is currently being expended by commercial and academic laboratories to understand the parameters that influence the therapeutic index of antimicrobial peptides and to discover how to optimize both potency and safety (Zasloff, 2001, 2002, 2003).

Diverse applications have been demonstrated for antimicrobial peptides as anti-infective agents. The broad antimicrobial spectrum of antimicrobial peptides positions them for consideration as "chemical condoms" to limit the spread of sexually transmitted diseases, including *Neisseria*, *Chlamydia*, human immunodeficiency virus (HIV), and herpes simplex virus (Yasin et al., 2000). Tachyplesin has been shown to have surprising activity against HIV via a specific blockade of the CXCR4 receptor (Xu et al., 1999). The affinity of antimicrobial peptides for microbial membranes has encouraged their evaluation as imaging probes for bacterial and fungal infections (Welling et al., 2000; Lupetti et al., 2003). Their ability to effectively bind to LPS has suggested their use in experimental models of septic shock (Nagaoka et al., 2002; Ghiselli et al., 2002). Antimicrobial peptides have been shown to enhance the potency of existing antibiotics in vivo, likely by facilitating access of antibiotics into the bacterial cell (Darveau et al., 1991) and through neutralization of LPS (Giacometti et al., 2002), phenomena previously recognized for the cationic peptide component of polymyxin. Numerous studies by Scalise and associates have confirmed the utility of this approach in vitro for both gram-negative and gram-positive bacterial species (Giacometti et al., 2000).

Microbial colonization and growth on the surfaces of synthetic polymeric materials is a problem that complicates the use of medical devices such as intravenous catheters. One novel solution has been suggested by the successful demonstration that magainin peptides, covalently bound to insoluble polymeric beads, retain antimicrobial activity (Haynie et al., 1995). Use of antimicrobial peptides as sterilants in corneal preservation media has been suggested (Mannis, 2002). Introduction of antimicrobial genes into both plants and animals has been successful in transferring some benefit against disease. Agricultural uses have progressed most extensively, as demonstrated in tobacco (Jaynes et al., 1993; Ponti et al., 2003), bananas (Chakrabarti et al., 2003), and potatoes (Osusky et al., 2000). The possibility of alleviating the pulmonary bacterial infections associated with cystic fibrosis by transferring in a genetic construct capable of expressing superphysiological levels of LL-37 has been demonstrated in an animal model (Bals et al., 1999). The potential of reengineering human macrophages to express β-defensins, to enhance their efficacy against *Mycobacterium tuberculosis*, has recently been proposed (Kisich et al., 2001).

The inducible nature of many antimicrobial peptide genes suggests that new therapeutics will be developed to enhance the expression of such peptides in settings that might provide therapeutic benefit. Hence, it might be possible to prevent those infections that arise because of a kinetic advantage possessed by an organism over the inducible response by administering an antimicrobial peptide inducer prior to pathogen exposure. Diseases such as Crohn's disease, atopic dermatitis, and certain forms of bacterial dysentery might be treatable through administration of substances that enhance antimicrobial peptide, circumventing the circuits depressed in the disease states. The discovery that the essential amino acid isoleucine can pharmacologically stimulate β-defensin gene expression in isolated enteric cells, operating through an NF-κB pathway, suggests that new classes of safe therapeutics could be developed based on their ability to turn on endogenous antimicrobial peptides (Fehlbaum et al., 2000; Schauber et al., 2003).

CONCLUSION

Antimicrobial peptides permit plants and animals, including humans, to live in harmony with microbes. As I have written elsewhere (Zasloff, 2002), it is hard to imagine (especially after reading a classical immunology text!) that most of the animals now alive, such as insects or creatures like the octopus or starfish, rely heavily on antimicrobial peptides for defense against microbes, and do so quite effectively without the help of lymphocytes, a thymus, or antibodies. A growing body of data suggests that antimicrobial peptides, in addition to functioning as "simple" antimicrobial agents, also participate in signaling the existence of injury or infection to the adaptive immune system. In addition, the recent discovery of the suppressive effects of cholinergic agonists on macrophage expression of inflammatory mediators such as IL-1β provides a novel functional linkage between the autonomic nervous system and epithelial antimicrobial peptide expression (Wang et al., 2003). If the story regarding diversity continues to unfold based on our current views, we might well discover that every species, and perhaps every distinct "ecological" niche in an organism available to microbes, will be found to express a specific collection of antimicrobial peptides designed to defend against microorganisms that it will predictably encounter. Antimicrobial peptides will continue to inspire new generations of anti–infective therapeutics based on antimicrobial strategies proven efficacious over the millennia. In addition, therapeutically valuable properties associated with these peptides, such as immunoadjuvant activity and proangiogenic activity (Li et al., 2000), will stimulate development in relevant therapeutic directions. Diseases that are associated with defects in expression of antimicrobial peptides will continue to be uncovered, and therapeutic intervention will likely be designed to correct—directly or indirectly— these deficits. Finally, as we continue to learn more about the intracellular circuitry involved

in regulation of expression of antimicrobial peptides, new therapeutics will be developed to either suppress or stimulate expression of these endogenous antibiotics.

REFERENCES

Aarbiou, J., M. Ertmann, S. Van Wetering, P. van Noort, D. Rook, K. F. Rabe, S. V. Litvinov, J. H. van Krieken, W. I. de Boer, and P. S. Hiemstra. 2002. Human neutrophil defensins induce lung epithelial proliferation in vitro. *J. Leukoc. Biol.* **72:**167–174.

Agerberth, B., J. Y. Lee, T. Berman, M. Carlquist, H. G. Boman, V. Mutt, and H. Jornvall. 1991. Amino acid sequence of PR39. Isolation of pig intestine of a new member of the family of proline arginine rich antibacterial peptides. *Eur. J. Biochem.* **202:** 849–854.

Albrect, M. T., W. Wang, O. Shamova, R. I. Lehrer, and N. L. Schiller. 2002. Binding of protegrin-1 to *Pseudomonas aeruginosa* and *Burkholderia cepacia. Respir. Res.* **3:**18.

Andersson, E., O. E. Sorensen, B. Frohm, N. Borregaard, A. Egesten, and J. Malm. 2002. Isolation of human cationic antimicrobial protein-18 from seminal plasma and its association with prostasomes. *Hum. Reprod.* **17:**2529–2534.

Andra, J., R. Herbst, and M. Leippe. 2003. Ameobapores, archaic effectors of protozoan origin, are discharged into phagosomes and kill bacteria by permeabilizing their membranes. *Dev. Comp. Immunol.* **27:**291–304.

Arrighi, R. B., C. Nakamura, J. Miyake, H. Hurd, and J. G. Burgess. 2002. Design and activity of antimicrobial peptides against sporoponic stage parasites causing murine malarias. *Antimicrob. Agents Chemother.* **46:**2104–2110.

Avrahami, D., and Y. Shai. 2002. Conjugation of a magainin analogue with lipophilic acids controls hydrophobicity, solution assembly, and cell selectivity. *Biochemistry* **41:**2254–2263.

Ayabe, T., D. P. Satchell, C. L. Wilson, W. C. Parks, M. E. Selsted, and A. J. Ouellette. 2000. Secretion of microbicidal α-defensins by intestinal Paneth cells in response to bacteria. *Nat. Immunol.* **1:**113–118.

Bajaj-Elliot, M., P. Fedeli, G. V. Smith, P. Domizio, L. Maher, R. S. Ali, A. G. Quinn, and M. J. Farthing. 2002. Modulation of host antimicrobial peptide (beta defensin 1 and 2) expression during gastritis. *Gut* **51:**356–361.

Bals, R., D. J. Weiner, A. D. Moscioni, R. L. Meegalla, and J. M. Wilson. 1999. Augmentation of innate host defense by expression of a cathelicidin antimicrobial peptide. *Infect. Immun.* **67:**6084–6089.

Bechinger, B., M. Zasloff, and S. J. Opella. 1993. Structure and orientation of the antibiotic peptide magainin in membranes by solid-state nuclear magnetic resonance spectroscopy. *Protein Sci.* **2**:2077–2084.

Becker, M. N., G. Diamond, M. W. Verghese, and S. H. Randell. 2000. CD14-dependent lipopolysaccharide-induced β-defensin-2 expression in human tracheobronchial epithelium. *J. Biol. Chem.* **275**:29731–29736.

Bera, A., S. Singh, R. Nagaraj, and T. Vaidya. 2003. Induction of autophagic cell-death in Leishmania donovani by antimicrobial peptides. *Mol. Biochem. Parisitol.* **127**:23–35.

Berrocal-Lobo, M., A. Segura, M. Moreno, G. Lopez, F. Garcia-Olmedo, and A. Molina. 2002. Snakin-2, an antimicrobial peptide from potato whose gene is locally induced by wounding and responds to pathogen infection. *Plant Physiol.* **128**:951–961.

Bierbaum, G., and H.-G. Sahl. 1985. Induction of autolysis of staphylococci by the basic peptide antibiotics pep5 and nisin and their influence on the activity of autolytic enzymes. *Arch. Microbiol.* **141**:249–254.

Biragyn, A., P. A. Ruffini, C. A. Leifer, E. Klyushnenkova, A. Shakhov, O. Chertov, A. K. Shirakawa, J. M. Farber, D. M. Segal, J. J. Oppenheim, and L. W. Kwak. 2002. Toll-like receptor 4-dependent activation of dendritic cells by beta-defensin 2. *Science* **298**:1025–1029.

Birchler, T., R. Seibl, K. Buchner, S. Loeliger, R. Seger, J. P. Hossle, A. Aguzzi, and R. P. Lauener. 2001. Human Toll-like receptor 2 mediates induction of the antimicrobial peptide human beta-defensin 2 in response to bacterial lipoprotein. *Eur. J. Immunol.* **31**:3131–3137.

Boman, H. G. 2000. Innate immunity and the normal microflora. *Immunol. Rev.* **173**:5–16.

Boulanger, N., R. Brun, L. Ehret-Sabatier, C. Kunz, and P. Bulet. 2002. Immunopeptides in the defense reactions of *Glossina morsitans* to bacterial and *Trypanosoma brucei brucei* infections. *Insect Biochem. Mol. Biol.* **32**:369–375.

Brey, P. T., W. J. Lee, M. Yamakawa, Y. Koizumi, S. Perrot, M. Franquis, and M. Ashida. 1993. Role of the integument in insect immunity: epicuticular abrasion and induction of cecropin synthesis in cuticular epithelial cells. *Proc. Natl. Acad. Sci. USA* **90**:6275–6279.

Brotz, H., M. Josten, L. Wiedeman, U. Schneider, F. Gotz, G. Bierbaum, and H.-G. Sahl. 1998. Role of lipid-bound peptidoglycan precursors in the formation of pores by nisin, epidermin and other lantibiotics. *Mol. Microbiol.* **30**:317–327.

Bulet, P., J. Dimarcq, C. Hetru, M. Lageux, M. Charlet, G. Hegy, A. Van Dorsselaer, and J. A. Hoffmann. 1993. A novel inducible antibacterial peptide of *Drosophila* carries an O-glycosylated substitution. *J. Biol. Chem.* **268**:14893–14897.

Chakrabarti, A., T. R. Ganapathi, P. K. Mukherjee, and V. A. Bapat. 2003. MSI-99, a mag-

ainin analogue, imparts enhanced disease resistance in transgenic tobacco and banana. *Planta* **216**:587–596.

Chen, J., T. J. Falla, H. Liu, M. A. Hurst, C. A. Fujii, D. A. Mosca, J. R. Embree, D. J. Loury, P. A. Radel, C. Cheng Chang, L. Gu, and J. C. Fiddes. 2000. Development of protegrins for the treatment and prevention of oral mucositis: structure-activity relationships of synthetic protegrin analogues. *Biopolymers* **55**:88–98.

Chertov, O., D. Yang, O. M. Howard, and J. J. Oppenheim. 2000. Leukocyte granule proteins mobilize innate host defenses and adaptive immune responses. *Immunol. Rev.* **177**:68–78.

Cho, J. H., I. Y. Park, M. S. Kim, and S. C. Kim. 2002. Matrix metalloproteinase 2 is involved in the regulation of antimicrobial peptide parasin I production in catfish skin mucosa. *FEBS Lett.* **531**:459–463.

Choe, K. M., T. Werner, S. Stoven, D. Hultmark, and K. V. Anderson. 2002. Requirement for a peptidoglycan recognition protein (PGRP) in Relish activation and antibacterial immune responses in Drosophila. *Science* **296**:359–362.

Circo, R., B. Skerlavaj, R. Gennaro, A. Amoroso, and M. Zanetti. 2002. Structural and functional characterization of hBD-1(ser35) peptide deduced from a DEFB1 polymorphism. *Biochem. Biophys. Res. Commun.* **293**:586–592.

Cole, A. M., H. I. Liao, O. Stuchlik, J. Tilan, J. Pohl, and T. Ganz. 2002. Cationic polypeptides are required for antibacterial activity of human airway fluid. *J. Immunol.* **169**:6985–6991.

Com, E., F. Bourgeon, B. Evrard, T. Ganz, D. Colleu, B. Jegou, and C. Pineau. 2003. Expression of antimicrobial defensins in the male reproductive tract of rats, mice, and humans. *Biol. Reprod.* **68**:95–104.

Corzo, G., E. Villegas, F. Gomez-Lagunas, L. D. Possani, O. S. Belokoneva, and T. Nakajima. 2002. Oxyopinin, large amphipathic peptides isolated from the venom of the wolf spider *Oxyopes kitabensis* with cytolytic properties and positive insecticidal cooperativity with spider neurotoxins. *J. Biol. Chem.* **277**:23627–23637.

Cudic, M., and L. Otvos, Jr. 2002. Intracellular targets of antibacterial peptides. *Curr. Drug Targets* **3**:101–106.

Cunliffe, R. N., M. Kamal, F. R. Rose, P. D. James, and Y. R. Mahida. 2002. Expression of antimicrobial neutrophil defensins in epithelial cells of active inflammatory bowel disease mucosa. *J. Clin. Pathol.* **55**:298–304.

Cuthbertson, B. J., E. F. Shepard, R. W. Chapman, and P. S. Gross. 2002. Diversity of the penaeidin antimicrobial peptides in two shrimp species. *Immunogenetics* **54**:442–445.

Dagan, A., L. Efron, L. Gaidukov, A. Mor, and H. Ginsburg. 2002. In vitro antiplasmodium effects of dermaseptin S4 derivatives. *Antimicrob. Agents Chemother.* **46:**1059–1066.

Dangl, J. L., and J. D. Jones. 2001. Plant pathogens and integrated defence responses to infection. *Nature* **411:**826–833.

Darveau, R. P., M. D. Cunningham, C. L. Seachord, L. Cassiano-Clough, W. L. Cosand, J. Blake, and C. S. Watkins. 1991. β-Lactam antibiotics potentiate Magainin 2 antimicrobial activity in vitro and in vivo. *Antimicrob. Agents Chemother.* **35:**1153–1159.

Del Pero, M., M. Boniotto, D. Zuccon, P. Cervella, A. Spano, A. Amoroso, and S. Crovella. 2002. Beta defensin 1 gene variability among non-human primates. *Immunogenetics* **53:**907–913.

Diamond, G., M. Zasloff, H. Eck, M. Brasseur, W. L. Maloy, and C. L. Bevins. 1991. Tracheal antimicrobial peptide, a novel cysteine-rich peptide from mammalian tracheal mucosa: peptide isolation and cloning of a cDNA. *Proc. Natl. Acad. Sci. USA* **88:** 3952–3956.

Di Nardo, A., A. Vitiello, and R. L. Gallo. 2003. Cutting edge: mast cell antimicrobial activity is mediated by expression of cathelicidin antimicrobial peptide. *J. Immunol.* **170:**2274–2278.

Droemann, D., T. Goldmann, D. Branscheid, R. Clark, K. Dalhoff, P. Zabel, and E. Vollmer. 2003. Toll like receptor 2 is expressed by alveolar epithelial cells type II and macrophages in the human lung. *Histochem. Cell Biol.* **119:**103–108.

Duda, T. F., Jr., D. Vanhoye, and P. Nicholas. 2002. Roles of diversifying selection and coordinated evolution in the evolution of amphibian antimicrobial peptides. *Mol. Biol. Evol.* **19:**858–864.

Efron, L., A. Dagan, L. Gaidukov, H. Ginsburg, and A. Mor. 2002. Direct inactivation of dermaseptin S4 aminoheptanoyl derivative with intraerythrocytic malaria parasite leading to increased specific antiparasitic activity in culture. *J. Biol. Chem.* **277:**24067–24072.

Engström, Y., L. Kadalayil, S.-C. Sun, C. Samakovlis, D. Hultmark, and I. Faye. 1993. κB like motifs regulate the induction of immune genes in *Drosophila. J. Mol. Biol.* **232:**327–333.

Epand, R. F., N. Umezawa, E. A. Porter, S. H. Gellman, and R. M. Epand. 2003. Interactions of the antimicrobial beta-peptide beta-17 with phospholipids vesicles differ from membrane interactions of magainins. *Eur. J. Biochem.* **270:**1240–1248.

Ernst, R. K., E. C. Yi, L. Guo, K. B. Lim, J. L. Burns, M. Hackett, and S. I. Miller. 1999. Specific lipopolysaccharide found in cystic fibrosis airway *Pseudomonas aeruginosa. Science* **286:**1561–1565.

Fahlgren, A., S. Hammarstrom, A. Danielsson, and M. L. Hammarstrom. 2003. Increased expression of antimicrobial peptides and lysozyme in colonic epithelial cells of patients with ulcerative colitis. *Clin. Exp. Immunol.* **131:**90–101.

Fehlbaum, P., M. Rao, M. Zasloff, and G. M. Anderson. 2000. An essential amino acid induces epithelial β-defensin expression. *Proc. Natl. Acad. Sci. USA* **97:**12723–12728.

Fernandez-Lopez, S., H.-S. Kim, E. C. Choi, M. Delgado, J. R. Granja, A. Khasanov, K. Kraehenbuel, G. Long, D. A. Weinberger, K. Wilcoxen, and M. R. Ghadziri. 2001. Antibacterial agents based on the cyclic D,L-α peptide architecture. *Nature* **412:**452–455.

Ge, Y., D. L. MacDonald, K. J. Holroyd, C. Thornsberry, H. Wexler, and M. Zasloff. 1999. In vitro antibacterial properties of Pexiganan, an analog of Magainin. *Antimicrob. Agents Chemother.* **43:**782–788.

Ghiselli, R., A. Giacometti, O. Cirioni, F. Mocchegiani, C. Viticchi, G. Scalise, and V. Saba. 2002. Cationic peptides combined with beta lactams reduce mortality from peritonitis in experimental rat model. *J. Surg. Res.* **108:**107–111.

Ghosh, D., E. Porter, B. Shen, S. K. Lee, D. Wilk, J. Drazba, S. P. Yadav, J. W. Crabb, T. Ganz, and C. L. Bevins. 2002. Paneth cell trypsin is the processing enzyme for human defensin-5. *Nat. Immunol.* **3:**583–590.

Ghosh, J. K., D. Shaool, P. Guillaud, L. Ciceron, D. Mazier, I. Kustanovich, Y. Shai, and A. Mor. 1997. Selective cytotoxicity of dermaseptin S3 toward intraerythrocytic *Plasmodium falciparum* and the underlying molecular basis. *J. Biol. Chem.* **272:**31609–31616.

Giacometti, A., O. Cirioni, F. Barchiesi, and G. Scalise. 2000. In-vitro activity and killing effect of polycationic peptides on methicillin-resistant *Staphylococcus aureus* and interactions with clinically used antibiotics. *Diagn. Microbiol. Infect. Dis.* **8:**115–118.

Giacometti, A., O. Cirioni, R. Ghiselli, F. Mocchegiani, M. S. Del Prete, C. Viticchi, W. Kamysz, E. Lempicka, V. Saba, and G. Scalise. 2002. Potential therapeutic role of cationic peptides in three experimental models of septic shock. *Antimicrob. Agents Chemother.* **46:**2132–2136.

Goldman, M. J., G. M. Anderson, E. D. Stolzenberg, U. P. Kari, M. Zasloff, and J. M. Wilson. 1997. Human β-defensin-1 is a salt-sensitive antibiotic in lung that is inactivated in cystic fibrosis. *Cell* **88:**553–560.

Gottar, M., V. Gobert, T. Michel, M. Belvin, G. Duyk, J. A. Hoffmann, D. Ferrandon, and J. Royet. 2002. The Drosophila immune response against Gram-negative bacteria is mediated by a peptidoglycan recognition protein. *Nature* **416:**640–644.

Grieco, P., C. Rossi, G. Colombo, S. Gatti, E. Novellino, J. M. Lipton, and A. Catania. 2003. Novel alpha melanocyte stimulating hormone peptide analogue with high candidacidal activity. *J. Med. Chem.* **46:**850–855.

Groisman, E. A. 1995. How bacteria resist killing by host defense peptides. *Trends Microbiol.* **2:**444–449.

Groisman, E. A. 1998. The ins and outs of virulence gene expression: Mg^{2+} as a regulatory signal. *Bioessays* **20**:96–101.

Gunn, J. S., S. S. Ryan, J. C. Van Velkinburgh, R. K. Ernst, and S. I. Miller. 2000. Genetic and functional analysis of a PmrA-PmrB-regulated locus necessary for lipopolysaccharide modification, antimicrobial peptide resistance, and oral virulence of *Salmonella enterica* serovar *typhimurium*. *Infect. Immun.* **68**:6139–6146.

Hamamoto, K., Y. Kida, Y. Zhang, T. Shimizu, and K. Kuwano. 2002. Antimicrobial activity and stability to proteolysis of small linear cationic peptides with D-amino acid substitutions. *Microbiol. Immunol.* **46**:741–749.

Hampe, J., J. Grebe, S. Nikolaus, C. Solberg, P. J. Croucher, S. Mascheretti, J. Jahnsen, B. Moum, B. Klump, M. Krawczak, M. M. Mirza, U. R. Foelsch, M. Vatn, and S. Schreiber. 2002. Association of NOD2 (CARD 15) genotype with clinical course of Crohn's disease: a cohort study. *Lancet* **359**:1661–1665.

Hamuro, Y., J. P. Schneider, and W. F. DeGrado. 1999. De novo design of antibacterial β-peptides. *J. Am. Chem. Soc.* **121**:12200–12201.

Hancock, R. E. W., T. Falla, and M. Brown. 1995. Cationic bactericidal peptides. *Adv. Microb. Physiol.* **37**:135–175.

Harder, J., J. Bartels, J. Christophers, and J. M. Schroder. 1997. A peptide antibiotic from human skin. *Nature* **387**:861.

Harder, J., U. Meyer-Hoffert, L. M. Teran, L. Schwichtenberg, J. Bartels, S. Maune, and J. M. Schroder. 2000. Mucoid *Pseudomonas aeruginosa*, TNF-α, and IL-1β, but not IL-6, induce human β defensin-2 in respiratory epithelia. *Am. J. Respir. Cell Mol. Biol.* **22**:714–721.

Haynie, S. L., G. A. Crum, and B. A. Doele. 1995. Antimicrobial activities of amphiphilic peptides covalently bonded to a water-insoluble resin. *Antimicrob. Agents Chemother.* **39**:301–307.

Hein, M., E. V. Valore, R. B. Helmig, N. Uldbjerg, and T. Ganz. 2002. Antimicrobial factors in the cervical mucous plug. *Am. J. Obstet. Gynecol.* **187**:137–144.

Helmerhorst, E. J., W. van't Hoft, P. Breeuwer, E. C. Veerman, T. Abee, R. F. Troxler, A. V. Amerongen, and F. G. Oppenheim. 2001. Characterization of histatin 5 with respect to amphipathicity, hydrophobicity, and effects on cell and mitochondrial membrane integrity excludes a candidacidal mechanism of pore formation. *J. Biol. Chem.* **276**:5643–5649.

Hendengren, M., B. Åsling, M. S. Dushay, L. Ando, S. Ekengren, M. Wihlborg, and D. Hultmark. 1999. Relish, a central factor in the control of humoral but not cellular immunity in *Drosophila*. *Mol. Cell* **4**:1–20.

Hieshima, K., H. Ohtani, M. Shibano, D. Izawa, T. Nakayama, Y. Kawasaki, F. Shiba, M. Shiota, F. Katou, T. Saito, and O. Yoshie. 2003. CCL28 has dual roles in mucosal immunity as a chemokine with broad spectrum antimicrobial activity. *J. Immunol.* **170**:1452–1461.

Hirakura, Y., S. Kobayashi, and K. Matsuzaki. 2002. Specific interactions of the antimicrobial peptide cyclic beta-sheet tachyplesin I with lipopolysaccharides. *Biochim. Biophys. Acta* **1562**:32–36.

Hoffmann, J. A., and J. M. Reichhart. 2002. Drosophila innate immunity: an evolutionary perspective. *Nat. Immunol.* **3**:121–126.

Hong, R. W., M. Shchepetov, J. N. Weiser, and P. H. Axelsen. 2003. Transcriptional profile of the E. coli response to the antimicrobial insect peptide Cecropin A. *Antimicrob. Agents Chemother.* **47**:1–6.

Hoover, D. M., C. Boulegue, D. Yang, J. J. Oppenheim, K. Tucker, W. Lu, and J. Lubkowski. 2002. The structure of human macrophage inflammatory protein-3 alpha/CCL20. Linking antimicrobial and CC chemokine receptor 6 binding activities with human beta defensins. *J. Biol. Chem.* **277**:37647–37654.

Huh, W. K., T. Oono, Y. Shirafuji, H. Akiyama, J. Arata, M. Sakaguchi, N. H. Huh, and K. Iwatsuki. 2002. Dynamic alteration of human beta-defensin 2 localization from cytoplasm to intercellular space in psoriatic skin. *J. Mol. Med.* **80**:678–684.

Hui, L., K. Leung, and H. M. Chen. 2002. The combined effects of antimicrobial peptide cecropin A and anti-cancer agents on leukemia cells. *Anticancer Res.* **22**:2811–2816.

Iijima, N., N. Tanimoto, Y. Emoto, Y. Morita, K. Uematsu, T. Murakami, and T. Nakai. 2003. Purification and characterization of three isoforms of chrysophsin, a novel antimicrobial peptide in the gills of the sea bream, Chrysophrys major. *Eur. J. Biochem.* **270**:675–686.

Imler, J. L., and J. A. Hoffmann. 2000. Signaling mechanisms in the antimicrobial host defense of *Drosophila*. *Curr. Opin. Microbiol.* **3**:16–22.

Imler, J. L., and J. A. Hoffmann. 2002. Toll receptors in Drosophila: a family of molecules regulating development and immunity. *Curr. Top. Microbiol. Immunol.* **270**:63–79.

Isaacson, T., A. Soto, S. Iwamuro, F. C. Knoop, and J. M. Conlon. 2002. Antimicrobial peptides with atypical structural features from the skin of the Japanese brown frog *Rana japonica*. *Peptides* **23**:419–425.

Islam, D., L. Bandholtz, J. Nilsson, H. Wigzell, B. Christensson, B. Agerberth, and G. Gudmundsson. 2001. Down-regulation of bactericidal peptides in enteric infections: a novel immune escape mechanism with bacterial DNA as a potential regulator. *Nat. Med.* **7**:180–185.

Iwanaga, S. 2002. The molecular basis of innate immunity in the horseshoe crab. *Curr. Opin. Immunol.* **14:**87–95.

Iwanaga, S., and S. Kawabata. 1998. Evolution and phylogeny of defense molecules associated with innate immunity in horseshoe crab. *Front. Biosci.* **3:**D973–D984.

Jacob, L., and M. Zasloff. 1994. Potential therapeutic applications of magainins and other antimicrobial agents of animal origin. *Ciba Found. Symp.* **186:**197–216.

Jacobs, T., H. Bruhn, I. Gaworski, B. Fleischer, and M. Leippe. 2003. NK-lysin and its shortened analog NK-2 exhibit potent activities against *Trypanosoma cruzi. Antimicrob. Agents Chemother.* **47:**607–613.

Jaynes, J. M., P. Nagpala, I. Destafano-Beltran, J. H. Huang, J. H. Kim, T. Denny, and S. Centiner. 1993. Expression of a cecropin β-lytic peptide analog in transgenic tobacco confers enhanced resistance to bacterial wilt caused by *Ps. solanacearium. Plant Sci.* **85:**43–54.

Jennings, C., J. West, C. Waine, D. Craik, and M. Anderson. 2001. Biosynthesis and insecticidal properties of plant cyclotides: the cyclic knotted proteins from *Oldenlandia affinis. Proc. Natl. Acad. Sci. USA* **98:**10614–10619.

Jurevic, R. J., P. Chrisman, L. Mancl, R. Livingston, and B. A. Dale. 2002. Single nucleotide polymorphisms and haplotype analysis in beta-defensin genes in different ethnic populations. *Genet. Test.* **6:**261–269.

Jurevic, R. J., M. Bai, R. B. Chadwick, T. C. White, and B. A. Dale. 2003. Single nucleotide polymorphisms in human beta-defensin 1: high throughput SNP assays and association with Candida carriage in Type I diabetics and non-diabetic controls. *J. Clin. Microbiol.* **41:**90–96.

Kao, C. Y., Y. Chen, Y. H. Zhao, and R. Wu. 2003. Orfeome based search of airway epithelial cell-specific novel human beta-defensins. *Am. J. Respir. Cell Mol. Biol.* (Epub ahead of print)

Kappler, C., M. Meister, M. Lagueux, E. Gateff, J. A. Hoffmann, and J. M. Reichhart. 1993. Insect immunity. Two 17 bp repeats nesting a kappa β-related sequence confer inducibility to the diptericin gene and bind a polypeptide in bacteria-challenged *Drosophila. EMBO J.* **12:**1561–1568.

Kieffer, A. E., Y. Goumon, O. Ruh, S. Chasserot-Golaz, G. Nullans, C. Gasnier, D. Aunis, and M. H. Metz-Boutigue. 2003. The N and C-terminal fragments of ubiquitin are important for the antimicrobial activities. *FASEB J.* **17:**776–778.

Kim, H. S., H. Yoon, C. B. Park, W. T. Lee, M. Zasloff, and S. C. Kim. 2000. Pepsin mediated processing of the cytoplasmic histone 2A to the strong antimicrobial peptide Buforin I. *J. Immunol.* **165:**3268–3274.

Kim, H. S., J. H. Cho, H. W. Park, H. Yoon, M. S. Kim, and D. S. C. Kim. 2002. Endotoxin neutralizing antimicrobial proteins of the human placenta. *J. Immunol.* **168:**2356–2364.

Kim, S. T., H. E. Cha, D. Y. Kim, G. C. Han, Y. S. Chung, Y. J. Lee, Y. J. Hwang, and H. M. Lee. 2003. Antimicrobial peptide LL-37 is upregulated in chronic nasal inflammatory disease. *Acta Otolaryngol.* **123:**81–85.

Kimbrell, D. A., and B. Beutler. 2001. The evolution and genetics of innate immunity. *Nat. Rev. Genet.* **2:**256–267.

King, A. E., D. C. Fleming, H. O. Critchley, and R. W. Kelly. 2002. Regulation of natural antibiotic expression by inflammatory mediators and mimics of infection in human endometrial epithelial cells. *Mol. Hum. Reprod.* **4:**341–349.

Kisich, K. O., L. Heifets, M. Higgins, and G. Diamond. 2001. Antimycobacterial agent based on mRNA encoding human β-Defensin 2 enables primary macrophages to restrict growth of *Mycobacterium tuberculosis. Infect. Immun.* **69:**2692–2699.

Konovalov, O., I. Myagkov, B. Struth, and K. Lohner. 2002. Lipid discrimination in phospholipid monolayers by the antimicrobial frog skin peptide PGLa. A synchrotron X-ray grazing incidence and reflectivity study. *Eur. Biophys. J.* **31:**428–437.

Kowalska, K., D. B. Carr, and A. W. Lipkowski. 2002. Direct antimicrobial properties of substance P. *Life Sci.* **71:**747–750.

Kragol, G., S. Lovas, G. Varadi, B. A. Condie, R. Hoffmann, and L. Otvos, Jr. 2001. The antibacterial peptide pyrrhocoricin inhibits the ATPase actions of DnaK and prevents chaperone-assisted protein folding. *Biochemistry* **40:**3016–3026.

Kragol, G., R. Hoffmann, M. A. Chattergoon, S. Lovas, M. Cudic, P. Bulet, B. A. Condie, K. J. Rosengren, L. J. Montaner, and L. Otvos, Jr. 2002. Identification of crucial residues for the antibacterial activity of the proline-rich peptide, pyrrhocoricin. *Eur. J. Biochem.* **269:**4226–4237.

Krijgsveld, J., S. A. Zaat, J. Meeldijk, P. A. van Vellan, G. Fang, B. Poolman, E. Brandt, J. E. Ehlert, A. J. Kuijpers, G. H. M. Engbers, J. Feijen, and J. Dankert. 2000. Thrombocidins, microbiocidal proteins from human blood platelets are C-terminal delection products of CXC chemokines. *J. Biol. Chem.* **275:**20374–20381.

Krisanaprakornkit, S., J. R. Kimball, A. Weinberg, R. P. Darveau, B. W. Bainbridge, and B. A. Dale. 2000. Inducible expression of human β-defensin 2 by *Fusobacterium nucleatum* in oral epithelial cells: multiple signaling pathways and role of commensal bacteria in innate immunity and the epithelial barrier. *Infect. Immun.* **68:**2907–2915.

Kuhn-Nentwig, L., J. Muller, J. Schaller, A. Walz, M. Dathe, and W. J. Nentwig. 2002. Cupiennin I, a new family of highly basic antimicrobial peptides in the venom of the spider *Cupiennius saliei* (Ctenidae). *J. Biol. Chem.* **277**:11208–11216.

Kutta, H., P. Steven, G. Kohla, B. Tillmann, and F. Paulsen. 2002. The human false vocal folds—an analysis of antimicrobial defense mechanisms. *Anat. Embryol.* **205**:315–332.

Kylsten, P., C. Samakovlis, and D. Hultmark. 1990. The cecropin locus in *Drosophila*: a compact gene cluster involved in response to infection. *EMBO J.* **9**:217–224.

Laederbach, A., A. H. Andreotti, and D. B. Fulton. 2002. Solution and micelle bound structures of tachyplesin I and its aromatic linear derivatives. *Biochemistry* **41**:12359–12368.

Lai, J. R., B. R. Huck, B. Weisblum, and S. H. Gellman. 2002. Design of non-cysteine containing antimicrobial beta-hairpins: structure-activity relationship studies with linear protegrin-1 analogues. *Biochemistry* **41**:12835–12842.

Lambert, R. W., K. Campton, W. Ding, H. Ozawa, and R. D. Granstein. 2002. Langerhans cell expression of neuropeptide Y and peptide YY. *Neuropeptides* **36**:246–251.

Lee, S. H., J. E. Kim, H. H. Lim, H. M. Lee, and J. O. Choi. 2002. Antimicrobial defensin peptides of the human nasal mucosa. *Ann. Otol. Rhinol. Laryngol.* **111**:135–141.

Lehmann, J., M. Retz, J. Hader, M. Krams, U. Kellner, J. Hartmann, K. Hohgrawe, U. Raffenberg, M. Gerber, T. Loch, K. Weichert-Jacobsen, and M. Stockle. 2002. Expression of human beta-defensins 1 and 2 in kidneys with chronic bacterial infection. *BMC Infect. Dis.* **18**:20.

Lemaitre, B., E. Nicholas, L. Michaut, J. M. Reichert, and J. A. Hoffmann. 1996. The dorsoventral regulatory gene cassette spätzle/Toll/cactus controls the potent antifungal response in *Drosophila* adults. *Cell* **86**:973–983.

Levashina, E. A., E. Langley, C. Green, D. Gubb, M. Ashburner, J. A. Hoffmann, and J. M. Reichhart. 1999. Constitutive activation of toll-mediated antifungal defenses in serpin-deficient *Drosophila*. *Science* **285**:1917–1919.

Li, J., M. Post, R. Volk, Y. Gao, M. Li, C. Metais, K. Sato, J. Tsai, W. Aird, R. D. Rosenberg, T. G. Hampton, F. Sellke, P. Carmeliet, and M. Simons. 2000. PR39, a peptide regulator of angiogenesis. *Nat. Med.* **6**:49–55.

Ligoxygakis, P., N. Pelte, J. A. Hoffmann, and J. M. Reichhart. 2002. Activation of Drosophila Toll during fungal infection by a blood serine protease. *Science* **297**:114–116.

Liu, A. Y., D. Destoumieux, A. V. Wong, C. H. Park, E. V. Valore, L. Liu, and T. Ganz. 2002. Human beta-defensin 2 production in keratinocytes is regulated by interleukin-1, bacteria, and the state of differentiation. *Invest. Dermatol.* **118**:275–281.

Liu, L., L. Wang, C. Zhao, H. H. Q. Heng, B. C. Schutte, and P. B. McCray, Jr. 1998. Structure and mapping of the human β-defensin 2 gene and its expression at sites of inflammation. *Gene* **222**:237–244.

Liu, L., A. A. Roberts, and T. Ganz. 2003. By IL-1 signalling, monocytes cderived cells dramatically enhance the epidermal antimicrobial response to lipopolysaccharide. *J. Immunol.* **170**:575–580.

Luders, T., G. A. Birkemo, G. Fimland, J. Nissen-Mayer, and I. F. Nes. 2003. Strong synergy between a eukaryotic antimicrobial peptide and bacteriocins from lactic acid bacteria. *Appl. Environ. Microbiol.* **69**:1797–1799.

Lupetti, A., P. H. Nibbering, M. M. Welling, and E. K. Pauwels. 2003. Radiopharmaceuticals: new antimicrobial agents. *Trends Biotechnol.* **21**:70–73.

Lysenko, E. S., J. Gould, R. Bals, J. M. Wilson, and J. N. Weiser. 2000. Bacterial phosphorylcholine decreases susceptibility to the antimicrobial peptide LL-37/hCAP18 expressed in the upper respiratory tract. *Infect. Immun.* **68**:1664–1671.

Mak, P., J. Pohl, A. Dubin, M. S. Reed, S. E. Bowers, M. T. Fallon, and W. M. Shafer. 2003. The increased bactericidal activity of a fatty acid modified synthetic antimicrobial peptide of human cathepsin G correlates with its enhanced capacity to interact with model membranes. *Int. J. Antimicrob. Agents* **21**:13–19.

Maloy, W. L., and U. P. Kari. 1995. Structure-activity studies on Magainins and other host defense peptides. *Biopolymers* **37**:105–122.

Mandal, M., and R. Nagaraj. 2002. Antibacterial activities and conformations of synthetic alpha-defensin HNP-1 and analogs with one, two, and three disulfide bridges. *J. Pept. Res.* **59**:95–104.

Mangoni, M. L., R. Miele, T. G. Renda, D. Barra, and M. Simmaco. 2001. The synthesis of antimicrobial peptides in the skin of *Rana esculenta* is stimulated by microorganisms. *FASEB J.* **8**:1431–1432.

Mannis, M. J. 2002. The use of antimicrobial peptides in ophthalmology: an experimental study in corneal preservation and the management of bacterial keratitis. *Trans. Am. Opthalmol. Soc.* **100**:243–271.

Matsushita, I., K. Hasegawa, K. Nakata, K. Yasuda, K. Tokunaga, and N. Keicho. 2002. Genetic variants of human beta-defensin 1 and chronic obstructive pulmonary disease. *Biochem. Biophys. Res. Commun.* **15**:17–22.

Matsuzaki, K. 1999. Why and how are peptide-lipid interactions utilized for self-defense? Magainins and tachyplesins as archetypes. *Biochim. Biophys. Acta* **1462**:1–10.

Melmed, G., L. S. Thomas, N. Lee, S. Y. Tesfay, K. Lukasek, K. S. Michelsen, Y. Zhou, B. Hu, M. Arditi, and M. T. Abreu. 2003. Human intestinal epithelial cells are broadly unresponsive to Toll-like receptor 2-dependent bacterial ligands: implications for host-microbial interactions in the gut. *J. Immunol.* **170:**1406–1415.

Michel, T., J. M. Reichhart, J. A. Hoffmann, and J. Royet. 2001. Drosophila Toll is activated by Gram-positive bacteria through a circulating peptidoglycan recognition protein. *Nature* **414:**756–759.

Morrison, G., F. Kilanowski, D. Davidson, and J. Dorin. 2002a. Characterization of the mouse defensin 1, Defb1, mutant mouse model. *Infect. Immun.* **70:**3053–3060.

Morrison, G. M., M. Rolfe, F. M. Kilanowski, S. H. Cross, and J. R. Dorin. 2002b. Identification and characterization of a novel murine beta-defensin related gene. *Mamm. Genome* **13:**445–451.

Morrison, G. M., C. A. Semple, F. M. Kilanowski, R. E. Hill, and J. R. Dorin. 2003. Signal sequence conservations and mature peptide divergence within subgroups of the murine beta-defensin gene family. *Mol. Biol. Evol.* **20:**460–470.

Moser, C., D. J. Weinder, E. Lysenko, R. Bals, J. N. Weiser, and J. M. Wilson. 2002. Beta-defensin 1 contributes to pulmonary innate immunity in mice. *Infect. Immun.* **70:**3068–3072.

Muhle, S. A., and J. P. Tam. 2001. Design of gram-negative selective antimicrobial peptides. *Biochemistry* **40:**5777–5785.

Munoz, M., F. Vandenbulcke, Y. Gueguen, and E. Bachere. 2003. Expression of penaedin antimicrobial peptides in early larval stages of the shrimp *Penaeus vannamei. Dev. Comp. Immunol.* **27:**283–289.

Murakami, M., T. Ohtake, R. A. Dorschner, and R. L. Gallo. 2002a. Cathelicidin antimicrobial peptides are expressed in salivary glands and saliva. *J. Dent. Res.* **81:**845–850.

Murakami, M., T. Ohtake, R. A. Dorschner, B. Schittek, C. Garbe, and R. L. Gallo. 2002b. Cathelicidin anti-microbial peptide expression in sweat, an innate defense system for the skin. *J. Invest. Dermatol.* **119:**1090–1095.

Murphy, J. E., C. Robert, and T. S. Kupper. 2000. Interleukin-1 and cutaneous inflammation: a crucial link between innate and acquired immunity *J. Invest. Dermatol.* **114:**602–608.

Nagaoka, I., S. Hirota, F. Niyonsaba, M. Hirata, Y. Adachi, H. Tamura, S. Tanaka, and D. Heumann. 2002. Augmentation of the lipopolysaccharide-neutralizing activities of human cathelicidin CAP18/LL37 derived antimicrobial peptides by replacement with hydrophobic and cationic amino acid residues. *Clin. Diagn. Lab. Immunol.* **9:**972–982.

Nagpal, S., K. J. Kaur, D. Jain, and D. M. Salunke. 2002. Plasticity in structure and interactions is critical for the action of indolicidin, an antibacterial peptide of innate immune origin. *Protein Sci.* **11:**2158–2167.

Naitza, S., C. Rosse, C. Kappler, P. Georgel, M. Belvin, D. Gubb, J. Camojnis, J. A. Hoffmann, and J. M. Reichhart. 2002. The Drosophila immune

defense against gram-negative infection requires the death protein dFADD. *Immunity* **17:**575–581.

Nakajima, Y., K. Ogihara, D. Taylor, and M. J. Yamakawa. 2003. Antibacterial hemoglobin fragments from the midgut of the soft tick, *Ornithodoros moubata (Acari:Argasidae). Med. Entomol.* **40:**78–81.

Nicolas, G., M. Bennoun, I. Devaux, C. Beaumont, B. Grandchamp, A. Kahn, and S. Vaulont. 2001. Lack of hepcidin gene expression and severe tissue iron overload in upstream stimulatory factor 2 (USF2) knockout mice. *Proc. Natl. Acad. Sci. USA* **98:**8780–8785.

Niyonsaba, F., K. Iwabuchi, A. Someya, M. Hirata, H. Matsuda, H. Ogawa, and I. Nagaoka. 2002. A cathelicidin family of human antibacterial peptide LL-37 induces mast cell chemotaxis. *Immunology* **106:**20–26.

Nizet, V., X. Ohtake, J. Trowbridge, J. Rudisill, R. A. Dorschner, V. Pestonjamasp, J. Piraino, K. Huttner, and R. L. Gallo. 2001. An antimicrobial peptide protects mice from invasive bacterial infection. *Nature* **414:**454–457.

Noland, B. W., J. M. Newman, J. Hendle, J. Badger, J. A. Christopher, J. Tresser, M. D. Buchanan, T. A. Wright, M. E. Rutter, W. E. Sanderson, H. J. Muller-Dieckmann, K. S. Gajiwala, and S. G. Buchanan. 2002. Structural studies of *Salmonella typhimurium* ArnB(PmrH) aminotransferase: a 4-amino-4-deoxy-L-arabinose lipopolysaccharide-modifying enzyme. *Structure* **10:** 1569–1580.

O'Neil, D. A., E. M. Porter, D. Elewaut, G. M. Anderson, L. Eckmann, T. Ganz, and M. F. Kagnoff. 1999. Expression and regulation of the human beta-defensins HBD-1 and HBD-2 in intestinal epithelium. *J. Immunol.* **163:**6718–6724.

Ong, P., T. Ohtake, C. Brandt, I. Strickland, M. Boguniewicz, T. Ganz, R. L. Gallo, and D. Y. M. Leung. 2002. Endogenous antimicrobial peptides and skin infections in atopic dermatitis. *New Engl. J. Med.* **347:**1151–1160.

Oren, Z., and Y. Shai. 2000. Cyclization of a cytolytic amphipathic α-helical peptide and its diastereomer: effect on structure, interaction with model membranes, and biological function. *Biochemistry* **39:** 6103–6114.

Orlov, D. S., T. Nguyen, and R. I. Lehrer. 2002. Potassium release, a useful tool for studying antimicrobial peptides. *J. Microbiol. Methods* **49:**325–328.

Osusky, M., G. Zhou, L. Osuska, R. E. Hancock, W. W. Kay, and S. Misra. 2000. Transgenic plants expressing cationic peptide chimeras exhibit broad-spectrum resistance to phytopathogens. *Nat. Biotechnol.* **18:**1162–1166.

Oulette, A. J., and C. L. Bevins. 2001. Paneth cell defensins and innate immunity of the small bowel. *Inflamm. Bowel Dis.* **7:**43–50.

Pacor, S., A. Giangaspero, M. Bacac, G. Sava, and A. Tossi. 2002. Analysis of the cytotoxicity of synthetic antimicrobial peptides on mouse leukocytes: implications for systemic use. *J. Antimicrob. Chemother.* 50:339–348.

Palladino, M. A., A. Mallonga, and M. S. Mishra. 2003. mRNA expression for the antimicrobial peptides beta-defensin 1 and beta defensin 2 in the male rat reproductive tract: beta defensin 1 mRNA in initial segment and caput epididymidis is regulated by androgens and not bacterial lipopolysaccharides. *Biol. Reprod.* 68:509–515.

Paone, G., A. Wada, L. A. Stevens, A. Matin, T. Hirayama, R. L. Levine, and J. Moss. 2002. ADP ribosylation of human neutrophil peptide 1 regulates its biological properties. *Proc. Natl. Acad. Sci. USA* 99:8231–8235.

Papo, N., Z. Oren, U. Pag, H. G. Sahl, and Y. Shai. 2002. The consequence of sequence alteration of an amphipathic alpha-helical antimicrobial peptide and its diasteriomers. *J. Biol. Chem.* 277:33913–33921.

Park, C. H., E. V. Valore, A. J. Waring, and T. Ganz. 2001. Hepcidin, a urinary antimicrobial peptide synthesized in the liver. *J. Biol. Chem.* 276:7806–7810.

Park, H. C., Y. H. Kang, H. J. Chun, and J. C. Koo. 2002. Characterization of a stamen-specific cDNA encoding a novel plant defensin in Chinese cabbage. *Plant Mol. Biol.* 50:59–69.

Patrzykat, A., C. L. Friedrich, L. Zhang, V. Mendoza, and R. E. Hancock. 2002. Sublethal concentrations of pleurocidin derived antimicrobial peptides inhibit macromolecular synthesis in E. coli. *Antimicro. Agents Chemother.* 46:605–614.

Perregaux, D. G., K. Bhavsar, L. Contillo, J. Shi, and C. A. Gabel. 2002. Antimicrobial peptides initiate IL-1 beta posttranslational processing: a novel role beyond innate immunity. *J. Immunol.* 168:3024–3032.

Peschel, A. 2002. How do bacteria resist human antimicrobial peptides? *Trends Microbiol.* 10:179–186.

Peschel, A., R. W. Jack, M. Otto, L. V. Collins, P. Staubitz, G. Nicholson, H. Kalbacher, W. F. Nieuwenhuizen, G. Jung, A. Tarkowski, K. P. van Kessel, and J. A. van Strijp. 2001. Staphylococcus aureus resistance to human defensins and evasion of neutrophil killing via the novel virulence factor MprF is based on modification of membrane lipids with l-lysine. *J. Exp. Med.* 193:1067–1076.

Phadke, S. M., V. Lazarevic, C. C. Bahr, K. Islam, D. B. Stolz, S. Watkins, S. B. Tencza, H. J. Vogel, R. C. Montelaro, and T. A. Mietzner. 2002. Lentivirus lytic peptide 1 perturbs both outer and inner membranes of Serratia marcescens. *Antimicrob. Agents Chemother.* 46:2041–2045.

Ponti, D., M. L. Mamgoni, G. Mignongna, M. Simmaco, and D. Barra. 2003. An amphibian antimicrobial peptide variant expressed in Nictiana tabacum confers resistance to phytopathogens. *Biochem. J.* 370:121–127.

Porter, E. A., X. Wang, H. S. Lee, B. Weisblum, and S. H. Gellman. 2000. Non-haemolytic β-amino acid oligomers. *Nature* 404:565.

Putsep, K. G. Carlsson, H. G. Boman, and M. Andersson. 2002. Deficiency of antibacterial peptides in patients with Morbus Kostmann: an observation study. *Lancet* 360:1144–1149.

Rinaldi, A. C. 2002. Antimicrobial peptides from amphibian skin: an expanding scenario. *Curr. Opin. Chem. Biol.* 6:799–804.

Risso, A., E. Braidot, M. C. Sordano, A. Vianello, F. Macri, B. Skerlavaj, M. Zanetti, R. Gennaro, and P. Bernardi. 2002. BMAP-28 an antibiotic peptide of innate immunity, induces cell death through opening of the mitochondrial permeability pore. *Mol. Cell. Biol.* 22:1926–1935.

Rodig, S. J., D. Jones, A. Shahsafaei, and D. M. Dorfman. 2002. CCR6 is a functional chemokine receptor that serves to identify select B-cell non-Hodgkin's lymphomas. *Hum. Pathol.* 33:1227–1233.

Roetto, A., G. Papanikolaou, M. Politou, F. Alberti, D. Girelli, J. Christakis, D. Loukopoulos, and C. Camaschella. 2003. Mutant antimicrobial peptide hepcidin is associated with severe juvenile hemochromatosis. *Nat. Genet.* 33:21–22.

Rollins-Smith, L. A., C. Carey, J. Longcore, J. K. Doersam, A. Boutte, J. E. Bruzgal, and J. M. Conlon. 2002a. Activity of antimicrobial skin peptides from ranid frogs against Batrachochytrium dendrobatidis, the chytrid fungus associated with global amphibian declines. *Dev. Comp. Immunol.* 26:471–479.

Rollins-Smith, L. A., J. K. Doersam, J. E. Longcore, S. K. Taylor, J. C. Shamblin, and M. Zasloff. 2002b. Antimicrobial peptide defenses against pathogens associated with global amphibian declines. *Dev. Comp. Immunol.* 26:63–72.

Rollins-Smith, L. A., L. K. Reinert, V. Miera, and J. M. Conlon. 2002c. Antimicrobial peptide defenses of the Tarahumara frog, Rana tarahumarae. *Biochem. Biophys. Res. Commun.* 297:361–367.

Romeo, D., B. Skerlavaj, M. Bolognesi, and R. Gennaro. 1988. Structure and bactericidal activity of an antibiotic dodecapeptide purified from bovine neutrophils. *J. Biol. Chem.* 263:9573–9575.

Russell, J. P., G. Diamond, A. P. Tarver, T. F. Scanlin, and C. L. Bevins. 1996. Coordinate induction of two antibiotic genes in tracheal epithelial cells exposed to the inflammatory mediators LPS and tumor necrosis factor α. *Infect. Immun.* 64:1565–1568.

Sadler, K., K. D. Eom, J. L. Yang, Y. Dimitrova, and J. P. Tam. 2002. Translocating proline-rich peptides from the antimicrobial peptide bactenecin 7. *Biochemistry* 41:150–157.

Salzman, N. H., M. M. Chou, H. deJong, L. Liu, E. M. Porter, and Y. Paterson. 2003a. Enteric salmonella infection inhibits Paneth cell antimicrobial peptide expression. *Infect. Immun.* 3:1109–1115.

Salzman, N. H., D. Ghosh, K. M. Huttner, Y. Paterson, and C. L. Bevins. 2003b. Protection against enteric salmonellosis in transgenic mice expressing a human intestinal defensin. *Nature* **422:**522–526.

Sawai, M. V., A. J. Waring, W. R. Kearney, P. McRay, Jr., W. R. Forsyth, R. I. Lehrer, and B. F. Tack. 2002. Impact of single residue mutations on the structure and function of ovispirin/novispirin antimicrobial peptides. *Protein Eng.* **15:**225–232.

Schaller-Bals, S., A. Schulze, and R. Bals. 2002. Increased levels of antimicrobial peptides in tracheal aspirates of newborn infants during infection. *Am. J. Respir. Crit. Care Med.* **165:**992–995.

Schauber, J., C. Svanholm, S. Termen, K. Iffland, T. Menzel, W. Scheppach, R. Melcher, B. Agerberth, H. Lührs, and G. H. Gudmundsson. 2003. Expression of the cathelicidin LL-37 is modulated by short chain fatty acids in colonocytes: relevance of signalling pathways. *Gut* **52:**735–741.

Scheetz, T., J. A. Bartlett, J. D. Walters, B. C. Schutte, T. L. Casavant, and P. B. McCray, Jr. 2002. Genomics based approaches to gene discovery in innate immunity. *Immunol. Rev.* **190:**137–145.

Schibili, D. J., H. N. Hunter, V. Aseyev, T. D. Starner, J. M. Wiencek, P. B. McCray, Jr., B. F. Tack, and H. J. Vogel. 2002a. The solution structures of the human beta-defensins lead to a better understanding of the potent bactericidal activity of HBD3 against *Staphylococcus aureus. J. Biol. Chem.* **277:**8279–8289.

Schibili, D. J., R. F. Epand, H. J. Vogel, and R. M. Epand. 2002b. Tryptophan-rich antimicrobial peptides: comparative properties and membrane interactions. *Biochem. Cell Biol.* **80:**667–677.

Schmidtchen, A., I. M. Frick, E. Andersson, H. Tapper, and L. Bjorck. 2002. Proteinase of common pathogenic bacteria degrade and inactivate the antibacterial peptide LL-37. *Mol. Microbiol.* **46:**157–168.

Schonwetter, B. S., E. D. Stolzenberg, and M. Zasloff. 1995. Epithelial antibiotics induced at sites of inflammation. *Science* **267:**1645–1648.

Scott, M. G., D. J. Davidson, M. R. Gold, D. Bowdish, and R. E. Hancock. 2002. The human antimicrobial peptide LL-37 is a multifunctional modulator of innate immune responses. *J. Immunol.* **169:** 3883–3891.

Selsted, M. E., S. S. L. Harwig, T. Ganz, J. W. Schilling, and R. I. Lehrer. 1985. Primary structure of three human neutrophil defensins. *J. Clin. Invest.* **76:**1436–1439.

Selsted, M. E., M. J. Novotny, W. L. Morris, Y. Q. Tang, W. Smith, and J. S. Cullor. 1992. Indolicidin, a novel bactericidal tridecapeptide amide from neutrophils. *J. Biol. Chem.* **267:**4292–4295.

Shai, Y. 1999. Mechanism of the binding, insertion and destabilization of phospholipid bilayer membranes by α-helical antimicrobial and cell non-selective membrane-lytic peptides. *Biochim. Biophys. Acta* **1462:** 55–70.

Shanahan, F. 2002. Crohn's disease. *Lancet* **359:**62–69.

Shepherd, C. M., H. J. Vogel, and D. P. Tieleman. 2003. Interactions of the designed antimicrobial peptide MB21 and truncated dermaseptin S3 with lipid bilayers: molecular-dynamics simulations. *Biochem. J.* **370:**233–243.

Shike, H., X. Lauth, M. E. Westerman, V. E. Ostland, J. M. Carlberg, J. C. Van Olst, C. Shimizu, P. Bulet, and J. C. Burns. 2002. Bass hepcidin is a novel antimicrobial peptide induced by bacterial challenge. *Eur. J. Biochem.* **269:**2232–2237.

Shin, S. W., V. Kokoza, I. Lobkov, and A. S. Rakiel. 2003. Relish mediated immune deficiency in the transgenic mosquito *Aedes aegypt. Proc. Natl. Acad. Sci. USA* **100:**2616–2621.

Shinnar, A. E., T. Uzzell, M. N. Rao, E. Spooner, W. S. Lane, and M. Zasloff. 1996. New family of linear antimicrobial peptides from hagfish intestine contains bromotryptophan as novel amino acid, p. 189–191. *In* P. Kaumaya and R. Hodges (ed.), *Peptides: Chemistry and Biology. Proceedings of the 14th American Peptide Symposium.* Mayflower Scientific Ltd., Leiden, The Netherlands.

Simmaco, M., G. Mignogna, and D. Barra. 1998. Antimicrobial peptides from amphibian skin: what do they tell us? *Biopolymers* **47:**35–50.

Singh, P. K., H. P. Jia, K. Wiles, J. Hesselberth, L. Liu, B. A. Conway, E. P. Greenberg, E. V. Valore, M. J. Welsh, T. Ganz, B. F. Tack, and P. B. McCray, Jr. 1998. Production of β-defensins by human airway epithelia. *Proc. Natl. Acad. Sci. USA* **95:** 14961–14966.

Smith, J. J., S. M. Travis, E. P. Greenberg, and M. J. Welsh. 1996. Cystic fibrosis airway epithelia fail to kill bacteria because of abnormal airway surface fluid. *Cell* **85:**229–236.

Steiner, H., D. Hultmark, A. Engstrom, H. Bennich, and H. G. Boman. 1981. Sequence and specificity of two antibacterial proteins involved in insect immunity. *Nature* **292:**246–268.

Stoven, S., I. Ando, L. Kadalayil, Y. Engstrom, and D. Hultmark. 2000. Activation of the *Drosophila* NF-κB factor relish by rapid endoproteolytic cleavage. *EMBO Rep.* **1:**347–352.

Strom, M. B., B. E. Haug, O. Rekdal, M. L. Skar, W. Stensen, and J. S. Svendsen. 2002. Important structural features of 15 residue lactoferricin derivatives and methods for improvement of antimicrobial activity. *Biochem. Cell Biol.* **80:**65–74.

Takeshima, K., A. Chikushi, K. K. Lee, S. Yonehara, and K. Matsuzaki. 2003. Translocation of analogues of the antimicrobial peptides magainin and buforin across human cell membranes. *J. Biol. Chem.* **278:**1310–1315.

Tam, J. P., Y. A. Lu, J. L. Yang, and K. W. Chiu. 1999. An unusual structural motif of antimicrobial peptides containing end-to-end macrocycle and cystine-knot disulfides. *Proc. Natl. Acad. Sci. USA* **96:** 8913–8918.

Tam, J. P., Y. A. Lu, and J. L. Yang. 2002. Antimicrobial dendrimeric peptides. *Eur. J. Biochem.* **269:**923–932.

Tamayo, R., S. S. Ryan, A. J. McCoy, and J. S. Gunn. 2002. Identification and genetic characteristics of PmrA regulated genes and genes involved in polymyxin B resistance in *Salmonella enterica* serovar *typhimurium. Infect. Immun.* **70:**6770–6778.

Tang, Y. Q., J. Yuan, G. Osapay, K. Osapay, D. Tran, C. J. Miller, A. J. Ouellette, and M. E. Selsted. 1999. A cyclic antimicrobial peptide produced in primate leukocytes by the ligation of two truncated α-defensins. *Science* **286:**498–502.

Tang, Y. Q., M. R. Yeaman, and M. E. Selsted. 2002. Antimicrobial peptides from human platelets. *Infect. Immun.* **70:**6524–6533.

Tarver, A. P., D. P. Clark, G. Diamond, J. P. Russell, H. Erdjüment-Bromage, P. Tempst, K. S. Cohen, D. E. Jones, R. W. Sweeney, M. Wines, S. Hwang, and C. L. Bevins. 1998. Enteric β-defensin: molecular cloning and characterization of a gene with inducible intestinal epithelial cell expression associated with *Cryptosporidium parvum* infection. *Infect. Immun.* **66:**1045–1056.

Tasiemki, A., H. Hammad, F. Vandenbulcke, C. Breton, T. J. Bilfinger, J. Pestel, and M. Salzet. 2002. Presence of Chromogranin derived antimicrobial peptides in plasma during coronary artery bypass surgery and evidence of an immune origin of these peptides. *Blood* **100:**553–559.

Termen, S., M. Tollin, B. Olsson, T. Svenberg, B. Agerberth, and G. H. Gudmundsson. 2003. Phylogeny, processing and expression of the rat cathelicidin rCRAMP: a model for innate antimicrobial peptides. *Cell. Mol. Life Sci.* **60:**536–549.

Terras, F. R., H. M. Schoofs, M. F. De Bolle, F. Van Leuven, S. B. Rees, J. Vanderleyden, B. P. Cammue, and W. F. Broekaert. 1992. Analysis of two novel classes of plant antifungal proteins from radish (*Raphanus sativus* L.) seeds. *J. Biol. Chem.* **267:** 15301–15309.

Tew, G. N., D. Liu, B. Chen, R. J. Doerksen, J. Kaplan, P. J. Carroll, M. L. Klein, and W. F. DeGrado. 2002. De novo design of biomimetic antimicrobial polymers. *Proc. Natl. Acad. Sci. USA* **99:** 5110–5114.

Thevissen, K., B. P. Cammue, K. Lemaire, J. Winderickx, R. C. Dickson, R. L. Lester, K. K. Ferket, F. Van Even, A. H. Parret, and W. F. Broekaert. 2000. A gene encoding a sphingolipid biosynthesis enzyme determines the sensitivity of *Saccharomyces cerevisiae* to an antifungal plant defensin from dahlia (*Dahlia merckii*). *Proc. Natl. Acad. Sci. USA* **97:**9531–9536.

Thomma, B. P., B. P. Cammue, and K. Thevissen. 2003. Mode of action of plant defensins

suggests therapeutic potential. *Curr. Drug Targets Infect. Disord.* **3:**1–8.

Tincu, J. A., L. P. Menzel, R. Azimov, J. Sands, T. Hong, A. J. Waring, S. W. Taylor, and R. I. Lehrer. 2003. Plictamide, an antimicrobial octapeptide from *Styela plicata* hemocytes. *J. Biol. Chem.* **278:**13546–13553.

Tomasinsig, L., M. Scocchi, C. Di Loreto, D. Artico, and M. Zanetti. 2002. Inducible expression of an antimicrobial peptide of the innate immunity in polymorphonuclear leukocytes. *J. Leukoc. Biol.* **72:** 1003–1010.

Tossi, A., L. Sandri, and A. Giangaspero. 2000. Amphipathic, alpha-helical antimicrobial peptides. *Biopolymers* **55:**4–30.

Tzou, P., J. M. Reichhart, and B. Lemaitre. 2002. Constitutive expression of a single antimicrobial peptide can restore wild-type resistance to infection in immunodeficient Drosophila mutants. *Proc. Natl. Acad. Sci. USA* **99:**2152–2157.

Uehara, N., A. Yagihashi, K. Kondoh, N. Tsuji, T. Fujita, H. Hamada, and N. Watanabe. 2003. Human beta-defensin-2 induction in Helicobacter pylori-infected gastric mucosal tissues: antimicrobial effect of overexpression. *J. Med. Microbiol.* **52:**41–45.

Ulvatne, H., and L. H. Vorland. 2001. Bactericidal kinetics of three lactoferricins against *S. aureus* and *E. coli. Scand. J. Infect. Dis.* **33:**507–511.

Van Heusden, H. E., B. de Kruijff, and E. Breukink. 2002. Lipid II induces a transmembrane orientation of the pore-forming peptide lantibiotic, Nisin. *Biochemistry* **41:**12171–12178.

Vila-Perello, M., A. Sanchez-Vallet, F. Garcia-Olmedo, A. Molina, and D. Andreu. 2003. Synthetic and structural studies on *Pyrularia pubera* thionin: a single residue mutation enhances activity against Gram-negative bacteria. *FEBS Lett.* **536:**215–219.

Vizioli, J., and M. Salzet. 2002. Antimicrobial peptides versus parasitic infections? *Trends Parasitol.* **18:** 475–476.

Vogel, H. J., D. J. Schibli, W. Jing, E. M. Lohmeier-Vogel, R. F. Epand, and R. M. Epand. 2002. Towards a structure-function analysis of bovine lactoferricin and related tryptophan and arginine containing peptides. *Biochem. Cell Biol.* **80:**49–63.

VonHorsten, H. H., A. Derr, and C. Kirchoff. 2002. Novel antimicrobial peptide of human epididymal duct origin. *Biol. Reprod.* **67:**804–813.

Wang, H., M. Yu, M. Ochani, C. A. Amella, M. Tanovic, S. Susarla, J. H. Li, H. Wang, H. Yang, L. Ulloa, Y. Al-Abed, C. J. Czura, and K. J. Tracey. 2003. Nicotinic acetylcholine receptor alpha7 subunit is an essential regulator of inflammation. *Nature* **421:** 384–388.

Wang, X., C. Moser, J. P. Louboutin, E. S. Lysenko, D. J. Weiner, J. N. Weiser, and J. N. Wilson. 2002. Toll-like receptor 4 mediates immune responses to *Haemophilius influenzae* infection in mouse lung. *J. Immunol.* **168**:810–815.

Wehkamp, J., K. Fellermann, K. R. Herrlinger, S. Baxmann, K. Schmidt, B. Schwind, M. Duchrow, C. Wohlschlager, A. C. Feller, and E. F. Stange. 2002. Human beta-defensin 2 but not beta-defensin 1 is expressed preferentially in colonic mucosa of inflammatory bowel disease. *Eur. J. Gastroenterol. Hepatol.* **14**:745–752.

Weiner, D. J., R. Bucki, and P. A. Janmey. 2003. The antimicrobial activity of cathelicidin LL37 is inhibited by F-actin and restored by gelsolin. *Am. J. Respir. Cell Mol. Biol.* **28**:738–745.

Welling, M. M., A. Paulusma-Annema, H. S. Balter, E. K. Pauwels, and P. H. Nibbering. 2000. Technetium-99m labeled antimicrobial peptides discriminate between bacterial infections and sterile inflammations. *Eur. J. Nucl. Med.* **27**:292–301.

Westerhoff, H. V., D. Juretic, R. W. Hendler, and M. Zasloff. 1989. Magainins and the disruption of membrane-linked free-energy transduction. *Proc. Natl. Acad. Sci. USA* **86**:6597–6601.

Wilson, C. L., A. J. Ouellette, D. P. Satchell, T. Ayabe, Y. S. Lopez-Boado, J. L. Stratman, S. J. Hultgren, L. M. Matrisian, and W. C. Parks. 1999. Regulation of intestinal α-defensin activation by the metalloproteinase matrilysin in innate host defense. *Science* **286**:113–117.

Wu, T., M. R. Yeaman, and A. S. Bayer. 1994. In vitro resistance to platelet microbicidal protein correlates with endocarditis source among staphylococcal isolates. *Antimicrob. Agents Chemother.* **38**:729–732.

Xu, Y., H. Tamamura, R. Arakaki, H. Nakashima, X. Zhang, N. Fujii, T. Uchiyama, and T. Hattori. 1999. Marked increase in anti-HIV activity as well as inhibitory activity against HIV entry mediated by CXCR4, linked to enhancement of the binding ability of tachyplesin analogs to CXCR4. *AIDS Res. Hum. Retrov.* **15**:419–427.

Yamaguchi, Y., T. Nagase, R. Makita, S. Fukuhara, T. Tomita, T. Tominaga, H. Kurihara, and Y. Ouchi. 2002. Identification of multiple novel epididymis-specific beta-defensin isoforms in humans and mice. *J. Immunol.* **169**:2516–2523.

Yang, D., Q. Chen, A. P. Schmidt, G. M. Anderson, J. M. Wang, J. Wooters, J. J. Oppenheim, and O. Chertov. 2000a. LL-37, the neutrophil granule and epithelial cell-derived cathelicidin, utilizes formyl

peptide receptor-like 1 (FRPL1) as a receptor to chemoattract human peripheral blood neutrophils, monocytes and T cells. *J. Exp. Med.* **192**:1069–1074.

Yang, L., T. M. Weiss, R. I. Lehrer, and H. W. Huang. 2000b. Crystallization of antimicrobial pores in membranes: magainin and protegrin. *Biophys. J.* **79**:2002–2009.

Yasin, B., M. Pang, J. S. Turner, Y. Cho, N. N. Dinh, A. J. Waring, R. I. Lehrer, and E. A. Wagar. 2000. Evaluation of the inactivation of infectious *Herpes simplex* virus by host-defense peptides. *Eur. J. Clin. Microbiol. Infect. Dis.* **19**:87–94.

Yoshio, H., M. Tollin, G. H. Gudmundsson, H. Lagercrantz, H. Jornval, G. Marchini, and B. Agerberth. 2003. Antimicrobial polypeptides of human vernix caseosa and amniotic fluid: implications for newborn innate defense. *Pediatr. Res.* **53**:211–216.

Yu, K., K. Park, S. W. Kang, S. Y. Shin, K. S. Hahm, and Y. J. Kim. 2002. Solution structure of a cathelicidin derived antimicrobial peptide, CRAMP as determined by NMR spectroscopy. *Peptide Res.* **60**:1–9.

Zanetti, M., R. Genaro, M. Scocchi, and B. Skerlavaj. 2000. Structure and biology of cathelicins. *Adv. Exp. Med. Biol.* **479**:203–218.

Zasloff, M. 1987. Magainins, a class of antimicrobial peptides from *Xenopus* skin: isolation, characterization of two active forms, and partial cDNA sequence of a precursor. *Proc. Natl. Acad. Sci. USA* **84**:5449–5453.

Zasloff, M. 2001. The commercial development of the antimicrobial peptide, Pexiganan, p. 261–270. *In* K. Lohner (ed.), *From Development of Novel Antimicrobial Agents: Emerging Strategies.* Horizon Scientific Press, Wymondham, United Kingdom.

Zasloff, M. 2002. Antimicrobial peptides of multicellular organisms. *Nature* **415**:389–395.

Zasloff, M. 2003. Amphibian antimicrobial peptides, p. 243–287. *In* C. J. Dutton, M. A. Haxwell, H. A. I. McArthur, and R. G. Wax (ed.), *Peptide Antibiotics: Discovery, Modes of Action, and Applications.* Marcel Dekker, New York, N.Y.

Zasloff, M., B. Martin, and H. C. Chen. 1988. Antimicrobial activity of synthetic magainin peptides and several analogues. *Proc. Natl. Acad. Sci. USA* **85**:910–913.

Zhao, H., and P. K. Kinnunen. 2003. Modulation of the activity of secretory phospholipase A2 by antimicrobial peptides. *Antimicrob. Agents Chemother.* **47**:965–971.

ANTIMICROBIAL PROTEINS

Tomas Ganz and Robert I. Lehrer

18

GENERAL PRINCIPLES

Since microbial effects on the host are often detrimental, antimicrobial defenses are ancient and essential functions. All life forms require host defenses that can repel or destroy potential parasites or greatly restrict their growth. This can be effected by denying nutrients essential for microbial function, or by physical or chemical attacks. Such tasks are a delicate balancing act because of the many structural and biochemical similarities between microbes and their potential hosts. Damage to the host is minimized by targeting microbe-specific structures and by sequestering the microbe before exposing it to antimicrobial substances.

The most prominent example of sequestration is phagocytosis, a process that confines microbes in specialized compartments (phagocytic vacuoles) where they can be exposed to very high local concentrations of antimicrobial substances. When phagocytes encounter targets too large to be ingested (e.g., fungi, protozoa, nematodes), the released microbicidal substances are concentrated within the contact zone between the phagocyte and its target.

Invertebrates as well as vertebrates often respond to pathogens by forming barriers composed of concentric layers of cells (encapsulation, nodulation, platelet aggregation, granuloma) or molecular meshworks generated by clotting. These complex responses also include the production of antimicrobial molecules (Tang et al., 2002; Hoffmann et al., 1999; Iwanaga et al., 1998).

Antimicrobial activity can be mediated by effectors ranging from inorganic molecules to polypeptides, carbohydrates, and lipids. However, in this chapter we focus on antimicrobial proteins, here defined as polypeptides larger than 10 kDa. As complement, coagulation, the generation of oxygen- and nitrogen-derived microbicides, and antimicrobial proteins of invertebrates are discussed elsewhere in this volume, our major emphasis is on antimicrobial proteins of mammalian phagocytes and epithelia, focusing on those that are not primarily involved in the production of reactive oxygen or nitrogen intermediates.

DISTRIBUTION

Antimicrobial proteins are widely distributed in host defense cells and secretions (Table 1). They are found in particularly high concentrations in specialized host defense cells of bone

Tomas Ganz and Robert I. Lehrer, CHS 37-055, Department of Medicine, David Geffen School of Medicine, University of California, Los Angeles, Los Angeles, CA 90095.

The Innate Immune Response to Infection
Ed. by S. H. E. Kaufmann, R. Medzhitov, and S. Gordon
©2004 ASM Press, Washington, D.C.

TABLE 1 Location of major antimicrobial proteins in cells and tissues

Cell or tissue	Location	Protein
Neutrophils	Granules	Lysozyme Lactoferrin (Lf) Serprocidins BPI Phospholipase A2 SLPI
Eosinophils	Granules	RNases (EDN, ECP) Eosinophil major basic protein (MBP) BPI
Cytotoxic lymphocytes	Granules	Granulysin
Paneth cells	Granules	Lysozyme Phospholipase A2 Angiogenin 4 (in mice, RNase)
Macrophages	Secreted product	Lysozyme SLPI
Epithelia	Secretions and surface associated	Lysozyme Lactoferrin (Lf) SLPI Phospholipase A2 BPI (lipoxin induced)

marrow (myeloid) origin, especially neutrophils (polymorphonuclear leukocytes) and eosinophils. In some animals, they are also prominent in Paneth cells (epithelial cells in the small intestine). In these cell types, many antimicrobial proteins are packaged at very high concentration in cytoplasmic organelles called granules. When the cells are appropriately stimulated (the specific pathways that result in degranulation are discussed elsewhere in this volume), the granules fuse to internalized cell membranes that enclose ingested microbes, or to the external plasma membrane that faces the pericellular space. Antimicrobial proteins are also abundant in the secretions of epithelia exposed to environmental microbes (e.g., in the skin, nose and bronchi, the mouth, and the surface of the eyes). Fluids lining or surrounding reproductive structures (e.g., the uterine cervical mucus, seminal fluid, avian egg white) are also rich sources of antimicrobial proteins, presumably protecting the germinal material. Milk, the secretory product of the mammary glands, contains high concentrations of lysozyme and lactoferrin, antimicrobial proteins also found in other epithelial secretions. Antimicrobial substances in milk may help to protect both the lactating breast and the gastrointestinal tract of the newborn.

METHODS

Classical characterization of antimicrobial proteins usually requires their extraction from the tissues or cells of origin, followed by activity-guided purification to homogeneity. Once pure, the protein can be tested against selected microbes in standardized microbicidal or growth inhibition assays. Although this approach is powerful, it also has serious limitations. The composition of the assay medium can modulate the antimicrobial activity of the purified protein as a consequence of pH, salt composition, the presence (or absence) of nutrients, and the presence of substances that bind or inactivate the protein tested. However, standard media cannot faithfully represent the milieu of the phagocytic vacuole, the thin layer of fluid lining the respiratory passages, or the multitude of other environments in which host defense takes place. Moreover, it is all too easy to miss molecules that require additional processing steps, such as limited proteolysis, before they become active. Furthermore, a focus on highly purified molecules is guaranteed to miss components that are effective only in combination—due to additive or synergistic effects. Finally, bacteria that are grown in standard nutrient-rich media express a phenotype quite different than they would in the far more stringent environment within the living host.

If these obstacles are overcome (or ignored) and a purified protein is found that manifests convincing evidence of antimicrobial activity, then the next level of complexity involves assessing its role in the antimicrobial activity of body fluids or isolated cell populations. The contribution of a specific protein can be assessed by neutralizing or specifically removing the protein from fluids or accessible cellular compartments using antibodies, or by decreasing the protein concentrations in cells or secretions by specific inhibitors of synthesis (antisense, inhibitor RNA, etc.). These techniques are especially problematic for antimicrobial proteins that are expressed at high concentrations. They also depend on identifying a combination of target organism and conditions that will unmask the deficiency, a process that often requires serendipity. Adding the protein to a compartment or fluid in which it is not usually expressed is generally less informative because of uncertainties about whether the environment and the protein concentrations reflect the physiologic conditions in vivo.

The *nonredundant* contribution of a protein to antimicrobial host defense in an intact organism can be assessed by studying patients or animals with isolated deficiency of the test protein, or by generating mice in which the gene or genes encoding the protein have been disrupted. Many genes encoding host defense proteins have undergone rapid evolution, so that the mouse may be a very imperfect model of host defense in humans or other mammals. Often antimicrobial proteins are coexpressed with other related proteins with overlapping activity, further complicating the ascertainment of their individual role in host defense.

MECHANISMS

Some antimicrobial proteins are enzymes (Table 2) that lyse the protein, lipid, carbohydrate, or perhaps nucleic acid components of microbes. Others disrupt microbial cell walls and membranes or inhibit microbial growth through nonenzymatic mechanisms (Table 3). In many cases, enzymatic and nonenzymatic activities coexist in the same molecule. A few antimicrobial molecules are catalytically inactive members of enzyme families, having presumably lost their catalytic activity as they evolved for host defense. Yet other antimicrobial molecules sequester or enzymatically inactivate nutrients that are essential to microbes. Because the discovery and study of antimicrobial proteins is an active area of investigation, this overview of the principal antimicrobial proteins should not be considered complete.

Lysozyme and Peptidoglycan-Binding Proteins

Lysozyme (Fleming, 1922) is a highly cationic 14-kDa enzyme that cleaves the glycosidic linkage between *N*-acetyl muramic acid and *N*-acetylglucosamine. Its natural substrate is peptidoglycan, the exoskeletal component of bacterial cell walls that provides bacteria with shape and mechanical rigidity. In gram-positive bacteria, the peptidoglycan is relatively exposed, but in gram-negative bacteria it is sandwiched between the outer and inner membranes. Some bacteria (e.g., *Micrococcus luteus* or *Bacillus subtilis*) are rapidly lysed and killed by lysozyme. However, most are at least partially resistant to lysozyme-mediated lysis due to either covalent modifications of their peptidoglycan or (in gram-negative bacteria) the ability of the outer membrane to keep lysozyme from reaching the peptidoglycan layer. In gram-negative bacteria, the effect of lysozyme can be potentiated by substances that disrupt the outer membrane. Human lysozyme has a pI of approximately 9.3, and as a highly

TABLE 2 Antimicrobial enzymes

Protein	Known substrates	Known antimicrobial effects in vitro under permissive conditions	Known nonredundant effects in experimental animals
Lysozyme	Peptidoglycan	(1) Bactericidal and bacteriolytic for susceptible gram-positive bacteria	Degrades peptidoglycan to terminate inflammation
		(2) Moderate broad antimicrobial activity	Bactericidal to susceptible gram-positive bacteria
Serprocidins (elastase, cathepsin G, proteinase 3)	Procathelicidins OmpA	(1) Direct broad antimicrobial activity (2) Activation of cathelicidins	(1) Bactericidal to gram-negative bacteria in mice (2) Fungicidal to *Aspergillus* in mice (3) Inhibition of *Staphylococcus epidermidis* in pig wounds (indirect effect via cathelicidin activation)
Phospholipase A2	Bacterial phospholipids	(1) Bactericidal for gram-positive bacteria (2) Synergy against gram-negative bacteria	C57BL/6J mice naturally deficient but relevant studies not reported
RNases	Single-stranded RNA	Some broadly cytotoxic, antimicrobial and antiviral	Not reported
IDO	Tryptophan	(1) Inhibition of intracellular bacteria and protozoa (2) Inhibition of T-lymphocyte activation	Induction of tolerance

cationic protein, lysozyme is also antimicrobial by a nonenzymatic mechanism, perhaps mediated in part by the ability of lysozyme and other highly cationic proteins to displace and activate autolytic bacterial cell wall enzymes that are required for peptidoglycan remodeling (Ginsburg, 1988).

Lysozyme is widely distributed in animal tissues. In humans, high concentrations of lysozyme are present in the cytoplasmic granules of neutrophils and Paneth cells and in cellular and secretory compartments of monocytes and macrophages. Lysozyme is found in many secretions, including tears, respiratory secretions, saliva, and cervical mucus. It is also produced by chondrocytes and is abundant in cartilage where its host defense role, if any, is uncertain. In humans and pigs, a single gene encodes the lysozyme found in all expressing tissues. Mice have two lysozyme genes, one (lysozyme M) expressed in myeloid cells and another (lysozyme P) expressed in Paneth cells. Although ruminants have up to 10 lysozyme genes, their tears—unlike those of humans—are lysozyme free. The expression of several lysozyme genes in the ruminant stomach may be driven by the need to digest the large volume of bacteria that ferment ingested plant materials.

The widespread distribution and abundance of lysozyme presents an apparent paradox, in view of its quite limited activity against microbial pathogens. Indeed, when the discoverer of lysozyme, Alexander Fleming, described this remarkable bacteriolytic enzyme to the Royal Society some 80 years ago, it received little attention—primarily because the bacteria most susceptible to its effects were non-

TABLE 3 Key interactions of nonenzymatic antimicrobial proteins

Protein	Known ligands	Known antimicrobial effects in vitro under permissive conditions	Known nonredundant effects in experimental animals
Lf	Iron	(1) Bactericidal for susceptible gram-negative bacteria	None yet (construction recent)
	LPS	(2) Bacteriostatic by iron deprivation	
		(3) Inhibits biofilm formation	
BPI	LPS	Bactericidal against some gram-negative bacteria	BPI protein is absent in mice
PGRP	Peptidoglycan	(1) Bacteriostatic for gram-positive bacteria (murine PGRP)	Not reported
		(2) Broadly microbicidal (bovine PGRP)	
SLPI	Serine proteases of neutrophils and mast cells	(1) Serine protease inhibitor	Impaired wound healing
		(2) Moderate broad-spectrum antimicrobial activity	
Calprotectin	Zinc	Bacteristatic and fungistatic	None yet (construction recent)

pathogens. It may be (and Fleming already raised this possibility) that resistance to this abundant and widely distributed antimicrobial enzyme is one of the prerequisites for pathogenicity.

Recent experiments in mice deficient in lysozyme M (Ganz et al., 2003) showed delayed killing of the lysozyme-sensitive *M. luteus* (which was called *Micrococcus lysodeikticus* in Fleming's era), but the major abnormality in these mice was the highly exaggerated inflammatory response to these bacteria and to peptidoglycan. Peptidoglycan is a potent inflammatory stimulus, in part through its binding to Toll-like receptor 2 and by peptidoglycan recognition proteins (PGRPs). Whatever lysozyme may contribute to antibacterial activity, it appears to be critically important for eliminating bacterial peptidoglycan and dousing the immunological conflagration caused by its prolonged presence.

More recently, another widely expressed group of proteins interacting with peptidoglycan was identified (Kang et al., 1998), the PGRPs. The proteins in this lectin family lack direct catalytic activity and were first characterized in insects, in which PGRPs provide the peptidoglycan recognition element of the proteolytic prophenoloxidase cascade. Contact of insect hemolymph with microbe-derived substances triggers this cascade, which cleaves the prophenoloxidase precursor and activates its phenoloxidase domain. Phenoloxidase, a copper-containing dioxygenase, can oxidize a variety of phenolic substances, generating products with antimicrobial activity, including hydrogen peroxide and melanin. Although the prophenoloxidase cascade does not exist in vertebrates, the PGRP family is represented in humans, mice, cows, and other mammals as 19-kDa three-disulfide proteins that bind peptidoglycan with high affinity but may also bind other bacterial determinants. PGRPs are found in neutrophils, and in cows they are also found in eosinophils. Recombinant murine PGRP was weakly bacteriostatic against selective gram-positive bacteria (Liu et al., 2000), but the highly abundant bovine form was more broadly microbicidal against a variety of bacteria and a fungus (Tydell et al., 2002).

sPLA2

Secretory group IIA phospholipase A2 (sPLA2) is a 14-kDa enzyme that catalyzes the removal of the fatty acid attached to the middle carbon in the glycerol backbone of phospholipids (Ganz and Weiss, 1997). The enzyme is found in the granules of phagocytes, but also in those of platelets, mast cells, and Paneth cells and in very high concentrations in tears (Qu and Lehrer, 1998) and seminal fluid. A member of a large family of phospholipases, sPLA2 appears to be particularly active against bacterial targets. This is not due to unique catalytic activity because other phospholipases that are not antimicrobial can also hydrolyze isolated bacterial phospholipids. Rather, this specialization may result from the unusually high net positive charge of sPLA2 and a cluster of positively charged residues near its N terminus that facilitate its interaction with bacteria and access to its phospholipid target (Weiss et al., 1991). In general, sPLA2 is much more active against gram-positive than gram-negative bacteria, but certain host defense proteins (e.g., complement or bactericidal permeability-inducing [BPI] protein) that disrupt the outer membrane greatly potentiate the activity of sPLA2 against gram-negative bacteria (Ganz and Weiss, 1997). In addition to its likely role in the killing of bacteria by phagocytes and epithelial secretions, sPLA2 may also contribute to the antibacterial properties of serum and plasma (Gronroos et al., 2002). C57BL/6J mice, a strain normally lacking sPLA2, showed increased resistance to *Staphylococcus aureus* or *Escherichia coli* peritonitis after transgenic expression of high levels of human sPLA2. However, these mice have other phenotypic abnormalities calling into question whether the high levels or sites of expression are physiologic.

RNases

Eosinophil-derived neurotoxin (EDN, also called RNase 2) and eosinophil cationic protein (ECP, also called RNase 3) were the first members of the RNase A family implicated in host defense (Gleich et al., 1986). Both are approximately 18-kDa cationic proteins that are among the principal components of the primary granules of human eosinophils. Of the two, ECP is more cationic, and it has demonstrated antibacterial activity and cytotoxic activity against helminths and mammalian cells. This activity is at least in part independent of the catalytic activity. Additional members of this family have been identified recently, including RNase 7, a highly cationic (pI, 9.73) antimicrobial component of healthy human skin (Harder and Schroder, 2002). RNase 6 (pI, 9.0) is expressed in neutrophils and monocytes, but it remains to be seen if it is antimicrobial. Angiogenin 4, another antimicrobial member of this family, is an abundant component of Paneth cell granules in the mouse. Although there is strong circumstantial evidence for host defense function of many members of this family, based on the pattern of tissue expression and their antimicrobial and antihelminthic properties, their specific contribution to host defense is not known.

Because these RNases are catalytically active against only single-stranded RNA, their high positive charge likely contributes more to their antimicrobial properties than does their enzymatic activity. Rosenberg et al. recently proposed that single-stranded RNA viruses may be an important target (Domachowske et al., 1998). EDN (RNase 2) does indeed show activity against respiratory syncytial virus, and catalytic activity is necessary but not sufficient for antiviral effect. However, it is not yet clear whether the virus or the host cell is the key target of the RNase. The study of this family of proteins is made challenging by its very rapid evolution and consequently extreme variability from one animal species to another, hindering the design and interpretation of murine gene disruption studies.

Serine Proteases ("Serprocidins")

Members of the serine protease family are very abundant in the primary (azurophil) granules of neutrophils and were named serprocidins (Gabay and Almeida, 1993) because of their antimicrobial activity in vitro. Neutrophil elastase, proteinase 3, and cathepsin G are catalytically active proteases but the fourth human serprocidin, azurocidin/"CAP37," is enzymatically inactive due to substitution of two of the three critical amino acids at the catalytic site. Mice lacking neutrophil elastase are susceptible to infections with gram-negative bacteria (Belaaouaj et al., 1998), and mice doubly deficient in neutrophil elastase and cathepsin G are susceptible to fungal infection with *Aspergillus fumigatus* and resistant to the endothelial injury seen in endotoxic shock, suggesting an important role for serprocidins in both host defense and its pathological consequences (Tkalcevic et al., 2000). The elastase and cathepsin G content of neutrophil granules is severely reduced in the human and murine Chediak–Higashi syndrome (Ganz et al., 1988), a condition accompanied by complex abnormalities of granule formation in neutrophils, NK cells, and other granule-containing cells and defective chemotaxis. Patients with this disease manifest delayed neutrophil-mediated microbicidal activity, frequent pyogenic infections, and infections with fungi and gram-negative bacteria; "beige mice," the murine counterpart of Chediak–Higashi syndrome, are less resistant to fungal and some bacterial infections than their normal counterparts.

The extent to which the catalytic activity of the proteases contributes to their antimicrobial function is not certain. The serprocidins are highly cationic amphipathic molecules that could disrupt microbial membranes by mechanisms similar to those of antimicrobial peptides (Bangalore et al., 1990). The most amphipathic of these molecules, azurocidin/CAP37, is active as an antimicrobial protein in vitro in the absence of any known catalytic activity. Similarly, the inhibition of the catalytic activity of purified cathepsin G does not interfere with its bactericidal action in vitro. However, in vivo experiments point to an important role for the protease function of serprocidins. Protease inhibitors decrease the killing of bacteria by murine neutrophils (Reeves et al., 2002), and the inhibition of neutrophil elastase interferes with the clearance of bacteria from pig skin wounds (Cole et al., 2001). In some models, the catalytic activity of serprocidins may potentiate the killing of microbes by proteolytic activation of cathelicidins, antimicrobial peptides that are stored in specific granules of neutrophils in an inactive precursor form. Neutrophil elastase is the biological activator of bovine and porcine cathelicidins (Panyutich et al., 1997), and proteinase 3 may serve this function in humans (Sorensen et al., 2001). Alternatively, proteases may kill bacteria by attacking important proteins on the bacterial surface. The killing of *E. coli* by elastase apparently requires the outer membrane protein OmpA, which undergoes proteolysis coincident with bacterial death (Belaaouaj, 2002). Neutrophil elastase may also digest *Shigella* virulence factors required for bacterial escape from phagosomes (Weinrauch et al., 2002).

Serine Protease Inhibitors

Both epithelia and phagocytes secrete protease inhibitors, of which the secretory leukoprotease inhibitor (SLPI) is the most abundant. SLPI is a 12-kDa disulfide-cross-linked cationic protein consisting of two similar domains. SLPI is particularly abundant in cervical mucus, and especially the cervical mucus plugs of pregnancy, but is also secreted by all other mucosal epithelia. SLPI is an inhibitor of neutrophil elastase, cathepsin G, and mast cell tryptase and chymase, all proteases that are associated with inflammation. Mice deficient in SLPI show impaired wound healing (Ashcroft et al., 2000; Zhu et al., 2002), but their response to infection has not been reported yet. In vitro, SLPI shows low-level activity against bacteria and fungi (Hiemstra, 2002) and has been also reported to have anti-human immunodeficiency virus activity. It is possible that the high concentrations of SLPI in many epithelial secretions compensate for its low intrinsic potency to make the antimicrobial activity biologically important.

BPI Protein

The BPI protein (Elsbach and Weiss, 1998) is a 55-kDa cationic protein and a member of a family of lipid-binding proteins, two of which (BPI and lipopolysaccharide [LPS]-binding protein) avidly bind to bacterial LPS. BPI protein is found in the azurophil (primary) granules of human and rabbit neutrophils but, like defensins, may be absent from mouse neutrophils. More recently, BPI protein was also identified as a component of human eosinophil granules and as a lipoxin-inducible protein in mucosal epithelia. In vitro studies suggest that BPI contributes to the killing of gram-negative bacteria in isolated epithelia and neutrophils. The structure of BPI protein consists of two structurally similar domains. The N-terminal domain is more cationic and preferentially binds LPS. It is not yet certain where the lipid A moiety of LPS interacts with BPI, but an apolar, phospholipid-binding pocket of BPI protein is a strong candidate (Beamer et al., 1999). The C-terminal domain binds to phagocytic cells, so that the holoprotein may act as an opsonin of gram-negative bacteria. In contrast, the closely related LPS-binding protein molecule delivers LPS to phagocytes in a form that functions as a potent stimulus of innate immunity by engaging the Toll-like receptor 4/CD14 receptor complex.

In vitro, BPI protein is specifically active against selected gram-negative bacteria at concentrations as low as nanomolar, and this activity is wholly contained in a 25-kDa amino-terminal fragment. The mechanism of activity of BPI against bacteria depends on the initial high-affinity interaction with LPS in the outer membrane. The resulting rapid permeabilization of the outer membrane is followed by a slower process that culminates in the disruption of the inner membrane of gram-negative bacteria with the attendant loss of viability (Wiese et al., 1997). Because of the antibacterial and LPS-neutralizing properties of BPI protein, it has become one of the templates for pharmaceutical development of agents for the treatment of sepsis, but these have not yet showed sufficient efficacy for clinical use.

Eosinophil MBP

Eosinophil major basic protein (MBP) is a highly cationic 14-kDa protein (pI of 11.4 and a net charge of 15.0 at neutral pH) that is very abundant in the primary granules of eosinophilic leukocytes, together with the RNases eosinophil cationic protein and eosinophil-derived neurotoxin (Gleich and Adolphson, 1986). MBP is also found in the placenta. It is a broad-spectrum cytotoxin active against mammalian cells, helminths, and bacteria (Lehrer et al., 1989). Like other highly cationic proteins, MBP disrupts microbial membranes. Structurally it is related to C-type lectins, including mannose-binding protein and lung surfactant protein SP-D, but it does not bind calcium (Swaminathan et al., 2001). Its interaction with heparin is stronger than that of other similarly cationic proteins, suggesting specific interactions with sulfated sugars.

Granulysin

Granulysin (Stenger et al., 1998) is a small protein (with 9- and 15-kDa forms) expressed in the granules of cytolytic T lymphocytes. Spanning a huge evolutionary distance, it is related to amoebapores, i.e., antibacterial and cytotoxic proteins from amoebae, which are unicellular organisms that feed on bacteria but are also capable of causing cytotoxic injury to their hosts. Granulysin is also related to NK lysin, a protein originally isolated from pig small intestine and found in porcine lymphocytes. The proteins have a structure similar to that of other five helical bundle proteins called saposins. Granulysin and its fragments display a broad spectrum of activity against many bacteria including *Mycobacterium tuberculosis*, and the protein has also been shown to contribute to CD8 T-cell-mediated killing of the yeast *Cryptococcus neoformans* (Ma et al., 2002). The mechanism of activity of granulysin may depend on permeabilization of target membranes and in this regard may be similar to that of other cationic proteins with amphipathic domains. The murine homolog of granulysin has not yet been identified, delaying the assessment of the contribution of granulysin to host defense.

Lf

Lactoferrin (Lf) (Brock, 2002; Ward et al., 2002) is a 78-kDa cationic protein consisting of two similar domains, both of which bind ferric iron without using heme or other prosthetic groups. Lf is a highly abundant component of milk, mucosal secretions, and the specific (secondary) granules of neutrophils. In these settings, lysozyme and Lf are present in similar amounts. In avian egg white, lysozyme is also paired with an iron-binding homolog of Lf called ovotransferrin. Although closely related to the plasma iron-carrier protein transferrin, Lf has a higher affinity for iron, and its iron binding is less affected by acid pH, supporting its proposed role as an iron-sequestering protein in mucosal secretions and inflammatory fluids. Iron is an essential metal for all living organisms, and restriction of iron availability is an effective means of inhibiting microbial growth. Iron starvation also interferes with bacterial biofilm formation. Even under conditions that otherwise promote biofilm formation, Lf-exposed bacteria remain in the planktonic form, so that the more mobile bacterial population can disperse and reach iron sources (Singh et al., 2002). Microbes have evolved other sophisticated mechanisms for obtaining iron even in very iron-deficient environments (Braun and Killmann, 1999), in part through the induction of low-molecular-weight iron-binding molecules, "siderophores," and import systems for iron–siderophore complexes. Other bacteria have adapted to a pathogenic lifestyle by developing systems that allow them to obtain iron from host-derived iron-binding proteins. Using a remarkable but poorly understood guerilla strategy, *Neisseria* spp. and *Haemophilus influenzae* can even get their iron from Lf.

Lf can also exert antimicrobial activity that is independent of its iron-binding ability. This mode of action resembles that of other cationic proteins, results in the disruption of the membranes of gram-negative bacteria, and may be mediated by the highly cationic N-terminal region of Lf. The N-terminal peptide "lactoferricin," generated by gastric pepsin cleavage of Lf, has a moderate affinity for LPS, perhaps accounting for the ability of Lf to disrupt outer membranes of gram-negative bacteria. Other proposed modes of action of Lf

involve its protease activity and its ability to release iron for the catalysis of oxygen radical-mediated cytotoxicity.

The initial description of the phenotype of the Lf knockout mouse (Ward et al., 2003) shows that these mice are viable and fertile. Mice lacking Lf and suckled on Lf-deficient milk did not develop any significant abnormalities of iron metabolism, presumably because murine milk contains much more transferrin than Lf, and the former may be more important as a source of iron for the newborn. It remains to be seen whether specific challenges with microbes can uncover host defense defects in the Lf-deficient mice.

Calprotectin

Calprotectin (also called myeloid-related protein or migration-inhibition factor-related protein MRP8/14, or S100A8/S100A9, or L1 protein, or calgranulin A and B) is a highly abundant cytoplasmic protein of neutrophils, monocytes, and squamous epithelial cells and is also present at high concentrations in inflammatory fluids. It is a dimer of two subunits, MRP8 (S100A8) and MRP14 (S100A9), whose sizes are about 8 and 13 kDa, respectively. Each of the subunits can bind two calcium ions and also can bind various fatty acids. Calprotectin is microbistatic against yeast and bacteria (Brandtzaeg et al., 1995; Sohnle et al., 1996), and this activity is inhibited by zinc. Nevertheless, at least with *Candida albicans*, zinc sequestration may not be responsible for the inhibition of growth (Murthy et al., 1993). Since calprotectin is not concentrated in cytoplasmic granules, it is probably released either by an unusual secretion process or from dying leukocytes and keratinocytes. The murine S100A8 protein (also called CP10 or MRP8) is chemotactic for myeloid cells, but this property is not shared by its human ortholog. Homozygous disruption of the S100A8 gene in mice results in abrupt embryonic death and resorption by day 9.5, but S100A9-deficient mice are viable and healthy (Manitz et al., 2003) even though their neutrophils lack not only S100A9 but also its dimerization partner

S100A8. Initial studies of these mice detected only very mild defects in neutrophil cytoskeletal organization and migration, but the antimicrobial functions of these neutrophils were not tested.

IDO

Many microbes are able to survive in intracellular compartments inside a variety of cell types, including macrophages. The cells' ability to restrict the multiplication of these intracellular microbes is greatly enhanced by exposure to gamma interferon (IFN-γ). The enzyme indoleamine-2,3-dioxygenase (IDO) is a heme-containing enzyme whose expression is induced by IFN-γ (Taylor and Feng, 1991). IDO catalyzes the breakdown of the essential amino acid tryptophan to kynurenine and N-formylkynurenine. The intracellular multiplication of several tryptophan-dependent microbes, including *Toxoplasma gondii* and *Chlamydia trachomatis*, is inhibited by IFN-γ, and in many cell types this effect is reversed by the addition of tryptophan. However, the contribution of IDO to IFN-γ-mediated restriction varies by cell type and the species of origin. In addition, IDO has an important tolerogenic function that is mediated by tryptophan deprivation of T lymphocytes by activated macrophages or in the placenta, allowing female mammals to tolerate their allogeneic fetuses (Mellor and Munn, 1999).

Nutritional restriction may be a common mode of host defense, as is suggested by the association of other nutrient-binding proteins with host defense cells or settings. Prominent examples include the biotin-binding protein avidin in the avian egg white and the vitamin B_{12}-binding protein in human neutrophils.

Other Antimicrobial Proteins

Antimicrobial function has been proposed for a number of other proteins whose locations and known other roles may obscure their contribution to antimicrobial processes in vivo. They include such highly cationic proteins as histones (Hirsch, 1958), ribosomal protein S30 (ubiquicidin) (Hiemstra et al., 1999), and even hemoglobin and its cationic fragments (Hobson and Hirsch, 1958). These and other proteins could contribute to antimicrobial activity of abscess fluids, or of macrophages in infected areas where widespread host cell destruction could result in high levels of these proteins in phagosomal vacuoles.

SUMMARY AND CONCLUSIONS

Many mammalian proteins plausibly qualify as antimicrobial proteins by virtue of their activity in vitro and abundance in host defense settings. The specific contribution of some of these proteins to the host defense process in vivo is beginning to be elucidated.

REFERENCES

Ashcroft, G. S., K. Lei, W. Jin, G. Longenecker, A. B. Kulkarni, T. Greenwell-Wild, H. Hale-Donze, G. McGrady, X. Y. Song, and S. M. Wahl. 2000. Secretory leukocyte protease inhibitor mediates non-redundant functions necessary for normal wound healing. *Nat. Med.* **6:**1147–1153.

Bangalore, N., J. Travis, V. C. Onunka, J. Pohl, and W. M. Shafer. 1990. Identification of the primary antimicrobial domains in human neutrophil cathepsin G. *J. Biol. Chem.* **265:**13584–13588.

Beamer, L. J., S. F. Carroll, and D. Eisenberg. 1999. The three-dimensional structure of human bactericidal/permeability-increasing protein: implications for understanding protein-lipopolysaccharide interactions. *Biochem. Pharmacol.* **57:**225–229.

Belaaouaj, A. 2002. Neutrophil elastase-mediated killing of bacteria: lessons from targeted mutagenesis. *Microb. Infect.* **4:**1259–1264.

Belaaouaj, A., R. McCarthy, M. Baumann, Z. Gao, T. J. Ley, S. N. Abraham, and S. D. Shapiro. 1998. Mice lacking neutrophil elastase reveal impaired host defense against gram negative bacterial sepsis. *Nat. Med.* **4:**615–618.

Brandtzaeg, P., T. O. Gabrielsen, I. Dale, F. Muller, M. Steinbakk, and M. K. Fagerhol. 1995. The leucocyte protein L1 (calprotectin): a putative nonspecific defence factor at epithelial surfaces. *Adv. Exp. Med. Biol.* **371A:**201–206.

Braun, V., and H. Killmann. 1999. Bacterial solutions to the iron-supply problem. *Trends Biochem. Sci.* **24:**104–109.

Brock, J. H. 2002. The physiology of lactoferrin. *Biochem. Cell Biol.* **80:**1–6.

Cole, A. M., J. Shi, A. Ceccarelli, Y. H. Kim, A. Park, and T. Ganz. 2001. Inhibition of neutrophil elastase prevents cathelicidin activation and impairs clearance of bacteria from wounds. *Blood* **97:**297–304.

Domachowske, J. B., K. D. Dyer, C. A. Bonville, and H. F. Rosenberg. 1998. Recombinant human eosinophil-derived neurotoxin/RNase 2 functions as an effective antiviral agent against respiratory syncytial virus. *J. Infect. Dis.* **177:**1458–1464.

Elsbach, P., and J. Weiss. 1998. Role of the bactericidal/permeability-increasing protein in host defence. *Curr. Opin. Immunol.* **10:**45–49.

Fleming, A. 1922. On a remarkable bacteriolytic element found in tissues and secretions. *Proc. R. Soc. London B Biol. Sci.* **93:**306–317.

Gabay, J. E., and R. P. Almeida. 1993. Antibiotic peptides and serine protease homologs in human polymorphonuclear leukocytes: defensins and azurocidin. *Curr. Opin. Immunol.* **5:**97–102.

Ganz, T., and J. Weiss. 1997. Antimicrobial peptides of phagocytes and epithelia. *Semin. Hematol.* **34:**343–354.

Ganz, T., J. A. Metcalf, J. I. Gallin, L. A. Boxer, and R. I. Lehrer. 1988. Microbicidal/cytotoxic proteins of neutrophils are deficient in two disorders: Chediak-Higashi syndrome and "specific" granule deficiency. *J. Clin. Invest.* **82:**552–556.

Ganz, T., V. Gabayan, H. I. Liao, L. Liu, A. Oren, T. Graf, and A. M. Cole. 2003. Increased inflammation in lysozyme M-deficient mice in response to *Micrococcus luteus* and its peptidoglycan. *Blood* **101:**2388.

Ginsburg, I. 1988. The biochemistry of bacteriolysis: paradoxes, facts and myths. *Microbiol. Sci.* **5:**137–142.

Gleich, G. J., and C. R. Adolphson. 1986. The eosinophilic leukocyte: structure and function. *Adv. Immunol.* **39:**177–253.

Gleich, G. J., D. A. Loegering, M. P. Bell, J. L. Checkel, S. J. Ackerman, and D. J. McKean. 1986. Biochemical and functional similarities between human eosinophil-derived neurotoxin and eosinophil cationic protein: homology with ribonuclease. *Proc. Natl. Acad. Sci. USA* **83:**3146–3150.

Gronroos, J. O., V. J. Laine, and T. J. Nevalainen. 2002. Bactericidal group IIA phospholipase A2 in serum of patients with bacterial infections. *J. Infect. Dis.* **185:**1767–1772.

Harder, J., and J. M. Schroder. 2002. RNase 7, a novel innate immune defense antimicrobial protein of healthy human skin. *J. Biol. Chem.* **277:**46779–46784.

Hiemstra, P. S. 2002. Novel roles of protease inhibitors in infection and inflammation. *Biochem. Soc. Trans.* **30:**116–120.

Hiemstra, P. S., M. T. van den Barselaar, M. Roest, P. H. Nibbering, and R. van Furth. 1999. Ubiquicidin, a novel murine microbicidal protein present in the cytosolic fraction of macrophages. *J. Leukoc. Biol.* **66:**423–428.

Hirsch, J. G. 1958. Bactericidal action of histone. *J. Exp. Med.* **108:**925–944.

Hobson, D., and J. G. Hirsch. 1958. The antibacterial activity of hemoglobin. *J. Exp. Med.* **107:**167–183.

Hoffmann, J. A., F. C. Kafatos, C. A. Janeway, and R. A. Ezekowitz. 1999. Phylogenetic perspectives in innate immunity. *Science* **284:**1313–1318.

Iwanaga, S., S. Kawabata, and T. Muta. 1998. New types of clotting factors and defense molecules found in horseshoe crab hemolymph: their structures and functions. *J. Biochem. (Tokyo)* **123:**1–15.

Kang, D., G. Liu, A. Lundstrom, E. Gelius, and H. Steiner. 1998. A peptidoglycan recognition protein in innate immunity conserved from insects to humans. *Proc. Natl. Acad. Sci. USA* **95:**10078–10082.

Lehrer, R. I., D. Szklarek, A. Barton, T. Ganz, K. J. Hamann, and G. J. Gleich. 1989. Antibacterial properties of eosinophil major basic protein and eosinophil cationic protein. *J. Immunol.* **142:**4428–4434.

Liu, C., E. Gelius, G. Liu, H. Steiner, and R. Dziarski. 2000. Mammalian peptidoglycan recognition protein binds peptidoglycan with high affinity, is expressed in neutrophils, and inhibits bacterial growth. *J. Biol. Chem.* **275:**24490–24499.

Ma, L. L., J. C. Spurrell, J. F. Wang, G. G. Neely, S. Epelman, A. M. Krensky, and C. H. Mody. 2002. CD8 T cell-mediated killing of *Cryptococcus neoformans* requires granulysin and is dependent on CD4 T cells and IL-15. *J. Immunol.* **169:**5787–5795.

Manitz, M. P., B. Horst, S. Seeliger, A. Strey, B. V. Skryabin, M. Gunzer, W. Frings, F. Schonlau, J. Roth, C. Sorg, and W. Nacken. 2003. Loss of S100A9 (MRP14) results in reduced interleukin-8-induced CD11b surface expression, a polarized microfilament system, and diminished responsiveness to chemoattractants in vitro. *Mol. Cell. Biol.* **23:**1034–1043.

Mellor, A. L., and D. H. Munn. 1999. Tryptophan catabolism and T-cell tolerance: immunosuppression by starvation? *Immunol. Today* **20:**469–473.

Murthy, A. R., R. I. Lehrer, S. S. Harwig, and K. T. Miyasaki. 1993. In vitro candidastatic properties of the human neutrophil calprotectin complex. *J. Immunol.* **151:**6291–6301.

Panyutich, A., J. Shi, P. L. Boutz, C. Zhao, and T. Ganz. 1997. Porcine polymorphonuclear leukocytes generate extracellular microbicidal activity by elastase-mediated activation of secreted proprotegrins. *Infect. Immun.* **65:**978–985.

Qu, X. D., and R. I. Lehrer. 1998. Secretory phospholipase A2 is the principal bactericide for staphylococci and other gram-positive bacteria in human tears. *Infect. Immun.* **66:**2791–2797.

Reeves, E. P., H. Lu, H. L. Jacobs, C. G. Messina, S. Bolsover, G. Gabella, E. O. Potma, A. Warley, J. Roes, and A. W. Segal. 2002. Killing activity of neutrophils is mediated through activation of proteases by K+ flux. *Nature* **416:**291–297.

Singh, P. K., M. R. Parsek, E. P. Greenberg, and M. J. Welsh. 2002. A component of innate immunity prevents bacterial biofilm development. *Nature* **417:** 552–555.

Sohnle, P. G., B. L. Hahn, and V. Santhanagopalan. 1996. Inhibition of *Candida albicans* growth by calprotectin in the absence of direct contact with the organisms. *J. Infect. Dis.* **174:**1369–1372.

Sorensen, O. E., P. Follin, A. H. Johnsen, J. Calafat, G. S. Tjabringa, P. S. Hiemstra, and N. Borregaard. 2001. Human cathelicidin, hCAP-18, is processed to the antimicrobial peptide LL-37 by extracellular cleavage with proteinase 3. *Blood* **97:**3951–3959.

Stenger, S., D. A. Hanson, R. Teitelbaum, P. Dewan, K. R. Niazi, C. J. Froelich, T. Ganz, S. Thoma-Uszynski, A. Melian, C. Bogdan, S. A. Porcelli, B. R. Bloom, A. M. Krensky, and R. L. Modlin. 1998. An antimicrobial activity of cytolytic T cells mediated by granulysin. *Science* **282:**121–125.

Swaminathan, G. J., A. J. Weaver, D. A. Loegering, J. L. Checkel, D. D. Leonidas, G. J. Gleich, and K. R. Acharya. 2001. Crystal structure of the eosinophil major basic protein at 1.8 A. An atypical lectin with a paradigm shift in specificity. *J. Biol. Chem.* **276:**26197–26203.

Tang, Y. Q., M. R. Yeaman, and M. E. Selsted. 2002. Antimicrobial peptides from human platelets. *Infect. Immun.* **70:**6524–6533.

Taylor, M. W., and G. S. Feng. 1991. Relationship between interferon-gamma, indoleamine 2,3-dioxygenase, and tryptophan catabolism [see comments]. *FASEB J.* **5:**2516–2522.

Tkalcevic, J., M. Novelli, M. Phylactides, J. P. Iredale, A. W. Segal, and J. Roes. 2000. Impaired immunity and enhanced resistance to endotoxin in the absence of neutrophil elastase and cathepsin G. *Immunity* **12:**201–210.

Tydell, C. C., N. Yount, D. Tran, J. Yuan, and M. E. Selsted. 2002. Isolation, characterization, and antimicrobial properties of bovine oligosaccharide-binding protein. A microbicidal granule protein of eosinophils and neutrophils. *J. Biol. Chem.* **277:**19658–19664.

Ward, P. P., S. Uribe-Luna, and O. M. Conneely. 2002. Lactoferrin and host defense. *Biochem. Cell Biol.* **80:**95–102.

Ward, P. P., M. Mendoza-Meneses, G. A. Cunningham, and O. M. Conneely. 2003. Iron status in mice carrying a targeted disruption of lactoferrin. *Mol. Cell. Biol.* **23:**178–185.

Weinrauch, Y., D. Drujan, S. D. Shapiro, J. Weiss, and A. Zychlinsky. 2002. Neutrophil elastase targets virulence factors of enterobacteria. *Nature* **417:**91–94.

Weiss, J., G. Wright, A. C. Bekkers, C. J. van den Bergh, and H. M. Verheij. 1991. Conversion of pig pancreas phospholipase A2 by protein engineering into enzyme active against *Escherichia coli* treated with the bactericidal/permeability-increasing protein. *J. Biol. Chem.* **266:**4162–4167.

Wiese, A., K. Brandenburg, B. Lindner, A. B. Schromm, S. F. Carroll, E. T. Rietschel, and U. Seydel. 1997. Mechanisms of action of the bactericidal/permeability-increasing protein BPI on endotoxin and phospholipid monolayers and aggregates. *Biochemistry* **36:**10301–10310.

Zhu, J., C. Nathan, W. Jin, D. Sim, G. S. Ashcroft, S. M. Wahl, L. Lacomis, H. Erdjument-Bromage, P. Tempst, C. D. Wright, and A. Ding. 2002. Conversion of proepithelin to epithelins. Roles of SLPI and elastase in host defense and wound repair. *Cell* **111:**867–878.

REACTIVE OXYGEN AND REACTIVE NITROGEN METABOLITES AS EFFECTOR MOLECULES AGAINST INFECTIOUS PATHOGENS

Christian Bogdan

19

The primary task of the immune system is the immediate recognition and efficient control of pathogenic infectious agents once they cause damage to the host organism. The cells that belong to the innate compartment of the immune system (e.g., macrophages, dendritic cells, alpha/beta interferon [IFN-α/β])-producing cells, natural killer [NK] cells) are equipped with surface or cytosolic receptors that serve to detect viral and microbial pathogens, such as C-type lectins (e.g., mannose receptor, dectin-1, DC-SIGN), Toll-like receptors, or NOD proteins (Figdor et al., 2002; Gordon, 2002; Inohara et al., 2002; Takeda et al., 2003). Ideally, these receptors mediate the endocytosis of the pathogens, induce the release of proinflammatory cytokines, and activate antiviral and/or antimicrobial effector mechanisms. The latter include (i) preformed peptides with direct cidal activity against bacteria and/or fungi (e.g., serprocidins, defensins) (Bevins, 2003); (ii) oxygen-independent constitutive or inducible mechanisms that deprive the microorganisms of essential nutrients (e.g.,

lactoferrin, which binds iron; indoleamine-2,3-dioxygenase, which depletes the amino acid tryptophan) or generate an acidic milieu within the phagolysosome via an ATPase-dependent proton pump (Caccavo et al., 2002; Däubener and MacKenzie, 1999; Nishi and Forgac, 2002); and (iii) oxygen-dependent inducible enzymes that produce reactive oxygen intermediates (ROIs) or reactive nitrogen intermediates (RNIs) (Bogdan et al., 2000b; DeGroote and Fang, 1999; Nathan and Shiloh, 2000). This chapter focuses on the sources, the regulation, the spectrum of activities, and the viral and microbial targets of ROIs and RNIs generated by mammalian host cells. Microbial mechanisms of evasion are also discussed.

SOURCES OF ROIs AND RNIs

With respect to the control of infectious agents, the two most important oxygen-dependent pathways for the generation of antiviral or antimicrobial effector molecules are the phagocyte NADPH oxidase (Phox) and the inducible nitric oxide synthase (iNOS) pathways. Both of them are found in phagocytes. Whereas Phox is prototypically expressed in neutrophils, iNOS is most abundant in tissue macrophages. Phox and iNOS also differ with respect to various aspects of

Christian Bogdan, Institute of Medical Microbiology and Hygiene, Department of Medical Microbiology and Hygiene, University of Freiburg, Hermann-Herder-Strasse 11, D-79104 Freiburg, Germany.

The Innate Immune Response to Infection
Ed. by S. H. E. Kaufmann, R. Medzhitov, and S. Gordon
©2004 ASM Press, Washington, D.C.

TABLE 1 Comparison of Phox and iNOS

Parameter	Phox	iNOS
Enzyme family	NOX family (NADPH oxidases)	Hemeprotein monooxygenase
Resting state	Two integral membrane components (p22^{phox}, gp91^{phox}) forming the flavocytochrome b Four cytosolic proteins (p40-p47-p67^{phox} complex, Rac)	Not expressed in strictly resting cells
Composition of the active enzyme	Enzyme complex consisting of at least six proteins	Homodimer with several bound cofactors (tetrahydrobiopterin, flavin nucleotides [FMN, FAD], heme, calmodulin)
Cellular distribution (examples)	Neutrophils; monocytes, macrophages	Macrophages, monocytes, neutrophils, hepatocytes, endothelial cells
Intracellular localization	Flavocytochrome b in neutrophils: ca. 90% specific granules, approximately 10% plasma membrane	iNOS in primary macrophages: ca. 50% vesicular, ca. 50% cytosolic
(Co-)substrate(s)	NADPH, O_2	L-Arginine, NADPH, O_2
Primary product(s)[a]	Superoxide (O_2^-)	Nitric oxide radical ($\cdot$NO), citrullin
Subsequent metabolites[a] (examples)	$^1O_2$, O_3, H_2O_2, hypohalites (e.g., HOCl), OH$^-$, $\cdot$OH,	NO$^+$, NO$^-$, NO$_2$, NO$_2^-$, N$_2$O$_3$, ONOO$^-$, N$_2$O$_4$, NO$_3^+$, S-nitrosothiols, nitrosyl-metal complexes
Mechanism of induction or activation	Phosphorylation of the cytosolic components Translocation to membrane Association with flavocytochrome	Transcriptional induction Posttranscriptional, translational, and posttranslational control
Inducing or activating stimuli	Phagocytosis of (opsonized) pathogens Microbial products Experimental: phorbol ester, F-Met-Leu-Phe	Cytokines (e.g., IFN-γ, IFN-α/β, TNF) Microbial products (e.g., LPS, flagellin, bacterial DNA) Cell-to-cell contact-dependent signals (e.g., CD40 and CD40L)
Onset and duration of production	Instantaneous (seconds) and brief (minutes to hours) ("oxidative burst")	Slow onset (hours) and prolonged release (hours to days)
Spectrum of activities	Antiviral Antibacterial Antiparasitic Regulation of cell growth, differentiation, function, and death Cytotoxic, tissue damaging	
Genetically determined diseases in humans	Chronic granulomatous disease (severe bacterial and/or fungal infections due to defects of NADPH oxidase components)	iNOS gene promoter polymorphisms with possibly enhanced susceptibility to certain infections (e.g., malaria)

[a]Collectively called ROIs or RNIs, respectively.

enzyme regulation (Table 1). These pathways show multiple interactions between each other as well as with the myeloperoxidase (MPO) pathway (Fig. 1).

ROIs

NADPH Oxidase.

History. In 1933, Baldridge and Gerard reported on the increased oxygen consumption ("extra respiration") of dog leukocytes following phagocytosis of the gram-positive bacterium *Sarcina lutea* (Baldridge and Gerald, 1933). Sbarra and Karnovsky (1959) described that the unusual process was not inhibitable by mitochondrial poisons. In 1961, Iyer et al. provided evidence for the production of hydrogen peroxide (H_2O_2) by guinea pig neutrophils following phagocytosis and for the involvement of an enzyme system that utilizes flavin and reduced pyridine nucleotides (Iyer et al., 1961). Cagan and Karnovsky (1964) postulated a NADH oxidase that contains flavin adenine dinucleotide (FAD). Holmes et al. (1967) noticed that neutrophils from patients with chronic granulomatous disease (CGD) did not undergo a burst of oxygen consumption upon phagocytosis of bacteria and had a reduced bactericidal activity (Quie et al., 1967). Curnette and Babior demonstrated the production of superoxide (O_2^-) by neutrophils and concluded that O_2^- is bactericidal based on the observation that granulocytes from CGD patients did not release O_2^- or other oxidizing radicals (Babior et al., 1973; Curnutte et al., 1974). Klebanoff (1968, 1970) discovered the MPO-H_2O_2-halide antibacterial system, which contributes to the microbicidal activity of intact neutrophils. In 1978 Segal and Jones identified a novel flavocytochrome b_{558} in the phagocytic vacuoles of human granulocytes (Segal and Jones, 1978), which was later shown by the same authors to be also present in human monocytes, macrophages, and eosinophils. Between 1987 and 1993, several groups discovered the two subunits of the flavocytochrome b as well as the four cytosolic components of the Phox and described their association with the different genetic forms of CGD (Abo et al., 1991; Knaus et al., 1991;

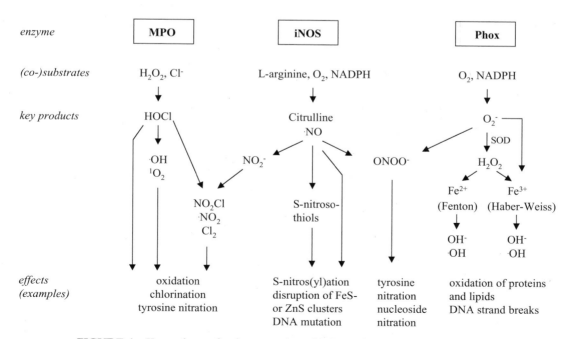

FIGURE 1 Key pathways for the generation of ROIs and RNIs (for details see text).

Nunoi et al., 1988; Parkos et al., 1987, 1988; Teahan et al., 1987; Volpp et al., 1998; Wientjes et al., 1993). In 1995, two transgenic mouse models for the analysis of Phox in vivo were established (Jackson et al., 1995; Pollock et al., 1995).

Enzymology and Intracellular Localization. Phox is a NADPH:O_2-oxidoreductase which transfers electrons from NADPH to molecular oxygen and generates superoxide anions (O_2^-) (Fig. 1 and 2). The rapid oxygen consumption ("respiratory or oxidative burst") is independent of mitochondrial respiration and requires the assembly of a multiprotein enzyme com-

plex either in the peripheral cell membrane or in the membrane of an intracellular compartment (Babior, 1999; Clark, 1999). The underlying processes have been primarily analyzed in human neutrophils. The catalytic core unit of Phox is a heterodimeric integral membrane protein (flavocytochrome b_{558}) that consists of a glycosylated 91-kDa protein (gp91[phox]) and a nonglycosylated 22-kDa subunit (p22[phox]). The gp91[phox] (Nox2) is a member of a new family of NADPH oxidases (termed "Nox/Duox family") (Lambeth, 2002) and contains all the prosthetic groups that are required to transfer electrons from NADPH to oxygen (two hemes, FAD, and a binding site for

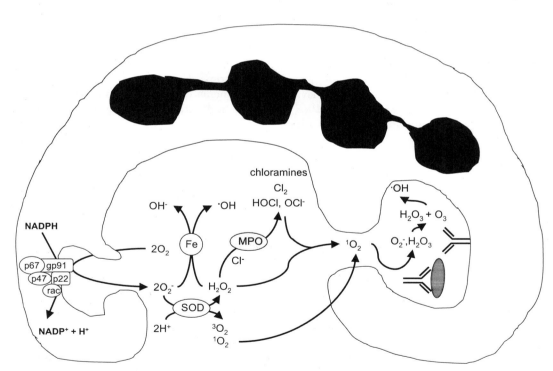

FIGURE 2 Enzymatic and nonenzymatic generation of ROIs in the phagosomes or exocytosed granules of neutrophils. The NADPH oxidase (Phox) is assembled in the plasma membrane (forming phagosomes) or in the membrane of specific granules (which can be exocytosed). The produced superoxide (O_2^-) enters the iron (Fe)-catalyzed Fenton–Weiss reaction (which leads to the release of hydroxyl radical [OH·] or hydroxyl anions [OH⁻]) or dismutates into hydrogen peroxide (H_2O_2) and molecular oxygen (in the triplet or singlet state). H_2O_2 is a substrate for the MPO, which leads to the generation of halogen-containing oxidants. Singlet oxygen ($^1O_2$), which is also derived from the reaction of H_2O_2 with OCl⁻, is transformed into ozone (O_3) and other ROIs by catalytic antibodies that are specifically bound to phagocytosed microbes or attached to the surface of neutrophils.

NADPH) (Rotrosen et al., 1992; Yu et al., 1998). From 70 to 90% of the flavocytochrome c of resting neutrophils is localized in the specific granules and 10 to 30% is localized in the plasma membrane (Borregard and Tauber, 1984; Clark et al., 1987; Jesaitis et al., 1990). Upon activation, at least four cytosolic proteins (p40[phox], p47[phox], p67[phox], small GTPase Rac) are translocated to the membrane, where they associate with the flavocytochrome to form the active Phox (reviewed by DeLeo and Quinn [1996]) (Fig. 2). Translocation involves specific phosphorylation events. Phosphorylation of p47[phox] is a prerequisite for the release of its autoinhibitory state and the formation and membrane translocation of the p40-p47-p67[phox] complex (Groemping et al., 2003).

According to standard views, the active Phox assembles on the plasma membrane. During phagocytosis it is internalized to the membrane of phagocytic vacuoles. Substantial assembly of active Phox, however, also takes place on intracellular membrane compartments such as specific granules, which subsequently fuse not only with forming phagosomes but also with the peripheral plasma membrane. Thus, O_2^- can be released by activated neutrophils through exocytosis of intracellular granules carrying active Phox (Kobayashi et al., 1998). Whereas the release of O_2^- into phagosomes is suitable to combat phagocytosed, intracellular pathogens, the extracellular accumulation might also cause severe damage to host tissues.

O_2^-, the primary product of the Phox reaction, can enter a spontaneous or superoxide dismutase (SOD)-catalyzed dismutation reaction:

$$O_2^- + O_2^- + 2H^+ \rightarrow {}^3O_2 \, ({}^1O_2) + H_2O_2$$

SODs are found in the cytosol (Cu,Zn-SOD) or in the matrix and inner membrane of mitochondria (Mn-SOD) (Okado-Matsumoto and Fridovich, 2001). They are not constitutive components of phagosomes or phagolysosomes, but can be introduced by intracellular pathogens (see Mechanisms of Evasion, below). However, spontaneous dismutation is optimal at a pH of 4.8 and therefore is likely to occur in the acidic milieu of phagolyso-

somes. It is assumed that part of the formed molecular dioxygen assumes an excited state (singlet oxygen, ${}^1O_2$) (Klebanoff, 1999). Both O_2^- and hydrogen peroxide (H_2O_2) exert antimicrobial activity, the extent of which varies with the presence of detoxifying systems in the microbial target organisms (see Mechanisms of Evasion, below).

Expression and Regulation. The oxidative burst of neutrophils (and macrophages) can be triggered by phagocytosis of pathogens, by internalization of immune complexes, by chemoattractants (interleukin-8 [IL-8], leukotriene B₄, C5a, platelet-activating factor), and by certain microbial products such as bacterial peptides (e.g., N-formyl-methionyl-leucyl-phenylalanine) and fungal cell wall components (e.g., zymosan). Experimentally, phorbol esters (e.g., phorbol myristate acetate [PMA]) efficiently activate the Phox through stimulation of protein kinase C and subsequent phosphorylation of p47[phox] (Babior, 1999; DeLeo and Quinn, 1996). The two membrane and four cytosolic components of the Phox are constitutively expressed in phagocytes. Nevertheless, they are subject to regulation by cytokines. The production of O_2^- in response to a triggering agent is significantly potentiated by prior treatment of macrophages or neutrophils with tumor necrosis factor (TNF), IFN-γ, or lipopolysaccharide (LPS) (see Ding et al., 1988; Philipps and Hamilton, 1989; Cassatella et al., 1990; and references therein). At least part of the enhanced oxidative burst after pretreatment of phagocytes with IFN-γ or TNF can be explained by increased mRNA expression of gp91[phox], p47[phox], p67[phox], and/or p22[phox] (Amezaga et al., 1992; Cassatella et al., 1990; Green et al., 1994; Newburger et al., 1988). The transcription factors PU-1, AP-1, interferon regulatory factor-1 (IRF-1), and IFN consensus sequence-binding protein were shown to participate in the upregulation of p67[phox] and/or gp91[phox] mRNA (Dusi et al., 2001; Eklund et al., 1998; Gauss et al., 2002). Phagocytes exposed to cytokines like transforming growth factor β (TGF-β), IL-4, and IL-10 exhibit a strongly decreased oxidative burst in response to phorbol esters (reviewed by Bogdan and Nathan [1993]), which was paralleled by a reduced mRNA expression of one or several Phox subunits (Kuga et al., 1996; Zhou et al., 1995).

Peroxidase-H_2O_2-Halide System. The primary (azurophilic) granules of neutrophils contain large amounts of MPO. The same enzyme is also in found in lysosomes of blood monocytes, whereas mature tissue macrophages usually lack granule peroxidases. A related enzyme encoded by a different gene, eosinophil peroxidase (EPO), is present in eosinophils. The human MPO consists of two heavy- and two light-chain protein subunits and two iron-containing prosthetic groups. During phagocytosis, the granules fuse with the forming phagosome and the MPO is either released into the phagosome or to the outside of the cell. The primary substrate of MPO is H_2O_2, which in phagocytes is derived either from the oxidative burst (see NADPH Oxidase, above) or from ingested catalase-negative bacteria (e.g., *Streptococcus* spp.) and from certain fungi (e.g., *Candida albicans*).

MPO converts H_2O_2 in the presence of halide anions ($Cl^- > Br^- > I^-$) to a variety of toxic products including hypohalous acids (e.g., HOCl), halogens (e.g., Cl_2), and other oxidants (e.g., chloramines, hydroxyl radical [OH^-], singlet oxygen [$^1O_2$]) (Fig. 1 and 2). For a detailed presentation of the MPO-H_2O_2-halide system, the reader is referred to a recent review by Klebanoff (1999).

The MPO system also interacts with nitrite. NO_2^- converts the inactive form of MPO (compound II, MPO-Fe[IV]) into the native enzyme (ground state, MPO-Fe[III]), thereby releasing $\cdot NO_2$ (a strong nitrating species). Furthermore, HOCl can also react with NO_2^-, which results in the formation of NO_2Cl, a compound that shows a strong chlorinating reactivity toward aromates (Eiserich et al., 1998) (Fig. 1).

Finally, there is also evidence that MPO can function as a sink of nitric oxide radicals ($\cdot NO$) by catalytic conversion (oxidation) of NO into nitrite (NO_2^-) (Abu-Soud and Hazen, 2000; Eiserich et al., 2002) (Fig. 1). In endotoxin-treated MPO-deficient mice the NO bioavailability was indeed higher than in the respective wild-type controls (Eiserich et al., 2002). To date, it is unknown whether this pathway could negatively affect the antimicrobial activity of iNOS in vivo. In human leukocytes, the NADPH oxidase, but not the MPO, was identified as the primary NO consumption pathway (Clark et al., 2002).

Formation of Hydroxyl Radical. H_2O_2 can be further reduced, which results in the formation of hydroxyl anion (OH^-) and hydroxyl radicals ($\cdot OH$). $\cdot OH$ radicals are strong oxidants and can be generated from H_2O_2 by at least three different mechanisms (Klebanoff, 1999):

(i) The Fenton reaction (in which ferrous iron [Fe^{2+}] functions as a reducing agent for H_2O_2):

$$H_2O_2 + Fe^{2+} \rightarrow Fe^{3+} + OH^- + \cdot OH$$

(ii) The Haber–Weiss reaction (in which Fe^{3+} is first reduced to Fe^{2+} by O_2^- before Fe^{2+} then enters the Fenton reaction):

$$Fe^{3+} + O_2^- \rightarrow Fe^{2+} + O_2$$
$$\underline{H_2O_2 + Fe^{2+} \rightarrow Fe^{3+} + OH^- + \cdot OH}$$
$$H_2O_2 + O_2^- \xrightarrow{Fe} O_2 + OH^- + \cdot OH$$

(iii) The MPO-H_2O_2-chloride system; using highly sensitive spin-trapping techniques, hydroxyl radical formation via this pathway was demonstrated within intact neutrophils (Ramos et al., 1992).

$$H_2O_2 + Cl^- \xrightarrow{MPO} HOCl + OH^-$$
$$HOCl + O_2^- \rightarrow Cl^- + O_2 + \cdot OH$$

Formation of Singlet Oxygen. In its ground state, molecular oxygen (dioxygen) exists as a triplet molecule with the two unpaired 2p electrons assuming the same spin orientation ($\uparrow$O=O$\uparrow$; $^3O_2$). Upon excitation, a spin inversion can occur and both electrons will occupy the same orbit (delta singlet dioxygen, O=O$\uparrow\downarrow$, $^1\Delta_gO_2$). Since the initial observations by Allen et al. (1972), there is now convincing evidence that this highly reactive and diffusible oxygen species is generated by neutrophils (Steinbeck et al., 1992; Wentworth et al., 2002) and participates in the killing of ingested bacteria (Tatsuzawa et al., 1999). The most likely sources of singlet oxygen are the spontaneous dismutation of O_2^- at acidic pH as found in phagolysosomes (see NADPH Oxidase, above) and the MPO-H_2O_2-halide system (Steinbeck et al., 1992; Tatsuzawa et al., 1999):

$$H_2O_2 + Cl^- \xrightarrow{MPO} HOCl + OH^- \rightarrow OCl^- + H_2O$$

$$H_2O_2 + OCl^- \rightarrow {}^1\Delta_gO_2 + H_2O + Cl^-$$

Generation of ROIs by Catalytic Antibodies. One of the most intriguing discoveries in the field of ROIs in recent years was the observation by Wentworth and colleagues that antibodies, independent of their source or antigen specificity, can catalyze the generation of ROIs. Due to an oxygen binding site within the variable region of the immunoglobulin light chain, they can convert singlet oxygen ($^1O_2$) (generated by activated neutrophils or by photochemical sources) and water (H_2O) into hydrogen peroxide (H_2O_2). The process of catalysis is very efficient (up to 500 mol eq of H_2O_2 are generated from $^1O_2$) and is thought to involve superoxide (O_2^-) (Wentworth et al., 2000) and dihydrogen trioxide (H_2O_3) as intermediates (Wentworth et al., 2001). Additional studies showed that this water-based oxidation pathway exerts bactericidal activity, most likely via the production of ozone (O_3) as well as other trioxygen species (e.g., hydrotrioxy radical [HO_3^-]) (Wentworth et al., 2002, 2003). Human neutrophils, which were coated with antibodies and activated with phorbol ester (PMA), generated O_3 based on the use of two different chemical probes (Babior et al., 2003). O_3 can react with H_2O_2,

which leads to the formation of hydroxyl radicals (Lerner and Eschenmoser, 2003) (Fig. 2). These findings have multiple implications. First, they illustrate a novel form of interaction between the innate (phagocyte) and adaptive (antibody, B cell) immune system. Second, they strongly suggest that the same molecule (antibody) can recognize and kill an infectious pathogen. They also provide an additional explanation as to why antibody-opsonized pathogens are more efficiently killed than the unopsonized counterparts. Third, they open up a new avenue for the generation of diverse species of ROIs. Fourth, the presence of a surface immunoglobulin on B cells (B-cell receptor), the binding of antibodies to cells other than neutrophils, and the fact that the α/β T-cell receptor was also capable of generating H_2O_2 catalytically (Wentworth et al., 2001) suggest that ROIs produced by the antibody-catalyzed pathway exert a broad spectrum of immunoregulatory and signaling functions, which might range from the transcriptional modulation of cytokine responses to the induction of cell death (Wentworth et al., 2002). Finally, antibody-catalyzed formation of ROIs might contribute to the pathogenesis of immune complex-mediated diseases as well as to the therapeutic effect of polyclonal as well as monoclonal antibodies in infectious diseases and certain autoimmune disorders.

Other Sources. In nonmyeloid cells (e.g., vascular smooth muscle cells, colon epithelial cells, proximal tubule epithelial cells of the kidney) a new family of NADPH oxidases (Nox/Duox), which are homologous to gp91[phox] (Nox2), was recently detected and characterized (Lambeth, 2002, 2004). In some cases, these proteins (Nox1, Nox3, Nox4, Nox5, Duox 1, Duox 2) were found to generate O_2^- upon expression in Nox2-negative target cells (Geiszt et al., 2000). Whether they also require interaction with cytosolic proteins and whether they exert antimicrobial activities is currently unknown. It is possible that they account for the production of ROIs by cell types that were previously found to lack gp91^{phox} (e.g., T and B lymphocytes) (Devadas et al., 2002; Reth, 2002). Other enzyme systems that generate ROIs include the NADPH cytochrome P450 reductase, the xanthine oxidase, the lipoxygenase, the cyclooxygenase family, the γ-glutamyl-transpeptidase, and the mitochondrial electron transport chain. With the exception of the ubiquitously expressed xanthine oxidase (Segal et al., 2000; Tubaro et al., 1980; Umezawa et al., 1997) that catalyzes the transformation of hypoxanthine to xanthine and further to uric acid and thereby generates H_2O_2 from H_2O and $^3O_2$, there is no evidence that the ROIs produced by these pathways participate in the control of infectious pathogens.

RNIs

iNOS.

History. In 1818, the British medical doctor William Prout reported on the presence of distinct traces of nitric acid (HNO_3) in the "pink sediment . . . deposited from the urine of those labouring under febrile and inflammatory conditions" (Prout, 1818). One hundred years later Mitchell and colleagues (1916) performed detailed experiments on men, rats, and pigs that strongly suggested that the animal body excretes more nitrate in the urine than is ingested with the food. These results were later confirmed and extended by Green and Tannenbaum, who analyzed the biosynthesis of nitrate in humans and germfree rats (Green et al., 1981a, 1981b). The excretion of nitrate strikingly increased during infections or after treatment of mice or rats with inflammatory stimuli (Green et al., 1981a; Wagner et al., 1983). In 1985 Stuehr and Marletta identified mouse macrophages as a source of nitrite and nitrate after stimulation with LPS, *Mycobacterium bovis* BCG, lymphokines, or IFN-γ (Stuehr and Marletta, 1985, 1987). In 1987, the amino acid L-arginine was shown to be required for the killing of schistosomula by macrophages (Malkin et al., 1987). In the same year and thereafter, Hibbs and colleagues demonstrated that macrophage cytotoxicity against tumor cells and fungi requires an L-arginine-dependent pathway which leads to the production of L-citrulline and nitrite (Granger et al., 1988; Hibbs et al., 1987a, 1987b). Subsequently, three groups provided evidence that nitric oxide (·NO) is a product of activated macrophages and exerts cytostatic activity (Hibbs et al., 1988; Marletta et al., 1988; Stuehr and Nathan, 1989). In 1989 and 1990, the NOS inhibitor N^G-monomethyl-L-arginine (L-NMMA) was used to demonstrate the antimicrobial activity of RNIs in macrophages and in mice (James and Glavin, 1989; Liew et al., 1990). In 1991, the enzyme underlying this pathway, iNOS (NOS2), was purified and identified as a flavoprotein (Hevel et al., 1991; Stuehr et al., 1991; Yui et al., 1991). One year later, the enzyme was cloned from mouse macrophages by the groups of Carl Nathan and Jim Cunningham (Lyons et al., 1992; Xie et al., 1992). In 1995, three groups reported on mice with a deletion of the iNOS gene (Laubach et al., 1995; MacMicking et al., 1995; Wei et al., 1995), one of which turned out to be incomplete (Niedbala et al., 1999; Wei et al., 1995).

Enzymology and Intracellular Localization. iNOS (like all other NO synthases) is a heme protein that is only active as a homodimer and catalyzes the oxidation of L-arginine to ·NO and L-citrulline (Fig. 3). Dimerization requires binding of calmodulin (which in the case of iNOS is irreversible and already occurs at Ca^{2+} concentrations found in resting cells) and incorporation of iron protoporphyrin IX (heme) and possibly Zn^{2+}. iNOS dimers are further stabilized by binding of (6R)-tetrahydrobiopterin (BH_4) and of the substrate L-arginine (Stuehr, 1999). The electron transfer during the redox reaction is complex and entails four redox active groups (FAD, flavin mononucleotide [FMN], heme, and BH_4). When the concentration of L-arginine ($\leq$100 μM) or BH_4 ($\leq$2 μM) drops below levels required for saturation of the enzyme, iNOS may generate both ·NO and O_2^-, which may

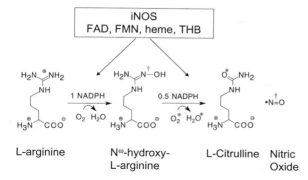

FIGURE 3 Substrates, intermediates, and products of the iNOS reaction (modified from Stuehr et al., 2001). L-Arginine is transformed into L-citrulline and nitric oxide (·NO) via the intermediate N^g-hydroxy-L-arginine (LOHA). The reaction involves a five-electron reduction of the guanidino-nitrogen of arginine, in which NADPH and four redox active groups (FAD, FMN, heme, and tetrahydrobiopterin [THB]) participate in the electron transport to oxygen (O_2).

combine to form peroxynitrite ($ONOO^-$) (Stuehr et al., 2001; Xia and Zweier, 1997).

Cytokine-activated macrophages express iNOS diffusely in the cytosol as well as in a membrane fraction. In IFN-γ- and LPS-stimulated mouse peritoneal macrophages, each compartment contains approximately 50% of the total cellular iNOS activity. Immunoelectron microscopy and confocal laser microscopy revealed that the iNOS protein is associated with small vesicles ("nitroxosomes"), which are different from lysosomes and peroxisomes and await further characterization (Vodovotz et al., 1995; Webb et al., 2001). In the RAW264.7 macrophage cell line, the iNOS protein was also detected adjacent to the peripheral cell membrane, where it colocalized with the cortical actin cytoskeleton (Webb et al., 2001). Unexpectedly, neither in primary macrophages nor in macrophage cell lines was iNOS recruited to phagosomes carrying inert particles (e.g., latex beads) or virulent pathogens (e.g., *Mycobacterium* spp., *Salmonella enterica* serovar Typhimurium, *Leishmania mexicana*, *Leishmania major*) (see also Mechanisms of Evasion, below) (Vodovotz et al., 1995; Webb et al., 2001; C. Bogdan, unpublished observations). However, this does not question a direct antimicrobial function of ·NO because as an uncharged radical ·NO is highly diffusible (Lancaster, 1997).

Expression and Regulation. iNOS mRNA protein and activity have been found in phagocytic cells (including macrophages, monocytes,

microglia, Kupffer cells, neutrophils, and eosinophils), mast cells, dendritic cells, and NK cells as well as other cells that participate in immune reactions and inflammatory processes (e.g., endothelial cells, epithelial cells, vascular smooth muscle cells, fibroblasts, keratinocytes, hepatocytes, and mesangial cells) (reviewed by Bogdan [2000] and Nathan [1992]). iNOS expression is regulated by transcriptional (mRNA synthesis), posttranscriptional (mRNA stability), translational (protein synthesis), and posttranslational (protein stability; availability of arginine and the cofactors of the enzyme) mechanisms. Prototypic inducers of iNOS are proinflammatory cytokines (e.g., IFN-γ, IFN-α/β, TNF) and microbial products (e.g., LPS, lipoteichoic acid, lipoproteins, flagellin, streptococcal beta-hemolysin, bacterial DNA) that either alone or in combination induce iNOS gene transcription via activation of transcription factors such as NF-κB, AP-1, STAT1α, IRF-1, and the high-mobility group-I(Y) protein (reviewed by Bogdan [2001a] and MacMicking et al. [1997a]) (Fig. 4). At least part of the upregulation of iNOS by bacterial products is due to the induction of endogenous cytokines with iNOS-stimulatory capacity (e.g., LPS and flagellin induce IFN-α/β) (Gao et al., 1998; Mizel et al., 2003). It is possible that the cytokine-induced iNOS mRNA stabilization is more important than the increase of iNOS gene transcription for the overall level of iNOS mRNA expression (Vodovotz et al., 1993). iNOS mRNA expression can also be negatively regulated by cytokines

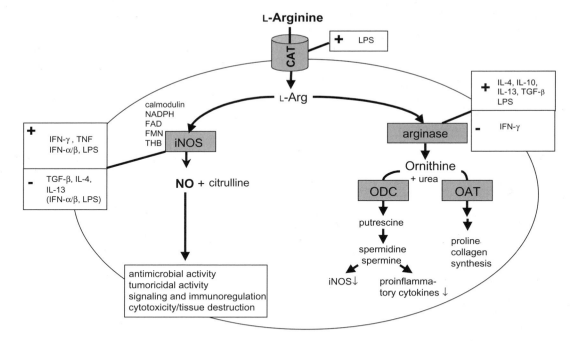

FIGURE 4 Cytokine regulation and function of iNOS and arginase as alternative arginine-consuming pathways. For the production of NO by iNOS, the cells (e.g., macrophages, fibroblasts) require the uptake of extracellular L-arginine via cationic amino acid transporters (CAT). Arginine can enter either the iNOS pathway or the arginase pathway. Arginase degrades arginine into urea and ornithine. Ornithine is a substrate for two enzymes: the ornithine-decarboxylase (ODC), which leads to the generation of polyamines that support cell proliferation but also exert immunosuppressive functions; and the ornithine aminotransferase (OAT), which leads to the production of proline, a precursor of collagen synthesis by fibroblasts. iNOS and arginase are regulated antagonistically by overlapping sets of cytokines and also fulfill complementary functions. THB, tetrahydrobiopterin.

(e.g., IL-4, TGF-β), which is crucial for the shutdown of the inflammatory response once an infection is under control (Bogdan, 2000, 2001a; Nathan, 2002) (Fig. 4).

Additional levels of iNOS regulation include the synthesis and stability of the iNOS protein. Some cytokines, whose expression during infections with certain intracellular pathogens correlates with a more severe course of the disease, have been shown to decrease iNOS protein synthesis and stability with (IL-4, TGF-β) or without (IL-13) simultaneous suppression of iNOS mRNA (Bogdan et al., 1997; Vodovotz et al., 1993) (Fig. 4). Recently, the depletion of arginine (≤10 μM) via the induction and/or activation of arginase was found to strongly and selectively impair the synthesis of iNOS protein in macrophages (El-Gayar et al., 2003) and astrocytes (Lee et al., 2003) and to account for the downregulation of iNOS protein by IL-13 (El-Gayar et al., 2003). In the astrocyte model, arginine deficiency correlated with an increased phosphorylation of the eukaryotic translation initation factor eIF2α, which thereby loses its ability to form the ternary translation initiation complex (Lee et al., 2003). In addition to arginine, tryptophan was also reported to be required for iNOS protein expression in IFN-γ-stimulated macrophages (Chiarugi et al., 2003). It is possible that in IFN-γ-activated macrophages tryptophan becomes limiting due to the simultaneous induction of indoleamine-2,3-dioxygenase (which metabolizes tryptophan) and of tryptophanyl-tRNA synthetase (which shuttles tryptophan into protein synthesis).

Independent of its effect on iNOS protein synthesis, depletion of arginine directly affects the high-output production of NO, because iNOS cannot access the intracellular arginine pools and strictly requires the uptake of extracellular arginine via a family of cationic amino acid transporter proteins (CAT1, -2A and -2B, and -3) (Chang et al., 1998a; Closs et al., 2000; Granger et al., 1990; Nicholson et al., 2001). The extracellular arginine concentration is strongly modulated by arginase. This enzyme, which can also be released into the extracellular space, degrades arginine to urea and ornithine and exists in at least two isoforms (cytosolic, "hepatic" arginase I and mitochondrial, extrahepatic arginase II). The induction or upregulation of arginase type I in macrophages (e.g., by IL-4/IL-10, IL-13) prior to the induction of iNOS (e.g., by IFN-γ plus TNF or LPS) will prevent NO production via substrate depletion (El-Gayar et al., 2003; Modolell et al., 1995; Rutschman et al., 2001), independent of additional effects on iNOS mRNA and protein expression (Fig. 4).

cNOS. In addition to iNOS, there are two other well-characterized NO synthases: the neuronal NO synthase (nNOS, NOS1) and the endothelial NO synthase (eNOS, NOS3). Unlike iNOS, both the nNOS and the eNOS proteins are constitutively expressed in a variety of cells such as neurons or endothelial cells (hence their description as "constitutive" NOS or cNOS). Brief Ca^{2+} influxes (e.g., triggered by neurotransmitters or by vascular shear stress) cause reversible binding of calmodulin with homodimerization and activation of the enzymes (MacMicking et al., 1997a). In general, nNOS and eNOS produce small amounts of NO over a short period of time and are much less subject to regulation by cytokines or microbial products than iNOS (Förstermann et al., 1998; Li et al., 2002a,

2002b). A number of studies suggest the expression of nNOS and/or eNOS in cells of the immune system (e.g., monocytes, macrophages, NK cells, B and T lymphocytes) and their participation in the regulation of cell death, cell adhesion, the expression of iNOS, or vascular permeability during inflammatory processes (Bogdan, 2001a). However, with a few exceptions (Connelly et al., 2003), direct proof of the expression of cNOS in immune cells does not exist, and convincing data on the control of infectious pathogens by cNOS-derived NO have not yet been published.

NOS-Independent Generation of RNIs. The NOS-independent generation of RNIs might be relevant for antimicrobial defense (i) in cells and/or tissues under steady-state conditions, when iNOS is not induced; (ii) in cells and/or tissues in which iNOS is not or only poorly inducible; and (iii) in organ cavities in which NO produced by iNOS–positive cells in the organ wall might not reach the microbial target organism.

Reduction of Nitrate and Nitrite. Ingested inorganic nitrate (NO_3^-) is rapidly absorbed in the stomach and intestine, concentrated in the salivary glands, and reduced to nitrite (NO_2^-) in the mouth by nitrate-reductase-positive bacteria on the posterior surface of the tongue of rats (e.g., *Streptococcus* spp., *Staphylococcus* spp.). Once swallowed, the nitrite is exposed to an acid (pH 1 to 2) milieu in the stomach and forms nitrous acid (HNO_2), which disintegrates into multiple reactive nitrogen species including NO, N_2O_3, NO_2, and nitrate. The nitrate is reabsorbed and completes the enterosalivary cycle (Duncan et al., 1995). Acidified nitrite has been repeatedly shown to exert strong toxic effects against various bacteria including *Salmonella* spp., *Yersinia* spp., *Shigella* spp., and enterohemorrhagic *Escherichia coli* (DeGroote and Fang, 1999). Thus, it was proposed that the enterosalivary circulation of nitrate provides an antimicrobial defense mechanism against infectious pathogens in the mouth and lower gut (Duncan et al., 1995,

1997). A similar chemical, nonenzymatic generation of NO is also likely to occur in the urinary tract. During urinary tract infections with nitrate reductase-positive bacteria (e.g., *E. coli*), the urine contains up to 700 μM nitrite. The antibacterial activity of nitrite-positive urine is drastically enhanced by acidification (pH 4.5 to 5.0) due to the generation of NO, which is further increased by the addition of ascorbic acid (which acts both as an acidifying and a reducing agent). These findings also explain why urease-positive pathogens (which generate NH_4^+ with a subsequent rise of the urinary pH) are protected against nitrite-mediated damage (Carlsson et al., 2001).

MPO-Mediated Generation of RNIs. In human neutrophils, the expression of iNOS and the production of NO are still controversial (Evans et al., 1996; Miles et al., 1995; Tse et al., 2001; and references therein). However, even if human neutrophils were unable to express iNOS themselves, they can still generate RNIs. Activated neutrophils were shown to convert nitrite (NO_2^-) into nitrogen dioxide ($\cdot NO_2$) and nitryl chloride (NO_2Cl) through MPO-dependent pathways (Eiserich et al., 1998) (see also Peroxidase-H_2O_2-Halide System, above) (Fig. 1). This pathway might be more important for the nitration of microbial and tissue targets during infections than peroxynitrite (see below).

iNOS-Independent Generation of RNIs from Arginine. L-Arginine and N^ω-hydroxy-L-arginine, substrate and intermediate of the iNOS reaction, can be oxidized to citrulline and NO by a number of heme proteins other than iNOS (such as peroxidases and cytochrome P450) as well as chemically by superoxide or peroxide (Nagase et al., 1997; Wu and Morris, 1998). This iNOS-independent process can also take place physiologically in phagocytic cells during the respiratory burst (Modolell et al., 1997) or in a pathophysiological situation, where antineutrophil cytoplasmic antibodies induce the production of reactive oxygen species by cross-linking pro-

teinase-3 or MPO with Fcγ receptors on neutrophils (Tse et al., 2001).

Chemical Reaction between NO and O_2^-. NO and O_2^- avidly react with each other under formation of peroxynitrite anions ($ONOO^-$). Whereas $ONOO^-$ is very stable at alkaline pH, it forms peroxynitrous acid ($ONOOH$) and spontaneously decomposes at physiological pH into molecular species that resemble hydroxyl radical ($OH\cdot$) and nitrogen dioxide ($\cdot NO_2$) (Beckman et al., 1990, 1994). In the presence of carbon dioxide, $ONOO^-$ is a potent nitrating agent that causes tyrosine nitration of proteins (Ischiropoulos and Beckman, 2003). Recently, there has been a vivid debate (i) whether $ONOO^-$ is formed in phagocytes (macrophages) at all and (ii) to what extent tyrosine nitration detected in macrophages or tissues is due to $ONOO^-$ or, alternatively, is caused by (myelo-)peroxidase-generated reactive nitrogen species (see above) (Brennan et al., 2002; Deen et al., 2002; Espey et al., 2002; Pfeiffer et al., 2001a, 2001b; Reiter et al., 2000; Sawa et al., 2000). At present, there are convincing studies with MPO- and EPO-deficient mice (Brennan et al., 2002) and with O_2^- scavengers (Pfeiffer et al., 2001b) as well as plausible arguments that both pathways will operate in vivo. First, in the presence of low concentrations of arginine, iNOS will produce both O_2^- and NO (Xia and Zweier, 1997). Second, there is no need for O_2^- and NO to be produced within the same cell. Considering that macrophages and neutrophils are frequently neighbors at inflammatory sites, the MPO pathway in neutrophils can utilize NO/NO_2^- produced by macrophages, and NO released by tissue macrophages (which are poor producers of O_2^-) can interact with O_2^- released by iNOS-negative neutrophils through exocytosis of intracellular granules. Third, nonoverlapping kinetics of NO and O_2^- production, as seen in vitro due to the use of inherently different and artificial stimuli (e.g., IFN-γ/LPS versus PMA) (Pfeiffer et al., 2001a), are unlikely to occur in vivo, also because the phagocyte populations are neither homogeneous nor synchronized with respect to their state of activation. Finally, whether the ONOO⁻- or the MPO-mediated pathway of tyrosine nitration predominates is also dependent on the production of O_2^- versus H_2O_2.

SPECTRUM OF ACTIVITIES IN THE IMMUNE SYSTEM

Overview

ROIs and RNIs are a heterogenous group of molecules that exert multiple functions in the immune system (as well as all other organ systems) far beyond their antimicrobial activities. Small, membrane-permeable, and short-lived species (e.g., ˙NO, H_2O_2) with a reactivity toward (heme-)proteins are perfect signaling molecules within and between cells. They regulate the ontogeny, proliferation, differentiation, function (e.g., cytokine and chemokine production, adhesion, migration and chemotaxis, endocytosis or antigen presentation), and death of T cells, B cells, granulocytes, macrophages, dendritic cells, NK cells, mast cells, and other immune cells by targeting cysteine residues and metal-sulfur centers of proteins (Bogdan, 2001a; Bogdan et al., 2000b; Marshall et al., 2000). To date, numerous target molecules of ROIs and RNIs have been identified. Examples are the soluble guanylyl cyclase, ion channels, components of the cytoskeleton (e.g., actin), intracellular signal transducers (e.g., heterotrimeric GTP-binding proteins, phospholipases, Janus and mitogen-activated protein kinases, Src kinases, members of the STAT family, caspases, protein phosphatases, metalloproteases), cell cycle proteins (e.g., cyclin D1), transcription factors (e.g., NF-κB, AP-1, Sp1, HIF-1), histone (de)acetylases, DNA methylases, regulators of mRNA stability and translation (e.g., iron regulatory proteins 1 and 2), and posttranslational processing enzymes (e.g., IL-1β-converting enzyme, TNF-converting enzyme). The molecular and phenotypic aspects of the signaling function of ROIs and RNIs have been covered by several recent in-depth reviews (Bogdan, 2001b; Forman and Torres, 2001; Nathan, 2003;

Nathan and Shiloh, 2000; Pfeilschifter et al., 2001; Reth, 2002; Sauer et al., 2001).

On the other hand, some ROI and RNI species exhibit strong oxidative and/or nitrosative capacity (e.g., ˙OH, HOCl, ONOO⁻, N_2O_3) and are therefore thought to account not only for the killing of infectious pathogens but also for immunosuppression, tissue damage (e.g., matrix degradation, increased apoptosis and necrosis of cells, vascular leakage), degeneration and aging processes, and mutagenesis (Bogdan, 1998, 2000; Brüne et al., 1999; Felley-Bosco, 1998; Klein and Ackerman, 2003; Kolb and Kolb-Bachofen, 1998; Nakano et al., 2003). It is evident from both in vitro and in vivo analyses that the benign signaling character of ROIs and RNIs (that helps to maintain the homeostasis of the macroorganism) cannot be segregated from their toxicity toward infectious agents or host cells, neither in terms of the underlying ROI or RNI species nor with respect to the underlying molecular pathways. As discussed below for infectious diseases, host-protective and host-damaging functions of ROIs and RNIs are not separate, but are parallel or consecutive events that are frequently required for the control of both the pathogen and the immune response.

Mechanisms of Antimicrobial Action

NADPH Oxidase and MPO. Although the chemical reactivities of the different ROIs are fairly well defined and in vitro systems generating the different ROIs have been used to assess their activity against infectious microorganisms, it has remained a formidable task to define which of the different ROI species are involved in the killing of microbial pathogens inside phagocytes. There have been two major obstacles. First, definitive proof of the production of some of the ROI species under physiological conditions has been difficult to obtain. Second, if a spectrum of different ROIs is released into or generated within the phagosomes, it is hard to determine which of the compounds is essential for the killing and/or clearance of the ingested microbes.

However, the application of new methods for the specific and sensitive detection of ROIs (Babior, 1999; Ramos et al., 1992; Steinbeck et al., 1992; Wentworth et al., 2002), the use of novel scavengers of defined ROI species, the generation of mutant microbes that hyperexpress or lack ROI quenchers, ROI-catabolizing enzymes (e.g., SOD or catalase mutants) or enzymatic DNA repair systems (Cox et al., 2003; Fang et al., 1999; Ghosh et al., 2003; Shiloh et al., 1999; Späth et al., 2003b; Tatsuzawa et al., 1999; van Diepen et al., 2002), and the study of phagocytes from NADPH oxidase- or MPO-deficient mice or humans (see below) have provided at least partial answers.

The current view is that Phox/O_2^- and the MPO-H_2O_2-halide system are important mediators of oxygen-dependent killing of viruses (e.g., human immunodeficiency virus type 1), bacteria (e.g., *Staphylococcus* spp., *Salmonella* spp.), parasites (e.g., *Leishmania tropica*, *Leishmania donovani*), fungi (e.g., *Candida* spp., *Aspergillus fumigatus*), and helminths (e.g., *Schistosoma mansoni* schistosomula) by neutrophils and macrophages (Cox et al., 2003; Fang et al., 1999; Ghosh et al., 2003; Klebanoff, 1999; Philippe et al., 2003). As a strong nonradical oxidant, HOCl is capable of oxidating thiol groups, iron-sulfur clusters, heme prosthetic groups, and sulfur-ether groups of proteins. Furthermore, it causes lipid peroxidation and chlorination of tyrosine residues and phenol groups and it inhibits DNA synthesis. Hydroxyl radical (˙OH) is presumably the most biologically reactive molecule known to exist and causes DNA strand breaks, inactivation of enzymes, and lipid peroxidation (Hampton et al., 1998; Klebanoff, 1999).

Whether O_2^- is directly bactericidal has been controversial (Hampton et al., 1998; Klebanoff, 1999). However, dismutation of O_2^- leads to the formation of H_2O_2 (which fuels the MPO pathway) and to the production of singlet oxygen ($^1O_2$), which is bactericidal in itself (Tatsuzawa et al., 1999) and, in the presence of antibodies, leads to the generation of ozone (O_3). O_3 induces holes in the cell wall and kills bacteria (Wentworth et al., 2002). In addition, the release of O_2^- into the endocytic vacuole necessitates an influx of cations into the vacuole to compensate for the negative intravacuolar charge produced by the electrogenic action of Phox (Geiszt et al., 2001). A recent study demonstrated that K^+ ions rather than protons are pumped into the vacuole during the activation of Phox. This leads to a rise of the intravacuolar pH, to the release of the granule proteases from their anionic proteoglycan matrix (which were jointly discharged into the vacuole during its fusion with specific granules), and thus to the activation of the cationic proteases (elastase, cathepsin G). Based on experiments with granulocytes from protease-deficient mice, the use of protease inhibitors, and the application of a K^+ channel blocker, it was concluded that O_2^- indirectly induces killing of *Staphylococcus aureus* and *C. albicans* by activation of granule proteases via a surge of K^+ ions (Reeves et al., 2002; Ahluwalla et al., 2004).

iNOS. The strong antiviral and antimicrobial properties of RNIs were demonstrated by the use of NO-generating compounds, by the positive correlation between iNOS expression and RNI production, and the killing of pathogens in cell cultures and in infected mammalian organisms, as well as by the inhibition of pathogen clearance in host cells and in mice that were treated with (i)NOS inhibitors or lacked the iNOS gene (Bogdan, 1997; DeGroote and Fang, 1999). Members of all groups of infectious pathogens (viruses, bacteria, protozoa, helminths, and fungi) were found to be controlled by RNIs. Despite an impressive number of phenotypic studies (see also Results from the Mouse Models and Results from the Human Model, below), it is still unclear to what extent the protective function of RNIs is due to direct and indirect effects.

Direct Antiviral and Antimicrobial Effects. The direct antiviral and antimicrobial activity of NO is thought to result from mutation of DNA; inhibition of DNA repair and synthesis; alteration of proteins by S-nitrosylation, ADP-ribosylation or tyrosine nitration; inactivation of enzymes by disruption of Fe-S clusters, zinc fingers or heme groups; and/or peroxidation of membrane lipids (Bogdan et al., 2000b; DeGroote and Fang, 1999). For several infectious pathogens, target molecules have been defined that are inactivated by RNIs, e.g., the active site of the viral protease 3C of coxsackievirus B3 (Saura et al., 1999), the protease 2A of coxsackievirus B4 (Badorff et al., 2002), the ferredoxin of *Clostridium pasteurianum* (Stuehr et al., 1989), the RING fingerlike domain of the cochaperone DnaJ of *E. coli* (Kröncke et al., 2001), and most likely DNA-binding zinc metalloproteins of *S. enterica* serovar Typhimurium (Shapiro et al., 2003). The ultimate effector molecules that operate in vivo remain ill-defined, but most likely include free ˙NO (Pacelli et al., 1995), ˙NO_2 (Eiserich et al., 1998), *S*-nitrosoalbumin (Mnaimneh et al., 1997), *S*-nitrosoglutathione (Venketaraman et al., 2003) and peroxynitrite ($ONOO^-$) (Hickman-Davis et al., 1999). Even if the host cell does not produce ˙NO and O_2^- at the same time (see NOS-Independent Generation of RNIs, above), $ONOO^-$ might still be formed within the host cell or the microbial organism due to the reaction of host-derived ˙NO with pathogen-derived O_2^- as postulated for *Helicobacter pylori* and *E. coli* (Nagata et al., 1998; St. John et al., 2001).

There is also evidence that RNIs affect the development and stage conversion of parasites and fungi (Bogdan, 1997). IFN-γ-activated murine macrophages killed conidia of the fungus *Paracoccidioides brasiliensis*, but also inhibited the transformation of conidia into the tissue yeast cell form (Gonzalez et al., 2000).

Indirect Antimicrobial Effects. The antimicrobial activity of the iNOS pathway might also be totally unrelated to the direct toxic effects of the generated RNIs. Two groups reported that iNOS-derived RNIs inhibited the formation of the mature, phagolysosome-like, large acidified vacuoles in *Coxiella burnetii*-infected macrophages, in which the bacterium normally replicates (Howe et al., 2002; Zamboni and Rabinovitch, 2003). It is possible that NO inhibits the vacuolar H^+-ATPase and thereby disturbs the environment that is required for the replication of this pathogen (Forgac, 1999).

Several infectious pathogens (e.g., *Trypanosoma cruzi*, African trypanosomes, *Giardia lamblia, S. mansoni*) are dependent on exogenous arginine, which they require for the synthesis of polyamines and cell proliferation. Therefore, local arginine depletion by induction of iNOS in macrophages or other cells of the host organism can lead to growth inhibition or death of these parasites (Eckmann et al., 2000; Olds et al., 1980; Piacenza et al., 2001). As another possible mechanism of iNOS-dependent but RNI-independent control, it was recently suggested that N^ω-hydroxy-L-arginine, the primary intermediate of the L-arginine-iNOS-NO pathway, contributes to the killing of intracellular *Leishmania* by blocking the arginase activity within the parasite and/or the macrophage. This leads to a reduction of the synthesis of ornithine and subsequently to a lack of polyamines that are thought to be essential for the growth of *Leishmania* and other trypanosomatidae (Iniesta et al., 2001).

Multiple indirect antimicrobial effects of the iNOS pathway can also result from the numerous immunomodulatory functions of RNIs. Thus, in mouse cutaneous leishmaniasis the iNOS-dependent early upregulation of IFN-γ was required for the prevention of early parasite spreading (Diefenbach et al., 1998). In human cerebral malaria, the disease-protective effects of iNOS-derived RNIs might be due to the suppression of the production of disease-mediating, proinflammatory cytokines, the inhibition of the cytoadherence of the parasite, and/or the reduction of the adhesion and sequestration of infected erythrocytes in the microvasculature (Hobbs et al., 2002).

Results from the Mouse Models

$iNOS^{-/-}$ Mice: Overview. The discovery of the substrate analog N^G-monomethyl-L-arginine as a competitive inhibitor of all isoforms of NO synthases allowed the definition of iNOS for the first time as the critical control and killing mechanism of dozens of pathogens in macrophages and in mice (Bogdan, 1997; DeGroote and Fang, 1999; James and Glavin, 1989; Liew et al., 1990). Further progress became possible with the availability of iNOS-specific antisera for in situ immunohistochemical analyses (Bogdan et al., 2000a; Stenger et al., 1996, 1994; Xie et al., 1992), the application of iNOS-selective NO inhibitors (Stenger et al., 1996), and the generation of iNOS$^{-/-}$ mice (Laubach et al., 1995; MacMicking et al., 1995). The analysis of iNOS$^{-/-}$ mice in more than 50 infectious disease models revealed that, depending on species and strain of the infectious pathogen, the infection dose and the pathogen entry route, iNOS-derived RNIs were indispensable or helped to control the infection, had no discernible effect, or even worsened the disease (Table 2). Today we know that iNOS-derived NO comes into play during virtually all phases of infection, not only as an antimicrobial but also as an immunoregulatory molecule. It affects the function or differentiation of cells of the innate and adaptive arms of the immune response (e.g., IFN-γ production and cytotoxic activity of NK cells, release of IL-12 by macrophages, differentiation of Th1 cells) (Diefenbach et al., 1999; Niedbala et al., 2002).

iNOS and Pathogen Persistence. A prominent role of iNOS was observed during healed local or systemic infections with intracellular bacteria (e.g., *Mycobacterium tuberculosis*) or protozoa (e.g., *L. major*) that are characterized by the lifelong persistence of small numbers of pathogens despite clinical cure of the disease. In these cases, suppression of iNOS activity led to a rapid increase of pathogen replication and the reappearance of clinical disease (Botha and Ryffel, 2002; Flynn et al., 1998; MacMicking et al., 1997b; Stenger et al., 1996). However, reactivation of disease by inhibition of iNOS was not observed in all models of latent murine tuberculosis (Scanga et al., 1999). Furthermore, reactivation of latent tuberculosis after depletion of CD4$^+$ T cells was not associated with a decrease of IFN-γ or iNOS expression, which illustrates that CD4$^+$

T cells control persisting mycobacteria also by factors other than IFN-γ- and iNOS-derived RNIs (Scanga et al., 2000).

Persistence of *Chlamydia trachomatis* in the female genital tract after resolution of the acute infection frequently gave rise to hydrosalpinx formation in iNOS$^{-/-}$, but not in iNOS$^{+/+}$ mice. After treatment with cyclophosphamide, viable *Chlamydia* became detectable only in iNOS$^{-/-}$ mice. This supports the concept that iNOS confers protection against chronic chlamydial infections (Ramsey et al., 2001a).

iNOS and Immunopathology. The significant improvement of certain infectious diseases after inhibition or genetic deletion of iNOS, which was without negative effects on the pathogen clearance, was unexpected (Table 2). It can be explained by the inhibition of T-cell proliferation or induction of T-cell apoptosis via iNOS-positive suppressor cells (macrophages and dendritic cells) or by the tissue-damaging properties of RNIs (Bogdan, 2000). Especially during lung infections with viruses (e.g., influenza virus, Sendai virus), much of the histopathology, protein, and nucleic acid damage directly resulted from the expression of iNOS as illustrated by the strong formation of 3-nitrotyrosine and 8-nitroguanosine in wild-type mice and the reduced mortality and pathology in iNOS$^{-/-}$ mice (Akaike et al., 2003; Karupiah et al., 1998a). In chlamydial infections of the lung, only partial but not complete inhibition of iNOS activity abolished pulmonary disease in Th1-prone C57BL/6 mice, suggesting that high doses of NO cause tissue damage, whereas low doses are still required for the control of the pathogen (Huang et al., 2002).

There are also examples for the reverse situation, where iNOS protected against immunopathology by downregulating the immune response. In staphylococcal enterotoxin B-induced shock or in *M. avium*-induced pulmonary granulomatosis, iNOS activity helped to limit the inflammatory processes (Ehlers et al., 2001; Florquin et al., 1994).

TABLE 2 The effect of iNOS deficiency on the control of infectious pathogens and the course of infections[a]

Role of iNOS	Category of pathogens	Infectious disease model[b]	Reference(s)
Dispensable for pathogen control	Viruses	Lymphocytic choriomeningitis virus (i.v., liver and spleen; i.cr, CNS)	Bartholdy et al. (1999)
		Mouse hepatitis virus (i.cr.; brain)	Chen and Lane (2002), Wu et al. (2000)
		Sendai virus (by inhalation; lung)	Akaike et al. (2000, 2003)
		Vaccinia virus (i.p.; ovaries)	van den Broek et al. (2000)
	Bacteria	Anaplasma phagocytophilum (HGE agent) (i.p.; spleen, liver, blood)	von Loewenich et al. (2004)
		Borrelia burgdorferi (s.c.; arthritis)	Brown and Reiner (1999)
		Chlamydia trachomatis (MoPn strain)(i.vg.; local cervicovaginal infection)	Perry et al. (1998), Ramsey et al. (1998)
		Escherichia coli (i.ves.; urinary tract infection [kidney, bladder])	Poljakovic and Persson (2003)
		Helicobacter pylori (gastritis)	Blanchard et al. (2003)
		Mycobacterium leprae (s.c.; footpad)	Adams et al. (2000)
		Shigella flexneri (i.n.)	Way and Goldberg (1998)
		Streptococcus pneumoniae (i.ci.)	Winkler et al. (2001)
	Protozoa	Eimeria vermiformis (i.g.; fecal oocyst excretion)	Smith and Hayday (2000)
		Plasmodium berghei (i.v.; blood-stage or cerebral malaria)	Favre et al. (1999), Yoneto et al. (1999)
		Plasmodium chabaudi (i.p.; blood-stage malaria)	van der Heyde et al. (2000)
		Trypanosoma brucei rhodesiense (LouTat1) (i.p.; parasitemia)	Hertz and Mansfield (1999)
	Helminths	Brugia malayi (i.p.)	Ganley et al. (2001)
		Schistosoma mansoni (p.c.; parasitemia)	James et al. (1998)
Essential for pathogen control	Viruses	Coxsackievirus B3 (i.p.; myocarditis)	Zaragoza et al. (1998)
		Coxsackievirus B3 (i.p.; pancreatitis)	Zaragoza et al. (1999)
		Coxsackievirus B4 (i.p.; pancreatitis, hepatitis)	Flodstrom et al. (2001)
		Murine cytomegalovirus (intermediate dose) (i.p.; lung, salivary gland, spleen, and liver)	Noda et al. (2001)
		Ectromelia virus (i.v.; mouse pox; lung, liver, spleen)	Karupiah et al. (1998b)
	Bacteria	Chlamydia trachomatis (i.vg.; chronic urogenital disease)	Ramsey et al. (2001b)
		Mycobacterium avium (aerosol; caseating pulmonary necrosis)[c]	Ehlers et al. (2001, 1999)
		Mycobacterium bovis (i.v.; lung, liver, spleen)	Garcia et al. (2000)
		Mycobacterium tuberculosis (Erdman, H37Rv, clinical isolates) (i.v.; lung, liver, spleen)	Adams et al. (1997), MacMicking et al. (1997b), Scanga et al. (2001)
		Mycobacterium tuberculosis (Erdman, H37Rv, clinical isolates (by inhalation; lung, liver, spleen)	Cooper et al. (2000a), Jung et al. (2002), Scanga et al. (2001)
		Rhodococcus equi (i.v.; lung, liver, spleen)	Darrah et al. (2000)

(continued)

TABLE 2 The effect of iNOS deficiency on the control of infectious pathogens and the course of infections[a] *(continued)*

Role of iNOS	Category of pathogens	Infectious disease model[b]	Reference(s)
Essential for pathogen control *(continued)*	Protozoa	*Salmonella enterica* serovar Typhimurium (i.v.; spleen, liver)	Alam et al. (2002), Mastroeni et al. (2000), Shiloh et al. (1999)
		Leishmania donovani (i.v.; liver)	Murray and Nathan (1999)
		Leishmania major (s.c.; skin and lymph node)	Diefenbach et al. (1998)
		Toxoplasma gondii (i.p. or p.o.; CNS)	Scharton-Kersten et al. (1997)
		Trypanosoma cruzi (Tulahuen strain; Y strain) (i.p.; blood stage, spleen, liver, heart)	Hölscher et al. (1998), Martins et al. (2001)
Contributory to pathogen control	Viruses	Hepatitis B virus (transgenic expression; liver)	Guidotti et al. (2000)
		Lymphocytic choriomeningitis virus (i.v.; liver)	Guidotti et al. (2000)
		Murine cytomegalovirus (high dose; i.v.; lung, liver, spleen)	Noda et al. (2001)
	Bacteria	*Anaplasma phagocytophilum* (HGE agent) (i.p.; spleen)	Banerjee et al. (2000)
		Brucella abortus (i.p.; lung, liver, spleen)	Ko et al. (2002)
		Chlamydia pneumoniae (i.n.; pneumonitis)	Rottenberg et al. (1999)
		Chlamydia trachomatis (MoPn strain) (i.vg.; spread to lung and spleen)	Igietseme et al. (1998)
		Listeria monocytogenes (i.v. or i.p.; liver, spleen)	MacMicking et al. (1995), Shiloh et al. (1999)
		Listeria monocytogenes (i.n.; nose, trigeminal ganglion, brain)	Jin et al. (2001)
		Mycoplasma pulmonis (i.n.; pneumonia)	Hickman-Davis et al. (1999)
		Porphyromonas gingivalis (s.c.; chamber model)	Gyurko et al. (2003)
	Protozoa	*Cryptosporidium parvum* (i.g.; fecal oocyst excretion)	Leitch and He (1999)
		Entamoeba histolytica (i.h.; liver abscesses)	Seydel et al. (2000)
Detrimental to the host	Viruses	Influenza virus (i.n. or by inhalation; pneumonitis)	Akaike et al. (2003), Karupiah et al. (1998a)
		Mouse hepatitis virus (i.c.; brain)	Chen et al. (2002)
		Sendai virus (by inhalation; lungs)	Akaike et al. (2003)
	Bacteria	*Mycobacterium avium* (i.v.; lung, liver, spleen)	Gomes et al. (1999)
		Streptococcus pneumoniae (i.ci.)	Winkler et al. (2001)
	Protozoa	*Toxoplasma gondii* (p.o.; small intestine and liver)	Khan et al. (1997)
		Trypanosoma cruzi (Brazil strain) (i.p.; heart)	Huang et al. (1999)

[a]iNOS is regarded as essential if any of the following applies: iNOS[−/−] mice die, control mice survive; nonhealing disease in iNOS[−/−], healing of the disease in iNOS[+/+] mice; uncontrolled pathogen replication in iNOS[−/−], pathogen control in iNOS[+/+] mice. iNOS is regarded as contributory if iNOS[−/−] die earlier than control mice and/or if the pathogen burden in iNOS[−/−] mice is higher than in control mice. iNOS[−/−] mice have more severe organ lesions, die earlier from immunopathology, or have a higher pathogen burden in the tissue than iNOS[−/−] mice. Listed are only those studies that were performed with iNOS[−/−] mouse strains that were proven to have a complete lack of iNOS activity (Laubach et al., 1995; MacMicking et al., 1995).

[b]CNS, central nervous system; HGE, human granulocytic ehrlichiosis (anaplasmosis); i.ci., intracisternal; i.cr., intracranial; i.g., intragastric; i.h., intrahepatic; i.n., intranasal; i.p., intraperitoneal; i.t., intratracheal; i.v., intravenous; i.ves., intravesical; i.vg., intravaginal; p.c., percutaneous; p.o., per os; s.c., subcutaneous.

[c]In the aerosol *M. avium* model, iNOS deficiency caused severe immunopathology (advanced pulmonary insufficiency) without increased bacterial load in the lung.

Stage and Organ Specificity of iNOS.
Depending on the infectious pathogen and the route of infection, the antimicrobial and host-protective functions of iNOS/NO can be restricted to certain organs and/or stages of the infection. Examples are infections of the liver with *L. donovani*, of the liver and spleen with *S. enterica* serovar Typhimurium, and aerosol-induced infections of the lungs with *M. tuberculosis*, in each of which iNOS is critical during the late but not during the early phase of infection (Cooper et al., 2000a; Jung et al., 2002; Mastroeni et al., 2000; Murray and Nathan, 1999); intravaginal infections with *C. trachomatis*, which in the absence of iNOS spread to visceral organs (lung, spleen) despite clinical resolution of the vaginal infection; oral infections with *Toxoplasma gondii*, where iNOS causes significant immunopathological lesions and enhances the severity of the disease in the intestine (Khan et al., 1997), but contributes to the control of the pathogen in the central nervous system (Scharton-Kersten et al., 1997); infections with *L. major*, in which iNOS is essential for the killing of the parasite in the skin and draining lymph node, but not in the spleen (Blos et al., 2003); and infections with *Trypanosoma cruzi* (Tulahuen strain), in which iNOS is required for the control of the parasites during the acute but not during the chronic (latent) phase of infection (Saeftel et al., 2001). Interestingly, in some of these cases Phox appears to confer the complementary part of protection. In *L. major*-infected mice, Phox was critical for the defense against *L. major* in the spleen (Blos et al., 2003), and in mice infected with *L. donovani*, *S. enterica* serovar Typhimurium, or *M. tuberculosis*, Phox-dependent pathogen control was seen during the early but not during the late phase of the acute infection (Cooper et al., 2000b; Mastroeni et al., 2000; Murray and Nathan, 1999) (see also below).

Disease Susceptibility of Phox- or MPO-Deficient Mice. Two different transgenic mouse strains have been established for the in vivo analysis of Phox function. Mice lacking the cytosolic p47^{phox} component of Phox spontaneously developed severe skin, ear, and lung infections (caused by commensal bacteria such as coagulase-negative staphylococci) similar to patients with CGD (Jackson et al., 1995). This was not the case in mice deficient for the gp91^{phox} membrane component of Phox (Pollock et al., 1995), which suggests an association of p47^{phox} with other members of the NADPH oxidase (Nox) family in addition to gp91^{phox}. p47$^{phox-/-}$ and/or gp91$^{phox-/-}$ mice have been used for the study of infections with specific (intracellular) pathogens, which include bacteria, protozoa, and fungi (Table 3). In the *Listeria monocytogenes* infection model, lethality was observed in intravenously (i.v.) infected p47$^{phox-/-}$ mice (Endres et al., 1997), but not in intraperitoneally infected gp91$^{phox-/-}$ mice (Dinauer et al., 1997; Shiloh et al., 1999). This points to a possible influence of undiagnosed opportunistic infections in p47$^{phox-/-}$ mice and/or to the route of infection as a factor that determines whether Phox activity is required as a defense mechanism. Evidence for the latter also comes from the *M. tuberculosis* mouse models. In gp91$^{phox-/-}$ (or p47$^{phox-/-}$) mice the course of an airborne infection with virulent *M. tuberculosis* was essentially the same as in wild-type mice. In contrast, in the i.v. infection model an increased bacterial load was observed in the lungs and the spleen of gp91$^{phox-/-}$ mice, but all mice were still alive after 180 days. iNOS deficiency, on the other hand, led to progressive bacterial growth in all organs (lung, spleen, and liver) and in most cases to the death of the mice, independent of the route of infection (Adams et al., 1997; Cooper et al., 2000a; Jung et al., 2002; MacMicking et al., 1997b; Scanga et al., 2001). gp91$^{phox-/-}$ mice were highly susceptible to i.v. infections with *S. enterica* serovar Typhimurium (Mastroeni et al., 2000; Shiloh et al., 1999). All gp91$^{phox-/-}$ mice died within 5 days, whereas iNOS-deficient mice successfully controlled the bacteria for 7 to 12 days and survived for up to 25 days (Mastroeni et al., 2000).

Short-term intranasal or intratracheal infection of MPO-deficient mice with a variety of fungi or bacteria revealed (i) a severely impaired killing of *C. albicans, Candida tropicalis, Trichosporon ashaii*, and *Pseudomonas aeruginosa*; (ii) a slightly delayed clearance of *Aspergillus fumigatus* and *Klebsiella pneumoniae*; and (iii) an unaltered capacity to control *Candida glabrata, Cryptococcus neoformans, Staphylococcus aureus*, and *Streptococcus pneumoniae* (Aratani et al., 2000).

Thus, the nature of the pathogen and its route of entry are decisive factors that determine the primary antimicrobial defense mechanism (iNOS versus Phox versus MPO) which will initially operate in the host organism. The molecular and cellular basis for the observed pathogen specificity, organ specificity, and stage-dependent activation of the effector pathways is currently unknown.

Phox and Immunopathology. Even in the absence of effects on the pathogen load, Phox was found to increase or inhibit the inflammatory response and tissue damage in several infectious disease models. Phox-derived ROIs mediated the microvascular injury in the lungs of mice with an *E. coli* sepsis and accounted at least partially for the urogenital disease (hydrosalpinx formation) of mice chronically infected with *Chlamydia trachomatis* (Gao et al., 2002; Ramsey et al., 2001b). In contrast, Phox activity was associated with reduced inflammation and tissue protection in *M. tuberculosis*- or *H. pylori*-infected mice (Blanchard et al., 2003; Cooper et al., 2000b). Thus, similar to iNOS-derived, RNI Phox-derived ROIs are capable of exerting pro- or anti-inflammatory effects.

Interaction between Phox and iNOS. Mice deficient for both iNOS and Phox revealed that the two pathways can act synergistically (Shiloh et al., 1999). However, there is also evidence that ROIs can impede the production and/or activity of RNIs (e.g., by modulation of iNOS expression or by scavenging of ·NO) (Ramsey et al., 2001b). The killing of certain microorganisms (e.g., *E. coli*, *Senterica* serovar Typhimurium, *Brucella abortus*) was unimpaired or only partially affected in

TABLE 3 The effect of Phox gene deficiency on the course of infections in mice

Mouse model	Infectious agent	Route of infection[a]; form of disease	Role of Phox for pathogen control[b]	Reference(s)
gp47[phox]−/−	Bacteria			
	Burkholderia cepacia	i.p.; systemic infection (blood, liver, peritoneum)	Essential	Segal et al. (2003)
	Chlamydia trachomatis	i.vg.; chronic urogenital disease	Dispensable	Ramsey et al. (2001b)
	Chromobacterium violaceum	i.p.; systemic infection (blood, liver, peritoneum)	Essential	Segal et al. (2003)
	Commensal staphylococci (and fungi)	Spontaneus development of lethal deep infections; CGD mouse model	Essential	Jackson et al. (1995)
	Escherichia coli	i.p.; systemic infection (lung, blood)	Contributory	Gao et al. (2002)
		i.v.; systemic infection (liver)	Dispensable	Segal et al. (2000)
	Listeria monocytogenes	i.v.; listeriosis (liver, spleen)	Contributory	Endres et al. (1997)
	Mycobacterium avium	i.p. and i.v.; mycobacteriosis of spleen and lung	Dispensable	Segal et al. (1999)
	Mycobacterium tuberculosis	Aerosol; pulmonary tuberculosis	Contributory (transient)	Cooper et al. (2000b)

gp91[phox−/−]

	Route; disease model	Role	References
Bacteria			
Anaplasma phagocytophilum	i.p.; systemic infection (spleen, liver, blood)	Dispensable	Banerjee et al. (2000), von Loewenich et al. (2004)
Brucella abortus	i.p.; systemic infection (spleen, liver)	Contributory (transient)	Ko et al. (2002)
Escherichia coli	i.p.; systemic infection	Contributory	Gao et al. (2002)
Helicobacter pylori	p.o.; gastritis	Inhibitory	Blanchard et al. (2003)
Listeria monocytogenes	i.p.; listeriosis (liver, spleen)	Contributory (transient)	Dinauer et al. (1997), Shiloh et al. (1999)
Mycobacterium tuberculosis	i.v.; systemic (spleen, liver, lungs)	Contributory	Adams et al. (1997)
Mycobacterium tuberculosis	Aerosol; systemic (spleen, liver, lungs)	Dispensable	Jung et al. (2002)
Rhodococcus equi	i.v.; systemic (liver, spleen, lung)	Essential	Darrah et al. (2000)
Salmonella enterica serovar Typhimurium	i.p.; systemic infection	Essential	De Groote et al. (1997), Mastroeni et al. (2000), Shiloh et al. (1999)
Staphylococcus aureus	CGD mouse model	Essential	Pollock et al. (1995)
Protozoa			
Leishmania donovani	i.v.; visceral leishmaniasis	Contributory (transient)	Murray and Nathan (1999)
Leishmania major	s.c.; cutaneous leishmaniasis	Contributory, essential[c]	Blos et al. (2003)
Fungi			
Aspergillus fumigatus	i.t.; pulmonary aspergillosis	Essential	Morgenstern et al. (1997)
Aspergillus nidulans	i.n.; pulmonary aspergillosis	Essential	Chang et al. (1998b)
Candida glabrata	i.v.; systemic infection (spleen, liver, kidney)	Essential	Ju et al. (2002)

[a] i.n., intranasal; i.p., intraperitoneal; i.t., intratracheal; i.v., intravenous; i.vg., intravaginal; p.o., per os; s.c., subcutaneous.
[b] Phox is regarded as essential if any of the following applies: Phox−/− mice die, control mice survive; nonhealing disease in Phox−/−, healing of the disease in Phox+/+ mice; uncontrolled pathogen replication in Phox−/−, pathogen control in Phox+/+ mice.
[c] Skin lesions initially healed, but spontaneously relapsed; high parasite loads in the tissue including spleen.

the simultaneous absence of Phox and iNOS. This clearly demonstrates that, in addition to iNOS and Phox, other bactericidal effector mechanisms must exist (Ko et al., 2002; Shiloh et al., 1999).

Results from the Human Model

CGD. Transgenic mouse models have been extremely helpful to elucidate the relative contributions of ROIs and RNIs for the control of infectious pathogens. However, only the discovery of genetic defects in patients with certain clinical phenotypes provided direct evidence for the relevance of the different antimicrobial effector mechanisms in humans. This "human model" (Casanova and Abel, 2002) clearly showed that Phox is critical for the control of certain bacteria and fungi in vitro and in vivo. CGD is due to an X-linked mutation of the gp91[phox] gene (approximately 60% of cases) or to autosomal recessively inherited mutations of the p47[phox] (approximately 30%), p67[phox] (approximately 5%), or p22[phox] (approximately 5%) gene and the absence (or, rarely, the inactivity) of the respective proteins (Lekstrom-Himes and Gallin, 2003). Patients with CGD suffer from recurrent infections of the soft tissues, mucous membranes, lungs, liver, brain, and bones which are characterized by granulomatous infiltrations and abscesses and are typically caused by catalase-positive microorganisms such as *Staphylococcus* spp., *Burkholderia cepacia*, *Serratia marcescens*, *Nocardia* spp., and *Aspergillus* spp. Infections with catalase-negative organisms are uncommon (Lekstrom-Himes and Gallin, 2003; Smith and Curnette, 1991). The previous theory that catalase-negative organisms are less virulent in CGD patients due to the endogenous production of H_2O_2 (which is then utilized by the MPO pathway for the generation of hypochlorous acid [HOCl]) (Geiszt et al., 2001) was recently questioned by the results of studies with p47[phox] knockout mice. These were found to be equally susceptible to infections with catalase-positive and catalase-negative strains of *S. aureus* or *Aspergillus nidulans* (Chang et al., 1998b; Messina et al., 2002). Furthermore, no evidence was obtained that the small amounts of H_2O_2 produced by catalase-negative bacteria (approximately 1,000-fold less compared with neutrophils) are sufficient to cause MPO-mediated halogenation in the absence of Phox activity (Messina et al., 2002). Thus, the high prevalence of infections with catalase-positive bacteria in CGD patients remains currently without conclusive molecular explanation.

MPO Deficiency. MPO deficiency is regarded as the most common inherited disorder of neutrophils (incidence, 1:2,000 to 1:4,000). Although MPO-deficient neutrophils exhibit a clear defect in the killing of various microorganisms, patients with a partial or complete MPO deficiency usually do not suffer from an increased frequency of infections. Cases of disseminated candidiasis were observed in MPO-deficient patients who at the same time suffered from diabetes mellitus (Lanza, 1998; Nauseef, 1998). The unexpected benign clinical phenotype of MPO deficiency does not question the importance of the MPO-H_2O_2-halide pathway under normal conditions. It rather reflects the fact that only neutrophils and circulating monocytes, but not eosinophils, mast cells, and tissue macrophages, are affected. Furthermore, MPO-deficient neutrophils and monocytes show an enhanced phagocytosis, degranulation, and generation of H_2O_2 (presumably because H_2O_2 does not enter the MPO pathway) (Klebanoff, 1999; Locksley et al., 1983; Nauseef et al., 1983). Thus, compensatory mechanisms exist in MPO-deficient patients, whereas in CGD patients not only the Phox but also the MPO pathway is defective.

iNOS Activity and Gene Polymorphism in Humans. Much of the data on iNOS in macrophages discussed above were derived from studies with rodents, notably mice. Consequently, the past 12 years have seen a debate about whether these results also pertain to humans (Albina, 1995; Chan et al., 2001; Fang and Vazquez-Torres, 2002; MacMicking et al., 1997a; Murray and Teitelbaum, 1992; Schneemann et al., 2002, 1993; Weinberg, 1998). There is no doubt that there are species-specific differences in the iNOS promoter, the synthesis and availability of iNOS cofactors, and the stimulation requirements for the induction of iNOS in monocytes, macrophages, and other cell types. However, based on a number of different experimental approaches it is now clear that not only human hepatocytes, chondrocytes, keratinocytes, and epithelial cells but also human monocytes and macrophages can be activated for the expression of iNOS and that iNOS plays a role in the control of infectious pathogens in humans (Bogdan, 2000; Kröncke et al., 1998). First, iNOS was most potently induced in human blood monocytes and macrophages by stimuli other than IFN-γ plus LPS, e.g., by IL-4 plus cross-linking of Fcε receptors (Vouldoukis et al., 1997, 1995), by IFN-α (Sharara et al., 1997), by chemokines (Villalta et al., 1998), or by surfactant protein A (Hickman-Davis et al., 2002). Second, iNOS-positive macrophages were detected in patients with various infectious disease states, e.g., in the bronchoalveolar lavage and lung tissue of patients with tuberculosis (Chan et al., 2001; Choi et al., 2003; Nicholson et al., 1996), in the peritoneal fluid of a patient with gas gangrene and septic shock (Annane et al., 2000), in the peripheral blood monocytes of patients with hepatitis C (Sharara et al., 1997) or malaria (Anstey et al., 1996), or in the oral mucosa and lymph nodes of patients with paracoccidioidomycosis (Neworal et al., 2003). Third, human macrophages killed intracellular pathogens such as *Klebsiella pneumoniae* (Hickman-Davis et al., 2002), *Mycobacterium avium* (Denis, 1991), *L. major* (Vouldoukis et al., 1995), *Leishmania infantum* (Vouldoukis et al., 1997), and *Leishmania chagasi* (Grantt et al., 2001) in an iNOS-dependent fashion. Fourth, the severity of various diseases and/or the

pathogen load was correlated inversely with the degree of iNOS expression in the tissues of patients with cutaneous leishmaniasis (Qadoumi et al., 2002), leprosy (Khanolkar-Young et al., 1998), or cerebral malaria (Anstey et al., 1996). Fifth, treatment of human immunodeficiency virus-negative patients suffering from pulmonary tuberculosis with arginine led to significant clinical and microbiological improvement of the disease (Schön et al., 2003). Finally, there is now evidence that three different polymorphisms in the promoter of the human iNOS gene [−954 G→C; $(CCTTT)_n$ microsatellite repeats ($n = 11$); −1173 C→T] are more frequent among patients with a less severe course of *Plasmodium falciparum* malaria (Burgner et al., 1998; Hobbs et al., 2002; Kun et al., 2001, 1998).

The biological effect of these polymorphisms is far from being clear. An association with an increased production of NO in vivo was demonstrated only for two of these polymorphisms (Hobbs et al., 2002; Kun et al., 2001). To date, the mechanism of the beneficial effect of NO remains unknown. Furthermore, the protective effect of the polymorphisms is restricted to certain areas and populations. For example, the -954G→C and the long ($n = 11$) $(CCTTT)_n$ microsatellite repeats protect patients against severe malaria in Gabon and The Gambia, respectively, but not in Tanzania (Levesque et al., 1999). In Thailand, long ($n ≥ 15$) $(CCTTT)_n$ microsatellite repeats do not confer protection, but are associated with more severe courses of *P. falciparum* malaria (Ohashi et al., 2002). Importantly, the course of another infection with a NO-sensitive pathogen (chronic *Trypanosoma cruzi* infection in a Peruvian population) was not affected by the $(CCTTT)_n$ microsatellite repeat of any given length (Calzada et al., 2002). In contrast to Phox and MPO, an iNOS gene deficiency has not yet been detected in humans. Therefore, to date it is impossible to judge the importance of iNOS relative to other antimicrobial effector mechanisms for the control of infections in humans.

MECHANISMS OF EVASION

Viruses, bacteria, parasites, and fungi have developed multiple strategies to evade killing by oxygen-dependent effector mechanisms. These include the suppression of the synthesis of ROIs and RNIs, the avoidance of colocalization with Phox or iNOS, the scavenging of ROIs and RNIs, the consumption or degradation of ROIs and RNIs by detoxifying enzymes, and the induction of repair genes.

Suppression of ROI and RNI Synthesis

Polypeptides encoded by the adenoviral E1A gene inhibited the transcription of the iNOS gene in macrophages by blocking the nuclear translocation of NF-κB and the transactivation of the iNOS promoter (Cao et al., 2003). Exposure of macrophages to bacterial LPS prior to stimulation with cytokines or triggering with PMA blocked the activation of Phox and suppressed the mRNA and protein expression of iNOS (Bogdan et al., 1993). Parasites such as *Leishmania* spp., *Trypanosoma cruzi*, and *Toxoplasma gondii* can enter neutrophils, macrophages, and other host cells without eliciting an oxidative burst. This "silent entry" can be further facilitated if the parasites are coated with antibodies and cross-link inhibitory Fcγ receptors or induce phagocyte-deactivating cytokines (Mosser, 2003). Furthermore, parasite products (e.g., lipophosphoglycan and glycoinositolphospholipids of *Leishmania* spp.) were reported to suppress the induction of iNOS by IFN-γ and the production of ROIs (O_2^- and H_2O_2), although the latter finding was called into question by a recent report that studied *L. major* parasites deficient for lipophosphoglycan (Bogdan and Röllinghoff, 1998; Mauël, 1996; Späth et al., 2003a). *C. albicans* strongly decreased the protein expression and activity of iNOS in macrophages without affecting the levels of iNOS mRNA (Schröppel et al., 2001).

In addition to these transcriptional and posttranscriptional modes of interference with the production of RNIs there is also evidence that microbial pathogens affect the availability of arginine. In a peritoneal *Trypanosoma brucei brucei* infection model, arginase expression was upregulated in the inflammatory macrophages, but parasite killing could be restored after application of arginine (Gobert et al., 2000). Likewise, wild-type *H. pylori*, but not an arginase-deficient mutant, inhibited the production of NO by activated macrophages (Gobert et al., 2001). However, the physiological relevance of the later finding is not yet clear, because *H. pylori* and its urease were also shown to induce iNOS mRNA, protein, and activity (Gobert et al., 2002).

Avoidance of Colocalization with Phox or iNOS

Some pathogens manage to survive in host cells despite an unaltered overall expression of iNOS protein and activity in the tissue. In clinically healed mice infected with *L. major* the parasites persist in the lymph node draining the former skin lesion. The majority of these parasites reside and survive within iNOS-negative fibroblasts. However, the rapid reactivation of the disease illustrates that they are still under control of iNOS, which is expressed abundantly in neighboring macrophages and dendritic cells (Bogdan et al., 2000a; Stenger et al., 1996). A related observation was recently made with the murine enteric pathogen *Citrobacter rodentium*, which preferentially colocalized with iNOS-negative epithelial cells in the colon (Vallance et al., 2002).

The products of the pathogenicity island 2 (SPI2) of virulent strains of *S. enterica* serovar Typhimurium inhibited the translocation of Phox- or iNOS-containing vesicles toward the phagosomes. In contrast, phagosomes carrying SPI2 mutants colocalized extensively with Phox and iNOS. Furthermore, SPI2 mutants, which were rapidly eliminated by wild-type macrophages and wild-type mice, regained virulence in gp91[phox−/−] and iNOS[−/−] mice (Chakravortty et al., 2002; Vazquez-Torres et al., 2000). In the case of Phox, the trafficking of the oxidase-positive vesicles to the phagosomes carrying the salmonellae was shown to be dependent on TNF-receptor signaling (Vazquez-Torres et al., 2001).

Constitutive and Inducible Antioxidants

The cell wall of bacteria, parasites, and fungi is equipped with a number of structures that are capable of scavenging ROIs and RNIs. The phenolic glycolipid of *Mycobacterium leprae*, the lipo- and proteophosphoglycans of *L. donovani*, and the fungal melanin (e.g., of pigmented *Cryptococcus neoformans*) have all been shown to confer protection against ROIs and/or RNIs (Chan et al., 1989; Jacobson and Tinnell, 1993; Späth et al., 2003a, 2003b; Wang and Casadevall, 1994).

Several intracellular pathogens (including *E. coli*, *S. enterica* serovar Typhimurium, *M. tuberculosis*, *H. pylori*, *Neisseria meningitidis*, *Nocardia asteroides*, *Leishmania* spp., and *Cryptococcus neoformans*) express or secrete SODs and/or catalase (peroxidase) which detoxify O_2^- and H_2O_2 associated with the virulence of these pathogens (Cox et al., 2003; DeGroote et al., 1997; Ghosh et al., 2003; Manca et al., 1999; Mauël, 1996; Piddington et al., 2001). Through dismutation of O_2^- the periplasmic Cu/Zn-SOD of *S. enterica* serovar Typhimurium impeded the formation of peroxynitrite (ONOO$^-$) and thereby protected the bacteria against O_2^- and NO (DeGroote et al., 1997).

Contact with host cell products leads to a transcriptional response in both extracellular and intracellular pathogens, which helps them to survive despite a hostile environment. In *E. coli*, exposure to O_2^- activates a distinct set of antioxidant genes that are under the control of the SoxRS regulon (e.g., manganese-containing SOD [*sodA*], oxidative DNA repair enzyme endonuclease IV [*nfo*], and glucose-6-phosphate dehydrogenase [*zwf*]). Similarly, H_2O_2 stimulates the thiol-containing transcriptional activator OxyR, which controls the expression of catalase/hydroperoxidase (*katG*), glutathione reductase (*gorA*), and peroxiredoxins in *E. coli* and *S. enterica* serovar Typhimurium (Chen et al., 1998; Hausladen et al., 1996). Peroxiredoxins (e.g., of *E. coli*, serovar

Typhimurium, *M. tuberculosis*, *H. pylori*, and *Leishmania chagasi*) not only enzymatically reduce hydrogen peroxide, alkyl hydroperoxides, and hydroxyl radicals, but also are efficient peroxynitrite reductases that rapidly and quantitatively detoxify ONOO$^-$ to nitrite (NO_2^-) (Barr and Gedamu, 2003; Bryk et al., 2000). Interestingly, both the *soxRS* and the OxyR regulon are also responsive to NO or S-nitrosothiols, suggesting a common defense strategy against nitrosative and oxidative stress (Chen et al., 1998; Hausladen et al., 1998, 1996). In *M. tuberculosis* residing in the phagosome of IFN-γ-activated macrophages, a limited set of antioxidant genes (e.g., alkyl hydroperoxidase reductase subunit C [*ahpC*] of the peroxynitrite reductase) was induced in an iNOS/NO-dependent manner, which was largely identical to the set of genes upregulated after exposure to exogenous ·NO or H_2O_2 (Schnappinger et al., 2003).

Recently, several other genes and proteins were identified that confer protection against ROIs and/or RNIs in *E. coli*, *S. enterica* serovar Typhimurium, *M. tuberculosis*, and other bacteria as shown by gene overexpression or by complementation of mutants. These include (i) flavohemoglobin (*hmp*), which exhibits a nitric oxide dioxygenase activity (i.e., detoxifies ·NO to NO_3^-) and is induced by ·NO via inactivation of an iron-dependent repressor (Crawford and Goldberg, 1998; Gardner et al., 1998; Hausladen et al., 1998); (ii) the truncated hemoglobin HbN of *Mycobacterium bovis* and *M. tuberculosis*, which metabolizes NO to nitrate (NO_3^-) (Pathania et al., 2002; Quellet et al., 2002); (iii) the bifunctional enzyme aspartokinase II-homoserine dehydrogenase II (*metL*), which is critical for the synthesis of homocysteine, an antagonist of S-nitrosothiols in serovar Typhimurium (DeGroote et al., 1996); (iv) the peptide methionine sulfoxide reductases (MsrA/B), which can be translocated from their regular cytoplasmic position to the outer membrane and protect against H_2O_2 and against nitrite or S-nitrosoglutathione, which under acidic and aerobic conditions become bactericidal due to the generation of peroxynitrite (ONOO$^-$) (Skaar et al., 2002; St. John et al., 2001); and (v) two novel genes (*noxR1* and *noxR3*) that were isolated from *M. tuberculosis*, which protect against both RNIs and ROIs by an as yet unknown mechanism and are not expressed in nonpathogenic or opportunistic mycobacteria (Ruan et al. [1999] and references therein). Thus, pathogenic bacteria are most likely equipped with a whole array of mechanisms that mediate resistance to oxidative and nitrosative effector molecules of the host.

CONCLUSIONS AND OUTLOOK

ROIs and RNIs are indispensable components of the innate and adaptive immune system for the control of infectious pathogens. Based on studies with gene-deleted mice as well as on the clinical phenotype of patients with CGD, RNIs appear to be most important for the defense against intracellular pathogens that reside in macrophages, whereas ROIs are crucial for the killing of extra- and intracellular bacteria and fungi by neutrophils. There are several interactions between ROIs and RNIs that can lead to the generation of effector molecules (e.g., peroxynitrite [ONOO$^-$], nitrogen dioxide radical [$^\cdot$NO$_2$], and hydroxyl radical [$^\cdot$OH]; hypochlorite [OCl$^-$]; nitryl chloride [NO$_2$Cl]) that are more potent antimicrobials than the primary products of the Phox and iNOS pathway, superoxide (O$_2^-$), and nitric oxide ($^\cdot$NO). In addition to their antimicrobial properties, both ROIs and RNIs also exert immunoregulatory, pro- or anti-inflammatory, as well as tissue-protective or cytotoxic effects, which in the mouse models were shown to positively or negatively influence the course of infections. The functional diversity of ROIs and RNIs makes systemic applications of ROI or RNI donors for the treatment of infections a rather hazardous adventure because the clinical consequences are hardly predictable. Current research projects aim at the development of ROI or RNI precursors that enter only certain types of host cells and are activated by the infectious pathogens themselves.

REFERENCES

Abo, A., E. Pick, A. Hall, N. Totty, C. G. Teahan, and A. W. Segal. 1991. Activation of the NADPH oxidase involves the small GTP-binding protein p21rac1. *Nature* **353**:668–670.

Abu-Soud, H. M., and S. L. Hazen. 2000. Nitric oxide is a physiological substrate for mammalian peroxidases. *J. Biol. Chem.* **275**:37524–37532.

Adams, L. B., M. C. Dinauer, D. E. Morgenstern, and J. L. Krahenbuhl. 1997. Comparison of the roles of reactive oxygen and nitrogen intermediates in the host response to *Mycobacterium tuberculosis* using transgenic mice. *Tuber. Lung Dis.* **78**:237–246.

Adams, L. B., C. K. Job, and J. L. Krahenbuhl. 2000. Role of inducible nitric oxide synthase in resistance to *Mycobacterium leprae* in mice. *Infect. Immun.* **68**:5462–5465.

Ahluwalla, J., A. Tinker, L. H. Clapp, M. R. Duchen, A. Y. Abramor, S. Pope, M. Nobles, and A. W. Segal. 2004. The large-conductance Ca^{2+}-activated K$^+$ channel is essential for innate immunity. *Nature* **427**:853–858.

Akaike, T., S. Fujii, A. Kato, J. Yoshitake, Y. Miyamoto, T. Sawa, S. Okamoto, M. Suga, M. Asakawa, Y. Nagai, and H. Maeda. 2000. Viral mutation accelerated by nitric oxide production during infection *in vivo*. *FASEB J.* **14**:1447–1454.

Akaike, T., S. Okamoto, T. Sawa, J. Yoshitake, F. Tamura, K. Ichimori, K. Miyazaki, K. Sasamoto, and H. Maeda. 2003. 8-Nitroguanosine formation in viral pneumonia and its implication for pathogenesis. *Proc. Natl. Acad. Sci. USA* **100**:685–690.

Alam, M. S., T. Akaike, S. Okamoto, T. Kubota, J. Yoshitake, T. Sawa, Y. Miyamoto, F. Tamura, and H. Maeda. 2002. Role of nitric oxide in host defense in murine salmonellosis as a function of its antibacterial and antiapoptotic activities. *Infect. Immun.* **70**:3130–3142.

Albina, J. E. 1995. On the expression of nitric oxide synthase by human macrophages. Why no NO? *J. Leukoc. Biol.* **58**:643–649.

Allen, R. C., R. L. Stjernholm, and R. H. Steele. 1972. Evidence for the generation of an electronic excitation state(s) in human polymorphonuclear leukocytes and its participation in bactericidal activity. *Biochem. Biophys. Res. Commun.* **47**:679–684.

Amezaga, M. A., F. Bazzoni, C. Sorio, F. Rossi, and M. A. Cassatella. 1992. Evidence for the involvement of distinct signal transduction pathways in the regulation of constitutive and interferon-g-dependent gene expression of NADPH oxidase components (gp91[phox], p47[phox] and p22[phox]) and high-affinity receptor for IgG (FcγRI) in human polymorphonuclear leukocytes. *Blood* **79**:735–744.

Annane, D., S. Sanquer, V. Sebille, A. Faye, D. Djuranovic, J.-C. Raphael, P. Gajdos, and E. Bellisant. 2000. Compartmentalized inducible nitric-oxide synthase activity in septic shock. *Lancet* **355**:1143–1148.

Anstey, N. M., J. B. Weinberg, M. Y. Hassanali, E. D. Mwaikambo, D. Manyenga, M. A. Misukonis, D. R. Arnelle, D. Hollis, M. I. McDonald, and D. L. Granger. 1996. Nitric oxide in Tanzanian children with malaria: inverse relationship between malaria severity and nitric oxide production/nitric oxide synthase type 2 expression. *J. Exp. Med.* **184**:557–567.

Aratani, Y., F. Kura, H. Watanabe, H. Akagawa, Y. Takano, K. Suzuki, N. Maeda, and H. Koyama. 2000. Differential host susceptibilities to pulmonary infections with bacteria and fungi in mice deficient in myeloperoxidase. *J. Infect. Dis.* **182**:1276–1279.

Babior, B. M. 1999. NADPH oxidase: an update. *Blood* **93**:1464–1476.

Babior, B., R. Kipnes, and J. Curnette. 1973. Biological defense mechanisms. The production by leukocytes of superoxide, a potential bactericidal agent. *J. Clin. Invest.* **52**:741–744.

Babior, B. M., C. Takeuchi, J. M. Ruedi, A. Gutierrez, and P. J. Wentworth. 2003. Investigating antibody-catalyzed ozone generation by human neutrophils. *Proc. Natl. Acad. Sci. USA* **100**:3031–3034.

Badorff, C., B. Fichtlscherer, A. Muelsch, A. M. Zeiher, and S. Dimmeler. 2002. Selective delivery of nitric oxide to a cellular target: a pseudosubstrate-coupled dinitrosyl-iron complex inhibits the enteroviral protease 2A. *Nitric Oxide* **6**:305–312.

Baldridge, C. W., and R. W. Gerard. 1933. The extra respiration of phagocytosis. *Am. J. Physiol.* **103**:235–236.

Banerjee, R., J. Anguita, and E. Fikrig. 2000. Granulocytic ehrlichiosis in mice deficient in phagocyte oxidase or inducible nitric oxide synthase. *Infect. Immun.* **68**:4361–4362.

Barr, S. D., and L. Gedamu. 2003. Role of peroxidoxins in *Leishmania chagasi* survival. Evidence of an enzymatic defense against nitrosative stress. *J. Biol. Chem.* **278**:10816–10823.

Bartholdy, C., A. Nansen, J. E. Christensen, O. Marker, and A. R. Thomsen. 1999. Inducible nitric oxide synthase plays a minimal role in LCMV-induced, T cell–mediated protective immunity and immunopathology. *J. Gen. Virol.* **80**:2997–3005.

Beckman, J. S., T. W. Beckman, J. Chen, P. A. Marshall, and B. A. Freeman. 1990. Apparent hydroxyl radical production by peroxynitrite: implications for endothelial injury from nitric oxide and superoxide. *Proc. Natl. Acad. Sci. USA* **87**:1620–1624.

Beckman, J. S., J. Chen, H. Ischiropoulos, and J. P. Crow. 1994. Oxidative chemistry of peroxinitrite. *Methods Enzymol.* **233**:229–240.

Bevins, C. L. 2003. Antimicrobial peptides as effector molecules of mammalian host defense. *Contrib. Microbiol.* **10**:106–148.

Blanchard, T. G., F. Yu, C. L. Hsieh, and R. W. Redline. 2003. Severe inflammation and reduced bacteria load in murine helicobacter infection caused by lack of phagocyte oxidase activity. *J. Infect. Dis.* **187**:1609–1615.

Blos, M., U. Schleicher, F. J. Rocha, U. Meissner, M. Röllinghoff, and C. Bogdan. 2003. Organ-specific and stage-dependent control of *Leishmania major* infection by inducible nitric oxide synthase and phagocyte NADPH oxidase. *Eur. J. Immunol.* **33**:1224–1234.

Bogdan, C. 1997. Of microbes, macrophages and NO. *Behring Inst. Res. Commun.* **99**:58–72.

Bogdan, C. 1998. The multiplex function of nitric oxide in (auto)immunity. *J. Exp. Med.* **187**:1361–1365.

Bogdan, C. 2000. The function of nitric oxide in the immune system, p. 443–492. *In* B. Mayer (ed.), *Handbook of Experimental Pharmacology: Nitric Oxide.* Springer, Heidelberg, Germany.

Bogdan, C. 2001a. Nitric oxide and the immune response. *Nat. Immunol.* **2**:907–916.

Bogdan, C. 2001b. Nitric oxide and the regulation of gene expression. *Trends Cell Biol.* **11**:66–75.

Bogdan, C., and C. Nathan. 1993. Modulation of macrophage function by transforming growth factor-β, interleukin 4 and interleukin 10. *Ann. N.Y. Acad. Sci.* **685**:713–739.

Bogdan, C., and M. Röllinghoff. 1998. The immune response to *Leishmania*: mechanisms of parasite control and evasion. *Int. J. Parasitol.* **28**:121–134.

Bogdan, C., Y. Vodovotz, J. Paik, Q.-W. Xie, and C. Nathan. 1993. Traces of bacterial lipopolysaccharide suppress IFN-γ-induced nitric oxide synthase gene expression in primary mouse macrophages. *J. Immunol.* **151**:301–309.

Bogdan, C., H. Thüring, M. Dlaska, M. Röllinghoff, and G. Weiss. 1997. Mechanism of suppression of macrophage nitric oxide release by IL-13. *J. Immunol.* **159**:4506–4513.

Bogdan, C., N. Donhauser, R. Döring, M. Röllinghoff, A. Diefenbach, and M. G. Rittig. 2000a. Fibroblasts as host cells in latent leishmaniosis. *J. Exp. Med.* **191**:2121–2129.

Bogdan, C., M. Röllinghoff, and A. Diefenbach. 2000b. Reactive oxygen and reactive nitrogen intermediates in innate and specific immunity. *Curr. Opin. Immunol.* **12**:64–76.

Borregard, N., and A. I. Tauber. 1984. Subcellular localization of human neutrophil NADPH oxidase: b-cytochrome and associated flavoprotein. *J. Biol. Chem.* **259**:47–52.

Botha, T., and B. Ryffel. 2002. Reactivation of latent tuberculosis by an inhibitor of inducible nitric oxide synthase in an aerosol murine model. *Immunology* **107**:350–357.

Brennan, M. L., W. Wu, X. Fu, Z. Shen, W. Song, H. Frost, C. Vadseth, L. Narine, E. Lenkiewicz,

M. T. Borchers, A. J. Lusis, J. J. Lee, N. A. Lee, H. M. Abu-Soud, H. Ischiropoulos, and S. L. Hazen. 2002. A tale of two controversies: defining both the role of peroxidases in nitrotyrosine formation in vivo using eosinophil peroxidase and myeloperoxidase-deficient mice, and the nature of peroxidase-generated reactive nitrogen species. *J. Biol. Chem.* **277**:17415–17427.

Brown, C., and S. L. Reiner. 1999. Development of Lyme arthritis in mice deficient in inducible nitric oxide synthase. *J. Infect. Dis.* **179**:1573–1576.

Brüne, B., A. von Knethen, and K. B. Sandau. 1999. Nitric oxide (NO): an effector of apoptosis. *Cell Death Differ.* **6**:969–975.

Bryk, R., P. Griffin, and C. Nathan. 2000. Peroxynitrite reductase activity of bacterial peroxiredoxins. *Nature* **407**:211–215.

Burgner, D., W. Xu, K. Rockett, M. Gravenor, I. G. Charles, A. V. Hill, and D. Kwiatkowski. 1998. Inducible nitric oxide synthase polymorphism and fatal cerebral malaria. *Lancet* **352**:1193–1194.

Caccavo, D., N. M. Pellegrino, M. Altamura, A. Rigon, L. Amati, A. Amoroso, and E. Jirillo. 2002. Antimicrobial and immunoregulatory functions of lactoferrin and its potential therapeutic application. *J. Endotoxin Res.* **8**:403–417.

Cagan, R. H., and M. L. Karnovsky. 1964. Enzymatic basis of the respiratory stimulation during phagocytosis. *Nature* **204**:255–257.

Calzada, J. E., M. A. Lopez-Nevot, Y. Beraun, and J. Martin. 2002. No evidence for association of the inducible nitric oxide synthase promotor polymorphism with Trypanosoma cruzi infection. *Tissue Antigens* **59**:316–319.

Cao, W., C. Bao, and C. J. Lowenstein. 2003. Inducible nitric oxide synthase expression inhibition by adenovirus E1A. *Proc. Natl. Acad. Sci. USA* **100**:7773–7778.

Carlsson, S., N. P. Wiklund, L. Engstrand, E. Weitzberg, and J. O. N. Lundberg. 2001. Effects of pH, nitrite, and ascorbic acid on non-enzymatic nitric oxide generation and bacterial growth in urine. *Nitric Oxide* **5**:580–586.

Casanova, J.-L., and L. Abel. 2002. Genetic dissection of immunity to mycobacteria: the human model. *Annu. Rev. Immunol.* **20**:581–620.

Cassatella, M. A., F. Bazzoni, R. M. Flynn, S. Dusi, G. Trinchieri, and F. Rossi. 1990. Molecular basis of interferon-γ and lipopolysaccharide enhancement of phagocyte respiratory burst capability. *J. Biol. Chem.* **265**:20241–20246.

Chakravortty, D., I. Hansen-Wester, and M. Hensel. 2002. Salmonella pathogenicity island 2 mediates protection of intracellular Salmonella from reactive nitrogen intermediates. *J. Exp. Med.* **195**:1155–1166.

Chan, E. D., J. Chan, and N. W. Schluger. 2001. What is the role of nitric oxide in murine and human host defense against tuberculosis? *Am. J. Respir. Cell Mol. Biol.* **25**:606–612.

Chan, J., T. Fujiwara, P. Brennan, M. McNeil, S. J. Turco, J.-C. Sibille, P. Snapper, P. Aisen, and B. R. Bloom. 1989. Microbial glycolipids: possible virulence factors that scavenge oxygen radicals. *Proc. Natl. Acad. Sci. USA* **86**:2453–2457.

Chang, C., J. C. Liao, and L. Kuo. 1998a. Arginase modulates nitric oxide production in activated macrophages. *Am. J. Physiol.* **274**:H342–H348.

Chang, Y. C., B. H. Segal, S. M. Holland, G. F. Miller, and K. J. Kwon-Chung. 1998b. Virulence of catalase-deficient Aspergillus nidulans in p47phox−/− mice. Implications for fungal pathogenicity and host defense in chronic granulomatous disease. *J. Clin. Invest.* **101**:1843–1850.

Chen, B. P., and T. E. Lane. 2002. Lack of nitric oxide synthase type 2 (NOS2) results in reduced neuronal apoptosis and mortality following mouse hepatitis virus infection of the central nervous system. *J. Neurovirol.* **8**:58–63.

Chen, L., Q.-W. Xie, and C. Nathan. 1998. Alkyl hydroperoxide reductase subunit C (AhpC) protects bacterial and human cells against reactive nitrogen intermediates. *Mol. Cell* **1**:795–805.

Chiarugi, A., E. Rovida, P. D. Sbarba, and F. Moroni. 2003. Tryptophan availability selectively limits NO synthase induction in macrophages. *J. Leukoc. Biol.* **73**:172–177.

Choi, H. S., P. R. Rai, H. W. Chu, C. Cool, and E. D. Chan. 2003. Arginine as an adjuvant to chemotherapy improves clinical outcome in active tuberculosis. *Eur. Respir. J.* **21**:483–488.

Clark, R. A. 1999. Activation of the neutrophil respiratory burst oxidase. *J. Infect. Dis.* **179**(Suppl. 2):S309–S317.

Clark, R. A., K. G. Leidal, D. W. Pearson, and W. M. Nauseef. 1987. NADPH oxidase of human neutrophils. Subcellular localization and characterization of an arachidonate-activatable superoxide-generating system. *J. Biol. Chem.* **262**:4065–4074.

Clark, S. R., M. J. Coffey, R. M. Maclean, P. W. Collins, M. J. Lewis, A. R. Cross, and V. B. O'Donnell. 2002. Characterization of nitric oxide consumption pathways by normal, chronic granulomatous disease and myeloperoxidase-deficient human neutrophils. *J. Immunol.* **169**:5889–5896.

Closs, E. I., J.-S. Scheld, M. Sharafi, and U. Förstermann. 2000. Substrate supply for nitric oxide synthase in macrophages and endothelial cells: role of cationic amino acid transporters. *Mol. Pharmacol.* **57**:68–74.

Connelly, L., A. T. Jacobs, M. Palacios-Callender, S. Moncada, and A. J. Hobbs. 2003. Macrophage endothelial nitric oxide synthase autoregulates cellular activation and proinflammatory protein expression. *J. Biol. Chem.* **278**:26480–26487.

Cooper, A. M., J. E. Pearl, J. V. Brooks, S. Ehlers, and I. M. Orme. 2000a. Expression of nitric oxide synthase 2 gene is not essential for early control of *Mycobacterium tuberculosis* in the murine lung. *Infect. Immun.* **68:**6879–6882.

Cooper, A. M., B. H. Segal, A. A. Frank, S. M. Holland, and I. M. Orme. 2000b. Transient loss of resistance to pulmonary tuberculosis in p47$^{phox-/-}$ mice. *Infect. Immun.* **68:**1231–1234.

Cox, G. M., T. S. Harrison, H. C. McDade, C. P. Taborda, G. Heinrich, A. Casadevall, and J. R. Perfect. 2003. Superoxide dismutase influences the virulence of *Cryptococcus neoformans* by affecting growth within macrophages. *Infect. Immun.* **71:**173–180.

Crawford, M. J., and D. E. Goldberg. 1998. Regulation of the *Salmonella typhimurium* flavohemoglobin gene. A new pathway for bacterial gene expression in response to nitric oxide. *J. Biol. Chem.* **273:**34028–34032.

Curnutte, J. T., D. M. Whitten, and B. M. Babior. 1974. Defective superoxide production by granulocytes from patients with granulomatous disease. *N. Engl. J. Med.* **290:**593–597.

Darrah, P. A., M. K. Hondalus, Q. Chen, H. Ischiropoulos, and D. M. Mosser. 2000. Cooperation between reactive oxygen and nitrogen intermediates in killing of *Rhodococcus equi* by activated macrophages. *Infect. Immun.* **68:**3587–3593.

Däubener, W., and C. R. MacKenzie. 1999. IFN-gamma activated indoleamine 2,3-dioxygenase activity in human cells is an antiparasitic and an antibacterial effector mechanism. *Adv. Exp. Med. Biol.* **467:**517–524.

Deen, W. M., S. R. Tannenbaum, and J. S. Beckman. 2002. Protein tyrosine nitration and peroxynitrite. *FASEB J.* **16:**1144.

DeGroote, M. A., and F. C. Fang. 1999. Antimicrobial properties of nitric oxide, p. 231–261. *In* F. C. Fang (ed.), *Nitric Oxide and Infection.* Kluwer Academic, New York, N.Y.

DeGroote, M. A., T. Testerman, Y. Xu, G. Stauffer, and F. C. Fang. 1996. Homocysteine antagonism of nitric oxide-related cytostasis in *Salmonella typhimurium. Science* **272:**414–417.

DeGroote, M. A., U. A. Ochsner, M. Shiloh, J. M. McCord, M. C. Dinauer, S. J. Libby, A. Vazquez-Torres, Y. Xu, and F. C. Fang. 1997. Periplasmic superoxide dismutase protects *Salmonella* from products of phagocyte oxidase and nitric oxide synthase. *Proc. Natl. Acad. Sci. USA* **94:**13997–14001.

DeLeo, F. R., and M. T. Quinn. 1996. Assembly of the phagocyte NADPH oxidase: molecular interaction of oxidase proteins. *J. Leukoc. Biol.* **60:**677–691.

Denis, M. 1991. Tumor necrosis factor and granulocyte macrophage-colony stimulating factor stimulate human macrophages to restrict growth of virulent *Mycobacterium avium* and to kill avirulent *M. avium:* killing effector mechanism depends on the generation of reactive nitrogen intermediates. *J. Leukoc. Biol.* **49:**380–387.

Devadas, S., L. Zaritskaya, S. G. Rhee, L. Oberley, and M. S. Williams. 2002. Discrete generation of superoxide and hydrogen peroxide by T cell receptor stimulation: selective regulation of mitogen-activated protein kinase activation and Fas ligand expression. *J. Exp. Med.* **195:**59–70.

Diefenbach, A., H. Schindler, N. Donhauser, E. Lorenz, T. Laskay, J. MacMicking, M. Röllinghoff, I. Gresser, and C. Bogdan. 1998. Type 1 interferon (IFN-α/β) and type 2 nitric oxide synthase regulate the innate immune response to a protozoan parasite. *Immunity* **8:**77–87.

Diefenbach, A., H. Schindler, M. Röllinghoff, W. Yokoyama, and C. Bogdan. 1999. Requirement for type 2 NO-synthase for IL-12 responsiveness in innate immunity. *Science* **284:**951–955.

Dinauer, M. C., M. B. Deck, and E. R. Unanue. 1997. Mice lacking reduced nicotinamide adenine dinucleotide phosphate oxidase activity show increased susceptibility to early infection with *Listeria monocytogenes. J. Immunol.* **158:**5581–5583.

Ding, A. H., C. F. Nathan, and D. J. Stuehr. 1988. Release of reactive nitrogen intermediates and reactive oxygen intermediates from mouse peritoneal macrophages. Comparison of activating cytokines and evidence for independent production. *J. Immunol.* **141:**2407–2412.

Duncan, C., H. Dougall, P. Johnston, S. Green, R. Brogan, C. Leifert, L. Smith, M. Golden, and N. Benjamin. 1995. Chemical generation of nitric oxide in the mouth from the enterosalivary circulation of dietary nitrate. *Nat. Med.* **1:**546–551.

Duncan, C., H. Li, R. Dykhuizen, R. Frazer, P. Johnston, G. MacKnight, L. Smith, K. Lamza, H. McKenzie, L. Batt, D. Kelly, M. Golden, N. Benjamin, and C. Leifert. 1997. Protection against oral and gastrointestinal diseases: importance of dietary nitrate intake, orale nitrate reduction and enterosalivary nitrate ciruclation. *Comp. Biochem. Physiol. A* **118:**939–948.

Dusi, S., M. Donini, D. Lissandrini, P. Mazzi, V. D. Bianca, and F. Rossi. 2001. Mechanisms of expression of NADPH oxidase components in human cultured monocytes: role of cytokines and transcriptional regulators involved. *Eur. J. Immunol.* **31:**929–938.

Eckmann, L., F. Laurent, T. D. Langford, M. L. Hetsko, J. R. Smith, M. F. Kagnoff, and F. D. Gillin. 2000. Nitric oxide production by human intestinal epithelial cells and competition for arginine as potential determinants of host defense against the lumen-dwelling pathogen *Giardia lamblia. J. Immunol.* **164:**1478–1487.

Ehlers, S., S. Kutsch, J. Benini, A. Cooper, C. Hahn, J. Gerdes, I. Orme, and C. Martin. 1999. NOS2-derived nitric oxide regulates the size, quantity, and quality of granuloma formation in *Mycobacterium avium*-infected mice without affecting bacterial loads. *Immunology* **98**:313–323.

Ehlers, S., J. Benini, H.-D. Held, C. Roeck, G. Alber, and S. Uhlig. 2001. αβ T cell receptor-positive cells and interferon-γ, but not inducible nitric oxide synthase, are critical for granuloma necrosis in a mouse model of Mycobacteria-induced pulmonary immunopathology. *J. Exp. Med.* **194**:1847–1859.

Eiserich, J. P., M. Hristova, C. E. Cross, A. D. Jones, B. A. Freeman, B. Halliwell, and A. van der Vliet. 1998. Formation of nitric oxide-derived inflammatory oxidants by myeloperoxidase in neutrophils. *Nature* **391**:393–397.

Eiserich, J. P., S. Baldus, M.-L. Brennan, W. Ma, C. Zhang, A. Tousson, L. Castro, A. J. Lusis, W. M. Nauseef, C. R. White, and B. A. Freeman. 2002. Myeloperoxidase, a leukocyte-derived vascular NO synthase. *Science* **296**:2391–2394.

Eklund, E. A., A. Jalava, and R. Kakar. 1998. PU.1, interferon regulatory factor 1, and interferon consensus sequence-binding protein cooperate to increase gp91(phox) expression. *J. Biol. Chem.* **273**: 13957–13965.

El-Gayar, S., H. Thüring-Nahler, J. Pfeilschifter, M. Röllinghoff, and C. Bogdan. 2003. Translational control of inducible nitric oxide synthase by IL-13 and arginine availability in inflammatory macrophages. *J. Immunol.* **171**:4561–4568.

Endres, R., A. Luz, H. Schulze, H. Neubauer, A. Fütterer, S. M. Holland, H. Wagner, and K. Pfeffer. 1997. Listeriosis in p47phox$^{-/-}$ and TRp55$^{-/-}$ mice: protection despite absence of ROI and susceptibility despite presence of RNI. *Immunity* **7**:419–432.

Espey, M. G., S. Xavier, D. D. Thomas, K. M. Miranda, and D. A. Wink. 2002. Direct real-time evaluation of nitration with green fluorescent protein in solution and within human reveals the impact of nitrogen dioxide vs. peroxynitrite mechanisms. *Proc. Natl. Acad. Sci. USA* **99**:3481–3486.

Evans, T. J., L. D. K. Buttery, A. Carpenter, D. R. Springall, J. M. Polak, and J. Cohen. 1996. Cytokine-treated human neutrophils contain inducible nitric oxide synthase that produces nitration of ingested bacteria. *Proc. Natl. Acad. Sci. USA* **93**:9553–9558.

Fang, F. C., and A. Vazquez-Torres. 2002. Nitric oxide production by human macrophages: there's NO doubt about it. *Am. J. Physiol. Lung Cell. Mol. Physiol.* **282**:L941–L943.

Fang, F. C., M. DeGroote, J. Foster, A. Baumler, U. Ochsner, T. Testerman, S. Bearson, J. Giard, Y.

Xu, G. Campbell, and T. Laessig. 1999. Virulent *Salmonella typhimurium* has two periplasmic Cu,Zn-superoxide dismutases. *Proc. Natl. Acad. Sci. USA* **96**: 7502–7507.

Favre, N., B. Ryffel, and W. Rudin. 1999. The development of murine cerebral malaria does not require nitric oxide production. *Parasitology* **118**:135–138.

Felley-Bosco, E. 1998. Role of nitric oxide in genotoxicity: implication for carcinogenesis. *Cancer Metastasis Rev.* **17**:25–37.

Figdor, C. G., Y. van Kooyk, and G. J. Adema. 2002. C-type lectin receptors on dendritic cells and Langerhans cells. *Nat. Rev. Immunol.* **2**:77–84.

Flodstrom, M., M. S. Horwitz, A. Maday, D. Balakrishna, E. Rodriguez, and N. Sarvetnick. 2001. A critical role for inducible nitric oxide synthase in host survival following coxsackievirus B4 infection. *Virology* **281**:205–215.

Florquin, S., Z. Amraoui, C. Dubois, J. Decuyper, and M. Goldman. 1994. The protective role of endogenously synthesized nitric oxide in staphylococcal enterotoxin B-induced shock in mice. *J. Exp. Med.* **180**:1153–1158.

Flynn, J. L., C. A. Scanga, K. E. Tanaka, and J. Chan. 1998. Effects of Aminoguanidine on latent murine tuberculosis. *J. Immunol.* **160**:1796–1803.

Forgac, M. 1999. The vacuolar H$^+$-ATPase of clathrin-coated vesicles is reversibly inhibited by S-nitrosoglutathione. *J. Biol. Chem.* **274**:1301–1305.

Forman, H. J., and M. Torres. 2001. Redox signaling in macrophages. *Mol. Aspects Med.* **22**:189–216.

Förstermann, U., J. P. Boissel, and H. Kleinert. 1998. Expressional control of the "constitutive" isoforms of nitric oxide synthase (NOSI and NOSIII). *FASEB J.* **12**:773–790.

Ganley, L., S. Babu, and T. V. Rajan. 2001. Course of *Brugia malayi* infection in C57BL/6J NOS2$^{+/+}$ and $^{-/-}$ mice. *Exp. Parasitol.* **98**:35–43.

Gao, J. J., M. B. Filla, M. J. Fultz, S. N. Vogel, S. W. Russell, and W. J. Murphy. 1998. Autocrine/paracrine IFN-α/β mediates the lipopolysaccharide-induced activation of transcription factor Stat1α in mouse macrophages: pivotal role of Stat1α in induction of the inducible nitric oxide synthase gene. *J. Immunol.* **161**:4803–4810.

Gao, X.-P., T. J. Standiford, A. Rahman, M. Newstead, S. M. Holland, M. C. Dinauer, Q.-H. Liu, and A. B. Malik. 2002. Role of NADPH oxidase in the mechanism of lung neutrophil sequestration and microvessel injury induced by Gram-negative sepsis: studies in p47$^{phox-/-}$ and gp91$^{phox-/-}$ mice. *J. Immunol.* **168**:3974–3982.

Garcia, I., R. Guler, D. Vesin, M. L. Olleros, P. Vassalli, Y. Chvatchko, M. Jacobs, and B. Ryffel. 2000. Lethal *Mycobacterium bovis* Bacillus Calmette Guerin infection in nitric oxide synthase 2-deficient mice: cell-mediated immunity requires nitric oxide synthase 2. *Lab. Invest.* **80:**1385–1397.

Gardner, P. R., A. M. Gardner, L. A. Martin, and A. L. Salzman. 1998. Nitric oxide dioxygenase: an enzymatic function for flavohemoglobin. *Proc. Natl. Acad. Sci. USA* **95:**10378–10383.

Gauss, K. A., P. L. Bunger, and M. T. Quinn. 2002. AP-1 is essential for p67[phox] promotor activity. *J. Leukoc. Biol.* **71:**163–172.

Geiszt, M., J. B. Kopp, P. Varnai, and T. L. Leto. 2000. Identification of Renox, an NAD(P)H oxidase in kidney. *Proc. Natl. Acad. Sci. USA* **97:**8010–8014.

Geiszt, M., A. Kapus, and E. Ligeti. 2001. Chronic granulomatous disease: more than the lack of superoxide? *J. Leukoc. Biol.* **69:**191–196.

Ghosh, S., S. Goswami, and S. Adhya. 2003. Role of superoxide dismutase in survival of Leishmania within the macrophage. *Biochem. J.* **369:**447–452.

Gobert, A. P., S. Daulouede, M. Lepoivre, J. L. Boucher, B. Bouteille, A. Buguet, R. Cespuglio, B. Veyret, and P. Vincendeau. 2000. L-arginine availability modulates local nitric oxide production and parasite killing in experimental trypanosomiasis. *Infect. Immun.* **68:**4653–4657.

Gobert, A. P., D. J. McGee, M. Akhtar, G. L. Mendz, J. C. Newton, Y. Cheng, H. L. T. Mobley, and K. T. Wilson. 2001. *Helicobacter pylori* arginase inhibits nitric oxide production by eukaryotic cells: a strategy for bacterial survival. *Proc. Natl. Acad. Sci. USA* **98:**13844–13849.

Gobert, A. P., B. D. Mersey, Y. Cheng, D. R. Blumberg, J. C. Newton, and K. T. Wilson. 2002. Urease release by *Helicobacter pylori* stimulates macrophage inducible nitric oxide synthase. *J. Immunol.* **168:**6002–6006.

Gomes, M. S., M. Florido, T. F. Pais, and R. Appelberg. 1999. Improved clearance of *Mycobacterium avium* upon disruption of the inducible nitric oxide synthase gene. *J. Immunol.* **162:**6734–6739.

Gonzalez, A., W. de Gregori, D. Velez, A. Restrepo, and L. E. Cano. 2000. Nitric oxide participation in the fungicidal mechanism of gamma interferon-activated murine macrophages against *Paracoccidioides brasiliensis* conidia. *Infect. Immun.* **68:**2546–2552.

Gordon, S. 2002. Pattern recognition receptors: doubling up for the innate immune response. *Cell* **111:**927–930.

Granger, D. L., J. B. Hibbs, J. R. Perfect, and D. T. Durack. 1988. Specific amino acid (L-arginine) requirement for the microbiostatic activity of murine macrophages. *J. Clin. Invest.* **81:**1129–1136.

Granger, D. L., J. B. Hibbs, J. R. Perfect, and D. T. Durack. 1990. Metabolic fate of L-arginine in relation to microbiostatic capability of murine macrophages. *J. Clin. Invest.* **85:**264–273.

Grantt, K. R., T. L. Goldman, M. L. McCormick, M. A. Miller, S. M. B. Jeronimo, E. T. Nascimento, B. E. Britigan, and M. E. Wilson. 2001. Oxidative responses of human and murine macrophages during phagocytosis of *Leishmania chagasi.* *J. Immunol.* **167:**893–901.

Green, L. C., K. R. De Luzuriaga, D. A. Wagner, W. Rand, N. Istfan, V. R. Young, and S. R. Tannenbaum. 1981a. Nitrate biosynthesis in man. *Proc. Natl. Acad. Sci. USA* **78:**7764–7768.

Green, L. C., S. R. Tannenbaum, and R. Goldman. 1981b. Nitrate synthesis in the germfree and conventional rat. *Science* **212:**56–68.

Green, S. P., J. A. Hamilton, D. J. Uhlinger, and W. A. Philipps. 1994. Expression of p47[phox] and p67[phox] proteins in murine bone marrow-derived macrophages: enhancement by lipopolysaccharide and tumor necrosis factor α, but not colony stimulating factor 1. *J. Leukoc. Biol.* **55:**530–535.

Groemping, Y., K. Lapouge, S. J. Smerdon, and K. Rittinger. 2003. Molecular basis of phosphorylation-induced activation of the NADPH oxidase. *Cell* **113:**343–355.

Guidotti, L. G., H. McClary, J. Moorhead Loudis, and F. V. Chisari. 2000. Nitric oxide inhibits hepatitis B virus replication in the livers of transgenic mice. *J. Exp. Med.* **191:**1247–1252.

Gyurko, R., G. Boustany, P. L. Huang, A. Kantarci, T. E. van Dyke, C. A. Genco, and F. C. I. Gibson. 2003. Mice lacking inducible nitric oxide synthase demonstrate impaired killing of *Porphyromonas gingivalis.* *Infect. Immun.* **71:**4917–4924.

Hampton, M. B., A. J. Kettle, and C. C. Winterbourn. 1998. Inside the neutrophil phagosome: oxidants, myeloperoxidase and bacterial killing. *Blood* **92:**3007–3017.

Hausladen, A., C. T. Privalle, T. Keng, J. DeAngelo, and J. S. Stamler. 1996. Nitrosative stress: activation of the transcription factor oxyR. *Cell* **86:**719–729.

Hausladen, A., A. J. Gow, and J. S. Stamler. 1998. Nitrosative stress: metabolic pathway involving the flavohemoglobin. *Proc. Natl. Acad. Sci. USA* **95:**14100–14105.

Hertz, C. J., and J. M. Mansfield. 1999. IFN-γ-dependent nitric oxide production is not linked to resistance in experimental African trypanosomiasis. *Cell. Immunol.* **192:**24–32.

Hevel, J. M., K. A. White, and M. A. Marletta. 1991. Purification of the inducible murine macrophage nitric oxide synthase. Identification as a flavoprotein. *J. Biol. Chem.* **266:**22789.

Hibbs, J. B., R. R. Taintor, and Z. Vavrin. 1987a. Macrophage cytotoxicity: role of L-arginine deiminase and imino nitrogen oxidation to nitrite. *Science* **235:**473–476.

Hibbs, J. B., Z. Vavrin, and R. R. Taintor. 1987b. L-Arginine is required for expression of the activated macrophage effector mechanism causing selective metabolic inhibition in target cells. *J. Immunol.* **138:** 550–565.

Hibbs, J. B., R. R. Taintor, Z. Vavrin, and E. M. Rachlin. 1988. Nitric oxide: a cytotoxic activated macrophage effector molecule. *Biochem. Biophys. Res. Commun.* **157:**87–94.

Hickman-Davis, J., J. Gibbs-Erwin, J. R. Lindsey, and S. Matalon. 1999. Surfactant protein A mediates mycoplasmacidal activity of alveolar macrophages by production of peroxynitrite. *Proc. Natl. Acad. Sci. USA* **96:**4953–4958.

Hickman-Davis, J. M., P. O'Reilly, I. C. Davis, J. Teti-Peterdi, G. Davis, K. R. Young, R. B. Devlin, and S. Matalon. 2002. Killing of Klebsiella pneumoniae by human alveolar macrophages. *Am. J. Physiol. Lung Cell. Mol. Physiol.* **282:**L944–L956.

Hobbs, M. R., V. Udhayakumar, M. C. Levesque, J. Booth, J. M. Roberts, A. N. Tkachuk, A. Pole, H. Coon, S. Kariuki, B. L. Nahlen, E. D. Mwaikambo, A. L. Lai, D. L. Granger, N. M. Anstey, and J. B. Weinberg. 2002. A new NOS2 promotor polymorphism associated with increased nitric oxide production and protection from severe malaria in Tanzanian and Kenyan children. *Lancet* **360:** 1468–1475.

Holmes, B., A. R. Page, and R. A. Good. 1967. Studies of the metabolic activity of leukocytes from patients with a genetic abnormality of phagocyte function. *J. Clin. Invest.* **46:**1422–1432.

Hölscher, C., G. Köhler, U. Müller, H. Mossmann, G. A. Schaub, and F. Brombacher. 1998. Defective nitric oxide effector functions lead to extreme susceptibility of *Trypanosoma cruzi*-infected mice deficient in gamma interferon receptor or inducible nitric oxide synthase. *Infect. Immun.* **66:** 1208–1215.

Howe, D., L. F. Barrows, N. M. Lindstrom, and R. A. Heinzen. 2002. Nitric oxide inhibits *Coxiella burnetii* replication and parasitophorous vacuole maturation. *Infect. Immun.* **70:**5140–5147.

Huang, H., J. Chan, M. Wittner, L. A. Jelicks, S. A. Morris, S. M. Factor, L. M. Weiss, V. L. Braunstein, C. J. Bacchi, N. Yarlett, M. Chandra, J. Shirani, and H. B. Tanowitz. 1999. Expression of cardiac cytokines and inducible nitric oxide synthase (NOS2) in Trypanosoma cruzi-infected mice. *J. Mol. Cell. Cardiol.* **31:**75–88.

Huang, J., F. J. DeGraves, S. D. Lenz, D. Gao, P. Feng, D. Li, T. Schlapp, and B. Kaltenboeck. 2002. The quantity of nitric oxide released by macrophages regulates *Chlamydia*-induced disease. *Proc. Natl. Acad. Sci. USA* **99:**3914–3919.

Igietseme, J. U., L. L. Perry, G. A. Ananaba, I. M. Uriri, O. Ojior, S. N. Kumar, and H. D. Caldwell. 1998. Chlamydial infection in inducible nitric oxide synthase knockout mice. *Infect. Immun.* **66:**1282–1286.

Iniesta, V., L. C. Gomez-Nieto, and I. Corraliza. 2001. The inhibition of arginase by Nw-hydroxy-L-arginine controls the growth of *Leishmania* inside macrophages. *J. Exp. Med.* **193:**777–783.

Inohara, N., Y. Ogura, and G. Nunez. 2002. Nods: a family of cytosolic proteins that regulate the host response to pathogens. *Curr. Opin. Microbiol.* **5:**76–80.

Ischiropoulos, H., and J. S. Beckman. 2003. Oxidative stress and nitration in neurodegeneration: cause, effect or association? *J. Clin. Invest.* **111:**163–169.

Iyer, G. Y. N., D. M. F. Islam, and J. H. Quastel. 1961. Biochemical aspects of phagocytosis. *Nature* **192:**535–541.

Jackson, S. H., J. I. Gallin, and S. M. Holland. 1995. The p47phox mouse knock-out model of chronic granulomatous disease. *J. Exp. Med.* **182:**751–758.

Jacobson, E. S., and S. B. Tinnell. 1993. Antioxidant function of fungal melanin. *J. Bacteriol.* **175:** 7102–7104.

James, S. L., and J. Glavin. 1989. Macrophage cytotoxicity against schistosomula of *Schistosoma mansoni* involves arginine-dependent production of reactive nitrogen intermediates. *J. Immunol.* **143:**4208–4212.

James, S. L., A. W. Cheever, P. Caspar, and T. A. Wynn. 1998. Inducible nitric oxide synthase-deficient mice develop enhanced type 1 cytokine-associated cellular and humoral immune responses after vaccination with attenuated *Schistosoma mansoni* cercariae but display partially reduced resistance. *Infect. Immun.* **66:**3510–3518.

Jesaitis, A. J., E. S. Buescher, D. Harrison, M. T. Quinn, C. A. Parkos, S. Livesey, and J. Linner. 1990. Ultrastructural localization of cytochrome b in the membranes of resting and phagocytosing human granulocytes. *J. Clin. Invest.* **85:**821–835.

Jin, Y., L. Dons, K. Kristensson, and M. E. Rottenberg. 2001. Neural route of cerebral *Listeria monocytogenes* murine infection: role of immune response mechanisms in controlling bacterial neuroinvasion. *Infect. Immun.* **69:**1093–1100.

Ju, J. Y., C. Polhamus, K. A. Marr, S. M. Holland, and J. E. Bennett. 2002. Efficacies of fluconazole, caspofungin and amphotericin B in *Candida glabrata*-infected p47[phox−/−] knockout mice. *Antimicrob. Agents Chemother.* **46:**1240–1245.

Jung, Y.-J., R. LaCourse, L. Ryan, and R. J. North. 2002. Virulent, but not avirulent *Mycobacterium tuberculosis* can evade the growth inhibitory action of a T helper 1-dependent, nitric oxide synthase 2-independent defense in mice. *J. Exp. Med.* **7:**991–998.

Karupiah, G., J.-H. Chen, S. Mahalingam, C. F. Nathan, and J. D. MacMicking. 1998a. Rapid interferon γ-dependent clearance of influenza A virus and protection from consolidating pneumonitis in nitric oxide 2-deficient mice. *J. Exp. Med.* **188:**1541–1546.

Karupiah, G., J. H. Chen, C. F. Nathan, S. Mahalingam, and J. D. MacMicking. 1998b. Identification of nitric oxide synthase 2 as an innate resistance locus against ectromelia virus infection. *J. Virol.* **72:**7703–7706.

Khan, I. A., J. D. Schwartzman, T. Matsuura, and L. H. Kasper. 1997. A dichotomous role for nitric oxide during acute *Toxoplasma gondii* infection in mice. *Proc. Natl. Acad. Sci. USA* **94:**13955–13960.

Khanolkar-Young, S., D. Snowdon, and D. N. J. Lockwood. 1998. Immunocytochemical localization of inducible nitric oxide synthase and transforming growth factor-β (TGF-β) in leprosy lesions. *Clin. Exp. Immunol.* **113:**438–442.

Klebanoff, S. J. 1968. Myeloperoxidase-halide-hydrogen peroxide antibacterial system. *J. Bacteriol.* **95:** 2131–2138.

Klebanoff, S. J. 1970. Myeloperoxidase: contribution to the microbicidal activity of intact leukocytes. *Science* **169:**1095–1097.

Klebanoff, S. J. 1999. Oxygen metabolites from phagocytes, p. 721–768. *In* J. I. Gallin and R. Snyderman (ed.), *Inflammation: Basic Principles and Clinical Correlates.* Lippincott Williams & Wilkins, Philadelphia, Pa.

Klein, J. A., and S. L. Ackerman. 2003. Oxidative stress, cell cycle, and neurodegeneration. *J. Clin. Invest.* **111:**785–793.

Knaus, U. G., P. G. Heyworth, T. Evans, J. T. Curnutte, and G. M. Bokoch. 1991. Regulation of phagocyte oxygen radical production by the GTP-binding protein Rac2. *Science* **254:**1512–1515.

Ko, J., A. Gendron-Fitzpatrick, and G. A. Splitter. 2002. Susceptibility of IFN regulatory factor-1 and IFN consensus sequence binding protein-deficient mice to brucellosis. *J. Immunol.* **168:**2433–2440.

Kobayashi, T., J. M. Robinson, and H. Seguchi. 1998. Identification of intracellular sites of superoxide production in stimulated neutrophils. *J. Cell Sci.* **111:**81–91.

Kolb, H., and V. Kolb-Bachofen. 1998. Nitric oxide in autoimmune disease: cytotoxic or regulatory mediator. *Immunol. Today* **19:**556–561.

Kröncke, K.-D., K. Fehsel, and V. Kolb-Bachofen. 1998. Inducible nitric oxide synthase in human diseases. *Clin. Exp. Immunol.* **113:**147–156.

Kröncke, K.-D., H. Haase, D. Beyersmann, V. Kolb-Bachofen, and M. K. Hayar-Hartl. 2001. Nitric oxide inhibits the cochaperone activity of the RING finger-like protein DnaJ. *Nitric Oxide* **5:**289–295.

Kuga, S., T. Otsuka, H. Niiro, H. Nunoi, Y. Nemoto, T. Nakano, T. Ogo, T. Umei, and Y. Niho. 1996. Suppression of superoxide anion production by interleukin-10 is accompanied by a downregulation of the genes for subunit proteins of NADPH oxidase. *Exp. Hematol.* **24:**151–157.

Kun, J. F. J., B. Mordmüller, B. Lell, L. G. Lehman, D. Luckner, and P. G. Kremsner. 1998. Polymorphism in promotor region of inducible nitric oxide synthase gene and protection against malaria. *Lancet* **351:**265–266.

Kun, J. F., B. Mordmüller, D. J. Perkins, J. May, O. Mercereau-Puijalon, M. Alpers, J. B. Weinberg, and P. G. Kremsner. 2001. Nitric oxide synthase 2[Lambarene] (G-954C), increased nitric oxide production, and protection against malaria. *J. Infect. Dis.* **184:**330–336.

Lambeth, J. D. 2002. Nox/Duox family of nicotinamide adenine dinucleotide (phosphate) oxidases. *Curr. Opin. Hematol.* **9:**11–17.

Lambeth, J. D. 2004. NOX enzymes and the biology of reactive oxygen. *Nat. Rev. Immunol.* **4:**181–189.

Lancaster, J. R. J. 1997. A tutorial on the diffusibility and reactivity of free nitric oxide. *Nitric Oxide* **1:**18–30.

Lanza, F. 1998. Clinical manifestations of myeloperoxidase deficiency. *J. Mol. Med.* **76:**676–681.

Laubach, V. E., E. G. Shesely, O. Smithies, and P. A. Sherman. 1995. Mice lacking inducible nitric oxide synthase are not resistant to lipopolysaccharide-induced death. *Proc. Natl. Acad. Sci. USA* **92:**10688–10692.

Lee, J., H. Ryu, R. J. Ferrante, S. M. Morris, and R. R. Ratan. 2003. Translational control of inducible nitric oxide synthase expression by arginine can explain the arginine paradox. *Proc. Natl. Acad. Sci. USA* **100:**4843–4848.

Leitch, G. J., and Q. He. 1999. Reactive nitrogen and oxygen species ameliorate experimental cryptosporidiosis in the neonatal BALB/c mouse model. *Infect. Immun.* **67:**5885–5891.

Lekstrom-Himes, J. A., and J. I. Gallin. 2003. Immunodeficiency diseases caused by defects in phagocytes. *N. Engl. J. Med.* **343:**1703–1714.

Lerner, R. A., and A. Eschenmoser. 2003. Ozone in biology. *Proc. Natl. Acad. Sci. USA* **100:**3013–3015.

Levesque, M. C., M. R. Hobbs, N. M. Anstey, T. N. Vaughn, J. A. Chancellor, A. Pole, D. J. Perkins, M. A. Misukonis, S. J. Chanock, D. L. Granger, and J. B. Weinberg. 1999. Nitric oxide synthase type 2 promotor polymorphisms, nitric oxide production, and disease severity in Tanzanian children with malaria. *J. Infect. Dis.* **180:**1994–2002.

Li, H., T. Wallerath, and U. Förstermann. 2002a. Physiological mechanisms regulating the expression of endothelial-type NO synthase. *Nitric Oxide* **7:**132–147.

Li, H., T. Wallerath, T. Münzel, and U. Förster-mann. 2002b. Regulation of endothelial-type NO synthase expression in pathophysiology and in response to drugs. *Nitric Oxide* **7:**149–164.

Liew, F. Y., S. Millott, C. Parkinson, R. M. Palmer, and S. Moncada. 1990. Macrophage killing of *Leishmania* parasite *in vivo* is mediated by nitric oxide from L-arginine. *J. Immunol.* **144:**4794–4797.

Locksley, R. M., R. M. Wilson, and S. J. Klebanoff. 1983. Increased respiratory burst in myeloperoxidase-deficient monocytes. *Blood* **62:**902–909.

Lyons, C. R., G. J. Orloff, and J. M. Cunningham. 1992. Molecular cloning and functional expression of an inducible nitric oxide synthase from a murine macrophage cell-line. *J. Biol. Chem.* **267:**6370–6374.

MacMicking, J. D., C. Nathan, G. Hom, N. Chartrain, D. S. Fletcher, M. Trumbauer, K. Stevens, Q.-W. Xie, K. Sokol, N. Hutchinson, H. Chen, and J. S. Mudgett. 1995. Altered responses to bacterial infection and endotoxic shock in mice lacking inducible nitric oxide synthase. *Cell* **81:**641–650.

MacMicking, J., Q.-W. Xie, and C. Nathan. 1997a. Nitric oxide and macrophage function. *Annu. Rev. Immunol.* **15:**323–350.

MacMicking, J. D., R. J. North, R. LaCourse, J. S. Mudgett, S. K. Shah, and C. F. Nathan. 1997b. Identification of nitric oxide synthase as a protective locus against tuberculosis. *Proc. Natl. Acad. Sci. USA* **94:**5243–5248.

Malkin, R., E. Flescher, J. Lengy, and Y. Keisari. 1987. On the interactions between macrophages and the developmental stages of *Schistosoma mansoni:* the cytotoxic mechanism involved in macrophage-mediated killing of schistosomula in vitro. *Immunobiology* **176:** 63–72.

Manca, C., S. Paul, C. E. Barry, V. H. Freedman, and G. Kaplan. 1999. *Mycobacterium tuberculosis* catalase and peroxidase activities and resistance to oxidative killing in human monocytes in vitro. *Infect. Immun.* **67:**74–79.

Marletta, M. A., P. S. Yoon, R. Iyengar, C. D. Leaf, and J. S. Wishnok. 1988. Macrophage oxidation of L-arginine to nitrite and nitrate: nitric oxide is an intermediate. *Biochemistry* **27:**8706–8711.

Marshall, H. E., K. Merchant, and J. S. Stamler. 2000. Nitrosation and oxidation in the regulation of gene expression. *FASEB J.* **14:**1889–1900.

Martins, G. A., S. B. Petkova, F. S. Machado, R. N. Kitsis, L. M. Weiss, M. Wittner, and H. B. Tanowitz. 2001. Fas-FasL interaction modulates nitric oxide production in *Trypanosoma cruzi*-infected mice. *Immunology* **103:**122–129.

Mastroeni, P., A. Vazquez-Torres, F. C. Fang, Y. Xu, S. Khan, C. E. Hormaeche, and G. Dougan. 2000. Antimicrobial actions of the NADPH phagocyte oxidase and inducible nitric oxide synthase in experi-mental salmonellosis. II. Effects of microbial prolifera-tion and host survival in vivo. *J. Exp. Med.* **192:**237–247.

Mauël, J. 1996. Intracellular survival of protozoan parasites with special reference to *Leishmania* spp., *Toxoplasma gondii*, and *Trypanosoma cruzi*. *Adv. Parasitol.* **38:**1–51.

Messina, C. G. M., E. P. Reeves, J. Roes, and A. W. Segal. 2002. Catalase negative *Staphylococcus aureus* retain virulence in mouse model of chronic granulomatous disease. *FEBS Lett.* **518:**107–110.

Miles, A. M., M. W. Owens, S. Milligan, G. G. Johnson, J. Z. Fields, T. S. Ing, V. Kottapalli, A. Keshavarzian, and M. B. Grisham. 1995. Nitric oxide synthase in circulating vs. extravasated polymor-phonuclear leukocytes. *J. Leukoc. Biol.* **58:**616–622.

Mitchell, H. H., H. A. Shonle, and H. S. Grindley. 1916. The origin of the nitrates in the urine. *J. Biol. Chem.* **24:**461–490.

Mizel, S. B., A. N. Honko, M. A. Moors, P. S. Smith, and A. P. West. 2003. Induction of macrophage nitric oxide production by Gram-nega-tive flagellin involves signaling via heterodimeric Toll-like receptor 5/Toll-like receptor 4 complexes. *J. Im-munol.* **170:**6217–6223.

Mnaimneh, S., M. Geffard, B. Veyret, and P. Vincendeau. 1997. Albumin nitrosylated by activated macrophages possesses antiparasitic effects neutralized by anti-NO-acetylated-cysteine antibodies. *J. Immunol.* **158:**308–314.

Modolell, M., I. M. Corraliza, F. Link, G. Soler, and K. Eichmann. 1995. Reciprocal regulation of the nitric oxide synthase/arginase balance in mouse bone marrow-derived macrophages by Th1 and Th2 macrophages. *Eur. J. Immunol.* **25:**1101–1104.

Modolell, M., K. Eichmann, and G. Soler. 1997. Oxidation of N(G)-hydroxy-L-arginine to nitric oxide mediated by respiratory burst: an alternative pathway to NO synthesis. *FEBS Lett.* **401:**123–126.

Morgenstern, D. E., M. A. C. Gifford, L. L. Li, C. M. Doerschuk, and M. C. Dinauer. 1997. Absence of respiratory burst in X-linked chronic granulomatous disease mice leads to abnormalities in both host defense and inflammatory response to *Aspergillus fumigatus. J. Exp. Med.* **185:**207–218.

Mosser, D. M. 2003. The many faces of macrophage activation. *J. Leukoc. Biol.* **73:**209–212.

Murray, H. W., and C. F. Nathan. 1999. Macrophage microbicidal mechanisms in vivo: reactive nitrogen vs. oxygen intermediates in the killing of intracellular visceral *Leishmania donovani. J. Exp. Med.* **189:**741–746.

Murray, H. W., and R. F. Teitelbaum. 1992. L-argi-nine-dependent reactive nitrogen intermediates and the antimicrobial effect of activated human mononu-clear phagocytes. *J. Infect. Dis.* **165:**513–517.

Nagase, S., K. Takemura, A. Ueda, A. Hirayama, K. Aoyagi, M. Kondoh, and A. Koyama. 1997. A novel non-enzymatic pathway for the generation of nitric oxide by the reaction of hydrogen peroxide and D- or L-arginine. *Biochem. Biophys. Res. Commun.* **233**:150–153.

Nagata, K., H. Yu, M. Nishikawa, M. Kashiba, A. Nakamura, E. F. Sato, T. Tamura, and M. Inoue. 1998. *Helicobacter pylori* generates superoxide radicals and modulates nitric oxide metabolism. *J. Biol. Chem.* **273**:14071–14073.

Nakano, T., H. Terato, K. Asagoshi, A. Masaoka, M. Mukuta, Y. Ohyama, T. Suzuki, K. Makino, and H. Ide. 2003. DNA-protein cross-link formation mediated by oxanine. *J. Biol. Chem.* **278**:25264–25272.

Nathan, C. 1992. Nitric oxide as a secretory product of mammalian cells. *FASEB J.* **6**:3051–3064.

Nathan, C. 2002. Points of control in inflammation. *Nature* **420**:846–852.

Nathan, C. 2003. Specificity of a third kind: reactive oxygen and nitrogen intermediates in cell signaling. *J. Clin. Invest.* **111**:769–778.

Nathan, C., and M. U. Shiloh. 2000. Reactive oxygen and nitrogen intermediates in the relationship between mammalian hosts and microbial pathogens. *Proc. Natl. Acad. Sci. USA* **97**:8841–8848.

Nauseef, W. M. 1998. Insights into myeloperoxidase biosynthesis from its inherited deficiency. *J. Mol. Med.* **76**:661–668.

Nauseef, W. M., J. A. Metcalf, and R. K. Root. 1983. Role of myeloperoxidase in the respiratory burst of human neutrophils. *Blood* **61**:483–492.

Newburger, P. E., R. A. B. Ezekowitz, C. Whitney, J. Wright, and S. H. Orkin. 1988. Induction of phagocyte cytochrome b heavy chain gene expression by interferon-γ. *Proc. Natl. Acad. Sci. USA* **85**:5215–5219.

Neworal, E. P., A. Altemani, A. Mamoni, I. L. Noronha, and M. H. Blotta. 2003. Immunocytochemical localization of cytokines and inducible nitric oxide synthase (iNOS) in oral mucosa and lymph nodes of patients with paracoccidioidomycosis. *Cytokine* **21**:234–241.

Nicholson, B., C. K. Manner, J. Kleeman, and C. L. MacLeod. 2001. Sustained nitric oxide production in macrophages requires the arginine transporter CAT2. *J. Biol. Chem.* **276**:15881–15885.

Nicholson, S., M. da Gloria Bonecini-Almeida, J. R. Lapa e Silva, C. Nathan, Q.-W. Xie, R. Mumford, J. R. Weidner, J. Calaycay, J. Geng, N. Boechat, C. Linhares, W. Rom, and J. L. Ho. 1996. Inducible nitric oxide synthase in pulmonary alveolar macrophages from patients with tuberculosis. *J. Exp. Med.* **183**:2293–2302.

Niedbala, W., X.-Q. Wei, D. Piedrafita, D. Xu, and F. Y. Liew. 1999. Effects of nitric oxide on the induction and differentiation of Th1 cells. *Eur. J. Immunol.* **29**:2498–2505.

Niedbala, W., X.-Q. Wei, C. Campbell, D. Thomson, M. Komai-Koma, and F. Y. Liew. 2002. Nitric oxide preferentially induces type 1 T cell differentiation by selectively up-regulating IL-12 receptor β2 expression via cGMP. *Proc. Natl. Acad. Sci. USA* **99**:16186–16191.

Nishi, T., and M. Forgac. 2002. The vacuolar (H+)-ATPases—nature's most versatile proton pumps. *Nat. Rev. Mol. Cell Biol.* **3**:94–103.

Noda, S., K. Tanaka, S. Sawamura, M. Sasaki, T. Matsumoto, K. Mikami, Y. Aiba, H. Hasegawa, N. Kawabe, and Y. Koga. 2001. Role of nitric oxide synthase type 2 in acute infection with cytomegalovirus. *J. Immunol.* **166**:3533–3541.

Nunoi, H., D. Rotrosen, J. I. Gallin, and H. L. Malech. 1988. Two forms of autosomal chronic granulomatous disease lack distinct neutrophil cytosol factors. *Science* **242**:1298–1301.

Ohashi, J., I. Naka, J. Patarapotikul, H. Hananantachai, S. Looareesuwan, and K. Tokunaga. 2002. Significant association of longer forms of CCTTT microsatellite repeat in the inducible nitric oxide synthase promotor with severe malaria in Thailand. *J. Infect. Dis.* **186**:578–581.

Okado-Matsumoto, A., and I. Fridovich. 2001. Subcellular distribution of superoxide-dismutase (SOD) in rat liver. Cu,Zn-SOD in mitochondria. *J. Biol. Chem.* **42**:38388–38393.

Olds, G. R., J. J. Ellner, L. A. Kearse, J. W. Kazura, and A. A. F. Mahmoud. 1980. Role of arginase in killing of schistosomula of *Schistosoma mansoni. J. Exp. Med.* **151**:1557–1562.

Pacelli, R., D. A. Wink, J. A. Cook, M. C. Krishna, W. DeGraff, N. Friedman, M. Tsokos, A. Samuni, and J. B. Mitchell. 1995. Nitric oxide potentiates hydrogen peroxide-induced killing of *Escherichia coli. J. Exp. Med.* **182**:1469–1479.

Parkos, C. A., R. A. Allen, C. G. Cochrane, and A. J. Jesaitis. 1987. Purified cytochrome c from human granulocyte plasma membrane is composed of two polypeptides with relative molecular weights of 91,000 and 22,000. *J. Clin. Invest.* **80**:732–742.

Parkos, C. A., M. C. Dinauer, L. E. Walker, R. A. Allen, A. J. Jesaitis, and S. H. Orkin. 1988. Primary structure and unique expression of the 22 kDa light chain of human neutrophil cytochrome b. *Proc. Natl. Acad. Sci. USA* **85**:3319–3323.

Pathania, R., N. K. Navani, A. M. Gardner, P. R. Gardner, and K. L. Dikshit. 2002. Nitric oxide scavenging and detoxification by the *Mycobacterium tuberculosis* hemoglobin HbN in *Escherichia coli. Mol. Microbiol.* **45**:1303–1314.

Perry, L. L., K. Feilzer, and H. D. Caldwell. 1998. Neither interleukin-6 nor inducible nitric oxide synthase is required for clearance of *Chlamydia trachomatis* from the murine genital tract epithelium. *Infect. Immun.* **66**:1265–1269.

Pfeiffer, S., A. Lass, K. Schmidt, and B. Mayer. 2001a. Protein tyrosine nitration in cytokine-activated murine macrophages: involvement of a peroxidase/

nitrite pathway rather than peroxinitrite. *J. Biol. Chem.* **276:**34051–34058.

Pfeiffer, S., A. Lass, K. Schmidt, and B. Mayer. 2001b. Protein tyrosine nitration in mouse peritoneal macrophages activated in vitro and in vivo: evidence against an essential role of peroxynitrite. *FASEB J.* **15:**2355–2364.

Pfeilschifter, J., W. Eberhardt, and K.-F. Beck. 2001. Regulation of gene expression by nitric oxide. *Pflügers Arch. Eur. J. Physiol.* **442:**479–486.

Philippe, B., O. Ibrahim-Granet, M. C. Prevost, M. A. Gougerot-Pocidalo, M. Sanchez Perez, A. van der Meeren, and J. P. Latge. 2003. Killing of *Aspergillus fumigatus* by alveolar macrophages is mediated by reactive oxidant intermediates. *Infect. Immun.* **71:**3034–3042.

Philipps, W. A., and J. A. Hamilton. 1989. Phorbol ester-stimulated superoxide production by murine bone marrow-derived macrophages requires preexposure to cytokines. *J. Immunol.* **142:**2445–2449.

Piacenza, L., G. Peluffo, and R. Radi. 2001. L-arginine-dependent suppression of apoptosis in *Trypanosoma cruzi*: contribution of the nitric oxide and polyamine pathways. *Proc. Natl. Acad. Sci. USA* **98:** 7301–7306.

Piddington, D. L., F. C. Fang, T. Laessig, A. M. Cooper, I. M. Orme, and N. A. Buchmeier. 2001. Cu,Zn superoxide dismutase of *Mycobacterium tuberculosis* contributes to survival in activated macrophages that are generating an oxidative burst. *Infect. Immun.* **69:**4980–4987.

Poljakovic, M., and K. Persson. 2003. Urinary tract infection in iNOS-deficient mice with focus on bacterial sensitivity to nitric oxide. *Am. J. Physiol. Renal Physiol.* **284:**F22–F31.

Pollock, J. D., D. A. Williams, M. A. Gifford, L. L. Li, X. Du, J. Fisherman, S. H. Orkin, C. M. Doerschuk, and M. C. Dinauer. 1995. Mouse model of X-linked chronic granulomatous disease, an inherited defect in phagocyte superoxide production. *Nat. Genet.* **9:**202–209.

Prout, W. 1818. Further observations on the proximate principles of the urine. *Medico-Chirurgical Trans. (London)* **IX:**472–484.

Qadoumi, M., I. Becker, N. Donhauser, M. Röllinghoff, and C. Bogdan. 2002. Expression of inducible nitric oxide synthase in skin lesions of patients with American cutaneous leishmaniosis. *Infect. Immun.* **70:**4638–4642.

Quellet, H., Y. Quellet, C. Richard, M. Labarre, B. Wittenberg, J. Wittenberg, and M. Guertin. 2002. Truncated hemoglobin HbN protects *Mycobacterium bovis* from nitric oxide. *Proc. Natl. Acad. Sci. USA* **99:**5902–5907.

Quie, P. G., J. G. White, B. Holmes, and R. A. Good. 1967. In vitro bactericidal capacity of human polymorphonuclear leukocytes: diminished activity in chronic granulomatous disease of childhood. *J. Clin. Invest.* **46:**668–679.

Ramos, C. L., S. Pou, B. E. Britigan, M. S. Cohen, and G. M. Rosen. 1992. Spin trapping evidence for myeloperoxidase-dependent hydroxyl radical formation by human neutrophils and monocytes. *J. Biol. Chem.* **267:**8307–8312.

Ramsey, K. H., G. S. Miranpuri, C. E. Poulson, N. B. Marthakis, L. M. Braune, and G. I. Byrne. 1998. Inducible nitric oxide synthase does not affect resolution of murine chlamydial genital tract infections or eradication of chlamydiae in primary murine cell culture. *Infect. Immun.* **66:**835–838.

Ramsey, K. H., G. S. Miranpuri, I. M. Sigar, S. Quellette, and G. I. Byrne. 2001a. *Chlamydia trachomatis* persistence in the female mouse genital tract: inducible nitric oxide synthase and infection outcome. *Infect. Immun.* **69:**5131–5137.

Ramsey, K. H., I. M. Sigar, S. V. Rana, J. Gupta, S. M. Holland, and G. I. Byrne. 2001b. Role for inducible nitric oxide synthase in protection from chronic *Chlamydia trachomatis* urogenital disease in mice and its regulation by oxygen free radicals. *Infect. Immun.* **69:**7374–7379.

Reeves, E. P., H. Lu, H. L. Jacobs, C. G. M. Messina, S. Bolsover, G. Gabella, E. O. Potma, A. Warley, J. Roes, and A. W. Segal. 2002. Killing activity of neutrophils is mediated through activation of proteases by K^+ flux. *Nature* **416:**291.

Reiter, C. D., R.-J. Teng, and J. S. Beckman. 2000. Superoxide reacts with nitric oxide to nitrate tyrosine at physiological pH via peroxynitrite. *J. Biol. Chem.* **275:**32460–32466.

Reth, M. 2002. Hydrogen peroxide as second messenger in lymphocyte activation. *Nat. Immunol.* **3:**1129–1134.

Rotrosen, D., C. L. Yeung, T. L. Leto, H. L. Malech, and C. H. Kwong. 1992. Cytochrome b558: the flavin-binding component of the phagocyte NADPH oxidase. *Science* **256:**1459–1462.

Rottenberg, M. E., A. C. G. Rothfuchs, D. Gigliotti, C. Svanholm, L. Bandholtz, and H. Wigzell. 1999. Role of innate and adaptive immunity in the outcome of primary infection with *Chlamydia pneumoniae*, as analyzed in genetically modified mice. *J. Immunol.* **162:**2829–2836.

Ruan, J., G. S. John, S. Ehrt, L. Riley, and C. Nathan. 1999. *noxR3*, a novel gene from *Mycobacterium tuberculosis*, protects *Salmonella typhimurium* from nitrosative and oxidative stress. *Infect. Immun.* **67:**3276–3283.

Rutschman, R., R. Lang, M. Hesse, J. N. Ihle, T. A. Wynn, and P. J. Murray. 2001. Stat6-dependent substrate depletion regulates nitric oxide production. *J. Immunol.* **166:**2173–2177.

Saeftel, M., B. Fleischer, and A. Hoerauf. 2001. Stage-dependent role of nitric oxide in control of

Trypanosoma cruzi infection. *Infect. Immun.* **69:**2252–2259.

Sauer, H., M. Wartenberg, and J. Hescheler. 2001. Reactive oxygen species as intracellular messengers during cell growth and differentiation. *Cell. Physiol. Biochem.* **11:**173–186.

Saura, M., C. Zaragoza, A. McMillan, R. A. Quick, C. Hohenadl, J. M. Lowenstein, and C. J. Lowenstein. 1999. An antiviral mechanism of nitric oxide: inhibition of a viral protease. *Immunity* **10:**21–28.

Sawa, T., T. Akaike, and H. Maeda. 2000. Tyrosine nitration by peroxynitrite formed from nitric oxide and superoxide generated by xanthine oxidase. *J. Biol. Chem.* **275:**32467–32474.

Sbarra, A. I., and M. L. Karnovsky. 1959. The biochemical basis of phagocytosis. 1. Metabolic changes during the ingestion of particles by polymorphonuclear leukocytes. *J. Biol. Chem.* **234:**1355–1362.

Scanga, C. A., V. P. Mohan, H. Joseph, K. Yu, J. Chan, and J. L. Flynn. 1999. Reactivation of latent tuberculosis: variations on the Cornell murine model. *Infect. Immun.* **67:**4531–4538.

Scanga, C. A., V. P. Mohan, K. Yu, H. Joseph, K. Tanaka, J. Chan, and J. L. Flynn. 2000. Depletion of CD4+ T cells causes reactivation of murine persistent tuberculosis despite continued expression of IFN-γ and nitric oxide synthase 2. *J. Exp. Med.* **192:**347–358.

Scanga, C. A., V. P. Mohan, K. E. Tanaka, D. Alland, J. L. Flynn, and J. Chan. 2001. The inducible nitric oxide synthase locus confers protection against aerogenic challenge of both clinical and laboratory strains of *Mycobacterium tuberculosis* in mice. *Infect. Immun.* **69:**7711–7717.

Scharton-Kersten, T. M., G. Yap, J. Magram, and A. Sher. 1997. Inducible nitric oxide is essential for host control of persistent but not acute infection with the intracellular pathogen *Toxoplasma gondii. J. Exp. Med.* **185:**1261–1273.

Schnappinger, D., S. Ehrt, M. I. Voskuil, Y. Liu, J. A. Mangan, I. M. Monahan, G. Dolganov, B. Efron, P. D. Butcher, C. Nathan, and G. K. Schoolnik. 2003. Transcriptional adaptation of *Mycobacterium tuberculosis* within macrophages: insights into the phagosomal environment. *J. Exp. Med.* **198:**693–704.

Schneemann, M., G. Schoedon, S. Hofer, N. Blau, L. Guerrero, and A. Schaffner. 1993. Nitric oxide synthase is not a constituent of the antimicrobial armature of human mononuclear phagocytes. *J. Infect. Dis.* **167:**1358–1363.

Schneemann, M., G. Schoedon, and C. Bogdan. 2002. Species differences in macrophage NO production are important. *Nat. Immunol.* **3:**102.

Schön, T., D. Elias, F. Moges, E. Melese, T. Tessema, O. Stendahl, S. Britton, and T. Sundqvist. 2003. Arginine as an adjuvant to chemotherapy improves clinical outcome in active tuberculosis. *Eur. Respir. J.* **21:**483–488.

Schröppel, K., M. Kryk, M. Herrmann, E. Leberer, M. Röllinghoff, and C. Bogdan. 2001. Suppression of type 2 NO synthase activity in macrophages by *Candida albicans. Int. J. Med. Microbiol.* **290:**659–668.

Segal, A. W., and O. T. G. Jones. 1978. Novel cytochrome b system in phagocytic vacuoles from human granulocytes. *Nature (London)* **276:**515–517.

Segal, B. H., T. M. Doherty, T. A. Wynn, A. W. Cheever, A. Sher, and S. M. Holland. 1999. The p47phox$^{-/-}$ mouse model of chronic granulomatous disease has normal granuloma formation and cytokine responses to *Mycobacterium avium* and *Schistosoma mansoni* eggs. *Infect. Immun.* **67:**1659–1665.

Segal, B. H., N. Sakamoto, M. Patel, K. Maemura, A. S. Klein, S. M. Holland, and G. B. Bulkley. 2000. Xanthine oxidase contributes to host defense against *Burkholderia cepacia* in the p47$^{phox-/-}$ mouse model of chronic granulomatous disease. *Infect. Immun.* **68:**2374–2378.

Segal, B. H., L. Ding, and S. M. Holland. 2003. Phagocyte NADPH oxidase, but not inducible nitric oxide synthase, is essential for early control of *Burkholderia cepacia* and *Chromobacterium violaceum* infection in mice. *Infect. Immun.* **71:**205–210.

Seydel, K. B., S. J. Smith, and S. L. Stanley. 2000. Innate immunity to amebic liver abscess is dependent on gamma interferon and nitric oxide in a murine model of disease. *Infect. Immun.* **68:**400–402.

Shapiro, J. M., S. J. Libby, and F. C. Fang. 2003. Inhibition of bacterial DNA replication by zinc mobilization during nitrosative stress. *Proc. Natl. Acad. Sci. USA* **100:**8496–8501.

Sharara, A. I., D. J. Perkins, M. A. Misukonis, S. U. Chan, J. A. Dominitz, and B. J. Weinberg. 1997. Interferon-α activation of human blood mononuclear cells in vitro and in vivo for nitric oxide synthase (NOS) type 2 mRNA and protein expression: possible relationship of induced NOS2 to the anti-hepatitis C effects of IFN-α in vivo. *J. Exp. Med.* **186:**1495–1502.

Shiloh, M. U., J. D. MacMicking, S. Nicholson, J. E. Brause, S. Potter, M. Marino, F. Fang, M. Dinauer, and C. Nathan. 1999. Phenotype of mice and macrophages deficient in both phagocyte oxidase and inducible nitric oxide synthase. *Immunity* **10:**29–36.

Skaar, E. P., D. M. Tobiason, J. Quick, R. C. Judd, H. Weissbach, F. Etienne, N. Brot, and H. S. Seifert. 2002. The outer membrane localization of the *Neisseria gonorrhoeae* MsrA/B is involved in survival against reactive oxygen species. *Proc. Natl. Acad. Sci. USA* **99:**10108–10113.

Smith, A. L., and A. C. Hayday. 2000. Genetic dissection of primary and secondary responses to a widespread natural pathogen of the gut, *Eimeria vermiformis*. *Infect. Immun.* **68**:6273–6280.

Smith, R. M., and J. T. Curnette. 1991. Molecular basis of chronic granulomatous disease. *Blood* **77**:673–686.

Späth, G. F., L. A. Garraway, S. J. Turco, and S. M. Beverley. 2003a. The role(s) of lipophosphoglycan (LPG) in the establishment of *Leishmania major* infections in mammalian hosts. *Proc. Natl. Acad. Sci. USA* **100**:9536–9541.

Späth, G. F., L.-F. Lye, H. Segawa, D. L. Sacks, S. J. Turco, and S. M. Beverley. 2003b. Persistence without pathology in phosphoglycan-deficient *Leishmania major*. *Science* **301**:1241–1243.

St. John, G., N. Brot, J. Ruan, H. Erdjument-Bromage, P. Tempst, H. Weissbach, and C. Nathan. 2001. Peptide methionine sulfoxide reductase from *Escherichia coli* and *Mycobacterium tuberculosis* protects bacteria against oxidative damage from reactive nitrogen intermediates. *Proc. Natl. Acad. Sci. USA* **98**:9901–9906.

Steinbeck, M. J., A. U. Khan, and M. J. Karnovsky. 1992. Intracellular singlet oxygen generation by phagocytosing neutrophils in response to particles coated with a chemical trap. *J. Biol. Chem.* **267**: 13425–13433.

Stenger, S., H. Thüring, M. Röllinghoff, and C. Bogdan. 1994. Tissue expression of inducible nitric oxide synthase is closely associated with resistance to *Leishmania major*. *J. Exp. Med.* **180**:783–793.

Stenger, S., N. Donhauser, H. Thüring, M. Röllinghoff, and C. Bogdan. 1996. Reactivation of latent leishmaniasis by inhibition of inducible nitric oxide synthase. *J. Exp. Med.* **183**:1501–1514.

Stuehr, D. 1999. Mammalian nitric oxide synthases. *Biochim. Biophys. Acta* **1411**:217–230.

Stuehr, D. J., and M. A. Marletta. 1985. Mammalian nitrite biosynthesis: mouse macrophages produce nitrite and nitrate in response to *Escherichia coli* lipopolysaccharide. *Proc. Natl. Acad. Sci. USA* **82**: 7738–7742.

Stuehr, D. J., and M. A. Marletta. 1987. Induction of nitrite/nitrate synthesis in murine macrophages by BCG infection, lymphokines or interferon-γ. *J. Immunol.* **139**:518–525.

Stuehr, D. J., and C. F. Nathan. 1989. Nitric oxide: a macrophage product responsible for cytostasis and respiratory inhibition in tumor cell growth. *J. Exp. Med.* **169**:1543–1555.

Stuehr, D. J., S. S. Gross, I. Sakuma, R. Levi, and C. F. Nathan. 1989. Activated murine macrophages secrete a metabolite of arginine with the bioactivity of endothelium-derived relaxing factor and the chemical reactivity of nitric oxide. *J. Exp. Med.* **169**:1011–1020.

Stuehr, D. J., H. J. Cho, N. S. Kwon, M. F. Weise, and C. F. Nathan. 1991. Purification and characterization of the cytokine-induced macrophage nitric oxide synthase: an FAD- and FMN-containing flavoprotein. *Proc. Natl. Acad. Sci. USA* **88**:7773–7777.

Stuehr, D. J., S. Pou, and G. M. Rosen. 2001. Oxygen reduction by nitric oxide synthases. *J. Biol. Chem.* **276**:14533–14536.

Takeda, K., T. Kaisho, and S. Akira. 2003. Toll-like receptors. *Annu. Rev. Immunol.* **21**:335–376.

Tatsuzawa, H., T. Maruyama, K. Hori, Y. Sano, and M. Nakano. 1999. Singlet oxygen ($O_2{}^1\Delta_g$) as the principal oxidant in myeloperoxidase-mediated bacterial killing in neutrophil phagosome. *Biochem. Biophys. Res. Commun.* **262**:647–650.

Teahan, C., P. Rowe, P. Parker, N. Totty, and A. W. Segal. 1987. The X-linked chronic granulomatous disease gene codes for the beta-chain of cytochrome b-245. *Nature (London)* **327**:720–721.

Tse, W. Y., J. Williams, A. Pall, M. Wilkes, C. O. S. Savage, and D. Adu. 2001. Antineutrophil cytoplasm antibody-induced neutrophil nitric oxide production is nitric oxide synthase independent. *Kidney Int.* **59**: 593–600.

Tubaro, F., B. Lotti, C. Santiangeli, and G. Cavallo. 1980. Xanthine oxidase increase in polymorphonuclear leucocytes and macrophages in mice in three pathological situations. *Biochem. Pharmacol.* **29**: 1943–1948.

Umezawa, K., T. Akaike, S. Fujii, M. Suga, K. Setoguchi, A. Ozawa, and H. Maeda. 1997. Induction of nitric oxide synthesis and xanthine oxidase and their roles in the antimicrobial mechanism against *Salmonella typhimurium* in mice. *Infect. Immun.* **65**:2932–2940.

Vallance, B. A., W. Deng, M. de Grado, C. Chan, K. Jacobson, and B. B. Finlay. 2002. Modulation of inducible nitric oxide synthase expression by the attaching and effacing bacterial pathogen *Citrobacter rodentium* in infected mice. *Infect. Immun.* **70**:6424–6435.

van den Broek, M., M. F. Bachmann, G. Köhler, M. Barner, R. Escher, R. Zinkernagel, and M. Kopf. 2000. IL-4 and IL-10 antagonize IL-12-mediated protection against acute vaccinia virus infection with a limited role of IFN-γ and nitric oxide synthase-2. *J. Immunol.* **164**:371–378.

van der Heyde, H. C., Y. Gu, Q. Zhang, G. Sun, and M. B. Grisham. 2000. Nitric oxide is neither necessary nor sufficient for resolution of *Plasmodium chabaudi* malaria in mice. *J. Immunol.* **165**:3317–3323.

van Diepen, A., T. van der Straaten, S. M. Holland, R. Janssen, and J. T. van Dissel. 2002. A superoxide-hypersusceptible *Salmonella enterica* serovar typhimurium mutant is attenuated but regains virulence in p47$^{phox-/-}$ mice. *Infect. Immun.* **70**:2614–2621.

Vazquez-Torres, A., Y. Xu, J. Jones-Carson, D. W. Holden, S. M. Lucia, M. C. Dinauer, P. Mastroeni, and F. C. Fang. 2000. *Salmonella* pathogenicity island 2-dependent evasion of the phagocyte NADPH oxidase. *Science* **287:**1655–1658.

Vazquez-Torres, A., G. Fantuzzi, C. K. I. Edwards, C. G. Dinarello, and F. C. Fang. 2001. Defective localization of the NADPH oxidase to *Salmonella*-containing phagosomes in tumor necrosis factor p55 receptor-deficient macrophages. *Proc. Natl. Acad. Sci. USA* **98:**2561–2565.

Venketaraman, V., Y. K. Dayaram, A. G. Amin, R. Ngo, R. M. Green, M. T. Talaue, J. Mann, and N. D. Connelly. 2003. Role of glutathione in macrophage control of mycobacteria. *Infect. Immun.* **71:** 1864–1871.

Villalta, F., Y. Zhang, K. E. Bibb, J. C. Kappes, and M. F. Lima. 1998. The cysteine-cysteine family of chemokines RANTES, MIP-1α, and MIP-1β induce trypanocidal activity in human macrophages via nitric oxide. *Infect. Immun.* **66:**4690–4695.

Vodovotz, Y., C. Bogdan, J. Paik, Q.-W. Xie, and C. Nathan. 1993. Mechanisms of suppression of macrophage nitric oxide release by transforming growth factor-β. *J. Exp. Med.* **178:**605–613.

Vodovotz, Y., D. Russell, Q.-W. Xie, C. Bogdan, and C. Nathan. 1995. Vesicle membrane association of nitric oxide synthase in primary mouse macrophages. *J. Immunol.* **154:**2914–2925.

Volpp, B. D., W. M. Nauseef, and R. A. Clark. 1998. Two cytosolic neutrophil oxidase components absent in autosomal chronic granulomatous disease. *Science* **242:**1295–1297.

von Loewenich, F. D., D. G. Scorpio, U. Reischl, J. S. Dumler, and C. Bogdan. 2004. Control of *Anaplasma phagocytophilum*, an obligate intracellular pathogen, in the absence of inducible nitric oxide synthase, phagocyte NADPH oxidase, tumor necrosis factor, Toll-like receptor (TLR) 2 and 4, or the TLR adaptor molecule MyD88. *Eur. J. Immunol.* **34,** in press.

Vouldoukis, I., V. Riveros-Moreno, B. Dugas, F. Quaaz, P. Bécherel, P. Debré, S. Moncada, and M. D. Mossalayi. 1995. The killing of *Leishmania major* by human macrophages is mediated by nitric oxide induced after ligation of the FcεRII/CD23 surface antigen. *Proc. Natl. Acad. Sci. USA* **92:**7804–7808.

Vouldoukis, I., P.-A. Bécherel, V. Riveros-Moreno, M. Arock, O. da Silva, P. Debré, D. Mazier, and M. D. Mossalayi. 1997. Interleukin-10 and interleukin-4 inhibit intracellular killing of *Leishmania infantum* and *Leishmania major* by human macrophages by decreasing nitric oxide generation. *Eur. J. Immunol.* **27:**860–865.

Wagner, D. A., V. R. Young, and S. R. Tannenbaum. 1983. Mammalian nitrate biosynthesis: incorporation of $^{15}NH_3$ into nitrate is enhanced by endotoxin treatment. *Proc. Natl. Acad. Sci. USA* **80:** 4518–4521.

Wang, Y., and A. Casadevall. 1994. Susceptibility of melanized annd non-melanized *Cryptococcus neoformans*

to nitrogen- and oxygen-derived oxidants. *Infect. Immun.* **62:**3004–3007.

Way, S. S., and M. B. Goldberg. 1998. Clearance of *Shigella flexneri* infection occurs through a nitric oxide-independent mechanism. *Infect. Immun.* **66:** 3012–3016.

Webb, J. L., M. W. Harvey, D. W. Holden, and T. J. Evans. 2001. Macrophage nitric oxide synthase associates with cortical actin but is not recruited to phagosomes. *Infect. Immun.* **69:**6391–6400.

Wei, X.-Q., I. G. Charles, A. Smith, J. Ure, G.-J. Feng, F.-P. Huang, D. Xu, W. Müller, S. Moncada, and F. Y. Liew. 1995. Altered immune responses in mice lacking inducible nitric oxide synthase. *Nature* **375:**408–411.

Weinberg, J. B. 1998. Nitric oxide production and nitric oxide synthase type 2 expression by human mononuclear phagocytes: a review. *Mol. Med.* **4:**557–591.

Wentworth, A. D., L. H. Lones, P. Wentworth, K. D. Janda, and R. A. Lerner. 2000. Antibodies have the intrinsic capacity to destroy antigens. *Proc. Natl. Acad. Sci. USA* **97:**10930–10935.

Wentworth, P. J., L. H. Jones, A. D. Wentworth, X. Zhu, N. A. Larsen, I. A. Wilson, X. Xu, W. A. I. Goddard, K. D. Janda, A. Eschenmoser, and R. A. Lerner. 2001. Antibody catalysis of the oxidation of water. *Science* **293:**1806–1811.

Wentworth, P. J., J. E. McDunn, A. D. Wentworth, C. Takeuchi, J. Nieva, T. Jones, C. Bautista, J. M. Ruedi, A. Gutierrez, K. D. Janda, B. M. Babior, A. Eschenmoser, and R. A. Lerner. 2002. Evidence for antibody-catalyzed ozone formation in bacterial killing and inflammation. *Science* **298:**2195–2199.

Wentworth, P. J., A. D. Wentworth, X. Zhu, I. A. Wilson, K. D. Janda, A. Eschenmoser, and R. A. Lerner. 2003. Evidence for the production of trioxygen species during antibody-catalyzed chemical modification of antigens. *Proc. Natl. Acad. Sci. USA* **100:** 1490–1493.

Wientjes, F. B., J. J. Hsuan, N. F. Totty, and A. W. Segal. 1993. p40phox, a third cytosolic component of the activation complex of the NADPH oxidase to contain src homology 3 domains. *Biochem. J.* **296:**557–561.

Winkler, F., U. Koedel, S. Kastenbauer, and H. W. Pfister. 2001. Differential expression of nitric oxide synthases in bacterial meningitis: role of the inducible isoform for blood-brain barrier breakdown. *J. Infect. Dis.* **183:**1749–1759.

Wu, G., and S. M. Morris. 1998. Arginine metabolism: nitric oxide and beyond. *Biochem. J.* **336:**1–17.

Wu, G. F., L. Pewe, and S. Perlman. 2000. Coronavirus-induced demyelination occurs in the absence of inducible nitric oxide synthase. *J. Virol.* **74:** 7683–7686.

Xia, Y., and J. L. Zweier. 1997. Superoxide and peroxynitrite generation from inducible nitric oxide synthase in macrophages. *Proc. Natl. Acad. Sci. USA* **94:** 6954–6958.

Xie, Q.-W., H. J. Cho, J. Calaycay, R. A. Mumford, K. M. Swiderek, T. D. Lee, A. Ding, T. Troso, and C. Nathan. 1992. Cloning and characterization of inducible nitric oxide synthase from mouse macrophages. *Science* **256:**225–228.

Yoneto, T., T. Yoshimoto, C.-R. Wang, Y. Takahama, M. Tsuji, S. Waki, and H. Nariuchi. 1999. Gamma interferon production is critical for protective immunity to infection with blood-stage *Plasmodium berghei* XAT but neither NO production nor NK cell activation is critical. *Infect. Immun.* **67:** 2349–2356.

Yu, L., M. T. Quinn, A. R. Cross, and M. C. Dinauer. 1998. gp91[phox] is the heme binding subunit of the superoxide-generating NADPH oxidase. *Proc. Natl. Acad. Sci. USA* **95:**7993–7998.

Yui, Y., R. Hattori, K. Kosuga, H. Eizawa, K. Hiki, and C. Kawai. 1991. Purification of nitric oxide synthase from rat macrophages. *J. Biol. Chem.* **266:**12544.

Zamboni, D. S., and M. Rabinovitch. 2003. Nitric oxide partially controls *Coxiella burnetii* phase II infection in mouse primary macrophages. *Infect. Immun.* **71:**1225–1233.

Zaragoza, C., C. Ocampo, M. Saura, M. Leppo, X.-Q. Wei, R. Quick, S. Moncada, F. Y. Liew, and C. J. Lowenstein. 1998. The role of inducible nitric oxide synthase in the host response to Coxsackievirus myocarditis. *Proc. Natl. Acad. Sci. USA* **95:**2469–2474.

Zaragoza, C., C. J. Ocampo, M. Saura, C. Bao, M. Leppo, A. Lafond-Walker, D. R. Thiemann, R. Hruban, and C. J. Lowenstein. 1999. Inducible nitric oxide synthase protection against Coxsackievirus pancreatitis. *J. Immunol.* **163:**5497–5504.

Zhou, Y., G. Lin, and M. P. Murtaugh. 1995. Interleukin-4 suppresses the expression of macrophage NADPH oxidase heavy chain subunit (gp91[phox]). *Biochim. Biophys. Acta* **1265:**40–48.

CHEMOKINES

Bernhard Moser

20

CHEMOKINES, THE LARGEST FAMILY OF CYTOKINES

History

Interleukin-8 (IL-8, CXCL8), the first chemokine, was discovered 15 years ago on the basis of its neutrophil chemoattractant properties (Schmid and Weissmann, 1987; Walz et al., 1987; Yoshimura et al., 1987). The N-terminal two of four conserved Cys residues are separated by one amino acid, which typifies IL-8 as a CXC chemokine (Table 1). The monocyte chemoattractant protein MCP-1/CCL2 with the two N-terminal Cys residues in adjacent positions is a CC chemokine, is active on monocytes, and was discovered shortly after IL-8. At the time of these discoveries several "orphan" chemokines, i.e., proteins with amino acid similarity to IL-8 or MCP-1 but of unknown function, were already known. These include Mig/CXCL9, IP-10/CXCL10, I-309/CCL1, MIP-1α/CCL3, and MIP-1β/CCL4 (Table 1), and their chemoattractant properties were determined later. The large majority of chemokines fall into the group of either CXC or CC chemokines; there are only two C chemokines, Ltn-α/XCL1 and Ltn-β/XCL2, missing two of the four conserved Cys residues, and a single CX3C chemokine, fractalkine/CX3CL1, in which the N-terminal two Cys residues are separated by three additional amino acids. Today, over 40 human chemokines are known, and their traditional abbreviations as well as the corresponding systematic nomenclature (Zlotnik and Yoshie, 2000) are listed in Table 1 (http://cytokine.medic.kumamoto-u.ac.jp/ gives access to recent updates). In this overview, traditional abbreviations are appended by their systematic nomenclature at the first instance and then used on their own throughout the text. Of note, early progress was made for those chemokines with unique selectivity for cells of the innate immune system, giving the impression that T and B cells are poor targets for chemokines. Of course, it is now thoroughly established that chemokine selectivity reaches well beyond monocytes and phagocytes, embracing all types of leukocytes, including T and B cells as well as hematopoietic progenitor cells.

Chemokine Receptors

Chemokine receptors belong to the large family of seven-transmembrane domain receptors that couple to heterotrimeric GTP-binding

Bernhard Moser, Theodor-Kocher Institute, University of Bern, Freiestrasse 1, CH-3012 Bern, Switzerland.

The Innate Immune Response to Infection
Ed. by S. H. E. Kaufmann, R. Medzhitov, and S. Gordon
©2004 ASM Press, Washington, D.C.

TABLE 1 The human chemokine system

Systematic name[a]	Common name[b]		Receptor(s)[c]
CXC chemokines			
CXCL1	GROα	Growth-related protein α	CXCR2
CXCL2	GROβ	Growth-related protein β	CXCR2
CXCL3	GROγ	Growth-related protein γ	CXCR2
CXCL5	ENA-78	Epithelial cell-derived neutrophil activating peptide 78	CXCR2
CXCL6	GCP-2	Granulocyte chemotactic protein 2	CXCR1,-2
CXCL7	NAP-2	Neutrophil-activating peptide 2	CXCR2
CXCL8	IL-8	Interleukin 8	CXCR1,-2
CXCL9	Mig	Monocyte/macrophage-activating, IFN-γ-inducible protein	CXCR3
CXCL10	IP-10	IFN-γ-inducible 10-kDa protein	CXCR3
CXCL11	I-TAC	IFN-inducible T-cell alpha chemoattractant	CXCR3
CXCL12	SDF-1	Stromal cell-derived factor 1	CXCR4
CXCL13	BCA-1	B-cell attracting chemokine 1	CXCR5
CXCL14	BRAK	Breast and kidney chemokine	n.d.
CXCL16			CXCR6
CC chemokines			
CCL1	I-309	Intercrine-β glycoprotein 309	CCR8
CCL2	MCP-1	Monocyte chemoattractant protein 1	CCR2
CCL3	MIP-1α	Macrophage inflammatory protein α	CCR1,-5
CCL4	MIP-1β	Macrophage inflammatory protein β	CCR5
CCL5	RANTES	Regulated on activation normal T-cell expressed and secreted	CCR1,-3,-5
CCL7	MCP-3	Monocyte chemoattractant protein 3	CCR1,-2,-3
CCL8	MCP-2	Monocyte chemoattractant protein 2	CCR1,-2,-3,-5
CCL11	Eotaxin	Eosinophil chemoattractant protein	CCR3
CCL13	MCP-4	Monocyte chemoattractant protein 4	CCR2,-3
CCL14	HCC-1	Hemofiltrate CC chemokine 1	CCR1
CCL15	HCC-2	Hemofiltrate CC chemokine 2	CCR1,-3
CCL16	HCC-4	Hemofiltrate CC chemokine 4	n.d.
CCL17	TARC	Thymus- and activation-regulated chemokine	CCR4
CCL18	DC-CK1	Dendritic cell chemokine 1	n.d.
CCL19	ELC	Epstein-Barr virus-induced receptor (EBI1) ligand chemokine	CCR7
CCL20	LARC	Liver- and activation-regulated chemokine	CCR6
CCL21	SLC	Secondary lymphoid tissue chemokine	CCR7
CCL22	MDC	Macrophage-derived chemokine	CCR4
CCL23	MIP-3	Macrophage inflammatory protein 3	CCR1
CCL24	Eotaxin-2	Eosinophil chemoattractant protein 2	CCR3
CCL25	TECK	Thymus-expressed chemokine	CCR9
CCL26	Eotaxin-3	Eosinophil chemoattractant protein 3	CCR3
CCL27	CTACK	Cutaneous T-cell attracting chemokine	CCR10
CCL28	MEC	Mucosa-associated epithelial chemokine	CCR3,-10
C chemokines			
XCL1	Ltn-α	Lymphotactin α	XCR1
XCL2	Ltn-β	Lymphotactin β	XCR1
CX₃C chemokine			
CX₃CL1	Fractalkine		CX₃CR1

[a]Systematic nomenclature as defined in http://cytokine.medic.kumamoto-u.ac.jp. Numerical gaps designate positions for orphan chemokines (such as CXCL4/platelet factor 4) or mammalian chemokines with unknown human homologues.
[b]One of several traditional names that is frequently used in the literature.
[c]Agonistic receptor selectivity; n.d., not determined.

proteins (G proteins) (Pierce et al., 2002). Experiments with *Bordetella pertussis* toxin indicated that these receptors typically require G proteins of the G_i type for signal transduction (Baggiolini et al., 1997; Loetscher et al., 2000; Moser et al., 1998; Murphy et al., 2000; Murphy, 2002). Biochemical and functional analysis with IL-8 and related chemokines demonstrated that neutrophils express two types of IL-8 receptors, CXCR1 with selectivity for IL-8 and GCP-2, and CXCR2 with promiscuous binding of IL-8 and numerous other related CXC chemokines (Moser et al., 1991; Schnitzel et al., 1991), and the subsequent cloning of the corresponding cDNAs confirmed this observation (Holmes et al., 1991; Murphy and Tiffany, 1991). Incidentally, the cDNA for a rabbit IL-8 receptor was already published in 1990 but was originally mistaken for a rabbit formyl-peptide receptor. There are considerable species differences, as demonstrated by the presence of a single IL-8 receptor in rabbits and mice but not rats and humans and the lack of an IL-8 homologue in mice but not rabbits or humans.

Sequence information together with simple binding and functional assays led to the cloning of additional chemokine receptors, giving rise to a total of 18 currently known human chemokine receptors, which are abbreviated according to their ligand selectivity (Table 2).

Interestingly, structure conservation and chromosomal localization of the corresponding genes correlate with the expression profile of chemokine receptors in leukocyte subsets. CXC and CC chemokine receptors with function in effector leukocytes (monocytes, granulocytes, NK cells, and activated T cells) form two separate groups with highest amino acid identity, and their genes cluster on human chromosomes 2q34-35 and 3p21-24, respectively. By contrast, chemokine receptors that are not involved in the mobilization of inflammatory leukocytes show lowest amino acid sequence identity, and their genes are spread over many human chromosomes. Similar observations were made for genes encoding chemokines. Relatedness of chemokines and receptors with their function in inflammation

TABLE 2 Cellular distribution of human chemokine receptors

Receptor	Expression[a]	Function[b]
CXCR1,-2	Neutrophils (monocyte/macrophages, eosinophils, basophils, NK cells)	I
CXCR3	Activated T cells, Th1 > Th2 (B cells)	I
CXCR4	Hematopoietic precursors, mature leukocytes, plasma cells	H
CXCR5	B cells, T_{FH} cells	H
CXCR6	Activated T cells, Th1 > Th2	I/H
CCR1	Activated T cells, NK cells, DCs, monocyte/macrophages, eosinophils, basophils (neutrophils)	I
CCR2	Activated T cells, NK cells, B cells, monocyte/macrophages (neutrophils)	I
CCR3	Th2 cells, eosinophils, basophils	I
CCR4	T cells, DCs, NK cells, thymocytes	I/H
CCR5	Th1 cells, DCs, monocytes/macrophages	I
CCR6	T and B cells, DCs, hematopoietic precursors	I/H
CCR7	Naïve T cells, T_{CM} cells, B cells, DCs	H
CCR8	Activated T cells, thymocytes (B cells, monocytes/macrophages)	I/H
CCR9	Activated (gut-homing) T cells, thymocytes	I/H
CCR10	Activated (skin-homing) T cells	I/H
XCR1	Activated T cells, NK cells	I
CX₃CR1	Activated T cells, NK cells, monocytes/macrophages	I

[a]Chemokine receptor expression in leukocyte subsets; subsets of minor importance are in parentheses. Abbreviations: NK cells, natural killer cells.

[b]The broad classification of chemokine receptor involvement in homeostatic (H) or inflammatory (I) situations; I/H indicates dual or not fully defined functions.

is further underscored in the promiscuous chemokine receptor selectivity; i.e., inflammatory chemokine receptors bind more than one chemokine (up to nine chemokines for CCR1 and CCR3) and inflammatory chemokines frequently interact with more than one receptor. Again, this contrasts with chemokine systems controlling basal leukocyte traffic, which are frequently monogamous (Tables 1 and 2).

Chemokine Receptor Signaling

The principal signaling elements of G-protein-coupled receptors (GPCRs) are, as implied by their classification, heterotrimeric G proteins composed of one GTP-binding α subunit (out of 16), one β subunit (out of 5), and one γ subunit (out of 12). Typically, agonist binding induces conformational changes in GPCRs, which results in the exchange of GDP with GTP in receptor-associated G protein (Pierce et al., 2002). As such, chemokine receptors (as well as all other GPCRs) function in their active conformation as guanine nucleotide exchange factors. GTP-bound G_i proteins are in an active state, dislocate from the receptor, and dissociate into GTP-bound $G\alpha_i$ subunits and G$\beta\gamma$ heterodimers, which then stimulate a myriad of second messengers (Loetscher et al., 2000; Pierce et al., 2002; Thelen, 2001). For GTP-bound $G\alpha_i$ subunits these include adenylyl cyclase (inhibition) and c-Src-related nonreceptor tyrosine kinases; for G$\beta\gamma$ dimers these are phospholipase Cβ (PLCβ) isoforms, G-protein-coupled receptor kinases (GRKs), and phosphatidylinositol 3-kinase-γ (PI3Kγ). Activation of phosphatidylinositol-specific PLCβ isoforms results in the generation of inositol-1,3,5-triphosphate (InsP3) and diacylglycerol (DAG); InsP3 rapidly induces the release of Ca^{2+} from intracellular stores, which among other effects is required for modulating the adhesive properties of migrating cells, and DAG activates protein kinase C (PKC), which contributes to several cellular responses as well as negative feedback regulation of chemokine receptor function (see below). PLCβ is required for chemokine-mediated Ca^{2+} mobilization, a response widely used to evaluate chemokine receptor interaction and cellular desensitization (see below), whereas in vitro chemotactic migration does not depend on this enzyme. PI3Kγ, a key effector in chemokine receptor signal transduction, controls protein kinase B (PKB) activation, which leads to cellular desensitization, but also signals along the mitogen-activated protein kinase (MAPK) cascade via activation of extracellular signal-regulated protein kinase (ERK) (Loetscher et al., 2000; Thelen, 2001). PI3Kγ-null mice show severely impaired chemokine receptor signaling; however, chemotactic migration is only moderately affected, suggesting that alternative, perhaps G-protein-independent, signaling pathways control this prototype chemokine response (Thelen, 2001). Signal transmission by the GTP-bound $G\alpha_i$ subunits is terminated by the GTP-to-GDP hydrolysis action of regulators of G-protein signaling, a process known to affect the duration of signal transduction and, consequently, cellular responses to chemokines and other agonists of GPCRs. GDP-bound $G\alpha_i$ subunits and G$\beta\gamma$ dimers reassemble to form "resting" heterotrimeric G_i proteins for renewed receptor engagement.

Recent exciting progress focuses on the recognition that certain GPCRs also signal by G-protein-independent mechanisms (Pierce et al., 2002). By means of direct contact or via scaffolding or adaptor proteins, GPCRs activate c-Src kinase and Janus kinase (JAK), leading to ERK and MAPK and JAK signal transducers and activators of transcription (STAT) signaling. Also, β arrestins function as scaffolding proteins and, upon receptor binding (see below), induce the activation of two MAPK cascades via binding and stimulation of MAPK regulators c-Jun–amino-terminal kinase-3 (JNK3), ERK, Raf, and MEK (MAPK kinase [Pierce et al., 2002]). The β-arrestin signaling pathway is involved in the control of CXCR1-mediated granule release (Barlic et al., 2000). Some GPCRs are known to form homo- or heterodimers or even larger aggregates, but it is presently not clear if such structures are essential for chemokine-mediated signaling. In support, one group reported dimerization of chemokine receptors (such as CXCR4, CCR2, or CCR5) and suggested that higher-order structure formation is a prerequisite for chemokine receptor signaling (Rodriguez-Frade et al., 2001). Heterodimerization between CXCR4 and a mutant form of CCR2 (CCRbY139F) was proposed to account for the observed delay in disease progression in human immunodeficiency virus type 1 (HIV-1)-infected individuals carrying this genetic abnormality (Rodriguez-Frade et al., 2001).

Fine-Tuning of Chemokine Responses

Rapid initiation and short duration are hallmarks of chemokine-mediated cellular responses. Efficient mechanisms for termination of chemokine receptor signaling include receptor sequestration (cell surface depletion) and receptor downmodulation (internalization followed by lysosomal degradation). These negative-feedback regulatory mechanisms are responsible for fine-tuning cellular responses and occur even in the continuous presence of chemokines, a phenomenon known as cellular desensitization. Two types of cellular desensitization, both involving receptor phosphorylation, are recognized (Pierce et al., 2002). GRKs mediate homologous desensitization by phosphorylating Ser and/or Thr residues in the intracellular C-terminal regions of agonist-occupied but not free (inactive) receptors. GRK phosphorylation sites target β arrestins to the receptor, thereby preventing further G-protein activation. Subsequently, these agonist–receptor–β-arrestin complexes are internalized via clathrin-coated pits and directed to endosomal compartments for dephosphorylation and cell surface recycling or, alternatively, to lysosomal compartments for proteolytic degradation. As mentioned above and in addition to receptor desensitization, β arrestins contribute to cellular responses by linking agonist-occupied receptors with MAPK cascade elements. Protein kinase A and C also phosphorylate GPCRs, but these kinases inactivate, in addi-

tion to agonist-occupied receptors, alternative unoccupied receptors as well, a process termed heterologous desensitization. A novel mechanism of cellular desensitization was recently ascribed to the anti-inflammatory cytokine IL-10, which was shown to induce in monocytes and dendritic cells (DCs) the uncoupling of chemokine receptors from G proteins, thereby functioning as decoy (chemokine-neutralizing) receptors (D'Amico et al., 2000). Modulation of chemokine responses by altering chemokine receptor gene expression, transcript stability, or protein synthesis is a slow process and may not contribute to immediate changes in chemokine responses. Although chemokines directly influence cellular desensitization, induction of chemokine production for fine-tuning cellular responses in an autocrine or paracrine fashion is also time-consuming but may be an efficient method for leukocyte redirection in response to alternative chemokines (Foxman et al., 1997).

LEUKOCYTE MOBILIZATION AND OTHER CHEMOKINE FUNCTIONS

IL-8 was identified, purified, and sequenced on the basis of its potent in vitro neutrophil chemoattractant activity, and it is this functional property, together with a four-Cys-residue fingerprint arrangement, that prompted the term chemokines for "chemotactic cytokines" to embrace this group of cytokines (Lindley et al., 1991). Accordingly, a protein with structural similarity to chemokines but undefined chemoattractant function, such as platelet α-granule-derived platelet factor 4, is not a chemokine and at best is considered as a candidate or "orphan" chemokine. Also, "classical" chemoattractant agonists lacking the chemokine-typical structural motifs, such as complement component C5a, lipid derivatives leukotrienes and platelet-activating factor, and bacterial N-formylmethionyl peptides, do not belong to the chemokine family. Currently, there are only a few orphan chemokines left for functional characterization and these are not included in the official list of chemokines. As emphasized below, chemokines control

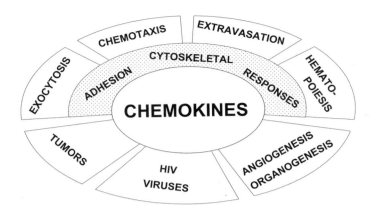

FIGURE 1 Remarkable diversity in chemokine function. Leukocyte chemotaxis is the prototype function of chemokines, which requires rapid and transient changes in cytoskeletal arrangements and adhesive interactions with extracellular matrices. Extravasation includes the transendothelial migration of bloodborne leukocytes, whereas chemotaxis is the directional movement of leukocytes along a chemoattractant gradient within the tissue. Chemokine-mediated cell migration as well as migration-unrelated functions may also affect hematopoiesis and aspects of exocytosis (and possibly other effector functions). Certain chemokines also function in tissue cells and may control, in part, secondary tumor formation, angiogenesis, and organogenesis. Finally, chemokines of viral or human origin play multiple roles in viral infections.

leukocyte mobility, but the functional diversity of many chemokines goes far beyond this prototypical effect on leukocytes (Fig. 1).

Leukocyte Recruitment and Localization

Mobility is a hallmark property of hematopoietic cells, and immunological defense largely depends on finely tuned orchestration of leukocyte mobilization and localization by chemokines. Today, it is clear that all types of hematopoietic cells respond to one or more chemokines, including neutrophils, eosinophils, basophils, mast cells, monocytes, T and B cells, and megakaryocytes and platelets (Baggiolini et al., 1994; Hamada et al., 1998; Lin et al., 2000; Loetscher et al., 2000; Moser et al., 1998; Moser and Loetscher, 2001). Typically, inflammatory leukocytes, as defined by their presence at sites of acute or chronic inflammation, express multiple chemokine receptors and respond to numerous chemokines, whereas "noneffector" leukocytes, such as resting T and B cells present in peripheral blood, primary lymphoid organs (bone marrow and thymus), or peripheral tissues, are

more restricted in their chemokine selectivity and generally do not respond to inflammatory chemokines. Because function and traffic pattern are interrelated, chemokines and their receptors have become highly useful tools for the functional characterization of leukocyte subsets, such as type 1 T-helper (Th1) and Th2 cells, which differ in the repertoire of chemokine receptors and responsiveness to chemokines (Loetscher et al., 2000; Moser and Loetscher, 2001; Sallusto et al., 2000). Other examples of leukocytes with distinct migration properties are DCs as well as subsets of T and B cells in peripheral blood and lymphoid tissues.

Relocation of circulating leukocytes involves extravasation, which is the migration of blood leukocytes across the vascular endothelium, and their subsequent migration to distinct microanatomical sites. Transendothelial migration and chemotaxis of leukocytes are highly complex processes, which are controlled by "inside-out" and "outside-in" signaling events during the adhesive interactions of leukocytes with tissue cells or extracellular matrix (Serrador et al., 1999). Many details are still poorly understood, but recent developments are beginning to shed light onto certain mechanistic aspects of cell movement. In essence, leukocyte chemotaxis can be summarized by the following sequential steps. (i) The cell forms a leading edge composed of actin polymerization-driven membrane protrusions called lamellae. Chemokines contribute to this cellular polarization, and chemokine receptors are frequently concentrated at the front of the moving cell. (ii) The cell attaches to the substratum by means of focal adhesions involving actin filaments, actin-binding proteins (vinculin, paxillin), adhesion receptors (integrins), and their extracellular ligands as well as kinases (focal adhesion kinase). (iii) Myosin-based motor forces are engaged to generate traction and polarized contractile motions. (iv) The rear end of the cell is released by disengagement of integrins and their extracellular ligands, which will allow the completion of the forward motion. In addition to the leading edge, a rear-end structure, called uropod, is recognized in the polarized (moving) lymphocytes. This stalklike cytoplasmic extension concentrates numerous adhesion molecules, microtubule-organizing center, and Golgi organelles and is believed to allow contact between moving cells (Serrador et al., 1999).

Early experiments in mice treated with *B. pertussis* toxin indicated that certain steps during leukocyte transendothelial migration are controlled by GPCRs, possibly chemokine receptors (Spangrude et al., 1984), and this was confirmed in recent studies (Campbell and Butcher, 2000). Transendothelial migration is initiated by the interaction of selectins (or low-affinity integrins) present on blood leukocytes with their ligands on endothelial cells, resulting in a tethering and rolling motion (Butcher et al., 1999; Springer, 1994). Leukocytes only come to a full stop through the action of integrins and their ligands on endothelial cells, and it is this adhesion step that is controlled by chemokines. Triggering of chemokine receptors in leukocytes by endothelia-associated chemokines induces a rapid and transient increase in integrin affinity and avidity, which results in firm leukocyte adhesion. The subsequent steps are not well understood and include the actual movement of adherent leukocytes across the endothelial cell layer and the underlying basement membrane and their "release" into the tissue. Of note, only those types of leukocytes which are capable of responding to the chemokines present on the local endothelium are able to transmigrate at a given vascular site. In other words, chemokines and their receptors largely determine the selectivity in leukocyte extravasation. For example, T and B cells with receptors for chemokines present in secondary lymphoid tissues will not be recruited to inflammatory sites but instead are destined to recirculate through spleen, lymph nodes (LNs), and Peyer's patches (PPs). By contrast, effector cells bearing receptors for inflammatory chemokines are efficiently recruited to sites of inflammation and disease. This leukocyte traffic control function forms the basis for the development of chemokine-based anti-inflammatory therapy (see below).

Hematopoiesis

Early reports provided evidence for a direct involvement of certain chemokines in the growth and differentiation of bone marrow progenitor cells (Broxmeyer et al., 1989). Today, however, the principal contributions of chemokines to hematopoiesis are believed to be their role as navigators of hematopoietic precursors. Considerable data highlight the important contribution by SDF-1/CXCL12, a chemokine constitutively produced by bone marrow stromal cells, in myelo- and B lymphopoiesis. Mice with defective SDF-1 or CXCR4 genes die at late embryonic stages (>E15.5) and present multiple severe abnormalities, including drastically impaired myelo- and B lymphopoiesis as well as defects in heart septum, nervous tissue, and intestinal blood vessel development (Nagasawa, 2000). T lymphopoiesis is not affected, which may be explained by the numerous chemokines shown to be involved in thymocyte development (see below). The SDF-1(CXCR4) system is monogamous, i.e., mice lacking either SDF-1 or CXCR4 show identical phenotypes, which is in contrast to the apparent functional redundancy in chemokine systems controlling inflammatory responses. SDF-1 is chemotactic for hematopoietic progenitor cells and lineage-restricted CD34$^+$ progenitor cells, which express CXCR4 (Aiuti et al., 1997; Deichmann et al., 1997; Wright et al., 2002). For B-lineage cells, SDF-1 is required during the earliest stage of B-cell development, targeting Lin$^-$ CD19$^-$ c-kit^+ IL-7Ra$^+$ B-cell precursors, and responsiveness to SDF-1 is gradually substituted toward late stages of B-cell development by newly acquired responsiveness to LN chemokines SLC/CCL21, ELC/CCL19, and BCA-1/CXCL13 (Bowman et al., 2000; D'Apuzzo et al., 1997; Egawa et al., 2001). Furthermore, SDF-1 controls the homing of adoptively transferred hematopoietic progenitor cells and newly generated plasma cells to the bone marrow, underscoring its unique role in the control of leukocyte traffic in this primary lymphoid tissue (Hargreaves et al., 2001; Kawabata et al., 1999; Ma et al., 1999; Onai et al., 2000).

Interestingly, numerous chemokines, including SDF-1, CXCL16, TARC/CCL17, ELC, SLC, MDC/CCL22, and TECK/CCL25, are present in the thymus and appear to contribute to thymocyte development (Ansel and Cyster, 2001; Kim and Broxmeyer, 1999; Savino et al., 2002). However, their roles must be overlapping since mice with deletions in single chemokine genes do not show abnormal T lymphopoiesis. The apparent redundancy in chemokine function within the thymus is striking and contrasts the singular importance of SDF-1 in myelo- and B lymphopoiesis. CD4$^-$CD8$^-$ double-negative T-cell lineage-committed bone marrow progenitor cells home to the subcapsular region of the thymic cortex, where they start to undergo sequential maturation steps. CD4$^+$CD8$^+$ double-positive thymocytes are the subsequent stage of development and undergo positive selection in the cortex. Surviving thymocytes move into the central region (medulla) of the thymus and turn into mature CD4$^+$ or CD8$^+$ single-positive cells. Finally, following elimination of autoreactive cells by negative selection, mature thymocytes bearing functional VαVβ or VγVδ T-cell antigen receptors exit the thymus at the corticomedullary junction. Obviously, the complex pattern of thymocyte relocation and contact formation with thymic DCs and stromal cells is tightly controlled by chemokines. SDF-1 is primarily involved in cortical functions, whereas TECK acts on both the cortical double-negative and the medullary double-positive cells, MDC and TARC attract negatively selected double- and single-positive cells in the medulla, and SLC and ELC are thought to enable the exit of mature thymocytes out of the thymus. The role of additional chemokines with expression in the thymus, including gamma interferon (IFN-γ)-inducible chemokines Mig/CXCL9, IP-10/CXCL10, and I-TAC/CXCL11 and the cell-associated chemokine CXCL16 and I-309/CCL1, is not clear at present.

Modulation of Leukocyte Effector Functions

Rapid and transient shape changes via cytoskeletal rearrangements and modulation of adhesion to integrin substrates are essential elements in leukocyte transendothelial migration and chemotaxis, and these responses were shown early on to be mediated by IL-8 in neutrophils. Today, modulation of integrin function is attributed to all chemokines. In addition, IL-8 was found to induce migration-unrelated neutrophil responses, such as granule exocytosis and respiratory burst activation (Baggiolini et al., 1994). It is clear that numerous chemokines are involved in shaping innate and adaptive immune responses by modulating effector functions, notably the release of preformed granule components in granulocytes, NK cells, and cytotoxic T cells (Fig. 1). Possibly, chemokines also contribute to differentiation and cytokine production in T cells, although these effects were seen only in the presence of other stimuli. Additional involvement of chemokines in leukocyte cell growth, survival, and apoptosis, which may depend on gene expression, needs further studies. Collectively, there is an increasing amount of evidence in support of a role for chemokines in the modulation of rapid and transient leukocyte effector functions, such as the release of preformed proteins and possibly cytokine synthesis.

Viral Chemokine and Chemokine Receptor Homologues

During coevolution of viruses and mammalian species, substantial exchange of genetic material occurred, resulting in accumulation of viral DNA in the genome of the host as well as in the "highjacking" of host DNA by viruses. From the point of view of viruses, their life cycles need to be optimized for efficient survival, i.e., invasion of the host should allow for efficient viral growth and dissemination while preserving the physiological integrity of the host. Herpes-, pox-, and retroviruses carry numerous genes for homologues (or "mimics") of chemokines and chemokine receptors as well as genes for unrelated (and presumably noncaptured) proteins with chemoattractant-related functions (McFadden and Murphy, 2000; Murphy, 2001). These virus-encoded proteins function either as leukocyte chemoattractants or receptors for chemoattractants, chemokine receptor antagonists, chemokine scavenger proteins, viral entry receptors or modulators of host cell physiology, and are thought to control evasion of the host immune system as well as viral replication and transmission, thereby critically determining viral infectivity and pathogenicity. For example, several herpesvirus-encoded proteins are bona fide chemokine receptors, including the IL-8 receptor ECRF3 in herpesvirus saimiri, or the highly promiscuous chemokine receptor US28 in human cytomegalovirus, which binds MIP-1α, MIP-1β, RANTES, MCP-1, MCP-3, and fractalkine as well as gp120 glycoprotein of HIV-1 (see below). The Kaposi's sarcoma-associated *ORF74* gene encodes a constantly active chemokine receptor, which may directly contribute to Kaposi's sarcoma pathology by means of its oncogenic and angiogenic function. Of note, the function of the ORF74 receptor is either enhanced or downmodulated by chemokines, suggesting that inhibitory chemokines may be used therapeutically. Interesting viral chemokine mimics include the herpesvirus 8-encoded vMIP-I and vMIP-III, which are agonistic, and the broad-range chemokine receptor antagonist vMIP-II. Several viral chemokine mimics are functionally related to chemokines that target cells of the innate immune system, suggesting that modulating the acute-phase antiviral response may be advantageous to the virus. Soluble chemokine scavengers of viral origin, such as herpesvirus 68-encoded M3 or poxvirus-encoded T1, M-T7, and vCBP-2, can neutralize certain chemokines and thus are of some therapeutic interest.

HIV Pathogenesis

In the mid-1980s the hypothesis of soluble, T-cell-derived HIV-1 suppressor factors was formulated (Walker et al., 1986). Similarly, it was known for a long time that CD4, the primary HIV-1 receptor on target cells, is required but not sufficient for mediating viral entry, indicating that alternative "coreceptors" need to be present (Maddon et al., 1986). It took 10 years of intensive investigation to discover that these critical elements are certain chemokines and chemokine receptors, a breakthrough that propelled the field of HIV research to new heights (Cairns and D'Souza, 1998; Loetscher et al., 2000; Moore, 1997; Moser, 1997). At the end of 1995 Cocchi and colleagues reported that the human T-cell-derived chemokines RANTES, MIP-1α, and MIP-1β blocked HIV-1 entry into CD4$^+$ target cells, and in early 1996 Berger's group identified the HIV-1 coreceptor activity of CXCR4 (Cocchi et al., 1995; Feng et al., 1996). In quick succession and unparalleled collaborative efforts, CXCR4 and CCR5 were demonstrated to be the major HIV-1 coreceptors, and the chemokines they bind (SDF-1 for CXCR4, and RANTES, MIP-1α, and MIP-1β for CCR5) were shown to block infection of target cells by HIV-1 (as well as HIV-2 and simian immunodeficiency virus [SIV]) (Fig. 2). Many more chemokine receptors function as HIV/SIV coreceptors in vitro but their importance in the pathophysiology of HIV-1 infection is questionable. Today, there is evidence for the existence of additional, chemokine-unrelated factors that modulate HIV-1 pathogenesis and disease progression, and structural and functional studies will be required to determine their importance in this disease. Clearly, CXCR4 and CCR5 are considered to be the major HIV-1 coreceptors. The distribution of CXCR4 and CCR5 among CD4$^+$ target cells determines viral tropism, i.e., the range of blood and tissue cells that may become infected by a particular type of virus. Consequently, HIV/SIV that require CCR5 for target cell entry are referred to as R5 viruses, those that are selective for CXCR4 are termed X4 viruses, and dual-tropic viruses that use either chemokine receptor as HIV/SIV coreceptors are designated as X4R5 viruses. R5 HIV-1 is far more infectious than X4 HIV-1 and predominates in newly infected individuals, whereas X4 HIV-1 particles are frequently observed in individuals with AIDS.

The importance of CCR5 in HIV-1 infection is underscored by the discovery of the mutant CCR5 gene *CCR5(Δ32)*, encoding a truncated, nonfunctional CCR5 variant (Cairns and D'Souza, 1998; Loetscher et al.,

2000; Moore, 1997; Moser, 1997). CD4$^+$ macrophages and T cells of individuals who are homozygous for this defect resist infection by R5 HIV-1 variants. Furthermore, exposed but noninfected individuals (e.g., certain sex workers or individuals with highly promiscuous sexual behavior) carry the *CCR5(Δ32)* allele more frequently than healthy, uninfected individuals, whereas the homozygous *CCR5(Δ32)* defect is not found among individuals with primary HIV-1 infections. These studies suggest that deletion of functional CCR5 correlates with protection from HIV-1 infection. In rare cases, individuals carrying the homozygous *CCR5(Δ32)* mutation were infected with X4 HIV-1 variants. Of interest, the *CCR5(Δ32)* allele is present in Caucasians but not Asians or Africans, and its exceptional high frequency suggests that it has evolved as recently as a few thousand years ago. Other less frequent genotypes affecting CCR5 function and thus infectivity by R5 viruses have also been described (Cairns and D'Souza, 1998; Loetscher et al., 2000; Moore, 1997; Moser, 1997). Genetic variations in the CXCR4 gene that may affect infection by X4 viruses, on the other hand, have not been found and, based on the severe defects in mice lacking this chemokine receptor, are unlikely to exist.

Two issues with regard to the role of chemokines in HIV-1 pathology need to be pointed out. First, the principal chemokine

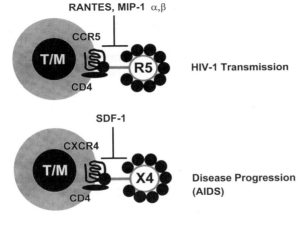

FIGURE 2 CCR5 and CXCR4 are the two major HIV-1 coreceptors. HIV-1 (as well as HIV-2 and SIV) requires CD4 and one of two chemokine receptors, termed HIV/SIV coreceptors, for entry into target cells, which include T cells and monocytes and macrophages (T/M). Coreceptor selectivity determines viral tropism; accordingly, CCR5 or CXCR4 usage defines R5 or X4 viruses. RANTES, MIP-1α, and MIP-1β with selectivity for CCR5, and SDF-1 with selectivity for CXCR4, inhibit target cell entry of R5 and X4 HIV/SIV, respectively, and are referred to as HIV/SIV suppressor factors. R5 HIV-1 particles predominate during viral transmission and the asymptomatic phase of the disease, whereas the appearance of X4 HIV-1 particles correlates with progression to AIDS.

function, the control of leukocyte traffic, is apparently of no relevance in this viral disease. Rather, HIV/SIV have learned to exploit some (but not all) chemokine receptors for gaining access to the proper target cells. Only secondarily, chemokines and their receptors may contribute to HIV-1 pathophysiology by controlling the dissemination of infected cells. It is still not clear why some other chemokine receptors with similar cellular distribution as CCR5 (such as CXCR3 or CCR2) do not function as principal HIV/SIV coreceptors. Second, CXCR4 and CCR5 differ fundamentally in terms of cellular distribution and function. CCR5 is thought to guide effector leukocytes, such as activated $CD4^+$ T cells, to inflammatory sites, whereas CXCR4 has multiple functions and is broadly expressed in all types of leukocytes, hematopoietic progenitor cells, and even many tissue cells. Perhaps the broad range of target cells for X4 viruses may explain the observed correlation between the appearance of X4 HIV-1 particles in infected individuals and disease acceleration (progression to AIDS).

Effects on Tissue Cells

The remarkable abnormalities in organogenesis in CXCR4 (or SDF-1)-deficient mice illustrate that chemokine functions can easily surpass the boundaries of immune processes. Yet this area of chemokine research is still in its infancy. Among the diverse chemokine effects observed in tissue cells, those affecting angiogenesis are best studied (Belperio et al., 2000). In essence, CXC chemokines are either angiogenic or angiostatic, whereas CC chemokines have no such activity. The angiogenic feature was attributed to the presence of the glutamine-leucine-arginine (ELR) sequence motif in the N-terminal region of IL-8 and related chemokines, and its absence in certain CXC chemokines, such as Mig and IP-10, was found to correlate with inhibition of angiogenesis. There is no evidence that mice lacking the corresponding chemokine receptors, CXCR2 or CXCR3, have altered wound healing or tumor growth properties, suggest-

ing that the observed effects were mediated by alternative receptors, such as proteoglycans or growth factor receptors. Yet tissue cells, such as endothelial cells, keratinocytes, neurons, and numerous tumor cells, were shown to express several chemokine receptors (in addition to the widespread CXCR4), but their contribution to tissue cell physiology remains to be determined. Possible functions include induction of apoptosis, as shown for CXCR4 in neurons, or cell survival, or regulation of cell proliferation and differentiation. For example, early reports documented a mitogenic role for melanoma growth-stimulatory activity, alternatively called GROα, for growth-regulated *GRO* gene product α (Dhawan and Richmond, 2002). Also, SDF-1 was originally described as pre-B-cell growth stimulating factor (Nagasawa et al., 1994), whereas IL-8 on the other hand was shown to inhibit proliferation of non-small cell cancer lines (Wang et al., 1996). Finally, recent reports demonstrated the involvement of chemokines in tumor metastasis, a finding that seems to be related to the chemokine-typical control of leukocyte traffic (Muller et al., 2001). Although tissue cell recruitment and localization may be fundamental roles played by chemokines in tissue remodeling and secondary tumor formation, elucidation of leukocyte mobilization–unrelated functions is one of the major topics in current chemokine research.

ROLE OF CHEMOKINES IN INITIATION OF IMMUNE RESPONSES

Our knowledge about the involvement of chemokines in acute and primary immune responses as well as inflammatory diseases is substantial and underscores the importance of chemokines in the control of leukocyte traffic (Gerard and Rollins, 2001; Godessart and Kunkel, 2001). In the remainder of this review I concentrate on exciting recent topics in chemokine research, including leukocyte recruitment and localization during the course of adaptive immune responses and secondary lymphoid tissue neogenesis.

Inflammatory and Homeostatic Chemokines

As an alternative to the structural motif-based chemokine classification (CXC, CC, C, and CX_3C chemokines), a function-based division into inflammatory and homeostatic chemokines turned out to be very practical for the discussion of diverse immune processes (Loetscher et al., 2000; Moser and Loetscher, 2001). It is not a strict classification and some chemokines appear to fulfill a dual function. For example, inflammatory chemokines (among other substances) that are present at inflammatory sites can drain to local LNs and even participate in the leukocyte recruitment process (Janatpour et al., 2001; Palframan et al., 2001). As such, secondary lymphoid tissues may adjust their cell recruitment profile accordingly to changes in the immune status of local tissues. Inflammatory chemokines are produced by almost all types of blood and tissue cells when exposed to inflammatory conditions, such as proinflammatory cytokines IL-1, tumor necrosis factor alpha, or bacterial endotoxins, or during immune engagement such as T-cell activation during antigen recognition. They target effector leukocytes of both the innate (granulocytes, monocytes, NK cells) and adaptive (Th1, Th2, cytotoxic T cells) immune system, which express the corresponding receptors. Importantly, changes in the diversity of local chemokines during ongoing inflammatory processes directly affect the composition of the inflammatory infiltrates and, as such, dictate disease evolution. By contrast, the production of homeostatic chemokines is inflammation independent and underlies constitutive control at discrete locations within primary (bone marrow, thymus) and secondary (LNs, PPs, spleen) lymphoid tissues and peripheral, extralymphoid tissues (skin, gastrointestinal tract). They target hematopoietic progenitor cells and resting mature leukocytes for homing to sites of differentiation, immune initiation, and immune surveillance. Generally, resting leukocytes, such as circulating T cells, loose the receptors for homeostatic chemokines during their development into effector cells, and this allows their redirection to inflammatory sites.

Control of Adaptive Immune Processes

Immediate responses to pathogen challenges involve the mobilization of cells of the innate immune system, which all express a variety of receptors for inflammatory chemokines. Typically, innate cells do not respond to homeostatic chemokines. Neutrophil granulocytes are often seen first, which agrees with the rapid induction of IL-8 and related chemokines in activated tissue cells, whereas effector T cells, which do not respond to these acute-phase chemokines, are typically late. Moreover, and by contrast to innate cells, effector T cells need to be specifically generated for optimal and selective neutralization of infectious particles, and this multiple-step process is time-consuming and occurs within secondary lymphoid tissues.

Substantial evidence from studies in mice argues for an essential role for SLC and ELC in the recruitment of $CCR7^+$ blood lymphocytes into the T zone of secondary lymphoid tissues (Fig. 3) (Campbell and Butcher, 2000; Cyster, 1999; Moser and Loetscher, 2001; Müller et al., 2002). Interestingly, B-cell recruitment is less affected than T-cell recruitment by genetic defects in this chemokine system, suggesting that other chemokines, including SDF-1 and BCA-1 (see below), may contribute to B-cell traffic control. Importantly, high endothelial venules-associated SLC triggers in blood $CCR7^+$ T cells firm adhesion to the endothelium and their subsequent high endothelial venule transmigration, and T-zone-expressed ELC and SLC localize freshly recruited $CCR7^+$ T cells in the antigen contact zone. Similarly, tissue DCs acquire an LN-homing program during pathogen-induced maturation, involving a switch from the prototypical antigen capture capabilities and responsiveness to inflammatory chemokines in immature DCs to expert antigen presentation and costimulation functions and CCR7 expression in mature DCs (Sallusto et

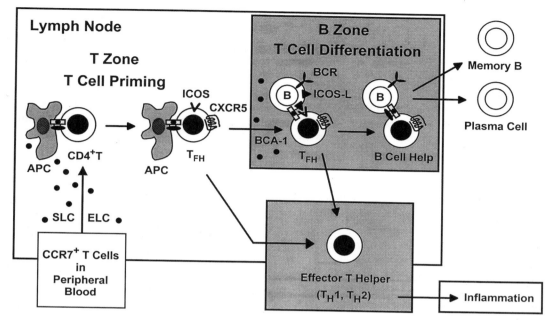

FIGURE 3 Central role of T_{FH} cells in the initiation of adaptive immune responses. The chemokines SLC and ELC direct the recruitment of CCR7-expressing peripheral blood T cells into secondary lymphoid tissues for colocalization in the T zone with CCR7+ antigen-presenting cells. Antigen recognition and costimulation result in CD4+ T-cell priming, characterized by expression of CXCR5 and certain costimulatory molecules, such as ICOS, and concomitant downmodulation of CCR7 and responsiveness to T-zone chemokines. CXCR5 characterizes T_{FH} cells, which are nonpolarized T-helper cells with unique homing properties for B-cell follicles. Through contact with antigen-presenting B cells, T_{FH} cells may develop into B helper T cells to support follicular B-cell activation and plasma cell or memory B-cell generation. Alternatively, contact with B cells induces differentiation of T_{FH} cells into effector T-helper cells, such as cytokine-producing Th1 and Th2 cells, with newly acquired homing capability for inflammatory sites. Abbreviations: APC, antigen-presenting cell; BCR, B-cell antigen receptor; ICOS, inducible costimulatory molecule; ICOS-L, ICOS ligand; T_{FH}, follicular B-helper T cell; T_H1, Th1 cell; T_H2, Th2 cell.

al., 2000). In addition, mature DCs produce high levels of ELC, which is thought to attract CCR7+ T cells for optimal antigen sampling and immune response initiation. CCR7, together with L-selectin, was proposed to serve as an address code for LN-homing T cells, which include all naive and the majority of memory αβ T cells (but not γδ T cells; see below) in peripheral blood (Sallusto et al., 1999). CCR7+ memory T cells, termed central memory T (T_{CM}) cells, are nonpolarized, i.e., have not yet acquired full effector functions, such as Th1- or Th2-type cytokine pro-

duction or target cell lysis. T_{CM} cells may form part of the long-lived memory T-cell pool, which relocate to LNs and other secondary lymphoid tissues and immediately differentiate into "second-wave" effector T cells in response to recall antigens. By contrast, the minor fraction of CCR7-negative memory T cells, termed effector memory T (T_{EM}) cells, represents terminally differentiated T cells with the full repertoire of effector functions and homing capabilities for inflammatory sites. Paradoxically, T-cell stimulation results in CCR7 expression, and CCR7+ T cells are readily detected in peripheral tissues, implying that the T_{CM}/T_{EM} cell paradigm applies primarily to resting, peripheral blood T cells.

Antigen recognition initiates a cascade of sequential steps, resulting eventually in antigen-specific effector and memory lymphocytes. Part of this process is controlled by the chemokine BCA-1 and its receptor CXCR5 (Fig. 3). BCA-1 is uniquely expressed in the B-cell follicles, predominantly in the follicular mantle and associated blood vessels, thereby differing clearly from the T-zone chemokines SLC and ELC, which are not present at these locations. BCA-1 (termed B-lymphocyte chemoattractant [BLC] in mice) was originally described as a selective chemoattractant for peripheral blood B cells, which uniformly express CXCR5 (Gunn et al., 1998; Legler et al., 1998). In addition to B cells, CXCR5 is present on a small subpopulation of CD4$^+$ memory T cells in peripheral blood, which is highly expanded in secondary lymphoid tissues, such as tonsils from patients with pharyngeal inflammation (Moser et al., 2002). Of note, CXCR5 marks recently primed, nonpolarized CD4$^+$ T cells, whereas this chemokine receptor is irreversibly lost in effector cells, such as Th1 and Th2 cells. CXCR5$^+$ T-helper cells respond well to BCA-1 and provide potent help to B cells for antibody production and, consequently, this subset of T-helper cells is now called follicular B-helper T (T_{FH}) cells (Moser et al., 2002). The fact that CXCR5 expression during antigen recognition is an early but general phenomenon in CD4$^+$ T-cell activation merits special attention and indicates that T_{FH} cells are precursors for the full range of effector T-helper cells. Furthermore, early induction of a follicular homing program (due to CXCR5 expression) suggests an unexpected role for the B-cell compartment in T-helper cell differentiation. Indeed, coculture of T_{FH} cells with B cells results not only in antibody production by newly generated plasma cells but also in subsets of T-helper cells with distinct cytokine (IFN-γ, IL-10) production profiles (L. Ebert and B. Moser, unpublished data). It is intriguing to speculate that B cells

make essential contributions to T-helper cell differentiation by presenting processed T-cell antigens in the context of appropriate costimulation (Bretscher, 1999). Following this scheme, SLC, ELC, and CCR7 would be principally involved in the recruitment of resting blood CD4$^+$ T cells and mature tissue DCs for colocalization within the T-zone, T-cell priming, and subsequent T_{FH} cell generation. Further steps in T-helper cell differentiation could be controlled in part by BCA-1, which recruits T_{FH} cells into the B-cell compartment. The large majority of CD8$^+$ T cells do not express CXCR5 and therefore are not influenced by follicular activities.

The mechanisms controlling the exit of lymphocytes within secondary lymphoid tissues are not well understood. Possibly, noninvolved T cells may become desensitized to T-zone chemokines, which allows their exit via medullary lymphatics. Plasma cell differentiation was shown to correlate with reduced responsiveness to T-zone and follicular chemokines but enhanced responsiveness to SDF-1, which may guide plasma cells to the bone marrow. Effector T cells express receptors for inflammatory chemokines and, again, by means of loss of responsiveness to LN chemokines, may relocate to pathogen-infected peripheral tissues. Similar to naive T cells, T_{CM} cells are characterized by their LN recirculation properties (CCR7$^+$, L-selectin$^+$) and may exit secondary lymphoid tissues by means of transient desensitization to LN chemokines.

LN Homing of $\gamma\delta$ T Cells

Due to their immediate cytokine production capability and NK cell-like lytic activity, peripheral blood $\gamma\delta$ T cells are regarded as members of the innate immune system (Carding and Egan, 2002). However, recent evidence supports an unexpected role for $\gamma\delta$ T cells in adaptive immunity (M. Brandes and B. Moser, unpublished data). The two major human subsets, the Vδ1$^+$ and Vδ2$^+$ T cells, differ in terms of tissue distribution and antigen selectivity. Vδ1$^+$ T cells are preferentially localized in the epithelial tissues and respond to stress-induced self-proteins and CD1-restricted lipid antigens, whereas V$\delta2^+$ T cells predominate in peripheral blood and respond to nonpeptide antigens of mostly microbial origin. In clear contrast to $\alpha\beta$ T cells, classical major histocompatibility complex molecules do not restrict antigen recognition by $\gamma\delta$ T cells. Furthermore, peripheral blood $\gamma\delta$ T cells are characterized by a uniform inflammatory migration program, which sets them clearly apart from $\alpha\beta$ T cells and fully supports their immediate (innate) involvement in inflammatory processes. Unexpectedly, antigen recognition triggers in $\gamma\delta$ T cells the expression of CCR7 and the downmodulation of the inflammatory chemokine receptors CCR2 and CCR5, which allows their redirection to local LNs where $\gamma\delta$ T cells were found to localize in the T zone and, notably, in the B-cell follicles (Brandes and Moser, unpublished data). Also, and similar to T_{FH} cells, activated $\gamma\delta$ T cells provide potent B-cell help, which may involve B-cell costimulatory molecules and suggests that $\gamma\delta$ T cells are capable of modulating humoral responses to microbial infections. Conceptually, $\gamma\delta$ T cells bridge innate and adaptive immunity by their rapid involvement in follicular (and possibly T-zone) activities, which precedes the contribution of $\alpha\beta$ T cells and B cells to antimicrobial defense.

LN Neogenesis

Follicular aggregates and LN-like structures are frequently observed at sites of chronic inflammation, such as rheumatoid arthritis, and are thought to contribute to the local inflammatory processes by means of the production of cytokines and antibodies (rheumatoid factor) (Godessart and Kunkel, 2001; Loetscher and Moser, 2002). It is interesting to note that BCA-1 was found in all extranodal lymphoid structures examined, including those present in rheumatoid arthritis, *Helicobacter pylori*-associated gastric diseases, and Sjögren's syndrome. In addition, ectopic expression of murine SLC, ELC, or BCA-1 transgenes resulted in vascularized LN-like structures with typical T-cell–B-cell partitions (Campbell and

Butcher, 2000; Cyster, 1999; Moser and Loetscher, 2001; Müller et al., 2002). Recently, murine PP ($CD3^-CD4^+$) anlage cells in mucosal tissues were found to express CXCR5 (Finke et al., 2002). BCA-1 stimulation induced cell surface lymphotoxin $\alpha1\beta2$ on PP anlage cells, which triggered lymphotoxin β receptor-positive stromal cells to initiate lymphoid tissue morphogenesis. Similarly, BCA-1 was shown to play an essential role in the development and maintenance of B-cell compartments within LNs (Ansel et al., 2000). Together, these findings provide strong evidence for critical contributions of BCA-1 and possibly the CCR7 chemokines SLC and ELC to LN activities that surpass by far the mere colocalization of lymphocytes and DCs during initiation of adaptive immune processes. Possibly, the LN morphogenic properties of certain chemokines may be exploited in the development of novel vaccination strategies.

STRUCTURE-ACTIVITY RELATION AND CHEMOKINE-BASED THERAPY

Early structure and activity relation studies have unraveled the critical role of the ELR (Glu-Leu-Arg) motif in the N-terminal region in IL-8 and related chemokines in receptor binding and induction of signaling (Clark-Lewis et al., 1995). The general importance of the N-terminal domain in other, non-ELR, chemokines was demonstrated subsequently. The ELR motif immediately precedes the first of the four conserved Cys residues and thus marks the border between the relatively free-folding N terminus of up to 12 amino acids and the rigid, globular structure of the rest of the protein (Baldwin et al., 1991; Clore et al., 1990). In IL-8, the N-terminal region by itself is not sufficient for receptor triggering. Other epitopes in the N-terminal loop region, defined by the second and the third Cys residues, were proposed to initiate interactions with the "closed" receptor, which lead to structural changes in the receptors and subsequent accommodation of the receptor "triggering" N-terminal region in IL-8 (Clark-

Lewis et al., 1995). Of note, structural variation in the N terminus of IL-8 resulted in the first IL-8 receptor antagonists and led the way for numerous synthetic chemokine variants with antagonistic activity for CXC and CC chemokine receptors. Of these the antagonists RANTES(8-68) and MetRANTES and the partial agonist aminooxypentane-RANTES attracted considerable attention because of their potent R5 HIV-1 blocking activity (Loetscher et al., 2000). In some other cases, such as SDF-1, N-terminal peptides are active on their own, suggesting that high concentrations of N-terminal epitopes may overcome the "closed" receptor conformation. Interesting new findings demonstrate that several natural chemokines also function as antagonists for "unrelated" chemokine receptors. These include Mig, IP-10, and I-TAC, the ligands for the Th1-cell-associated receptor CXCR3, which blocks the function of CCR3, a receptor involved in the control of cellular traffic during Th2-cell-driven inflammatory processes; therefore, these chemokines are thought to contribute to immune response polarization (Loetscher et al., 2001). On a similar note, the CCR3 ligand eotaxin was reported to inhibit CCR2 responses, which are associated with neuroinflammatory diseases, arthritis, and atherosclerosis (Ogilvie et al., 2001). It is possible that more chemokines with "cross-receptor" regulatory functions will be identified. It will be important to find out if individual chemokine systems, such as those operating at distinct inflammatory sites or during immune response development, in general neutralize opposing chemokine systems for gaining improved navigational control of their primary leukocyte targets.

Chemokines present in culture supernatants of activated blood or tissue cells often exist as a mixture of structure variants. Some chemokines, such as the isoforms SDF-1α and SDF-1β or Ltn-α and Ltn-β, show variations in their C-terminal domains, and these minor differences originate from gene isoforms, i.e., recently duplicated, highly homologous, and functional genes. Chemokines with N-termi-nal variations are much more frequent, and these changes are thought to be generated either during alternative processing of leader peptides or during postsecretory modifications by cell-bound or extracellular proteases. It should be emphasized that proteases may add an additional level of regulation in leukocyte traffic control because small variations in the N-terminal sequences have tremendous effects on chemokine function (Baggiolini et al., 1994, 1997; Loetscher et al., 2000). Many chemokines are characterized by a Pro residue at position 2 in their mature N terminus, making these chemokines a substrate for the dipeptidyl-peptidase CD26, which selectively cleaves off N-terminal X-P (any amino acid followed by Pro) motifs (Daelemans et al., 2000). CD26 is present on activated T cells and therefore may contribute to leukocyte infiltration at inflammatory sites by modulating local chemokine function. Other proteases that cleave chemokines include cathepsin G, matrix metalloproteinases MMP-2 and MMP-9, and plasmin; additional proteases are expected to modulate chemokine presentation, stability, potency, and receptor selectivity.

The pharmaceutical industry has elected chemokine receptors as a priority target for drug development for multiple reasons, including the recognition that the modulation of leukocyte traffic would directly affect inflammatory and autoimmune processes. Also, the function of several GPCRs (other than chemokine receptors) was already successfully blocked by small-molecular-weight compounds. The initial euphoric activities have been dampened by the discovery of numerous lead compounds with undesired cross-reactivity with other chemokine-unrelated GPCRs. Such compounds often resemble natural ligands of nonpeptide and protein receptors, such as the biogenic amine receptors (dopamine, histamine, acetylcholine receptors, adrenoreceptors, etc.), indicating that the chemokine receptor selectivity of these compounds needs to be validated on a large number of functionally distant GPCRs (Onuffer and Horuk, 2002). Also, because many inflammatory diseases involve multiple, apparently redundant chemokine systems, a single compound to a single chemokine receptor may not show drastic effects, and eventually combinatorial drug regimens need to be developed. Finally, mouse models do not faithfully reproduce many human inflammatory diseases; consequently, a large part of drug validation procedures requires costly and time-consuming primate experimentation. Still, despite these apparent setbacks, optimism prevails (as reflected by the industrial consensus to uphold chemokine receptor programs), and more encouraging results will undoubtedly be reported in the near future.

OUTLOOK

The field of chemokines has advanced with unbroken speed, as evidenced by the steady flow of original reports, from the early stages of monocyte and phagocyte recruitment to highly diverse activities in bone marrow-derived and tissue cells. It is clear that chemokines are powerful chemoattractants for leukocytes, and this function enables proper localization of leukocyte precursors during hematopoiesis in bone marrow and thymus, leukocyte contact for initiation of adaptive immunity, and effector cell recruitment to sites of inflammation. Major advances in chemokine research include the recognition that lymphocytes, in addition to monocytes and phagocytes, respond to chemokines, that HIV-1 entry into target cells and HIV-1 dissemination exquisitely depend on certain chemokine systems, and most recently that a separate network of homeostatic chemokines controls the highly complex pattern of inflammation-unrelated leukocyte traffic. It is unlikely that many new chemokines with principal function in leukocytes will be discovered in the near future, indicating that the present inventory of chemokines and their receptors will serve as an invaluable set of tools for global investigation of leukocyte relocation during all facets of immune activities and tissue remodeling processes. These studies will provide crucial information for defining therapeutic approaches for the treatment of autoimmune diseases, viral infections, and secondary tumor formation. In addition, chemokines may provide important coadjuvant functions in novel vaccination protocols. Future challenges in chemokine research are related to tissue cell responses to chemokines and include the potential effect of chemokines on tissue cell growth and differentiation during organogenesis and tissue repair.

REFERENCES

Aiuti, A., I. J. Webb, C. Bleul, T. Springer, and J. C. Gutierrez-Ramos. 1997. The chemokine SDF-1 is a chemoattractant for human CD34$^+$ hematopoietic progenitor cells and provides a new mechanism to explain the mobilization of CD34$^+$ progenitors to peripheral blood. *J. Exp. Med.* **185:**111–120.

Ansel, K. M., and J. G. Cyster. 2001. Chemokines in lymphopoiesis and lymphoid organ development. *Curr. Opin. Immunol.* **13:**172–179.

Ansel, K. M., V. N. Ngo, P. L. Hyman, S. A. Luther, R. Forster, J. D. Sedgwick, J. L. Browning, M. Lipp, and J. G. Cyster. 2000. A chemokine-driven positive feedback loop organizes lymphoid follicles. *Nature* **406:**309–314.

Baggiolini, M., B. Dewald, and B. Moser. 1994. Interleukin-8 and related chemotactic cytokines—CXC and CC chemokines. *Adv. Immunol.* **55:**97–179.

Baggiolini, M., B. Dewald, and B. Moser. 1997. Human chemokines: an update. *Annu. Rev. Immunol.* **15:**675–705.

Baldwin, E. T., I. T. Weber, R. St. Charles, J.-C. Xuan, E. Appella, M. Yamada, K. Matsushima, B. F. P. Edwards, G. M. Clore, A. M. Gronenborn, and A. Wlodawer. 1991. Crystal structure of interleukin 8: symbiosis of NMR and crystallography. *Proc. Natl. Acad. Sci. USA* **88:**502–506.

Barlic, J., J. D. Andrews, A. A. Kelvin, S. E. Bosinger, M. E. DeVries, L. Xu, T. Dobransky, R. D. Feldman, S. S. Ferguson, and D. J. Kelvin. 2000. Regulation of tyrosine kinase activation and granule release through beta-arrestin by CXCR1. *Nat. Immunol.* **1:**227–233.

Belperio, J. A., M. P. Keane, D. A. Arenberg, C. L. Addison, J. E. Ehlert, M. D. Burdick, and R. M. Strieter. 2000. CXC chemokines in angiogenesis. *J. Leukoc. Biol.* **68:**1–8.

Bowman, E. P., J. J. Campbell, D. Soler, Z. Dong, N. Manlongat, D. Picarella, R. R. Hardy, and E. C. Butcher. 2000. Developmental switches in chemokine response profiles during B cell differentiation and maturation. *J. Exp. Med.* **191:**1303–1318.

Bretscher, P. A. 1999. A two-step, two-signal model for the primary activation of precursor helper T cells. *Proc. Natl. Acad. Sci. USA* **96:**185–190.

Broxmeyer, H. E., B. Sherry, L. Lu, S. Cooper, C. Carow, S. D. Wolpe, and A. Cerami. 1989. Myelopoietic enhancing effects of murine macrophage inflammatory proteins 1 and 2 on colony formation in vitro by murine and human bone marrow granulocyte/macrophage progenitor cells. *J. Exp. Med.* **170:**1583–1594.

Butcher, E. C., M. Williams, K. Youngman, L. Rott, and M. Briskin. 1999. Lymphocyte trafficking and regional immunity. *Adv. Immunol.* **72:**209–253.

Cairns, J. S., and M. P. D'Souza. 1998. Chemokines and HIV-1 second receptors: the therapeutic connection. *Nat. Med.* **4:**563–568.

Campbell, J. J., and E. C. Butcher. 2000. Chemokines in tissue-specific and microenvironment-specific lymphocyte homing. *Curr. Opin. Immunol.* **12:**336–341.

Carding, S. R., and P. J. Egan. 2002. Gammadelta T cells: functional plasticity and heterogeneity. *Nat. Rev. Immunol.* **2:**336–345.

Clark-Lewis, I., K.-S. Kim, K. Rajarathnam, J.-H. Gong, B. Dewald, B. Moser, M. Baggiolini, and B. D. Sykes. 1995. Structure-activity relationships of chemokines. *J. Leukoc. Biol.* **57:**703–711.

Clore, G. M., E. Appella, M. Yamada, K. Matsushima, and A. M. Gronenborn. 1990. Three-dimensional structure of interleukin 8 in solution. *Biochemistry* **29:**1689–1696.

Cocchi, F., A. L. DeVico, A. Garzino-Demo, S. K. Arya, R. C. Gallo, and P. Lusso. 1995. Identification of RANTES, MIP-1α, and MIP-1β as the major HIV-suppressive factors produced by CD8+ T cells. *Science* **270:**1811–1815.

Cyster, J. G. 1999. Chemokines and cell migration in secondary lymphoid organs. *Science* **286:**2098–2102.

Daelemans, D., D. Schols, M. Witvrouw, C. Pannecouque, S. Hatse, S. Van Dooren, F. Hamy, T. Klimkait, E. De Clercq, and A. M. Vandamme. 2000. A second target for the peptoid Tat/transactivation response element inhibitor CGP64222: inhibition of human immunodeficiency virus replication by blocking CXC-chemokine receptor 4-mediated virus entry. *Mol. Pharmacol.* **57:**116–124.

D'Amico, G., G. Frascaroli, G. Bianchi, P. Transidico, A. Doni, A. Vecchi, S. Sozzani, P. Allavena, and A. Mantovani. 2000. Uncoupling of inflammatory chemokine receptors by IL-10: generation of functional decoys. *Nat. Immunol.* **1:**387–391.

D'Apuzzo, M., A. Rolink, M. Loetscher, J. A. Hoxie, I. Clark-Lewis, F. Melchers, M. Baggiolini, and B. Moser. 1997. The chemokine SDF-1, stromal cell-derived factor 1, attracts early stage B cell precursors via the chemokine receptor CXCR4. *Eur. J. Immunol.* **27:**1788–1793.

Deichmann, M., R. Kronenwett, and R. Haas. 1997. Expression of the human immunodeficiency virus type-1 coreceptors CXCR-4 (fusin, LESTR) and CKR-5 in CD34+ hematopoietic progenitor cells. *Blood* **89:**3522–3528.

Dhawan, P., and A. Richmond. 2002. Role of CXCL1 in tumorigenesis of melanoma. *J. Leukoc. Biol.* **72:**9–18.

Egawa, T., K. Kawabata, H. Kawamoto, K. Amada, R. Okamoto, N. Fujii, T. Kishimoto, Y. Katsura, and T. Nagasawa. 2001. The earliest stages of B cell development require a chemokine stromal cell-derived factor/pre-B cell growth-stimulating factor. *Immunity* **15:**323–334.

Feng, Y., C. C. Broder, P. E. Kennedy, and E. A. Berger. 1996. HIV-1 entry cofactor: functional cDNA cloning of a seven-transmembrane, G protein-coupled receptor. *Science* **272:**872–877.

Finke, D., H. Acha-Orbea, A. Mattis, M. Lipp, and J. Kraehenbuhl. 2002. CD4+CD3-cells induce Peyer's patch development: role of alpha4beta1 integrin activation by CXCR5. *Immunity* **17:**363–373.

Foxman, E. F., J. J. Campbell, and E. C. Butcher. 1997. Multistep navigation and the combinatorial control of leukocyte chemotaxis. *J. Cell Biol.* **139:**1349–1360.

Gerard, C., and B. J. Rollins. 2001. Chemokines and disease. *Nat. Immunol.* **2:**108–115.

Godessart, N., and S. L. Kunkel. 2001. Chemokines in autoimmune disease. *Curr. Opin. Immunol.* **13:**670–675.

Gunn, M. D., V. N. Ngo, K. M. Ansel, E. H. Ekland, J. G. Cyster, and L. T. Williams. 1998. A B-cell-homing chemokine made in lymphoid follicles activates Burkitt's lymphoma receptor-1. *Nature* **391:**799–803.

Hamada, T., R. Möhle, J. Hesselgesser, J. Hoxie, R. L. Nachman, M. A. S. Moore, and S. Rafii. 1998. Transendothelial migration of megakaryocytes in response to stromal cell-derived factor 1 (SDF-1) enhances platelet formation. *J. Exp. Med.* **188:**539–548.

Hargreaves, D. C., P. L. Hyman, T. T. Lu, V. N. Ngo, A. Bidgol, G. Suzuki, Y. R. Zou, D. R. Littman, and J. G. Cyster. 2001. A coordinated change in chemokine responsiveness guides plasma cell movements. *J. Exp. Med.* **194:**45–56.

Holmes, W. E., J. Lee, W.-J. Kuang, G. C. Rice, and W. I. Wood. 1991. Structure and functional expression of a human interleukin-8 receptor. *Science* **253:**1278–1280.

Janatpour, M. J., S. Hudak, M. Sathe, J. D. Sedgwick, and L. M. McEvoy. 2001. Tumor necrosis factor-dependent segmental control of MIG expression by high endothelial venules in inflamed lymph nodes regulates monocyte recruitment. *J. Exp. Med.* **194**:1375–1384.

Kawabata, K., M. Ujikawa, T. Egawa, H. Kawamoto, K. Tachibana, H. Iizasa, Y. Katsura, T. Kishimoto, and T. Nagasawa. 1999. A cell-autonomous requirement for CXCR4 in long-term lymphoid and myeloid reconstitution. *Proc. Natl. Acad. Sci. USA* **96**:5663–5667.

Kim, C. H., and H. E. Broxmeyer. 1999. Chemokines: signal lamps for trafficking of T and B cells for development and effector function. *J. Leukoc. Biol.* **65**:6–15.

Legler, D. F., M. Loetscher, R. S. Roos, I. Clark-Lewis, M. Baggiolini, and B. Moser. 1998. B cell-attracting chemokine 1, a human CXC chemokine expressed in lymphoid tissues, selectively attracts B lymphocytes via BLR1/CXCR5. *J. Exp. Med.* **187**:655–660.

Lin, T. J., T. B. Issekutz, and J. S. Marshall. 2000. Human mast cells transmigrate through human umbilical vein endothelial monolayers and selectively produce IL-8 in response to stromal cell-derived factor-1 alpha. *J. Immunol.* **165**:211–220.

Lindley, I. J. D., M. Ceska, and P. Peichl. 1991. NAP-1/IL-8 in rheumatoid arthritis. *Adv. Exp. Med. Biol.* **305**:147–156.

Loetscher, P., and B. Moser. 2002. Homing chemokines in rheumatoid arthritis. *Arthritis Res.* **4**:233–236.

Loetscher, P., B. Moser, and M. Baggiolini. 2000. Chemokines and their receptors in lymphocyte traffic and HIV infection. *Adv. Immunol.* **74**:127–180.

Loetscher, P., A. Pellegrino, J. H. Gong, I. Mattioli, M. Loetscher, G. Bardi, M. Baggiolini, and I. Clark-Lewis. 2001. The ligands of CXC chemokine receptor 3, I-TAC, Mig, and IP10, are natural antagonists for CCR3. *J. Biol. Chem.* **276**:2986–2991.

Ma, Q., D. Jones, and T. A. Springer. 1999. The chemokine receptor CXCR4 is required for the retention of B lineage and granulocytic precursors within the bone marrow microenvironment. *Immunity* **10**:463–471.

Maddon, P. J., A. G. Dalgleish, J. S. McDougal, P. R. Clapham, R. A. Weiss, and R. Axel. 1986. The T4 gene encodes the AIDS virus receptor and is expressed in the immune system and the brain. *Cell* **47**:333–348.

McFadden, G., and P. M. Murphy. 2000. Host-related immunomodulators encoded by poxviruses and herpesviruses. *Curr. Opin. Microbiol.* **3**:371–378.

Moore, J. P. 1997. Co-receptors for HIV-1 entry. *Curr. Opin. Immunol.* **9**:551–562.

Moser, B. 1997. Chemokines and HIV: a remarkable synergism. *Trends Microbiol.* **5**:88–90.

Moser, B., and P. Loetscher. 2001. Lymphocyte traffic control by chemokines. *Nat. Immunol.* **2**:123–128.

Moser, B., C. Schumacher, V. von Tscharner, I. Clark-Lewis, and M. Baggiolini. 1991. Neutrophil-activating peptide 2 and *gro*/melanoma growth-stimulatory activity interact with neutrophil-activating peptide 1/interleukin 8 receptors on human neutrophils. *J. Biol. Chem.* **266**:10666–10671.

Moser, B., M. Loetscher, L. Piali, and P. Loetscher. 1998. Lymphocyte responses to chemokines. *Int. Rev. Immunol.* **16**:323–344.

Moser, B., P. Schaerli, and P. Loetscher. 2002. CXCR5(+) T cells: follicular homing takes center stage in T-helper-cell responses. *Trends Immunol.* **23**:250–254.

Muller, A., B. Homey, H. Soto, N. Ge, D. Catron, M. E. Buchanan, T. McClanahan, E. Murphy, W. Yuan, S. N. Wagner, J. L. Barrera, A. Mohar, E. Verastegui, and A. Zlotnik. 2001. Involvement of chemokine receptors in breast cancer metastasis. *Nature* **410**:50–56.

Müller, G., U. E. Höpken, H. Stein, and M. Lipp. 2002. Systemic immunoregulatory and pathogenic functions of homeostatic chemokine receptors. *J. Leukoc. Biol.* **72**:1–8.

Murphy, P. M. 2001. Viral exploitation and subversion of the immune system through chemokine mimicry. *Nat. Immunol.* **2**:116–122.

Murphy, P. M. 2002. International Union of Pharmacology. XXX. Update on chemokine receptor nomenclature. *Pharmacol. Rev.* **54**:227–229.

Murphy, P. M., and H. L. Tiffany. 1991. Cloning of complementary DNA encoding a functional human interleukin-8 receptor. *Science* **253**:1280–1283.

Murphy, P. M., M. Baggiolini, I. F. Charo, C. A. Hebert, R. Horuk, K. Matsushima, L. H. Miller, J. J. Oppenheim, and C. A. Power. 2000. International Union of Pharmacology. XXII. Nomenclature for chemokine receptors. *Pharmacol. Rev.* **52**:145–176.

Nagasawa, T. 2000. A chemokine, SDF-1/PBSF, and its receptor, CXC chemokine receptor 4, as mediators of hematopoiesis. *Int. J. Hematol.* **72**:408–411.

Nagasawa, T., H. Kikutani, and T. Kishimoto. 1994. Molecular cloning and structure of a pre-B-cell growth-stimulating factor. *Proc. Natl. Acad. Sci. USA* **91**:2305–2309.

Ogilvie, P., G. Bardi, I. Clark-Lewis, M. Baggiolini, and M. Uguccioni. 2001. Eotaxin is a natural antagonist for CCR2 and an agonist for CCR5. *Blood* **97**:1920–1924.

Onai, N., Y. Zhang, H. Yoneyama, T. Kitamura, S. Ishikawa, and K. Matsushima. 2000. Impairment of lymphopoiesis and myelopoiesis in mice reconstituted with bone marrow-hematopoietic progenitor cells expressing SDF-1-intrakine. *Blood* **96**:2074–2080.

Onuffer, J. J., and R. Horuk. 2002. Chemokines, chemokine receptors and small-molecule antagonists: recent developments. *Trends Pharmacol. Sci.* **23**:459–467.

Palframan, R. T., S. Jung, G. Cheng, W. Weninger, Y. Luo, M. Dorf, D. R. Littman, B. J. Rollins, H. Zweerink, A. Rot, and U. H. Von Andrian. 2001. Inflammatory chemokine transport and presentation in HEV: a remote control mechanism for monocyte recruitment to lymph nodes in inflamed tissues. *J. Exp. Med.* **194**:1361–1373.

Pierce, K. L., R. T. Premont, and R. J. Lefkowitz. 2002. Seven-transmembrane receptors. *Nat. Rev. Mol. Cell Biol.* **3**:639–650.

Rodriguez-Frade, J. M., M. Mellado, and A. Martinez. 2001. Chemokine receptor dimerization: two are better than one. *Trends Immunol.* **22**:612–617.

Sallusto, F., D. Lenig, R. Förster, M. Lipp, and A. Lanzavecchia. 1999. Two subsets of memory T lymphocytes with distinct homing potentials and effector functions. *Nature* **401**:708–712.

Sallusto, F., C. R. Mackay, and A. Lanzavecchia. 2000. The role of chemokine receptors in primary, effector, and memory immune responses. *Annu. Rev. Immunol.* **18**:593–620.

Savino, W., D. A. Mendes-da-Cruz, J. S. Silva, M. Dardenne, and V. Cotta-de-Almeida. 2002. Intrathymic T-cell migration: a combinatorial interplay of extracellular matrix and chemokines? *Trends Immunol.* **23**:305–313.

Schmid, J., and C. Weissmann. 1987. Induction of mRNA for a serine protease and a β-thromboglobulin-like protein in mitogen-stimulated human leukocytes. *J. Immunol.* **139**:250–256.

Schnitzel, W., B. Garbeis, U. Monschein, and J. Besemer. 1991. Neutrophil activating peptide-2 binds with two affinities to receptor(s) on human neutrophils. *Biochem. Biophys. Res. Commun.* **180**:301–307.

Serrador, J. M., M. Nieto, and F. Sánchez-Madrid. 1999. Cytoskeletal rearrangement during migration and activation of T lymphocytes. *Trends Cell Biol.* **9**:228–232.

Spangrude, G. J., B. A. Braaten, and R. A. Daynes. 1984. Molecular mechanisms of lymphocyte extravasation. I. Studies of two selective inhibitors of lymphocyte recirculation. *J. Immunol.* **132**:354–362.

Springer, T. A. 1994. Traffic signals for lymphocyte recirculation and leukocyte emigration: the multistep paradigm. *Cell* **76**:301–314.

Thelen, M. 2001. Dancing to the tune of chemokines. *Nat. Immunol.* **2**:129–134.

Walker, C. M., D. J. Moody, D. P. Stites, and J. A. Levy. 1986. CD8+ lymphocytes can control HIV infection in vitro by suppressing virus replication. *Science* **234**:1563–1566.

Walz, A., P. Peveri, H. Aschauer, and M. Baggiolini. 1987. Purification and amino acid sequencing of NAF, a novel neutrophil-activating factor produced by monocytes. *Biochem. Biophys. Res. Commun.* **149**:755–761.

Wang, J. Y., M. Huang, P. Lee, K. Komanduri, S. Sharma, G. Chen, and S. M. Dubinett. 1996. Interleukin-8 inhibits non-small cell lung cancer proliferation: a possible role for regulation of tumor growth by autocrine and paracrine pathways. *J. Interferon. Cytokine Res.* **16**:53–60.

Wright, D. E., E. P. Bowman, A. J. Wagers, E. C. Butcher, and I. L. Weissman. 2002. Hematopoietic stem cells are uniquely selective in their migratory response to chemokines. *J. Exp. Med.* **195**:1145–1154.

Yoshimura, T., K. Matsushima, S. Tanaka, E. A. Robinson, E. Appella, J. J. Oppenheim, and E. J. Leonard. 1987. Purification of a human monocyte-derived neutrophil chemotactic factor that has peptide sequence similarity to other host defense cytokines. *Proc. Natl. Acad. Sci. USA* **84**:9233–9237.

Zlotnik, A., and O. Yoshie. 2000. Chemokines: a new classification system and their role in immunity. *Immunity* **12**:121–127.

LIPIDS

K. Frank Austen and Yoshihide Kanaoka

21

Lipids are an essential constituent of cell membranes and are sources of energy. Metabolites from membrane phospholipids, such as prostanoids, leukotrienes (LTs), platelet-activating factor (PAF), and lysophospholipids, including lysophosphatidic acids (LPAs) and sphingosine-1-phosphate (S1P), have been identified and characterized as mediators for various biological functions. The biosynthetic pathways and receptor systems of these lipid mediators are reviewed. The inflammatory response that follows the exposure of host receptors such as Toll-like receptors (TLRs) to microbial ligands is innate by definition. It arms the host for an adaptive immune response, which in turn utilizes further components of the inflammatory response. Thus, the inflammatory response effector functions precede and follow the adaptive immune response. Lipid mediator generation can be entirely innate or composite via an adaptive immune step. In this chapter we address only primary innate or exogenous signals assessed in vitro and in vivo. In vivo discussion is limited to studies in null

mouse strains for clarity. The activation of phospholipase A_2 (PLA_2) with release of arachidonic acid provides the substrate for all eicosanoids, namely, prostanoids and LTs. Although certain residual lysophospholipids by acetylation become PAF, other lysophospholipids are generated by more complex pathways. Each class of product operates through specific receptors. Thus, the assessment of innate responses in null strains (Table 1) encompasses both partners to the extent possible.

PLA_2

PLA_2 comprises a diverse family of enzymes that cleave the *sn*-2 position of glycerophospholipids to form a fatty acid and a lysophospolipid (Kudo and Murakami, 2002). PLA_2 is involved in the digestion of phospholipids in the diet and in the metabolism and turnover of phospholipids in cell membranes. In addition, PLA_2 is a key enzyme for the generation of various lipid mediators including PAF, prostaglandins, LTs, and lysophospholipids. Cytosolic PLA_2 ($cPLA_2$ or group IV PLA_2) is an 85-kDa protein that preferentially releases arachidonic acid (Clark et al., 1990; Sharp et al., 1991). In response to a signal transduction-initiated increase in intracellular calcium, $cPLA_2$ translocates to cellular membranes,

K. Frank Austen and Yoshihide Kanaoka, Department of Medicine, Harvard Medical School, Division of Rheumatology, Immunology and Allergy, Brigham and Women's Hospital, Boston, MA 02115.

The Innate Immune Response to Infection
Ed. by S. H. E. Kaufmann, R. Medzhitov, and S. Gordon
©2004 ASM Press, Washington, D.C.

TABLE 1 Innate immune responses in mice lacking eicosanoid synthetic enzymes and receptors[a]

Model	Disrupted gene	Response[a]	References
AA-induced ear inflammation			
Edema	PGHS-1	↓	Langenbach et al. (1995)
	PGHS-2	→	Morham et al. (1995), Dinchuk et al. (1995)
	EP3	↓	Tilley et al. (2001)
	5-LO	↓	Chen et al. (1994), Goulet et al. (1994)
	FLAP	↓	Byrum et al. (1997)
	LTA$_4$H	↓	Byrum et al. (1999)
	BLT1	↓	Haribabu et al. (2000)
Neutrophil infiltration	5-LO	↓	Chen et al. (1994), Goulet et al. (1994)
	FLAP	↓	Byrum et al. (1997)
	LTA$_4$H	↓	Byrum et al. (1999)
	BLT1	↓	Haribabu et al. (2000)
PMA-induced ear inflammation	PGHS-1	→	Langenbach et al. (1995)
	PGHS-2	→	Morham et al. (1995), Dinchuk et al. (1995)
	EP3	→	Tilley et al. (2001)
	5-LO	→	Chen et al. (1994), Goulet et al. (1994)
	FLAP	→	Byrum et al. (1997)
Zymosan-induced peritonitis			
Protein extravasation	5-LO	↓	Goulet et al. (1994)
	FLAP	↓	Byrum et al. (1997)
	LTA$_4$H	→	Byrum et al. (1999)
	LTC$_4$S	↓	Kanaoka et al. (2001)
	γ-GL	→	Shi et al. (2001)
	CysLT$_1$	↓	Maekawa et al. (2002)
Neutrophil infiltration	5-LO	↓	Goulet et al. (1994)
	FLAP	↓	Byrum et al. (1997)
	LTA$_4$H	↓	Byrum et al. (1999)
	LTC$_4$S	→	Maekawa et al. (2002)
	γ-GL	↓	Shi et al. (2001)
	CysLT$_1$	→	Maekawa et al. (2002)
Thioglycolate-induced peritonitis	BLT1	↓	Tager et al. (2000)

[a]↓ = attenuated; → = unchanged. Abbreviations: AA, arachidonic acid; PMA, phorbol myristate acetate; PGHS, prostaglandin endoperoxide synthase; EP, E-type prostanoid receptor; 5-LO, 5-lipoxygenase; FLAP, 5-LO activating protein; LTA$_4$H, leukotriene A$_4$ hydrolase; LTC$_4$S, leukotriene C$_4$ synthase; γ-GL, γ-glutamyl leukotrienase; BLT, leukotriene B$_4$ receptor; CysLT$_1$, cysteinyl leukotriene 1 receptor.

particularly endoplasmic and perinuclear membranes (Clark et al., 1991). Its activity is regulated by phosphorylation of Ser505 by the mitogen-activated protein kinase pathway. Peritoneal macrophages from cPLA$_2$ null mice do not produce prostaglandin (PG) E$_2$ (PGE$_2$), LTB$_4$, or LTC$_4$ in response to stimulation with either calcium ionophore or the TLR-active lipopolysaccharide (LPS) (Bonventre et al., 1997; Uozumi et al., 1997), indicating that cPLA$_2$ is responsible for providing arachidonic acid to the prostanoid and LT biosynthetic pathways (described below). Gijon and colleagues (2000) extended the role of cPLA$_2$ to signaling without calcium flux. Whereas arachidonic acid was liberated from the peritoneal macrophages of wild-type mice by stimulation with agonists that cause intracellular calcium mobilization, such as calcium ionophore and zymosan, as well as with those that do not such as phorbol ester and okadaic acid, the release of arachidonic acid from the peritoneal macrophages of $cPLA_2$ null mice stimulated with the same agents was substantially reduced or completely abolished. Furthermore, the production of PGE_2 and LTC_4 by these cells was almost completely dependent on $cPLA_2$. Thus, $cPLA_2$ plays a crucial role in the release of arachidonic acid and in the generation of terminal products in the arachidonic acid cascade.

Low-molecular-weight PLA_2s, or secretory PLA_2s ($sPLA_2$s), include groups of PLA_2 with features that differ from those of $cPLA_2$. $sPLA_2$s require millimolar concentrations of calcium for their activity, whereas $cPLA_2$ functions with less than 1 μM calcium. $sPLA_2$s have no strict fatty acid selectivity. At least 10 sPLAs have been identified in mammals, namely, IB, IIA, IIC, IID, IIE, IIF, III, V, X, and XII (Singer et al., 2002). Group I/II/V/X $sPLA_2$s, enzymes of 14 to 19 kDa with a highly conserved calcium-binding loop and a catalytic site, are closely related and characterized in terms of inflammatory responses. The group IB $sPLA_2$ ($sPLA_2$-IB) was originally identified as a pancreatic enzyme that digests glycerophospholipids in the diet, but its distribution in nondigestive organs, including lung and spleen, prompted identification of a novel function of $sPLA_2$-IB mediated through its specific PLA_2 receptor, or M (muscle)-type PLA_2 receptor (Ishizaki et al., 1994). This M-type PLA_2 receptor is a 180- to 200-kDa membrane glycoprotein that belongs to the C-type animal lectin family. The binding of $sPLA_2$-IB to the PLA_2 receptor is independent of its enzyme activity. PLA_2 receptor null mice were partially protected from LPS-induced shock, and that protection was considered to be due to the reduced production of tumor necrosis factor α (TNF-α) and interleukin 1β (IL-1β) after LPS treatment (Hanasaki et al., 1997). Another type of $sPLA_2$ receptor, N

(neuronal)-type receptor (Lambeau and Lazdunski, 1999), binds neurotoxic $sPLA_2$ from the venom of the Australian taipan snake, but its molecular structure and function in inflammatory responses are not known. $sPLA_2$-IIA has been implicated in inflammation; the levels of $sPLA_2$-IIA in sera or exudates are correlated with the severity of inflammatory diseases, and $sPLA_2$-IIA expression is induced by proinflammatory stimuli in various cells and tissues (Oka and Arita, 1991). In addition, $sPLA_2$-IIA has potent bactericidal activity against gram-positive bacteria (Weinrauch et al., 1996), and the overall positive charge of the $sPLA_2$-IIA is the dominant factor in the bactericidal potency (Koduri et al., 2002). $sPLA_2$-V and $sPLA_2$-X can release arachidonic acid from some types of cells more efficiently than $sPLA_2$-IB or $sPLA_2$-IIs. $sPLA_2$-V is expressed in several tissues, particularly heart and immune cells, and its expression is also induced by proinflammatory stimuli (Sawada et al., 1999). Exogenously added human $sPLA_2$-V can induce LTB_4 generation in human neutrophils by liberating fatty acids, including arachidonic acids and lysophosphocholine, from the plasma membrane and subsequently activating $cPLA_2$ (Kim et al., 2002). $sPLA_2$-X that has the capacity to release arachidonic acid and linoleic acid is expressed in immune, digestive, and testicular tissues. $sPLA_2$-X is another ligand for the M-type PLA_2 receptor (Yokota et al., 2000).

Mice lacking a particular $sPLA_2$ enzyme by targeted disruption have not been reported. $sPLA_2$-IIA is intrinsically disrupted in some strains of mice that are more susceptible to colorectal tumorigenesis. The relationship between $sPLA_2$-IIA and colon tumor is supported by the findings that transgenic mice overexpressing $sPLA_2$-IIA are resistant to colon tumorigenesis (Cormier et al., 1997), although the mechanisms are unknown.

PROSTANOIDS

Arachidonic acid cleaved by $cPLA_2$ is oxygenated by PG endoperoxide synthase-1 (PGHS-1; also called cyclooxygenase-1

[COX-1]) or PGHS-2 (COX-2) to form an unstable intermediate, PGH$_2$, which is a common precursor for all the PGs and thromboxane (Fig. 1). PGHS-1 is expressed constitutively in most cells. PGHS-2 is an inducible enzyme responsive to inflammatory stimuli such as LPS and proinflammatory cytokines. To differentiate the roles of the two PGHSs in inflammatory responses, enzyme null mutant mice were compared.

Arachidonic acid-induced ear edema is attenuated in PGHS-1 null mice (Langenbach et al., 1995) but not in PGHS-2 null mice (Morham et al., 1995; Dinchuk et al., 1995). 5-Lipoxygenase (5-LO) pathway products, namely, cysteinyl leukotrienes (cysLTs) and LTB$_4$, also participate in this response (described below). The contribution of prostan-oids generated by PGHS-1 to arachidonic acid-induced ear inflammation was also confirmed with 5-LO/PGHS-1 and 5-LO/PGHS-2 double null mice (Tilley et al., 2001). Phorbol ester-induced ear edema is not different in wild-type and PGHS-1 or PGHS-2 null mice. Although phorbol ester is a potent inducer of PGHS-2 expression in many types of cells, the mechanism of the inflammatory response to phorbol ester may be prostanoid independent and is probably related to proinflammatory cytokine induction. Carrageenan-induced PGE$_2$ production in the subdermal air pouch model is reduced by about 75 and 25%, respectively, in PGHS-2 and PGHS-1 null mice as compared with the wild type. Inflammatory cell infiltration, including apoptotic neutrophils in the air pouch exudates, is

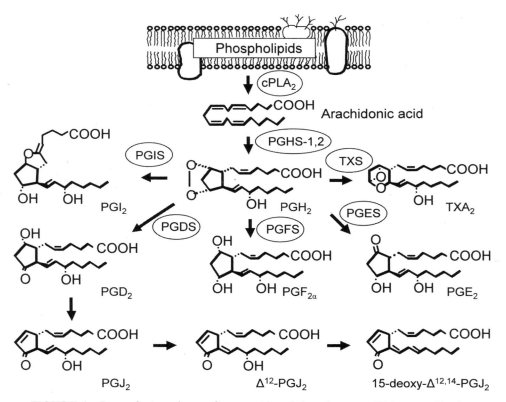

FIGURE 1 Biosynthetic pathway of prostanoids and thromboxanes. cPLA$_2$, cytosolic phospholipase A$_2$; PGHS, prostaglandin endoperoxide synthase; PGDS, prostaglandin D synthase; PGES, prostaglandin E synthase; PGFS, prostaglandin F synthase; PGIS, prostacyclin synthase; TXS, thromboxane synthase.

augmented in PGHS-2 null mice as compared with PGHS-1 null or wild-type mice, suggesting that PGE$_2$ generated by PGHS-2 is involved in the resolution of inflammation in this model (Langenbach et al., 1999).

To specify the role of each prostanoid in immune responses, null mice were generated for the biosynthetic terminal enzymes and their receptors. PGE$_2$ has been implicated in the pain, inflammation, and modulation of immune responses (Davies et al., 1984). Several enzymes that isomerize PGH$_2$ to PGE$_2$ have been identified. Microsomal PGE synthase-1 (mPGES-1), a member of the membrane-associated proteins in eicosanoid and glutathione metabolism superfamily, is a membrane protein whose expression is induced by proinflammatory cytokines such as IL-1 (Jakobsson et al., 1999). mPGES-1 has been implicated in adjuvant-induced arthritis (Mancini et al., 2001). Cytosolic μ-class glutathione S-transferases may be the major PGES in the normal brain (Beuckmann et al., 2000). Cytosolic PGES is a glutathione-dependent PGES and is functionally coupled with PGHS-1 (Tanioka et al., 2000). A second membrane-associated PGES (mPGES-2) has been cloned and characterized (Watanabe et al., 1999; Tanikawa et al., 2002).

Macrophages generate a large amount of PGE$_2$ in response to LPS and other inflammatory stimuli. PGE$_2$ acts on macrophages to modulate their functions for Th cell differentiation toward Th2 by suppressing the production of IL-12 and gamma interferon (IFN-γ) (van der Pouw Kraan et al., 1995; Hilkens et al., 1996). The mPGES-1 gene is one of the genes induced in mouse macrophages by stimulation with LPS, and the induction is TLR4 dependent and MyD88 dependent. No induction of mPGES-1 or production of PGE$_2$ was observed in peritoneal macrophages from mice null for nuclear factor for IL-6 expression (NF-IL-6). Thus, LPS-induced mPGES-1 expression and PGE$_2$ production depend on a TLR4/MyD88/NF-IL-6 signaling pathway (Uematsu et al., 2002). LPS-induced PGE$_2$ production in vitro was completely abolished

in peritoneal macrophages from mPGES-1 null mice and was not augmented in the serum of mPGES-1 null mice challenged systemically with LPS. However, the production of cytokines, such as TNF-α, IL-12, and IL-6, induced by LPS and/or IFN-γ and LPS-induced mortality were not reduced in mPGES-1 null mice compared with wild-type mice (Uematsu et al., 2002).

There are four subtypes of PGE$_2$ receptors, namely, E-type prostanoid (EP1), EP2, EP3, and EP4 (Narumiya and FitzGerald, 2001). EP1 is coupled to Gq and induces mobilization of intracellular calcium, whereas EP2 and EP4 are coupled to Gs and increase the level of cyclic AMP (cAMP). EP3 has multiple isoforms resulting from alternative splicing; one isoform is coupled to Gs and another isoform to Gi, which decreases the level of cAMP. Because the repertoire of EP receptors expressed by various cells and tissues differs, the role of each EP receptor in inflammatory responses can be elucidated only by the analysis of particular cells and tissues from mice null for each receptor subtype. Arachidonic acid-induced ear edema is mediated by PGE$_2$ through the EP3 receptor (Tilley et al., 2001). The EP4 receptor but not the EP2 receptor is involved in PGE$_2$-mediated inhibition of TNF-α and IL-12 production from macrophages in response to stimulation with LPS (Nataraj et al., 2001).

PGI$_2$, prostacyclin, is among the mediators that participate in the increased vascular permeability and edema at sites of inflammation (Davies et al., 1984). Paw swelling induced by carrageenan injection was reduced by half in wild-type mice pretreated with indomethacin and in IP receptor null mice, and indomethacin pretreatment of IP receptor null mice did not further reduce the paw edema. These results indicate that PGI$_2$ and the IP receptor provide the principal pathway for increased vascular permeability induced by carrageenan (Murata et al., 1997). The PGI$_2$ analog, carbacyclin, and PGE$_2$ reduced TNF-α production and augmented IL-10 production by zymosan-activated peritoneal macrophages

(Shinomiya et al., 2001). Macrophages from IP receptor null mice showed this cytokine modulation only in response to EP2 and EP4 receptor agonists or to PGE_2, but not to carbacyclin. By contrast, macrophages from EP2 and EP4 receptor null mice responded to PGE_2 or carbacyclin, but not to EP2 or EP4 receptor agonists. Thus, downregulation of TNF-α and upregulation of IL-10 by PGE_2 and PGI_2 are mediated redundantly through EP2, EP4, and IP receptors.

PGD_2 is a major arachidonic acid metabolite generated from activated mast cells. There are two receptors for PGD_2, namely, DP receptor (Narumiya and FitzGerald, 2001) and CRTH2 (Hirai et al., 2001). DP receptor null mice showed attenuated cellular infiltration and Th2 cytokine expression in the lung and reduced airway hyperresponsiveness to acetylcholine in an antigen-sensitized, aerosolized antigen-challenged acute lung injury model (Matsuoka et al., 2000). PGD_2 produced by the helminth parasite *Schistosoma mansoni* acts on the DP receptor expressed on epidermal dendritic cells to block their migration to regional lymph nodes (Angeli et al., 2001). The CRTH2 predominantly expressed in Th2 cells, eosinophils, and basophils is a chemoattractant receptor for these cells. The role of the CRTH2 in innate immune responses remains to be addressed. Nonenzymatic PGD_2 metabolites, Δ^{12}-PGJ_2 and 15-deoxy-$\Delta^{12,\,14}$-PGJ_2 (15-d-PGJ_2), act as ligands for peroxisome proliferator-activated receptor γ (PPAR-γ), a nuclear transcription factor, which was originally identified as a regulator of adipocyte differentiation and glucose and lipid metabolism. These PPAR-γ ligands downregulate the TNF-α and nitric oxide production from human peripheral blood monocytes (Jiang et al., 1998), and this downregulation may be due to the inhibition of the transcription factors AP-1, STAT, and NF-κB (Ricote et al., 1998). In addition, 15-d-PGJ_2 may directly inhibit the IκB kinase and subsequently block the translocation of NF-κB into the nucleus (Rossi et al., 2000; Straus et al., 2000).

The TP receptor is abundantly expressed by immature thymocytes, and thromboxane A_2 induces apoptosis of immature thymocytes in vitro (Ushikubi et al., 1993). However, the roles of thromboxane A_2 and the TP receptor in in vivo inflammatory responses using thromboxane synthase null or TP receptor null mice remain to be elucidated. FP receptor null mice show a defect in parturition (Sugimoto et al., 1997) but abnormalities in inflammatory responses have not been demonstrated.

LTs

Arachidonic acid is also converted to 5-hydroperoxyeicosatetraenoic acid (5-HPETE) and then to an epoxide intermediate, LTA_4, by 5-LO in the presence of the 5-LO activating protein (FLAP) (Dixon et al., 1988, 1990; Matsumoto et al., 1988; Miller et al., 1990). LTA_4 is processed either to the dihydroxy leukotriene, LTB_4, by LTA_4 hydrolase (Funk et al., 1987; Minami et al., 1987) or to LTC_4 through conjugation with reduced glutathione by LTC_4 synthase (LTC_4S) (Lam et al., 1994; Welsch et al., 1994). After carrier-mediated export of LTC_4 (Lam et al., 1992), glutamic acid and glycine are sequentially cleaved by γ-glutamyl transpeptidase (γ-GT) (Hammarstrom, 1981) or γ-glutamyl leukotrienase (γ-GL) (Carter et al., 1998) and dipeptidase (Lee et al., 1983) to form LTD_4 and LTE_4, respectively. LTC_4, LTD_4, and LTE_4 are collectively termed cysLTs (Fig. 2).

LTB_4 is a potent chemotactic factor for neutrophils, eosinophils, and macrophages. LTB_4 also stimulates adhesion of leukocytes to vascular endothelia and migration of the cells into adjacent tissues (Dahlen et al., 1981). Two cell surface receptors for LTB_4, BLT1 and BLT2, have been cloned and characterized (Yokomizo et al., 1997, 2000). Both are G-protein-coupled receptors. BLT1 receptor has a 1-log-higher affinity for LTB_4 than does the BLT2 receptor (K_d = 1.1 nM for the BLT1 receptor and 23 nM for the BLT2 receptor). The BLT2 receptor, 45.2% identical to the BLT1 receptor in amino acid sequence, is

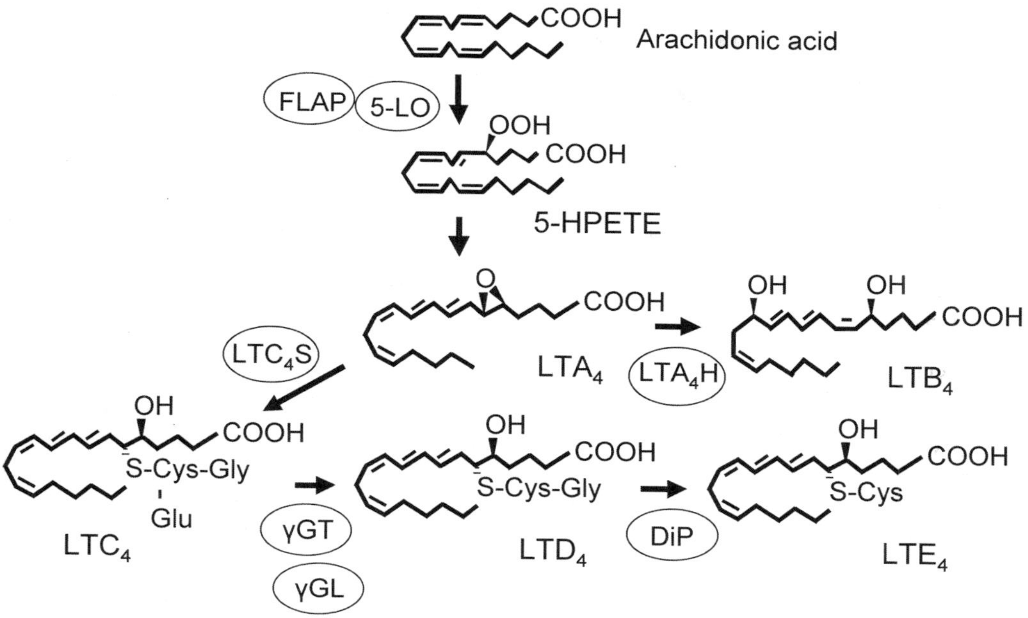

FIGURE 2 Biosynthetic pathway of leukotrienes. 5-LO, 5-lipoxygenase; FLAP, 5-LO activating protein; 5-HPETE, 5-hydroperoxyeicosatetraenoic acid; LT, leukotriene; LTA_4H, LTA_4 hydrolase; LTC_4S, LTC_4 synthase; γ-GT, γ-glutamyl transpeptidase; γ-GL, γ-glutamyl leukotrienase; DiP, dipeptidase.

located about 10 kb upstream in both the human and the mouse genes. Furthermore, LTB_4 binds to a nuclear transcription factor, PPAR-α, and promotes transcription of the acyl coenzyme A oxidase gene, a critical enzyme in the peroxisomal β-oxidation of fatty acids (Devchand et al., 1996).

The cysLTs act on airway and vascular smooth muscle to increase vascular permeability, promote mucus secretion, and attract inflammatory cells such as eosinophils. Human cysLT receptors, $CysLT_1$ and $CysLT_2$, have been cloned (Lynch et al., 1999; Heise et al., 2000). Both are G-protein-coupled receptors and share ~38% amino acid identity in humans (Lynch et al., 1999; Heise et al., 2000) and mice (Maekawa et al., 2001; Hui et al., 2001; Ogasawara et al., 2002). $CysLT_1$ receptor binds LTD_4 preferentially, and $CysLT_2$ receptor binds both LTC_4 and LTD_4 with similar affinity. However, the affinity for LTD_4 is 1 log

lower for $CysLT_2$ receptor than for $CysLT_1$ receptor based on the data from receptor-transfected cells. Human $CysLT_1$ receptor mRNA is expressed on airway smooth muscle, alveolar macrophages, peripheral blood monocytes, eosinophils, and endothelial cells (Lynch et al., 1999). Human $CysLT_2$ receptor mRNA is expressed on alveolar macrophages, airway smooth muscle, cardiac Purkinje cells, adrenal medulla cells, peripheral blood leukocytes, and brain cells (Heise et al., 2000).

Cord blood-derived human mast cells primed with IL-4 respond to the cysLTs with induction of gene products for proinflammatory and immunomodulatory cytokines and for chemokines in the absence of degranulation. Furthermore, this critical function seems to require IL-4 modulation of both $CysLT_1$ and $CysLT_2$ receptors for synergy via parallel signals or a heterodimeric receptor. That this response is shared with the nucleotide UDP links this early signal of tissue or microbial death to the inflammatory generation of the cysLTs with superimposed generation of proinflammatory cytokines such as TNF-α and chemokines to recruit more cell types (Mellor et al., 2002).

Mice deficient in 5-LO were generated by two different groups (Chen et al., 1994; Goulet et al., 1994). Because arachidonic acid is selectively released from cell membrane phospholipids when tissues are damaged or cells are activated by stimuli such as bacterial infection, arachidonic acid-induced ear inflammation was examined in 5-LO null mice to mimic such circumstances. Arachidonic acid-induced ear edema and subsequent neutrophil infiltration were attenuated in 5-LO null mice, whereas phorbol ester-induced ear edema, in which cytokine induction is considered to be involved, was not changed compared with wild-type mice. In addition, the 5-LO null mice were protected from PAF-induced shock. Essentially the same phenotypes were found in FLAP null mice (Byrum et al., 1997).

Byrum and colleagues generated LTA$_4$ hydrolase-deficient mice and compared their inflammatory responses with those of 5-LO null mice to reveal the role of LTB$_4$ and to indirectly differentiate the additional role of the cysLTs (Byrum et al., 1999). Zymosan, a carbohydrate component from the yeast cell wall, was used to stimulate LT generation from monocytes and macrophages in the peritoneal cavity (Rouzer et al., 1980; Rao et al., 1994). Plasma protein extravasation after zymosan injection was unchanged in LTA$_4$ hydrolase null mice as compared with wild-type mice, whereas 5-LO null mice showed a marked attenuation of the enhanced vascular permeability, implicating the cysLTs. Subsequent neutrophil recruitment was significantly reduced in LTA$_4$ hydrolase null mice, indicating a role for LTB$_4$, to a level between that of the 5-LO null mice and that of the wild-type controls. In addition, arachidonic acid–induced ear edema in LTA$_4$ hydrolase null mice was reduced to a level between the wild-type and

5-LO null mice, whereas neutrophil recruitment was reduced to the same extent as for 5-LO null mice.

Arachidonic acid-induced ear edema was reduced in BLT1 receptor null mice as assessed by both tissue weight and Evans blue dye extravasation. Histological examination revealed that neutrophil infiltration was diminished in BLT1 receptor null mice (Haribabu et al., 2000), suggesting that the edema is mediated via neutrophils. Intraperitoneal infiltration of neutrophils and macrophages after zymosan injection (Haribabu et al., 2000) and of eosinophils after thioglycolate injection (Tager et al., 2000) was significantly reduced in BLT1 receptor null mice as compared with wild-type mice. These observations in concert with those from LTA$_4$ hydrolase null mice indicate that LTB$_4$, acting through the BLT1 receptor, plays a role in leukocyte recruitment in peritoneal inflammation. The role of the BLT2 receptor in innate immune responses remains to be elucidated.

To investigate the direct role of cysLTs in inflammatory responses, LTC$_4$S-deficient mice were generated (Kanaoka et al., 2001). Targeted disruption of LTC$_4$S abolished conjugation of LTA$_4$ with reduced glutathione to form LTC$_4$ in all the tissues examined except testis, in which the likely enzyme was μ-class glutathione S-transferase (GST) or microsomal GST. The intraperitoneal injection of zymosan into LTC$_4$S null mice did not induce any detectable cysLT generation but produced amounts of LTB$_4$ comparable to wild-type mice. Plasma protein extravasation was reduced to about half, but neutrophil infiltration was unchanged (Maekawa et al., 2002) in LTC$_4$S null mice, indicating that cysLTs generated from activated monocytes and macrophages in the peritoneal cavity could alter vascular permeability induced through microbial insults.

Studies of γ-GT null mice, γ-GL null mice, and γ-GT/γ-GL double null mice revealed that γ-GL is responsible for more than 90% of the conversion of LTC$_4$ to LTD$_4$ in the spleen and uterus. The intraperitoneal injection of zymosan into γ-GL null mice and γ-GT/γ-GL double null mice led to the accumulation of LTC_4 in the peritoneal cavity (Shi et al., 2001). Plasma protein extravasation was not affected at any time points, 1 to 24 h after zymosan injection, but neutrophil infiltration was significantly reduced 2 to 4 h after the injection in γ-GL null mice. These findings suggest that LTC_4 is sufficient for increased vascular permeability and also plays a role in neutrophil recruitment.

Targeted disruption of the $CysLT_1$ receptor in mice demonstrated that this is the major cysLT receptor functioning in peritoneal macrophages as assessed in vitro by intracellular calcium mobilization. Plasma protein extravasation, but not neutrophil recruitment, induced by intraperitoneal injection of zymosan was 50 to 80% reduced in $CysLT_1$ receptor null mice as compared with wildtype mice (Maekawa et al., 2002). Thus, cysLTs acting through the $CysLT_1$ receptor play an important role in the enhancement of vascular permeability in this inflammatory response. The role of the $CysLT_2$ receptor in innate immune responses remains to be elucidated, but the findings with cultured cord blood-derived human mast cells suggest a function in the cellular component of the inflammatory response through cytokine and chemokine generation (Mellor et al., 2002).

LYSOPHOSPHOLIPIDS

LPA and S1P are bioactive lysophospholipids with cell functions that include growth, inhibition of apoptosis, differentiation, migration, and cytoskeletal rearrangement (Graler and Goetzl, 2002). LPA and S1P act via G-protein-coupled receptors, previously called endothelial differentiation gene EDG1-8 receptors. LPA_1 (EDG2), LPA_2 (EDG4), and LPA_3 (EDG7) are specific receptors for LPA, and $S1P_1$ (EDG1), $S1P_2$ (EDG5), $S1P_3$ (EDG3), $S1P_4$ (EDG6), and $S1P_5$ (EDG8) are receptors specific for S1P.

The major biosynthetic pathway of LPA is initiated by the action of phospholipase D on phospholipids to form phosphatidic acid and then the cleavage of the *sn*-2 position of the fatty acid by phosphatidic acid-specific PLA_2 to form LPA. An alternative pathway is through the action of $sPLA_2$ to liberate lysophosphatidylcholine (LPC) (Fourcade et al., 1995) and cleavage by lysophospholipase D to form LPA. Recently, lysophospholipase D was purified from human plasma. Lysophospholipase D is a soluble form of autaxin, a member of the ecto-nucleotide pyrophosphatase/ phosphodiesterase family (Tokumura et al., 2002). LPA is generated by activated platelets and is present in serum at concentrations of 2 to 20 μM in a largely albumin- and lipoprotein-bound form.

Sphingosine is the lipid component that forms the structural backbone of all sphingolipids. Sphingosine is converted to S1P by sphingosine kinase and alternatively to ceramide by ceramide synthase. S1P suppresses ceramide-induced apoptosis and stimulates mitogenic pathways; thus, the dynamic balance between S1P and ceramide forms a cellular rheostat (Le Stunff et al., 2002). S1P is degraded by S1P lyase, S1P phosphohydrolases, and lipid phosphate phosphohydrolases.

LPA promotes human monocyte migration (Zhou et al., 1995) and inhibits apoptosis of mouse macrophages via the phosphatidylinositol 3-kinase pathway (Koh et al., 1998). LPA and S1P both advance wound healing and modulate the expression of vascular cell adhesion molecules, including E-selectin and vascular adhesion molecule-1 (Xia et al., 1998; Lee et al., 1999). These adhesion molecules are important for the recruitment of leukocytes to the endothelium during inflammatory responses. The receptors for LPA and S1P are expressed on monocytes and macrophages from various tissues of human, mouse, and rat, but the pattern of expression is quite different. For example, human alveolar macrophages express LPA_1, LPA_2, LPA_3, and $S1P_1$ receptors; human peritoneal macrophages express LPA_1, $S1P_2$, and $S1P_3$ receptors; and mouse peritoneal macrophages express LPA_1, $S1P_1$, and $S1P_2$ receptors (Lee et al., 2002). LPA and S1P augment IL-1β and TNF-α secretion but suppress IL-2 expression from mouse peritoneal macrophages.

LPA$_1$ receptor null mice show 50% neonatal lethality due to craniofacial dysmorphism and a defect in suckling due to lack of olfactant detection (Contos et al., 2000). No gross movement and locomotion disorders were observed in LPA$_1$ receptor null mice even though apoptosis of sciatic nerve Schwann cells is increased. LPA$_2$ receptor null mice have no apparent phenotype (Contos et al., 2002). The role of LPA receptors in inflammatory responses remains to be elucidated.

Targeted disruption of the S1P$_1$ receptor in the mouse was shown to cause embryonic lethality due to defective vascular maturation (Liu et al., 2000). S1P$_2$ receptor null mice exhibited neuronal hyperexcitability with spontaneous seizures by 3 to 7 weeks of age (MacLennan et al., 2001). S1P$_3$ receptor null mice have no obvious phenotype (Ishii et al., 2001); a decrease in phospholipase C activation and adenyl cyclase inhibition was noted in ex vivo studies. The roles of LPA and S1P receptors in inflammatory responses remain to be elucidated with the use of gene knockout mice.

Two lysophospholipds containing lysophosphorylcholine, namely, sphingosylphosphorylcholine (SPC) and LPC, are involved in many biological processes including cell proliferation and growth inhibition (Xu, 2002). The biosynthetic pathway of SPC is unclear. A sphingomyelin deacylase, which converts sphingomyelin to SPC, was partially purified from the skin of patients with atopic dermatitis (Higuchi et al., 2000), but the role of this enzyme in the disease is unknown. SPC can bind S1P receptors but at a much higher concentration than S1P. Recently, an ovarian cancer G-protein-coupled receptor (ORG1) was found to be activated by nanomolar concentrations of SPC. The growth inhibitory effect of SPC on Jurkat T cells is considered to be mediated by ORG1. Furthermore, SPC can activate human neutrophils for the production of superoxide anions. LPC, produced by the action of sPLA$_2$ on phosphatidylcholine, shares structural features with SPC. SPC and LPC can specifically activate the G-protein-coupled receptors G2A and GPR4, which show close similarities to ORG1. G2A preferentially binds LPC, whereas GPR4 prefers SPC. G2A, a transcriptional target of the leukemogenic tyrosine kinase BCR-ABL in mouse B lymphoid progenitors, is expressed predominantly in hematopoietic cells, including T cells (Kabarowski et al., 2001). G2A null mice develop secondary lymphoid organ enlargement with expansion of T and B cells. The G2A null mice show late-onset systemic autoimmune syndrome including lymphocytic infiltration into various tissues, glomerular immune complex deposition, and antinuclear antibodies, similar to features of systemic lupus erythematosus (Le et al., 2001). It is speculated that G2A is also involved in innate immune responses of dendritic cells and macrophages that can modulate the T-cell response because LPC is likely produced at sites of inflammation. Although the signal transduction of GPR4 has been extensively investigated, the role of GPR4 in inflammatory responses is unknown.

CONCLUDING REMARKS

Lipid mediators per se are not encoded by genes, but their expression is regulated by the synthetic and catabolic enzyme cascades. Receptors for the extracellular lipid mediators are all G-protein-coupled, seven-transmembrane-type receptors, and the identification of the lipid ligands for orphan G-protein-coupled receptor is ongoing (Itoh et al., 2003). As compared with the extensive studies on signal transduction of these receptors, relatively little is known about the physiological function of each lipid mediator and its respective receptor. Their roles in inflammatory responses are being addressed. Inasmuch as most of the gene knockout animals have been generated and their initial phenotypic analyses completed, those with developmental effects have been recognized.

REFERENCES

Angeli, V., C. Faveeuw, O. Roye, J. Fontaine, E. Teissier, A. Capron, I. Wolowczuk, M. Capron, and F. Trottein. 2001. Role of the parasite-derived prostaglandin D_2 in the inhibition of epidermal Langerhans cell migration during schistosomiasis infection. *J. Exp. Med.* **193**:1135–1147.

Beuckmann, C. T., K. Fujimori, Y. Urade, and O. Hayaishi. 2000. Identification of mu-class glutathione transferases M2-2 and M3-3 as cytosolic prostaglandin E synthases in the human brain. *Neurochem. Res.* **25**: 733–738.

Bonventre, J. V., Z. Huang, M. R. Taheri, E. O'Leary, E. Li, M. A. Moskowitz, and A. Sapirstein. 1997. Reduced fertility and postischaemic brain injury in mice deficient in cytosolic phospholipase A_2. *Nature* **390**:622–625.

Byrum, R. S., J. L. Goulet, R. J. Griffiths, and B. H. Koller. 1997. Role of the 5-lipoxygenase-activating protein (FLAP) in murine acute inflammatory responses. *J. Exp. Med.* **185**:1065–1075.

Byrum, R. S., J. L. Goulet, J. N. Snouwaert, R. J. Griffiths, and B. H. Koller. 1999. Determination of the contribution of cysteinyl leukotrienes and leukotriene B_4 in acute inflammatory responses using 5-lipoxygenase- and leukotriene A_4 hydrolase-deficient mice. *J. Immunol.* **163**:6810–6819.

Carter, B. Z., Z. Z. Shi, R. Barrios, and M. W. Lieberman. 1998. Gamma-glutamyl leukotrienase, a gamma-glutamyl transpeptidase gene family member, is expressed primarily in spleen. *J. Biol. Chem.* **273**: 28277–28285.

Chen, X. S., J. R. Sheller, E. N. Johnson, and C. D. Funk. 1994. Role of leukotrienes revealed by targeted disruption of the 5-lipoxygenase gene. *Nature* **372**:179–182.

Clark, J. D., N. Milona, and J. L. Knopf. 1990. Purification of a 110-kilodalton cytosolic phospholipase A_2 from the human monocytic cell line U937. *Proc. Natl. Acad. Sci. USA* **87**:7708–7712.

Clark, J. D., L. L. Lin, R. W. Kriz, C. S. Ramesha, L. A. Sultzman, A. Y. Lin, N. Milona, and J. L. Knopf. 1991. A novel arachidonic acid-selective cytosolic PLA_2 contains a Ca^{2+}-dependent translocation domain with homology to PKC and GAP. *Cell* **65**:1043–1051.

Contos, J. J., N. Fukushima, J. A. Weiner, D. Kaushal, and J. Chun. 2000. Requirement for the lpA1 lysophosphatidic acid receptor gene in normal suckling behavior. *Proc. Natl. Acad. Sci. USA* **97**:13384–13389.

Contos, J. J., I. Ishii, N. Fukushima, M. A. Kingsbury, X. Ye, S. Kawamura, J. H. Brown, and J. Chun. 2002. Characterization of lpa₂ (Edg4) and lpa₁/lpa₂ (Edg2/Edg4) lysophosphatidic acid receptor knockout mice: signaling deficits without obvious phenotypic abnormality attributable to lpa₂. *Mol. Cell. Biol.* **22**:6921–6929.

Cormier, R. T., K. H. Hong, R. B. Halberg, T. L. Hawkins, P. Richardson, R. Mulherkar, W. F. Dove, and E. S. Lander. 1997. Secretory phospho-

lipase Pla2g2a confers resistance to intestinal tumorigenesis. *Nat. Genet.* **17**:88–91.

Dahlen, S. E., J. Bjork, P. Hedqvist, K. E. Arfors, S. Hammarstrom, J. A. Lindgren, and B. Samuelsson. 1981. Leukotrienes promote plasma leakage and leukocyte adhesion in postcapillary venules: in vivo effects with relevance to the acute inflammatory response. *Proc. Natl. Acad. Sci. USA* **78**: 3887–3891.

Davies, P., P. J. Bailey, M. M. Goldenberg, and A. W. Ford-Hutchinson. 1984. The role of arachidonic acid oxygenation products in pain and inflammation. *Annu. Rev. Immunol.* **2**:335–357.

Devchand, P. R., H. Keller, J. M. Peters, M. Vazquez, F. J. Gonzalez, and W. Wahli. 1996. The PPARalpha-leukotriene B_4 pathway to inflammation control. *Nature* **384**:39–43.

Dinchuk, J. E., B. D. Car, R. J. Focht, J. J. Johnston, B. D. Jaffee, M. B. Covington, N. R. Contel, V. M. Eng, R. J. Collins, P. M. Czerniak, S. A. Gorry, and J. M. Trzaskos. 1995. Renal abnormalities and an altered inflammatory response in mice lacking cyclooxygenase II. *Nature* **378**:406–409.

Dixon, R. A., R. E. Jones, R. E. Diehl, C. D. Bennett, S. Kargman, and C. A. Rouzer. 1988. Cloning of the cDNA for human 5-lipoxygenase. *Proc. Natl. Acad. Sci. USA* **85**:416–420.

Dixon, R. A., R. E. Diehl, E. Opas, E. Rands, P. J. Vickers, J. F. Evans, J. W. Gillard, and D. K. Miller. 1990. Requirement of a 5-lipoxygenase-activating protein for leukotriene synthesis. *Nature* **343**: 282–284.

Fourcade, O., M. F. Simon, C. Viode, N. Rugani, F. Leballe, A. Ragab, B. Fournie, L. Sarda, and H. Chap. 1995. Secretory phospholipase A_2 generates the novel lipid mediator lysophosphatidic acid in membrane microvesicles shed from activated cells. *Cell* **80**: 919–927.

Funk, C. D., O. Radmark, J. Y. Fu, T. Matsumoto, H. Jornvall, T. Shimizu, and B. Samuelsson. 1987. Molecular cloning and amino acid sequence of leukotriene A_4 hydrolase. *Proc. Natl. Acad. Sci. USA* **84**:6677–6681.

Gijon, M. A., D. M. Spencer, A. R. Siddiqi, J. V. Bonventre, and C. C. Leslie. 2000. Cytosolic phospholipase A_2 is required for macrophage arachidonic acid release by agonists that do and do not mobilize calcium. Novel role of mitogen-activated protein kinase pathways in cytosolic phospholipase A_2 regulation. *J. Biol. Chem.* **275**:20146–20156.

Goulet, J. L., J. N. Snouwaert, A. M. Latour, T. M. Coffman, and B. H. Koller. 1994. Altered inflammatory responses in leukotriene-deficient mice. *Proc. Natl. Acad. Sci. USA* **91**:12852–12856.

Graler, M. H., and E. J. Goetzl. 2002. Lysophospholipids and their G protein-coupled receptors in inflammation and immunity. *Biochim. Biophys. Acta* **1582:**168–174.

Hammarstrom, S. 1981. Metabolism of leukotriene C_3 in the guinea pig. Identification of metabolites formed by lung, liver, and kidney. *J. Biol. Chem.* **256:** 9573–9578.

Hanasaki, K., Y. Yokota, J. Ishizaki, T. Itoh, and H. Arita. 1997. Resistance to endotoxic shock in phospholipase A_2 receptor-deficient mice. *J. Biol. Chem.* **272:**32792–32797.

Haribabu, B., M. W. Verghese, D. A. Steeber, D. D. Sellars, C. B. Bock, and R. Snyderman. 2000. Targeted disruption of the leukotriene B_4 receptor in mice reveals its role in inflammation and platelet-activating factor-induced anaphylaxis. *J. Exp. Med.* **192:**433–438.

Heise, C. E., B. F. O'Dowd, D. J. Figueroa, N. Sawyer, T. Nguyen, D. S. Im, R. Stocco, J. N. Bellefeuille, M. Abramovitz, R. Cheng, D. L. Williams, Jr., Z. Zeng, Q. Liu, L. Ma, M. K. Clements, N. Coulombe, Y. Liu, C. P. Austin, S. R. George, G. P. O'Neill, K. M. Metters, K. R. Lynch, and J. F. Evans. 2000. Characterization of the human cysteinyl leukotriene 2 receptor. *J. Biol. Chem.* **275:**30531–30536.

Higuchi, K., J. Hara, R. Okamoto, M. Kawashima, and G. Imokawa. 2000. The skin of atopic dermatitis patients contains a novel enzyme, glucosylceramide sphingomyelin deacylase, which cleaves the N-acyl linkage of sphingomyelin and glucosylceramide. *Biochem. J.* **350:**747–756.

Hilkens, C. M., A. Snijders, H. Vermeulen, P. H. van der Meide, E. A. Wierenga, and M. L. Kapsenberg. 1996. Accessory cell-derived IL-12 and prostaglandin E_2 determine the IFN-gamma level of activated human CD4+ T cells. *J. Immunol.* **156:**1722–1727.

Hirai, H., K. Tanaka, O. Yoshie, K. Ogawa, K. Kenmotsu, Y. Takamori, M. Ichimasa, K. Sugamura, M. Nakamura, S. Takano, and K. Nagata. 2001. Prostaglandin D_2 selectively induces chemotaxis in T helper type 2 cells, eosinophils, and basophils via seven-transmembrane receptor CRTH2. *J. Exp. Med.* **193:**255–261.

Hui, Y., G. Yang, H. Galczenski, D. J. Figueroa, C. P. Austin, N. G. Copeland, D. J. Gilbert, N. A. Jenkins, and C. D. Funk. 2001. The murine cysteinyl leukotriene 2 (CysLT$_2$) receptor. cDNA and genomic cloning, alternative splicing, and in vitro characterization. *J. Biol. Chem.* **276:**47489–47495.

Ishii, I., B. Friedman, X. Ye, S. Kawamura, C. McGiffert, J. J. Contos, M. A. Kingsbury, G. Zhang, J. H. Brown, and J. Chun. 2001. Selective loss of sphingosine 1-phosphate signaling with no obvious phenotypic abnormality in mice lacking its G protein-coupled receptor, LP$_{B3}$/EDG-3. *J. Biol. Chem.* **276:**33697–33704.

Ishizaki, J., K. Hanasaki, K. Higashino, J. Kishino, N. Kikuchi, O. Ohara, and H. Arita. 1994. Molecular cloning of pancreatic group I phospholipase A_2 receptor. *J. Biol. Chem.* **269:**5897–5904.

Itoh, Y., Y. Kawamata, M. Harada, M. Kobayashi, R. Fujii, S. Fukusumi, K. Ogi, M. Hosoya, Y. Tanaka, H. Uejima, H. Tanaka, M. Maruyama, R. Satoh, S. Okubo, H. Kizawa, H. Komatsu, F. Matsumura, Y. Noguchi, T. Shinohara, S. Hinuma, Y. Fujisawa, and M. Fujino. 2003. Free fatty acids regulate insulin secretion from pancreatic beta cells through GPR40. *Nature* **422:**173–176.

Jakobsson, P. J., S. Thoren, R. Morgenstern, and B. Samuelsson. 1999. Identification of human prostaglandin E synthase: a microsomal, glutathione-dependent, inducible enzyme, constituting a potential novel drug target. *Proc. Natl. Acad. Sci. USA* **96:**7220–7225.

Jiang, C., A. T. Ting, and B. Seed. 1998. PPAR-gamma agonists inhibit production of monocyte inflammatory cytokines. *Nature* **391:**82–86.

Kabarowski, J. H., K. Zhu, L. Q. Le, O. N. Witte, and Y. Xu. 2001. Lysophosphatidylcholine as a ligand for the immunoregulatory receptor G2A. *Science* **293:**702–705.

Kanaoka, Y., A. Maekawa, J. F. Penrose, K. F. Austen, and B. K. Lam. 2001. Attenuated zymosan-induced peritoneal vascular permeability and IgE-dependent passive cutaneous anaphylaxis in mice lacking leukotriene C_4 synthase. *J. Biol. Chem.* **276:**22608–22613.

Kim, Y. J., K. P. Kim, S. K. Han, N. M. Munoz, X. Zhu, H. Sano, A. R. Leff, and W. Cho. 2002. Group V phospholipase A_2 induces leukotriene biosynthesis in human neutrophils through the activation of group IVA phospholipase A_2. *J. Biol. Chem.* **277:**36479–36488.

Koduri, R. S., J. O. Gronroos, V. J. Laine, C. Le Calvez, G. Lambeau, T. J. Nevalainen, and M. H. Gelb. 2002. Bactericidal properties of human and murine groups I, II, V, X, and XII secreted phospholipases A_2. *J. Biol. Chem.* **277:**5849–5857.

Koh, J. S., W. Lieberthal, S. Heydrick, and J. S. Levine. 1998. Lysophosphatidic acid is a major serum noncytokine survival factor for murine macrophages which acts via the phosphatidylinositol 3-kinase signaling pathway. *J. Clin. Invest.* **102:**716–727.

Kudo, I., and M. Murakami. 2002. Phospholipase A_2 enzymes. *Prostag. Other Lipid Mediat.* **68–69:**3–58.

Lam, B. K., X. Xu, M. B. Atkins, and K. F. Austen. 1992. Leukotriene C_4 uses a probenecid-sensitive export carrier that does not recognize leukotriene B_4. *Proc. Natl. Acad. Sci. USA* **89:**11598–11602.

Lam, B. K., J. F. Penrose, G. J. Freeman, and K. F. Austen. 1994. Expression cloning of a cDNA for human leukotriene C_4 synthase, an integral membrane protein conjugating reduced glutathione to leukotriene A$_4$. *Proc. Natl. Acad. Sci. USA* **91**:7663–7667.

Lambeau, G., and M. Lazdunski. 1999. Receptors for a growing family of secreted phospholipases A$_2$. *Trends Pharmacol. Sci.* **20**:162–170.

Langenbach, R., S. G. Morham, H. F. Tiano, C. D. Loftin, B. I. Ghanayem, P. C. Chulada, J. F. Mahler, C. A. Lee, E. H. Goulding, K. D. Kluckman, H. S. Kim, and O. Smithies. 1995. Prostaglandin synthase 1 gene disruption in mice reduces arachidonic acid-induced inflammation and indomethacin-induced gastric ulceration. *Cell* **83**:483–492.

Langenbach, R., C. Loftin, C. Lee, and H. Tiano. 1999. Cyclooxygenase knockout mice: models for elucidating isoform-specific functions. *Biochem. Pharmacol.* **58**:1237–1246.

Le, L. Q., J. H. Kabarowski, Z. Weng, A. B. Satterthwaite, E. T. Harvill, E. R. Jensen, J. F. Miller, and O. N. Witte. 2001. Mice lacking the orphan G protein-coupled receptor G2A develop a late-onset autoimmune syndrome. *Immunity* **14**:561–571.

Lee, C. W., R. A. Lewis, E. J. Corey, and K. F. Austen. 1983. Conversion of leukotriene D$_4$ to leukotriene E$_4$ by a dipeptidase released from the specific granule of human polymorphonuclear leucocytes. *Immunology* **48**:27–35.

Lee, H., J. J. Liao, M. Graeler, M. C. Huang, and E. J. Goetzl. 2002. Lysophospholipid regulation of mononuclear phagocytes. *Biochim. Biophys. Acta* **1582**:175–177.

Lee, M. J., S. Thangada, K. P. Claffey, N. Ancellin, C. H. Liu, M. Kluk, M. Volpi, R. I. Sha'afi, and T. Hla. 1999. Vascular endothelial cell adherens junction assembly and morphogenesis induced by sphingosine-1-phosphate. *Cell* **99**:301–312.

Le Stunff, H., C. Peterson, H. Liu, S. Milstien, and S. Spiegel. 2002. Sphingosine-1-phosphate and lipid phosphohydrolases. *Biochim. Biophys. Acta* **1582**: 8–17.

Liu, Y., R. Wada, T. Yamashita, Y. Mi, C. X. Deng, J. P. Hobson, H. M. Rosenfeldt, V. E. Nava, S. S. Chae, M. J. Lee, C. H. Liu, T. Hla, S. Spiegel, and R. L. Proia. 2000. Edg-1, the G protein-coupled receptor for sphingosine-1-phosphate, is essential for vascular maturation. *J. Clin. Invest.* **106**:951–961.

Lynch, K. R., G. P. O'Neill, Q. Liu, D. S. Im, N. Sawyer, K. M. Metters, N. Coulombe, M. Abramovitz, D. J. Figueroa, Z. Zeng, B. M. Connolly, C. Bai, C. P. Austin, A. Chateauneuf, R. Stocco, G. M. Greig, S. Kargman, S. B. Hooks, E. Hosfield, D. L. Williams, Jr., A. W. Ford-Hutchinson, C. T. Caskey, and J. F. Evans. 1999. Characterization of the human cysteinyl leukotriene CysLT$_1$ receptor. *Nature* **399**:789–793.

MacLennan, A. J., P. R. Carney, W. J. Zhu, A. H. Chaves, J. Garcia, J. R. Grimes, K. J. Anderson, S. N. Roper, and N. Lee. 2001. An essential role for the H218/AGR16/Edg-5/LP$_{B2}$ sphingosine 1-phosphate receptor in neuronal excitability. *Eur. J. Neurosci.* **14**:203–209.

Maekawa, A., Y. Kanaoka, B. K. Lam, and K. F. Austen. 2001. Identification in mice of two isoforms of the cysteinyl leukotriene 1 receptor that result from alternative splicing. *Proc. Natl. Acad. Sci. USA* **98**:2256–2261.

Maekawa, A., K. F. Austen, and Y. Kanaoka. 2002. Targeted gene disruption reveals the role of cysteinyl leukotriene 1 receptor in the enhanced vascular permeability of mice undergoing acute inflammatory responses. *J. Biol. Chem.* **277**:20820–20824.

Mancini, J. A., K. Blood, J. Guay, R. Gordon, D. Claveau, C. C. Chan, and D. Riendeau. 2001. Cloning, expression, and up-regulation of inducible rat prostaglandin E synthase during lipopolysaccharide-induced pyresis and adjuvant-induced arthritis. *J. Biol. Chem.* **276**:4469–4475.

Matsumoto, T., C. D. Funk, O. Radmark, J. O. Hoog, H. Jornvall, and B. Samuelsson. 1988. Molecular cloning and amino acid sequence of human 5-lipoxygenase. *Proc. Natl. Acad. Sci. USA* **85**:26–30.

Matsuoka, T., M. Hirata, H. Tanaka, Y. Takahashi, T. Murata, K. Kabashima, Y. Sugimoto, T. Kobayashi, F. Ushikubi, Y. Aze, N. Eguchi, Y. Urade, N. Yoshida, K. Kimura, A. Mizoguchi, Y. Honda, H. Nagai, and S. Narumiya. 2000. Prostaglandin D$_2$ as a mediator of allergic asthma. *Science* **287**:2013–2017.

Mellor, E. A., K. F. Austen, and J. A. Boyce. 2002. Cysteinyl leukotrienes and uridine diphosphate induce cytokine generation by human mast cells through an interleukin 4-regulated pathway that is inhibited by leukotriene receptor antagonists. *J. Exp. Med.* **195**:583–592.

Miller, D. K., J. W. Gillard, P. J. Vickers, S. Sadowski, C. Leveille, J. A. Mancini, P. Charleson, R. A. Dixon, A. W. Ford-Hutchinson, R. Fortin, J. Y. Gauthier, J. Rodkey, R. Rosen, C. Rouzer, I. S. Sigal, C. D. Strader, and J. F. Evans. 1990. Identification and isolation of a membrane protein necessary for leukotriene production. *Nature* **343**:278–281.

Minami, M., S. Ohno, H. Kawasaki, O. Radmark, B. Samuelsson, H. Jornvall, T. Shimizu, Y. Seyama, and K. Suzuki. 1987. Molecular cloning of a cDNA coding for human leukotriene A$_4$ hydrolase. Complete primary structure of an enzyme involved in eicosanoid synthesis. *J. Biol. Chem.* **262**:13873–13876.

Morham, S. G., R. Langenbach, C. D. Loftin, H. F. Tiano, N. Vouloumanos, J. C. Jennette, J. F. Mahler, K. D. Kluckman, A. Ledford, C. A. Lee, and O. Smithies. 1995. Prostaglandin synthase 2 gene disruption causes severe renal pathology in the mouse. *Cell* **83:**473–482.

Murata, T., F. Ushikubi, T. Matsuoka, M. Hirata, A. Yamasaki, Y. Sugimoto, A. Ichikawa, Y. Aze, T. Tanaka, N. Yoshida, A. Ueno, S. Oh-ishi, and S. Narumiya. 1997. Altered pain perception and inflammatory response in mice lacking prostacyclin receptor. *Nature* **388:**678–682.

Narumiya, S., and G. A. FitzGerald. 2001. Genetic and pharmacological analysis of prostanoid receptor function. *J. Clin. Invest.* **108:**25–30.

Nataraj, C., D. W. Thomas, S. L. Tilley, M. T. Nguyen, R. Mannon, B. H. Koller, and T. M. Coffman. 2001. Receptors for prostaglandin E₂ that regulate cellular immune responses in the mouse. *J. Clin. Invest.* **108:**1229–1235.

Ogasawara, H., S. Ishii, T. Yokomizo, T. Kakinuma, M. Komine, K. Tamaki, T. Shimizu, and T. Izumi. 2002. Characterization of mouse cysteinyl leukotriene receptors mCysLT$_1$ and mCysLT$_2$: differential pharmacological properties and tissue distribution. *J. Biol. Chem.* **277:**18763–18768.

Oka, S., and H. Arita. 1991. Inflammatory factors stimulate expression of group II phospholipase A$_2$ in rat cultured astrocytes. Two distinct pathways of the gene expression. *J. Biol. Chem.* **266:**9956–9960.

Rao, T. S., J. L. Currie, A. F. Shaffer, and P. C. Isakson. 1994. In vivo characterization of zymosan-induced mouse peritoneal inflammation. *J. Pharmacol. Exp. Ther.* **269:**917–925.

Ricote, M., A. C. Li, T. M. Willson, C. J. Kelly, and C. K. Glass. 1998. The peroxisome proliferator-activated receptor-gamma is a negative regulator of macrophage activation. *Nature* **391:**79–82.

Rossi, A., P. Kapahi, G. Natoli, T. Takahashi, Y. Chen, M. Karin, and M. G. Santoro. 2000. Anti-inflammatory cyclopentenone prostaglandins are direct inhibitors of IkappaB kinase. *Nature* **403:**103–108.

Rouzer, C. A., W. A. Scott, Z. A. Cohn, P. Blackburn, and J. M. Manning. 1980. Mouse peritoneal macrophages release leukotriene C in response to a phagocytic stimulus. *Proc. Natl. Acad. Sci. USA* **77:**4928–4932.

Sawada, H., M. Murakami, A. Enomoto, S. Shimbara, and I. Kudo. 1999. Regulation of type V phospholipase A$_2$ expression and function by proinflammatory stimuli. *Eur. J. Biochem.* **263:**826–835.

Sharp, J. D., D. L. White, X. G. Chiou, T. Goodson, G. C. Gamboa, D. McClure, S. Burgett, J. Hoskins, P. L. Skatrud, J. R. Sportsman, G. W. Becker, L. H. Kang, E. F. Roberts, and R. M. Kramer. 1991. Molecular cloning and expression of human Ca^{2+}-sensitive cytosolic phospholipase A$_2$. *J. Biol. Chem.* **266:**14850–14853.

Shi, Z. Z., B. Han, G. M. Habib, M. M. Matzuk, and M. W. Lieberman. 2001. Disruption of gamma-glutamyl leukotrienase results in disruption of leukotriene D$_4$ synthesis in vivo and attenuation of the acute inflammatory response. *Mol. Cell. Biol.* **21:**5389–5395.

Shinomiya, S., H. Naraba, A. Ueno, I. Utsunomiya, T. Maruyama, S. Ohuchida, F. Ushikubi, K. Yuki, S. Narumiya, Y. Sugimoto, A. Ichikawa, and S. Oh-ishi. 2001. Regulation of TNFalpha and interleukin-10 production by prostaglandins I$_2$ and E$_2$: studies with prostaglandin receptor-deficient mice and prostaglandin E-receptor subtype-selective synthetic agonists. *Biochem. Pharmacol.* **61:**1153–1160.

Singer, A. G., F. Ghomashchi, C. Le Calvez, J. Bollinger, S. Bezzine, M. Rouault, M. Sadilek, E. Nguyen, M. Lazdunski, G. Lambeau, and M. H. Gelb. 2002. Interfacial kinetic and binding properties of the complete set of human and mouse groups I, II, V, X, and XII secreted phospholipases A$_2$. *J. Biol. Chem.* **277:**48535–48549.

Straus, D. S., G. Pascual, M. Li, J. S. Welch, M. Ricote, C. H. Hsiang, L. L. Sengchanthalangsy, G. Ghosh, and C. K. Glass. 2000. 15-deoxy-delta^{12,14}-prostaglandin J$_2$ inhibits multiple steps in the NF-kappa B signaling pathway. *Proc. Natl. Acad. Sci. USA* **97:**4844–4849.

Sugimoto, Y., A. Yamasaki, E. Segi, K. Tsuboi, Y. Aze, T. Nishimura, H. Oida, N. Yoshida, T. Tanaka, M. Katsuyama, K. Hasumoto, T. Murata, M. Hirata, F. Ushikubi, M. Negishi, A. Ichikawa, and S. Narumiya. 1997. Failure of parturition in mice lacking the prostaglandin F receptor. *Science* **277:**681–683.

Tager, A. M., J. H. Dufour, K. Goodarzi, S. D. Bercury, U. H. von Andrian, and A. D. Luster. 2000. BLTR mediates leukotriene B4-induced chemotaxis and adhesion and plays a dominant role in eosinophil accumulation in a murine model of peritonitis. *J. Exp. Med.* **192:**439–446.

Tanikawa, N., Y. Ohmiya, H. Ohkubo, K. Hashimoto, K. Kangawa, M. Kojima, S. Ito, and K. Watanabe. 2002. Identification and characterization of a novel type of membrane-associated prostaglandin E synthase. *Biochem. Biophys. Res. Commun.* **291:**884–889.

Tanioka, T., Y. Nakatani, N. Semmyo, M. Murakami, and I. Kudo. 2000. Molecular identification of cytosolic prostaglandin E$_2$ synthase that is functionally coupled with cyclooxygenase-1 in immediate prostaglandin E$_2$ biosynthesis. *J. Biol. Chem.* **275:**32775–32782.

Tilley, S. L., T. M. Coffman, and B. H. Koller. 2001. Mixed messages: modulation of inflammation and immune responses by prostaglandins and thromboxanes. *J. Clin. Invest.* **108:**15–23.

Tokumura, A., E. Majima, Y. Kariya, K. Tominaga, K. Kogure, K. Yasuda, and K. Fukuzawa. 2002. Identification of human plasma lysophospholipase D, a lysophosphatidic acid-producing enzyme, as autotaxin, a multifunctional phosphodiesterase. *J. Biol. Chem.* **277**:39436–39442.

Uematsu, S., M. Matsumoto, K. Takeda, and S. Akira. 2002. Lipopolysaccharide-dependent prostaglandin E_2 production is regulated by the glutathione-dependent prostaglandin E_2 synthase gene induced by the Toll-like receptor 4/MyD88/NF-IL6 pathway. *J. Immunol.* **168**:5811–5816.

Uozumi, N., K. Kume, T. Nagase, N. Nakatani, S. Ishii, F. Tashiro, Y. Komagata, K. Maki, K. Ikuta, Y. Ouchi, J. Miyazaki, and T. Shimizu. 1997. Role of cytosolic phospholipase A_2 in allergic response and parturition. *Nature* **390**:618–622.

Ushikubi, F., Y. Aiba, K. Nakamura, T. Namba, M. Hirata, O. Mazda, Y. Katsura, and S. Narumiya. 1993. Thromboxane A_2 receptor is highly expressed in mouse immature thymocytes and mediates DNA fragmentation and apoptosis. *J. Exp. Med.* **178**:1825–1830.

van der Pouw Kraan, T. C., L. C. Boeije, R. J. Smeenk, J. Wijdenes, and L. A. Aarden. 1995. Prostaglandin-E_2 is a potent inhibitor of human interleukin 12 production. *J. Exp. Med.* **181**:775–779.

Watanabe, K., K. Kurihara, and T. Suzuki. 1999. Purification and characterization of membrane-bound prostaglandin E synthase from bovine heart. *Biochim. Biophys. Acta* **1439**:406–414.

Weinrauch, Y., P. Elsbach, L. M. Madsen, A. Foreman, and J. Weiss. 1996. The potent anti-*Staphylococcus aureus* activity of a sterile rabbit inflammatory fluid is due to a 14-kD phospholipase A_2. *J. Clin. Invest.* **97**:250–257.

Welsch, D. J., D. P. Creely, S. D. Hauser, K. J. Mathis, G. G. Krivi, and P. C. Isakson. 1994. Molecular cloning and expression of human leukotriene-C_4 synthase. *Proc. Natl. Acad. Sci. USA* **91**:9745–9749.

Xia, P., J. R. Gamble, K. A. Rye, L. Wang, C. S. Hii, P. Cockerill, Y. Khew-Goodall, A. G. Bert, P. J. Barter, and M. A. Vadas. 1998. Tumor necrosis factor-alpha induces adhesion molecule expression through the sphingosine kinase pathway. *Proc. Natl. Acad. Sci. USA* **95**:14196–14201.

Xu, Y. 2002. Sphingosylphosphorylcholine and lysophosphatidylcholine: G protein-coupled receptors and receptor-mediated signal transduction. *Biochim. Biophys. Acta* **1582**:81–88.

Yokomizo, T., T. Izumi, K. Chang, Y. Takuwa, and T. Shimizu. 1997. A G-protein-coupled receptor for leukotriene B_4 that mediates chemotaxis. *Nature* **387**:620–624.

Yokomizo, T., K. Kato, K. Terawaki, T. Izumi, and T. Shimizu. 2000. A second leukotriene B_4 receptor, BLT2. A new therapeutic target in inflammation and immunological disorders. *J. Exp. Med.* **192**:421–432.

Yokota, Y., K. Higashino, K. Nakano, H. Arita, and K. Hanasaki. 2000. Identification of group X secretory phospholipase A_2 as a natural ligand for mouse phospholipase A_2 receptor. *FEBS Lett.* **478**:187–191.

Zhou, D., W. Luini, S. Bernasconi, L. Diomede, M. Salmona, A. Mantovani, and S. Sozzani. 1995. Phosphatidic acid and lysophosphatidic acid induce haptotactic migration of human monocytes. *J. Biol. Chem.* **270**:25549–25556.

ROLE OF INNATE IMMUNITY IN BACTERIAL INFECTION

Peter Seiler, Ulrich Steinhoff, and Stefan H. E. Kaufmann

22

INTRODUCTION

The innate immune response is critical for the prompt combat of invading pathogens at their main ports of entry with skin as well as pulmonary and intestinal mucosae being misused as preferred sites of entry. Because of their different physiological functions, the defense mechanisms at skin and mucosa are quite different. Defense in the skin is unpretentious in that it is mostly based on impermeable mechanical shielding. Accordingly, microbial entrance through the skin barrier generally requires erosions of the skin, e.g., by injury, or injection through the skin, e.g., by insect bites. Defense strategies at the mucosa need to solve more complex obstacles. On the one hand, the intestinal and lung mucosae have to take care of nutrient uptake or gas exchange, respectively, and therefore have to supply appropriate permeability and translocation mechanisms. Unrestricted passage through this barrier is facilitated by a single-cell lining of specialized epithelial cells at the mucosal surface. On the other hand, this layer is highly vulnerable and the mucosa is not a sterile tissue, with the intestinal mucosa being heavily inhabited by microbes. To achieve host defense, mucosal tissues require a potent innate immune system that comprises sessile as well as mobile immune effector cells that are rapidly attracted by any assault.

Yet, despite several communalities, marked differences between lung and intestine exist. The deeper regions of the lung are virtually devoid of any commensal bacteria. Any microbe entering these alveolar regions has to be considered as dangerous by the host. In contrast, the intestine is inhabited by an enormous number of microbial organisms, with up to 10^{14} bacteria from approximately 500 different species in the large intestine. Hence, the intestine has to distinguish between the normal and the pathogenic flora to prevent pathogens from colonization or invasion, leaving the normal flora unaffected. In fact the enormous number of microbes in the gut renders the normal flora part of the host resistance because they compete with newly arising pathogens in numerous respects, notably for nutrients and attachment to the gut epithelia.

In this chapter we focus on innate immunity against bacterial pathogens with emphasis on the local response at the two major sites of entry, lung and gut. We use two microbes that

Peter Seiler, Ulrich Steinhoff, and Stefan H. E. Kaufmann, Max Planck Institute for Infection Biology, Schumannstr. 21/22, D-10117 Berlin, Germany.

The Innate Immune Response to Infection
Ed. by S. H. E. Kaufmann, R. Medzhitov, and S. Gordon
©2004 ASM Press, Washington, D.C.

have been well studied, namely, *Mycobacterium tuberculosis* and *Listeria monocytogenes,* which preferentially enter the host via the lung or gut, respectively. These two bacteria not only differ enormously with regard to their impact on human health: *M. tuberculosis* is one of the major threats worldwide, whereas *L. monocytogenes* plays only a minor role in human health morbidity and mortality statistics. They also differ with regard to virulence and course of infection. *L. monocytogenes* causes acute infection and is rapidly eliminated once the acquired immune response has been established. Innate immune mechanisms are critical in curtailing infection of this rapidly dividing bacterium. *M. tuberculosis,* in contrast, is a slow-growing microbe that causes chronic infection and disease and persists in the host even in the face of a fully activated acquired immune response. Although generally considered important, the role of innate immunity in control of tuberculosis is largely enigmatic. Hence, the two pathogens serve as different examples for discussing distinct and common mechanisms of antibacterial innate immune responses.

L. monocytogenes and Listeriosis

L. monocytogenes, a gram-positive bacterium, has proven to be remarkably well suited for studying various aspects of cellular microbiology and immunology. Although it rarely causes disease in humans, it provides an excellent experimental animal model for acute bacterial infections controlled by cell-mediated immunity. Yet neither the natural route of infection via the intestine nor the neuronal complications are fully reflected by the mouse model.

L. monocytogenes is a facultative intracellular bacterium with the ability to live and survive in macrophages, i.e., professional phagocytes that are well equipped to kill various microorganisms. Even more, this microbe has developed a number of mechanisms to exploit host cells for intracellular living without causing major damage to its habitat. Listeriosis is most common among newborn and immunocompromised individuals, and disease is mainly due to the ability of *L. monocytogenes* to enter the central nervous system and pass through the placenta (Huang et al., 2001). In immunocompetent adults listeriosis is rare (Schlech, 2000), and it has been estimated that approximately 5% of the population of the United States is asymptomatically colonized with *L. monocytogenes.* Yet when outbreaks of listeriosis occur, the fatalities exceed those of the notorious food-borne pathogen *Clostridium botulinum* (Havell et al., 1999).

Experimental infection is performed either intravenously or per os using high numbers of bacteria. Although *L. monocytogenes* is an enteroinvasive bacterial pathogen, oral infection of mice does not reflect fully the natural route of infection because mice lack the specific receptor that mediates the intestinal uptake. Therefore, although it is artificial, intravenous infection is generally employed and results in a rapid spread of the bacteria to the liver and spleen. In this part of the review we present data from mice and humans from the first contact of *L. monocytogenes* with the intestinal mucosa to systemic bacterial dissemination in the periphery.

M. tuberculosis and Tuberculosis

M. tuberculosis is a facultative intracellular, rod-shaped bacillus. The microorganism is shielded by a unique wax-rich cell wall that is composed of long-chain fatty acids, glycolipids, and other components (Brennan and Nikaido, 1995; Lee et al., 1996). This robust shell accounts for the acid fastness and contributes to the capacity of *M. tuberculosis* to survive in host phagocytes, primarily in alveolar macrophages. *M. tuberculosis* is a slow-growing organism, with a replication time of at least 20 h in the host. This slow growth forms the basis for the chronic nature of infection and disease (Kaufmann, 2001). Although tuberculosis can manifest itself at any tissue site, the lung represents both the main port of entry and the most frequent site of disease manifestation.

Extrapulmonary tuberculosis develops in less than 10% of all cases. Less than 10% of all infected individuals will develop clinical disease during their lifetime, but once disease does develop and remains untreated, it is fatal in 50% of patients. With approximately 2 million deaths annually, and with one third of the world's population, i.e., 2 billion people, infected, *M. tuberculosis* represents one of the most effective human pathogens (Kaufmann, 2001). Infection of a number of experimental animal species with *M. tuberculosis* provides suitable models for in vivo studies. In terms of the host response, most has been learned from the immunologically well-established mouse model employing the physiological route of infection via aerosols. The guinea pig compares better to humans in terms of lung pathology than the mouse, and this model thus provides valuable insights into pathology, disease susceptibility, and intervention strategies. Continuous comparison of experimental animal infection and clinical as well as histological data from human patients will not only better our understanding of *M. tuberculosis* infection, but also provide the basis for rational preventive and therapeutic measures.

INNATE IMMUNE RESPONSE AGAINST *L. MONOCYTOGENES*

The First Line of Defense: the Normal Gut Flora

The human gut flora comprises approximately 500 different bacterial species with up to 10^{11} microorganisms per g of feces and a total number of approximately 10^{14} microorganisms. Environmental bacteria are taken up in food and usually represent a transient flora. The dominant indigenous flora comprises four major groups, namely, *Bacteroides* spp., *Bifidobacterium* spp., *Eubacterium* spp., and *Peptostreptococcus* spp. The subdominant flora consists of bacteria belonging to the genera *Streptococcus*, *Lactobacillus* and *Enterococcus*, and *Clostridium* and *Bacillus*. Obviously the commensal flora competes for the adhesion at the intestinal epithelium and interferes with toxic products of pathogenic bacteria (Brook, 1999). Four different mechanisms of interference have been suggested: (i) consumption of limited

nutrients by the normal flora that restricts the growth of pathogens; (ii) inhibition of adhesion of pathogens to receptor sites, either by steric hindrance or by blockade of the receptor; (iii) generation of a restrictive physiological environment including volatile fatty acids, production of hydrogen sulfides, or alterations in the redox potential; and (iv) secretion of antimicrobial substances mainly by lactic acid bacteria (Falk et al., 1998).

Recently, angiogenins (ANGs), RNases released from Paneth cells, have been identified to discriminate between commensal and exogenous bacteria in the intestine. Commensal bacteria stimulate the release of ANGs, to which they are resistant themselves, that kill exogenous bacteria: *L. monocytogenes* is killed species specifically by the mouse ANG 4 and the human ANG in vitro (Ganz, 2003; Hooper et al., 2003).

Function of the Mucus

The mucosal surface of the gastrointestinal tract is covered by epithelial cells that are tightly joined absorptive cells called enterocytes, allowing the absorption of nutrients while preventing entry of pathogens. Interspersed among the epithelial cells are goblet cells that secrete mucus consisting of glycoproteins of various molecular sizes (Roussel et al., 1988). The mucus blanket of the human gastrointestinal tract is approximately 100 μm thick and serves at least two functions. First, it serves as a nutrient that positively influences intestinal colonization by adherent bacteria. Second, epithelial and Paneth cells that are located in the crypts of the villi secrete several antimicrobial defense molecules, including lactoferrin, lysozyme, cathelicidins, and secretory phospholipase A2, thus preventing bacterial adhesion and invasion (Ouellette, 1997).

Experiments with normal animals harboring an intestinal flora revealed that oral infection with 10^7 *L. monocytogenes* organisms is insufficient for establishing bacterial colonization in the gut. The exception are A/J mice, which bear the susceptible allele at the Hc locus and are characterized by severely impaired mobilization of inflammatory cells. These animals are highly susceptible to local and systemic infection with *L. monocytogenes* (Czuprynski et al., 2003). Similarly, in germfree animals, infection with 10^7 *L. monocytogenes* results in a systemic spread of high titers of *L. monocytogenes* even 6 days after oral infection (U. Steinhoff, unpublished results). Studies employing the ligated ileal loop system and in vitro experiments with cultured human intestinal cells revealed that infection with *L. monocytogenes* induces mucus secretion that facilitates association with and entry into epithelial cells (Coconnier et al., 1998; Pron et al., 1998). Mucus secretion is stimulated by the bacterial exotoxin listeriolysin O (LLO) that binds to a so far nonidentified brush border-associated receptor. In contrast to the intracellular lytic activity of LLO, which perforates the phagolysosomal membrane, allowing *L. monocytogenes* to escape into the cytosol of the host cell, LLO-stimulated mucus exocytosis is not related to membrane damage most likely because of its strict pH optimum at 5.5 (Geoffroy et al., 1987).

First Contact with Immune Receptors: TLRs

In mammalian cells, activation via Toll-like receptors (TLRs) results in stimulation of the innate immune system, including upregulation of cytokines, chemokines, costimulatory molecules, and oxidative burst. Ten members of the TLR family have been described, and for most of them the unique recognition specificity has been identified (Barton and Medzhitov, 2002). The important role of TLR signaling in innate immunity has been shown by microarray analysis of dendritic cells (DCs) infected with *Escherichia coli*. More than 160 genes were induced after infection with this gram-negative bacterium, with lipopolysaccharide accounting for the vast majority of the response (Huang et al., 2001).

Peptidoglycan is the major cell wall component of gram-positive bacteria, including *L. monocytogenes*, that interacts specifically with TLR-2. The proximal signal cascade of TLR is mediated via the common adapter MyD88, which in turn recruits interleukin-1 (IL-1)

receptor-associated kinase. Mutant mice deficient in TLR-2, infected with *L. monocytogenes*, did not show impaired resistance as compared with wild-type mice. However, mice deficient in the common adapter molecule MyD88 revealed a dramatically increased bacterial burden and diminished, although not absent, gamma interferon (IFN-γ), tumor necrosis factor alpha (TNF-α), and NO responses. Furthermore, in MyD88-deficient mice polymorphonuclear granulocyte as well as IL-1 and IL-18 responses were reduced. Although the reduced inflammatory reaction in MyD88 knockout (KO) mice temporarily increased resistance to a high bacterial load, mice ultimately succumbed to uncontrolled bacteremia (Edelson and Unanue, 2002). Thus, innate immune responses to *L. monocytogenes* comprise MyD88-dependent and -independent pathways of cytokine production.

TLR signaling by an MyD88-independent mechanism involving TIRAP (Toll-interleukin 1 receptor domain-containing adaptor protein) and TICAM-I (Toll-interleukin 1 receptor domain-containing adaptor molecule 1) has been described recently (Oshiumi et al., 2003). In vitro analyses demonstrated that TLR-2 was essential for stimulation of TNF-α, IL-12, and NO production by heat-killed *L. monocytogenes* but not by live bacteria (Edelson and Unanue, 2002). These findings suggest that *L. monocytogenes* stimulates the innate immune system by several pathogen-associated molecular patterns, including peptidoglycan, lipoteichoic acid, *L. monocytogenes* flagellin, and bacterial DNA employing TLR-2, -4, -5, -6 and -9, respectively (Ozinsky et al., 2000). The need for the central MyD88 adapter molecule in the resistance against *L. monocytogenes* emphasizes the redundancy of TLR-mediated recognition of a live microorganism, although further investigations are necessary to clarify the impact of individual TLRs in the defense against *L. monocytogenes*. Note that the expression pattern of TLRs shows species-specific variations. Although murine T cells express TLRs, human T cells lack the expression of these innate receptors (Matsuguchi et al., 2000).

Crossing the Intestinal Barrier and Uptake by Phagocytic Cells

Listeriosis is characterized by bacterial dissemination from the gut lumen to the central nervous system via the blood-brain barrier and to the fetus via the fetoplacental barrier (Lorber, 1997). Because the encounter between bacterial pathogen and professional phagocyte leads to the release of bacterial and host cell products that induce a strong inflammation, this step represents the heart of the innate immune response. A number of enteroinvasive pathogens including *Salmonella*, *Shigella*, and *Yersinia* translocate preferentially via M cells, highly specialized epithelial cells that sample the content of the gut lumen. Yet the mechanisms of translocation of *L. monocytogenes* through the epithelial barrier are still not fully understood (Pron et al., 2001). Although epithelial cells fail to spontaneously phagocytose, invasive bacteria can induce their own uptake. In vitro experiments with human epithelial cells have shown that the *L. monocytogenes* surface protein internalin A binds to E-cadherin, which mediates the formation of junctions between epithelial cells (Mengaud et al., 1996). This binding initiates listerial translocation through enterocytes. Mouse and rat E-cadherins do not bind to internalin, reflecting the minute translocation efficiency of *L. monocytogenes* after oral infection of mice. Because various cells express E-cadherin, it is most likely that the internalin–E-cadherin interaction is also critical for listerial spreading at later stages of infection. In addition, further host pathogen interactions that are not identified yet may contribute to the pathogenesis of listeriosis in the gastrointestinal tract as recently demonstrated in A/J mice (Czuprynski et al., 2003).

The paradox is that *L. monocytogenes* preferentially lives in macrophages and DCs, which are essential for the initiation of the acquired immune response. DCs migrate to the lymphoid organs, where they activate antigen-specific T cells. After capturing antigen, DCs undergo extensive transformation, referred to as maturation. While their phagocytic activity decreases, their T-cell stimulatory function increases, which is accompanied by the expression of costimulatory molecules and secretion of cytokines such as IL-12 and IL-18 (Austyn, 1996; Banchereau and Steinman, 1998; Guermonprez et al., 2002; Koski et al., 2001). Studies of the intestinal stage of listeriosis in rodents identified DCs in the subepithelial dome region of the Peyer's patches as first targets of *L. monocytogenes*. Thereafter, *L. monocytogenes* spreads to other intestinal cells via two distinct mechanisms, cell-to-cell spread by actin polymerization or by phagocytosis of free bacteria. Several hours after entry, *L. monocytogenes* is detected in DCs in the paracortical zone of the draining mesenteric lymph nodes (MLNs). *L. monocytogenes* obviously exploits the migratory capacity of DCs for transport from the intestinal lumen to the MLNs. After arrival in the MLNs, *L. monocytogenes* spreads from DCs to macrophages, where the bacteria rapidly replicate. Although the mechanism of bacterial transmission is incompletely understood, it appears ActA independent and most likely involves the death of DCs. Moreover, it is still controversial to what extent *L. monocytogenes* grows within DCs. Although several in vitro studies reported extensive growth, confocal analysis of infected tissues revealed limited replication, if any, and localization of the bacteria within phagosomes (Guzman et al., 1995; Kolb-Maurer et al., 2000). This is surprising because DCs possess only a weak oxidative burst and thus might be preferred by *L. monocytogenes* to macrophages, which are well equipped to destroy phagosomal listeriae. The observed differences could reflect the heterogeneity of DCs to support the replication of microbial agents. In conclusion, DCs seem to be the first cell type infected by *L. monocytogenes*, and the absent bacterial replication renders these cells a potent vector for transport to the draining lymph nodes and other tissue sites in the body.

Inside the Cell

After entering a host cell, *L. monocytogenes* multiplies intracellularly with an initial doubling time of approximately 40 min. The bacteria are first located in the phagosome, where they are killed unless they escape into the cytosol. The pore-forming protein LLO and two types of phospholipase Cs are responsible for vacuolar escape and thus represent an important virulence factor of *L. monocytogenes*. Mutants that lack LLO cannot escape from the phagosome or the secondary vacuole that is formed upon cell-to-cell spread (Gedde et al., 2000; Cossart et al., 1989).

Insertion of LLO into the phagosomal membrane serves two functions: first, to dissipate the pH gradient and thereby terminate phagosome maturation to a deadly trap for the bacteria, and second, to form a channel that allows proteins and enzymes to enter the cytoplasm that then achieve dissolution of the vacuole (Portnoy et al., 2002). LLO has its optimum at pH 5.5 and thus perforates the membrane of the phagosome but not the membrane surrounding the cell. The LLO includes a PEST (region enriched with Pro, Glu, Ser, and Thr)-like sequence characterized by N-terminal residues that are rich in proline, glutamate, serine, and threonine. Removal of this sequence does not affect the lytic activity of LLO, which is responsible for the vacuolar escape. In contrast, PEST-like sequence-deficient bacteria show increased virulence in vitro and decreased virulence in vivo (Decatur and Portnoy, 2000). How can this be explained? Early destruction of host cells results in release of extracellular bacteria that are readily killed by infiltrating monocytes and polymorphonuclear leukocytes (PMNs). This demonstrates on a molecular level how a successful pathogen has evolved sophisticated strategies to avoid destruction of the host cell in order to maintain the habitat for optimal growth and spread within its host organism.

Spread from Cell to Cell

Recently it was shown that a virulence-regulated hexose phosphate transporter is necessary for optimal cytosolic growth of *L. monocytogenes* (Chico-Calero et al., 2002). Having reached the cytosol, *L. monocytogenes* induces polymerization of host actin filaments to move, first within the cell and then from cell to cell. A single bacterial protein, ActA, is responsible for actin polymerization and actin-based motility. The exact process of how *L. monocytogenes* utilizes the cytoskeleton of the host cells is described in detail by Cameron et al. (2000). The critical impact of motility for resistance becomes most obvious in *L. monocytogenes*-immune mice. *L. monocytogenes* mutants that cannot polymerize actin show slightly reduced virulence in naive mice, but are highly impaired in immune mice (Auerbuch et al., 2001). Thus, efficient cell-to-cell spread is an important mechanism to evade the acquired immune response of the host.

Entering the Bloodstream: the Filter Function of the Spleen

Once a pathogen has overcome the local innate and adaptive immune response at the interface between environment and host, it will disseminate to other tissue sites via circulation. The highly organized microarchitecture of secondary lymphoid organs forms the basis for antigen trapping. The spleen is responsible for filtering blood-borne particles. Microanatomically, the spleen is separated into the white and red pulp separated by the marginal zone (Cyster, 2000; Kraal, 1992). The marginal zone consists of sinus-lining reticular cells, marginal zone B cells, DCs, marginal metallophilic macrophages (MMs), and marginal zone macrophages (MZMs). In the marginal zone the blood leaves the terminal arterioles and moves into open sinuses, the blood flow is slowed down, and blood-borne particles are entrapped. Recent data from our own group indicate that the MZMs and MMs are indispensable for particle trapping in the splenic marginal zone (Aichele et al., 2003). After selective depletion of these two macrophage subsets by clodronate-liposome treatment, microsphere beads or *L. monocytogenes* organisms were no longer entrapped. *L. monocytogenes* infection rapidly disseminated, and mice succumbed to infection. Yet antigen presentation still occurred independently of the trapping and the presence of MZMs and MMs. Normal T- and B-cell recall functions could be evoked. These data are in agreement with studies on various gene-deficient mice lacking an intact marginal zone organization: alymphoplastic (*aly/aly*) and osteopetrotic (*op/op*) mice and mouse mutants with targeted disruptions in TNF-α, TNF receptor-1, LT-α, LT-β, Pyk-2, RelB, NF-κB, or Bcl-3. The multiplicity of factors obviously involved in marginal zone formation underlines the importance of a specialized pathogen-trapping architecture and emphasizes the impact of pathogen trapping on innate immune defense.

In addition to their high phagocytic activity, the MZMs in particular are abundantly armed with a specialized and unique repertoire of opsonin-independent and -dependent surface receptors. Opsonin-independent phagocytosis is mediated by a variety of receptors including scavenger receptors type SR–AI and –II, MARCO (macrophage receptor with collagenous structure), and CD36 and pattern recognition receptors such as the TLR and the macrophage mannose receptor (MMR). Mutant KO mice deficient in type SR–AI and –II scavenger receptors are more susceptible to *L. monocytogenes* infection due to impaired capacity of macrophages to phagocytose and kill bacteria (Gough and Gordon, 2000).

Pathogen trapping in the splenic marginal zone is promoted by opsonins such as natural antibodies or collectins and complement factors. In mice genetically deficient of B cells, trapping of *L. monocytogenes* is highly compromised. It is likely that opsonization by antibodies enhances pathogen trapping in the splenic marginal zone. Complement components are also critically involved in the control of bacterial infections. MZMs express CR3 abundantly. Therefore, direct binding of C3 breakdown products to a pathogen promotes its trapping by MZMs (Ochsenbein and Zinkernagel, 2000).

The Liver Stage of Infection: Macrophages, Monocytes, PMNs, and NK Cells

The majority of *L. monocytogenes* organisms that reach the bloodstream soon end up in the liver. Analysis of this "liver-stage" infection

demonstrated the importance of innate immunity to control listerial replication during the first days (Cousens and Wing, 2000). After intravenous inoculation, more than 60% of the bacteria are taken up by the liver within 10 min (Gregory et al., 1996a; McGregor et al., 1973), and six hours later, hepatocytes harbor >90% of the *L. monocytogenes* organisms. Various cell types including monocytes, PMNs, NK cells, and Kupffer cells contribute to early control of infection (Cousens and Wing, 2000; Conlan and North, 1994; Unanue, 1996). In this subsection we mainly focus on two effector cells, the Kupffer cells and the PMNs.

Kupffer cells, the resident tissue macrophages of the liver, adhere to the endothelial cells of the liver sinusoids and are most densely accumulated in the periportal region. Accordingly, they are optimally located for the trapping of bacteria and other antigens that are transported from the gut to the liver via the portal vein (Fox et al., 1987). Because most *L. monocytogenes* organisms are found within hepatocytes and not Kupffer cells, it has been claimed that phagocytosis is not a critical issue. Evidence is growing that Kupffer cells clear the bacteria from the blood via lectin-mediated adherence rather than phagocytosis (Gregory et al., 1996a; Ofek and Sharon, 1988). In addition to their role in blood clearance, Kupffer cells may inhibit bacterial growth indirectly, although the exact mechanism remains unknown. Secretion of various soluble factors, including IL-6, IL-12, IL-1β, TNF-α, and nitric oxide, is known to induce inflammatory responses or to exhibit direct bacteriocidal activity (Ehlers et al., 1992; Gregory et al., 1998). Furthermore, Kupffer cells express the cell surface adhesion molecules ICAM-1 (intercellular adhesion molecule-1) and VCAM-1 (vascular cell adhesion molecule-1) that facilitate interactions with PMNs, indicating that both cell types collaborate in controlling the growth of *L. monocytogenes* (Gregory et al., 1996b). In support of this, recent studies demonstrated that *L. monocytogenes* is not directly killed by Kupffer cells but rather by immigrant PMNs which, in addition to colocalizing with Kupffer cells, are even found within these cells (Gregory and Wing, 2002).

Although hepatocytes and Kupffer cells serve as habitats for *L. monocytogenes*, PMNs and monocytes are the most potent effector cells of innate immunity (Rosen et al., 1989). Infected tissues are rich in PMNs, and depletion of these cells leads to rapid death of mice (Conlan and North, 1994; Rogers and Unanue, 1993). Recently, it was shown that LFA-1$^{-/-}$ mice are far more resistant to *L. monocytogenes*. Exacerbated listeriosis in the absence of LFA-1 (lymphocyte function-associated antigen-1) was due to neutrophilia that facilitated infiltration of PMNs into the liver, although this latter step itself was LFA-1 independent (Miyamoto et al., 2003). It is unlikely that PMNs kill infected hepatocytes; instead they seem to exert their antimicrobial activity by directly killing *L. monocytogenes* (Cousens and Wing, 2000). The importance of NK cells in innate immunity against *L. monocytogenes* has been largely defined in T-cell-deficient mice, and lysis of infected hepatocytes and production of IFN-γ and TNF-α have been revealed as the major effector mechanisms of this cell type (Gregory et al., 1996b; Guo et al., 1992).

Soluble Factors Secreted by Cells of the Innate Immune System: Cytokines and Chemokines

Infection with *L. monocytogenes* rapidly induces Th1-promoting cytokines, including IL-12, IFN-γ, and TNF-α. IL-12 is secreted by activated neutrophils and DCs in the early phase of infection and is essential for primary antilisterial responses. IL-12 synergizes with TNF-α in driving the IFN-γ production by NK cells, resulting in activation of macrophages. Two potent antimicrobial mechanisms of macrophages are production of reactive oxygen intermediates (ROIs) and reactive nitrogen intermediates (RNIs). Although resistance against *M. tuberculosis* infection is clearly RNI dependent, there is still some controversy about the impact of RNI and ROI metabo-

lites in the killing of *L. monocytogenes*. Approximately 50% of mutant mice double deficient in ROI and RNI generation revealed normal resistance to infection with *L. monocytogenes*, suggesting the existence of bacteriocidal mechanisms independent from phagocyte oxidase (Phox) and inducible nitric oxide synthase (iNOS) (Shiloh et al., 1999). It further appears that contributions of ROIs and RNIs to listerial killing differ between macrophages activated pre- and postinfection (Ohya et al., 1998).

IL-6 and IL-1 are required for resistance against *L. monocytogenes*, most likely by regulating the PMN response during the infection. IL-6-deficient mice suffer from increased bacterial growth in the liver, which correlated with inefficient blood neutrophilia (Dalrymple et al., 1995). IL-1 may contribute to antilisterial responses at various levels including activation of neutrophils, induction of chemokines, and expression of adhesion molecules on liver cells, both promoting neutrophil trafficking to sites of infection (Bevilacqua et al., 1985; Furie and McHugh, 1989).

Chemokines are critical mediators of leukocyte trafficking, including attraction to sites of inflammation. In addition, certain chemokines share characteristic features with defensins, including the cationic charge at neutral pH, size, disulfide bonding, and IFN-γ inducibility. Analysis of the antimicrobial activities of representative chemokines from all four families revealed that the monocyte-derived, IFN-γ-inducible chemokines MIG (CXCL9), IP-10 (CXCL10), and T-cell α chemoattractant ITAC (CXCL11) exhibit antilisterial activity comparable to that of the α-defensin human neutrophil peptide 1 (HNP-1) in vitro (Cole et al., 2001). Yet their contribution to growth restriction of *L. monocytogenes* in vivo remains to be tested. Note that the inflammatory chemokines macrophage inflammatory protein-1α (MIP-1α) (CCL3), MIP-1β (CCL4), RANTES (CCL5), and ATAC (activation-induced, T-cell-derived, and chemokine-related cytokine), which are secreted during early and late phases of *L. monocytogenes* infection, do not exhibit direct antimicrobial activity (Cole et al., 2001; Dorner et al., 2002). Accumulation of positively charged residues at the C terminus appears crucial for the antimicrobial effects of chemokines, explaining why IL-8 (CXCL8) and ENA-78 (epithelial neutrophil-activating peptide-78; CXCL5), both representatives of the CXC family, show no antimicrobial effects. The importance and potency of antimicrobial substances to locally restrict the growth of pathogenic bacteria in the gut was recently demonstrated. Transgenic mice expressing the human α-defensin (HD5) in Paneth cells revealed increased resistance against the intracellular bacterium *Salmonella typhimurium* (Salzman et al., 2003).

Remarks

Control and resolution of *L. monocytogenes* infection involve a variety of different cell types, cytokines, and chemokines. The major task of the soluble factors is the early mobilization and focusing of effector cells to the site of infection. Once *L. monocytogenes* has entered the bloodstream, bacteria are rapidly trapped in the liver, which is of critical importance for defense against systemic infection. There, host defense is mediated by the concerted action of monocytes, PMNs, and NK cells together with soluble factors. Although substantial progress has been made, further investigations will be needed to understand the complex regulation of innate immune responses.

INNATE IMMUNE RESPONSE AGAINST *M. TUBERCULOSIS*

Soluble Effectors in Mucus of the Upper Airways

In contrast to the gut, the lower respiratory system and the lung harbor no commensal flora. The immune system therefore does not have to discriminate between foreign and commensal bacteria, but it is destined to remove any inhaled particle and to eradicate any invading pathogen. Inhaled *M. tuberculosis* bacilli first face the viscous lung mucus in the upper airways and the lung surfactant in the lower airways,

the alveoli. Depending on the air speed, only particles >5 μm in size settle in the upper airways, i.e., only minute clumps of *M. tuberculosis* bacilli (Ferguson and Schlesinger, 2000; West, 1994). Most of this material is expelled by the mucociliary transport system. The importance of this system is often underestimated. Patients with abnormal mucus clearance, due to, for example, primary ciliary dyskinesia, cystic fibrosis, or pseudohypoaldosteronism, severely suffer from chronic airway infections (Knowles and Boucher, 2002). Increased incidences of tuberculosis have been reported in cystic fibrosis patients with perturbed mucus production and salt concentration and consequently perturbed mucociliary transport (Fauroux et al., 1997; Ferguson and Schlesinger, 2000).

Moreover, mucus contains a spectrum of soluble effector molecules including high concentrations of lysozyme and lactoferrin as well as trace amounts of secretory leukoprotease inhibitor and epithelial defensins and cathelicidins (Table 1). This combination of antibacterial agents enables control of most infectious agents, e.g., *Staphylococcus aureus*, *E. coli*, and *Pseudomonas aeruginosa*, during the first 2 to 6 h postentry, thus allowing for sufficient time for mucociliary clearance (Ganz, 2002a, 2002b; Knowles and Boucher, 2002; Lehrer and Ganz, 2002a, 2002b).

An impact of lysozyme on *M. tuberculosis* in vivo is very likely because mycobacteria are readily digested by lysozyme in vitro. Lactoferrin exhibits direct, so far uncharacterized, enzymatic microbicidal activity as well as indirect activity via iron chelation (Arnold et al., 1982; Ganz, 2002a). Recent results from our laboratory indicate a prominent effect of intracellular lactoferrin on mycobacterial growth in vitro as well as in vivo in mice at least in the presence of a high iron load (Schaible et al., 2002). Limiting the iron supply impaired mycobacterial replication but still allowed infected macrophages to generate host defense mechanisms. Reciprocally, iron overload favored mycobacteria over macrophages and exacerbated disease. Thus, control of intracellular iron supply represents a successful innate

TABLE 1 Secreted effector molecules in innate immune response against *M. tuberculosis*[a]

Effector	Source (human)	Effector function	References
Lysozyme	M, N, EC	Microbicidal in vitro	Ferguson and Schlesinger, 2000; Ganz, 2002a; McCormack and Whitsett, 2002
Lactoferrin	N, EC	Iron chelation, microbicidal	Ganz, 2002a; Schaible et al., 2002
SLPI	AII	Potentially microbicidal, to be tested on *M. tuberculosis*	Ganz, 2002a
MBL	Serum, M	Mannose binding, opsonization; complement activation via collectin pathway, to be tested on *M. tuberculosis*	McCormack and Whitsett, 2002; Thiel et al., 1997
Complement C1q	M, AII	Opsonization	McCormack and Whitsett, 2002
SP-A	AII, Clara cell	Opsonization and enhancement of bacterial uptake; overall upregulation of macrophage functions	Ferguson and Schlesinger, 2000; McCormack and Whitsett, 2002
SP-D	AII, Clara cell	Opsonization, overall downregulation of macrophage functions	Ferguson and Schlesinger, 2000; McCormack and Whitsett, 2002
SP-B/-D	AII, Clara cell	Downmodulation of TNF-α, IL-1β	Ferguson and Schlesinger, 2000; McCormack and Whitsett, 2002
α-Defensins	N, T; intestinal Paneth cell	Microbicidal at high concentrations in vitro; chemotactic, immune stimulatory, to be tested on *M. tuberculosis*	Ganz, 2002a; Ferguson and Schlesinger, 2000; Lehrer and Ganz, 2002a, 2002b; McCormack and Whitsett, 2002; Zhang et al., 2002
β-Defensins	N, EC	Not microbicidal, but colocalized in N-vacuoles; chemotactic, immune stimulatory, to be tested on *M. tuberculosis*	Ganz, 2002a; Lehrer and Ganz, 2002a, 2002b
Cathelicidins	N, EC, B, $\gamma\delta$T	Porcine cathelicidin microbicidal in vitro, human one not; chemotactic function to be tested	Ganz, 2002a; Lehrer and Ganz, 2002a, 2002b
Elastase	N	No effect in mouse	Seiler et al., unpublished data
Cathepsins	N	Microbicidal, to be tested on *M. tuberculosis*	Ganz, 2002a
Phospholipase A2	N	Microbicidal, to be tested on *M. tuberculosis*; Ag processing and presentation by CD1	Ferguson and Schlesinger, 2000; Fischer et al., 2001
Ig	B	Opsonization	Ferguson and Schlesinger, 2000
Complement C3	EC, AII, M, serum	Opsonization; assembly of membrane attack complex not effective on *M. tuberculosis*	Ferguson and Schlesinger, 2000
Surfactant	AII	Immune downmodulatory, effect on *M. tuberculosis* to be tested	Ferguson and Schlesinger, 2000

[a]M, monocyte/macrophage; N, PMN; EC, lung epithelial cell; AII, alveolar type II cells; T, T cell; B, B cell; Clara cell, lung epithelial cell line; Ig, immunoglobulin.

effector mechanism in the combat of tuberculosis. Human β-defensins HBD-1 to -3 and cathelicidin secreted by epithelial cells are present in the mucus in trace amounts (Ganz 2002a), probably too small to affect *M. tuberculosis* in vivo. Sufficient concentrations are probably reached only in vivo in vacuoles of PMNs (Kisich et al., 2002). The human cathelicidin LL-37 is ineffective against *M. tuberculosis* in vitro, whereas the porcine cathelicidins PR-39 and PG-1 exhibit weak antituberculous effects at high concentrations (Lehrer and Ganz, 2002a; Linde et al., 2001). Knowledge about antimycobacterial activities of epithelial β-defensins and cathelicidins is still scarce, and deeper insights are needed considering that neutrophil-derived α-defensins are involved in innate immune defense against *M. tuberculosis* (Ganz, 2002a; Lehrer and Ganz, 2002b).

Soluble Effectors in Surfactant of the Lower Airways

Only nonclumped single tubercle bacilli can settle in the lower airways due to the airway speed (Ferguson and Schlesinger, 2000; West, 1994). The first innate immune effectors that mycobacteria encounter in the alveoli are surfactant tubular myelin and the proteins contained in the lipid and aqueous phase of the surfactant (Ferguson and Schlesinger, 2000; McCormack and Whitsett, 2002). Surfactant itself appears to downmodulate immune functions in vitro (Ferguson and Schlesinger, 2000), most prominently proliferative lymphocyte responses, NK cell-mediated target cell lysis, and complement and Fc receptor expression, as well as antimicrobial activities of monocytes. This modulation is likely to affect the host responses against *M. tuberculosis*, although detailed experimental proof is missing so far.

Among the pulmonary collectins, surfactant proteins A, B, C, and D (SP-A to -D), the hydrophilic SP-A and -D opsonize mycobacteria promptly. Opsonization by SP-A upregulates and that by SP-D downmodulates phagocytosis of *M. tuberculosis* by macrophages in vitro. SP-A upregulates MMR expression on monocyte-derived macrophages, further enhancing uptake of mannosylated particles. The induction of RNIs in infected macrophages seems to be downmodulated by SP-A-opsonized *M. tuberculosis*. Overall, SP-A appears to enhance uptake of virulent *M. tuberculosis* by alveolar macrophages, and to downmodulate immune functions with a net benefit for the pathogen rather than the host. SP-D on the other hand seems to hamper uptake of *M. tuberculosis* by macrophages, thereby counteracting SP-A effects (Beharka et al., 2002; Ferguson and Schlesinger, 2000; Weikert et al., 2000). Recently, a collectin-induced pathway of complement activation has been discovered (Thiel et al., 1997). However, surfactant collectins, an exception among the collectins, do not activate this pathway. Any functions attributed to SP-A, therefore, are directly due to opsonization. It is unclear yet to what extent the mannose-binding lectin (MBL), a serum collectin that specifically recognizes mannose residues, is present in the surfactant or mucus. MBL activates complement via the collectin-dependent pathway. It is, therefore, of interest to learn more about MBL in surfactant and MBL in general. Does it play a role as a second collectin opsonin for *M. tuberculosis*, and does opsonization activate complement?

Natural antibodies are produced by type 1 B cells that preferentially home to the peritoneal and pleural cavities (Ansel et al., 2002; Ferguson and Schlesinger, 2000). Mycobacteria-specific antibodies are produced by type 2 B cells abundantly during active tuberculosis. Both types of antibodies are present in mucus and surfactant and they opsonize *M. tuberculosis*, thus enhancing its uptake by alveolar macrophages via Fc receptors. Finally, complement components, released from human alveolar type II cells and from alveolar macrophages, contribute to opsonization and uptake of *M. tuberculosis* (Schlesinger, 1998). Overall, during infection with *M. tuberculosis*, collectins, antibodies, and complement components act as opsonins, thus favoring colonization of the host rather than mobilizing host defense mechanisms.

First Cellular Encounter: Epithelial Cells, Alveolar Macrophages, and DCs

Epithelial cells and alveolar macrophages represent the first cellular encounter of mycobacteria in the lung (Table 2). Pathogen recognition involves pattern recognition receptors, scavenger receptors, and receptors for opsonins (Janeway and Medzhitov, 2002). Alveolar macrophages represent key effector cells of the immune response against *M. tuberculosis*. Recognition of mycobacterial lipoarabinomannan (LAM) and the secretory 19-kDa lipoprotein by TLR-2 and TLR-6 has been demonstrated in vitro (van Crevel et al., 2002).

An ill-defined culture supernatant component of *M. tuberculosis* is recognized by TLR-4, and mycobacterial DNA is recognized by TLR-9. However, data on the contribution of TLRs in vivo are conflicting to date. C3H/HeJ mice mutated in their TLR-4 intracellular signaling domain are compromised in the control of *M. tuberculosis* after low-dose aerosol infection (Abel et al., 2002). In contrast, mouse mutants lacking TLR-2 or TLR-4 due to gene KO mount normal responses to low-dose infection, but suffer from slightly higher mortality and increased lung pathology after high-dose infection with *M. tuberculosis* (Reiling et al., 2002). Very recently, TREM-1 (for triggering

TABLE 2 Surface effector molecules in innate immune response against *M. tuberculosis*[a]

Molecule	Source (human)	Effector function	Reference
TLR-2/6/1	M, DC, EC; basolateral	Recognition of LAM, 19-kDa protein; immune activation	Abel et al., 2002; Reiling et al., 2002; van Crevel et al., 2002
TLR-4/CD14	M, DC, EC; basolateral	Recognition of undefined, heat-labile culture supernatant factor, PIM4-6; immune activation	Abel et al., 2002; Ernst, 1998; Reiling et al., 2002; van Crevel et al., 2002
TLR-9	M, DC; intracellular	Recognition of bacterial DNA; to be tested on *M. tuberculosis*	van Crevel et al., 2002
TREM-1	M, DC	Synergistic recognition of TLR-2 and TLR-4 signaling pattern	Bleharski et al., 2003
MMR	M, DC	Opsonin-independent uptake; immune downmodulation	van Crevel et al., 2002
DC-SIGN	DC, alveolar M	Opsonin-independent uptake, MAN-LAM specific; immune downmodulation	Geijtenbeek et al., 2003; Kaufmann and Schaible, 2003; Tailleux et al., 2003
CR-1	M, DC	Opsonin-dependent uptake	van Crevel et al., 2002
CR-3	M, DC	Opsonin-dependent as well as opsonin-independent uptake	Ernst, 1998
SpA-R	M, N, AII	Opsonin-dependent uptake; R not identified yet	Ernst, 1998; van Crevel et al., 2002
SR-type A	M, alveolar M, DC; endothelia, smooth muscle	Opsonin-independent uptake	Gough and Gordon, 2000; van Crevel et al., 2002
FcγR	M, DC, N	Opsonin-dependent uptake	van Crevel et al., 2002
BPI	N, EC	Microbicidal; elevated in tuberculosis patient sera	Juffermans et al., 1998
CD44	M, N	Binding and phagocytosis	Leemans et al., 2003
Cholesterol	M	Internalization, phagosomal targeting	Pieters, 2001

[a]M, monocyte/macrophage; N, PMN; EC, lung epithelial cell; AII, alveolar type II cells; T, T cell; B, B cell; Clara cell, lung epithelial cell line; Ig, immunoglobulin.

receptor expressed on myeloid cells 1) and TLR have been shown to synergize with each other to trigger release of proinflammatory chemokines and cytokines (Bleharski et al., 2003). Efficacy of monocytes to phagocytose or kill *M. tuberculosis*, however, was not affected by TREM-1 signaling. Further investigations will have to clarify the precise role of different TLRs in control of tuberculosis.

The contribution of scavenger receptors to the antituberculous immune control is insufficiently defined as well. Because of their high affinity, but low specificity, these receptors bind a wide variety of chemically modified low-density lipoproteins (Gough and Gordon, 2000). Both SR-AI and SR-AII, which exhibit identical substrate-binding properties, are expressed on alveolar macrophages and bind *M. tuberculosis* in vitro. It is therefore likely that SR-A fulfills pattern recognition functions for *M. tuberculosis*, although direct in vivo proof is missing. Experimental data addressing the involvement of other scavenger receptors such as MARCO or SR-B, -C, -D, -E, or -F in mycobacterial recognition are not yet available.

The carbohydrate specificity of C-type lectins predestines this category of receptors for mycobacterial recognition. The MMR is involved in phagocytosis of *M. tuberculosis* (Beharka et al., 2002; Kang and Schlesinger, 1998). Microspheres coated with LAM from *M. tuberculosis* strain Erdman were phagocytosed in an MMR-dependent manner. The MMR expression by human monocyte-derived macrophages and subsequent phagocytosis of LAM-coated microspheres are enhanced by SP-A. It is possible that MMRs are exploited by virulent strains of *M. tuberculosis* to enter macrophages, thus bypassing their microbicidal activities (Astarie-Dequeker et al., 1999; Beharka et al., 2002; Schlesinger et al., 1996; Zimmerli et al., 1996). Very recently, an additional C-type lectin, DC-SIGN (DC-specific ICAM-3-grabbing nonintegrin), which is expressed on human DCs and alveolar macrophages and physiologically involved in DC extravasation and interactions with T cells, has

been found to bind mannose-capped LAM (MAN-LAM). This receptor is responsible for uptake of mycobacteria into DCs in vitro (Geijtenbeek et al., 2003; Kaufmann and Schaible, 2003; Tailleux et al., 2003). *M. tuberculosis* has been localized in DC-SIGN-positive cells in human granulomas and draining lymph nodes. Furthermore, MAN-LAM has been shown to suppress DC differentiation in vitro and to induce IL-10 secretion by DCs in vitro. Consistent with this, binding of MAN-LAM, e.g., shed from *M. tuberculosis*, is involved in immune suppression (Engering et al., 2002; Nigou et al., 2001). DC-SIGN seems to bind only MAN-LAM from slow-growing mycobacteria including *M. tuberculosis*. Arabinose-capped LAM (ARA-LAM) from fast-growing, nonvirulent mycobacteria does not induce immune downmodulation. Therefore, DCs present at submucosal and interstitial sites (Soilleux et al., 2002) could take up *M. tuberculosis* via DC-SIGN and transport it from the lung to the lymphatic system and to the circulation, serving as a Trojan horse for mycobacterial dissemination.

In addition to MMR and DC-SIGN, LAM is recognized directly by a third opsonin-independent receptor, CD11b/c, as part of complement receptor 3 (CR3) (Ehlers and Daffe, 1998). This interaction mediates uptake of *M. tuberculosis* into macrophages, bypassing their activation. Quantitatively, uptake via CR3 may represent the major way of macrophage entry for *M. tuberculosis*. Recently, CD44, a hyaluronate adhesion molecule, was found to bind *M. tuberculosis* opsonin independently and to be involved in phagocytosis by macrophages in vitro (Leemans et al., 2003). Lack of CD44 in gene KO mutant mice impaired antimycobacterial control and granuloma formation, and the survival of mice was significantly reduced compared with wild-type mice. Because CD44 is also expressed on T cells and PMNs, further analyses will have to unravel to what extent the in vivo results from the KO mutant mice reflect the in vitro macrophage experiments. Finally, cholesterol-rich lipid rafts are bound by *M.*

tuberculosis species specifically. If macrophages are depleted of cholesterol in vitro, *M. tuberculosis* is hampered in intracellular entry. Cholesterol-focused surface binding may enhance receptor-mediated internalization of *M. tuberculosis* and subsequent targeting to phagosomes, allowing intracellular survival of the bacilli (Pieters, 2001).

A variety of opsonin-dependent receptors enhance mycobacterial uptake by alveolar macrophages. Notably, CR1, but also CR3 and CR4, mediate uptake of complement-opsonized mycobacteria (Ernst, 1998; Schlesinger, 1998; Schorey et al., 1997). In addition, a total of three candidate SP-A receptors exist: (i) CR1 may recognize not only complement-but also SP-A-opsonized mycobacteria; (ii) C1qR, a 126-kDa protein expressed on monocytes, macrophages, neutrophils, and endothelial cells, may interact with SP-A and MBL; (iii) SPR210 expressed on macrophages and alveolar type II cells interacts with SP-A but not with C1q, and SP-A enhances uptake of *M. tuberculosis*, independently from the receptor involved.

Last but not least, engulfment of *M. tuberculosis* is promoted by the Fcγ receptor (FcγR) that interacts with antibody-opsonized mycobacteria. FcγR-mediated recognition appears to influence the intracellular trafficking of ingested mycobacteria. Phagosomes containing antibody-opsonized mycobacteria fuse with lysosomes more readily than those containing nonopsonized mycobacteria (Ernst, 1998; van Crevel et al., 2002). However, neither of the two intracellular trafficking pathways was found to influence intraphagosomal survival of *M. tuberculosis* (Ernst, 1998).

In conclusion, *M. tuberculosis* uses an impressive collection of receptors to enter macrophages. It is therefore challenging to consider this multitude of receptor-mediated uptake as beneficial for this pathogen. This notion is in line with the well-known strategy of interference with intracellular destruction. *M. tuberculosis* prevents maturation of the phagosome and subsequent fusion with lysosomes in order to evade intracellular killing (Pieters and Gatfield, 2002; Schaible et al., 1999).

Thus far, most of the studies on receptor-mediated uptake of *M. tuberculosis* have dealt with macrophages. However, evidence is accumulating that at the early stage of infection *M. tuberculosis* not only invades alveolar macrophages, but also epithelial cells, notably type II alveolar cells (Sato et al., 2002), and DCs (Jiao et al., 2002; Tailleux et al., 2003). Recent findings have stipulated the hypothesis that receptor-mediated uptake promotes transepithelial migration of *M. tuberculosis*, rendering the bacteria independent from macrophages and DCs for crossing the epithelial barrier (Russell, 2001). Such mechanisms could circumvent mycobacterial recognition by TLRs on epithelial cells. Epithelial cells express TLR-2, TLR-4, and TLR-5 on their basolateral surface (Fusunyan et al., 2001; Ganz, 2002b; Gewirtz et al., 2001). This basolateral expression restricts signaling to steps subsequent to bacterial penetration of epithelial layers. Given that mycobacteria transmigrate through epithelia, they can be missed by epithelial TLRs. Identification of DC-SIGN as a receptor for *M. tuberculosis* on DCs, however, has focused interest on these cells as shuttle carriers to the periphery as discussed above (Kaufmann and Schaible, 2003; Tailleux et al., 2003).

Encounter of mycobacteria with macrophages and epithelia induces secretion of TNF-α, IL-1, and IL-6 and hence marks the onset of inflammation. These proinflammatory cytokines induce ample immune effector functions including direct cytocidal effects on infected cells, vasodilatation, and secretion of effector molecules such as chemokines and epithelial defensins and also mark an important link to the adaptive immune response, e.g., IFN-γ induction by IL-6. Animal experiments have proven directly the importance of TNF-α in control of *M. tuberculosis* in vivo. Mice deficient in any component of the TNF-α/TNF receptor signaling cascade succumb to tuberculosis (Flynn and Chan, 2001; van Crevel et al., 2002). Consistent with this, rheumatoid arthritis patients treated with antibodies to block detrimental effects of TNF-α on rheumatoid arthritis are at risk of *M. tuberculosis* recrudescence (Gardam et al., 2003).

Direct impact of IL-1β on control of tuberculosis in vivo seems similarly important (van Crevel et al., 2002). IL-1α/β double-deficient and IL-1 receptor-deficient mouse KO mutants develop higher mycobacterial counts and succumb to *M. tuberculosis* infection more rapidly than wild-type mice. Inflammatory and granulomatous responses in these mutants are greatly delayed. In vitro type I IFNs are strongly induced in human peripheral blood mononuclear cell-derived DCs upon infection with *M. tuberculosis* (Remoli et al., 2002). IL-6-deficient KO mice suffer from higher bacterial load after aerosol infection compared with wild-type control mice at early time points postinfection and succumb to intravenous infection with *M. tuberculosis*, further emphasizing the unique importance of a proinflammatory cytokine response during innate immune control of tuberculosis (Ladel et al., 1997; Saunders et al., 2000).

Among the plethora of antimycobacterial effector mechanisms elicited in activated macrophages, production of RNIs and to a lesser extent ROIs is critical for controlling mycobacterial infection. Block of the iNOS exacerbates persistent *M. tuberculosis* infection in mice in vivo, as does the lack of iNOS due to gene KO technology (Flynn and Chan, 2001). Human peripheral blood monocytes and PMNs express small amounts of iNOS, and expression is not induced by microbial products and cytokines as it is in rodent peripheral blood monocytes. Hence, human peripheral blood monocytes and PMNs fail to kill mycobacteria in vitro by means of RNIs. However, macrophages and PMNs isolated from inflamed or infected sites express iNOS at higher levels than their blood-derived counterparts and at levels that enable them to kill mycobacteria (Nathan and Shiloh, 2000; Nozaki et al., 1997). Involvement of RNIs in control of human tuberculosis, therefore, is still under debate, although involvement is very likely (Nathan and Shiloh, 2000). Mouse KO

mutants deficient in gp47phox compromised in ROI production exhibited a transient loss of mycobacterial control, and mouse KO mutants deficient in gp91phox exhibited increased mycobacterial burden in some peripheral organs (Zahrt and Deretic, 2002). However, macrophages from chronic granulomatous disease patients deficient in Phox are not limited in antimycobacterial effector functions. To what extent, therefore, such pathways contribute to the control of tuberculosis in humans is still under debate (Nathan and Shiloh, 2000; Rich et al., 1997; Zahrt and Deretic, 2002).

Second Cellular Encounter: Infiltrating PMNs and Monocytes

Upon encounter with mycobacteria, macrophages and epithelial cells secrete chemokines that recruit PMNs and monocytes to the site of infection. In vitro, RANTES, MCP-1 (monocyte chemotactic protein-1), MIP-1α, IP-10, MIG, ITAC, and IL-8 in humans and MIP-1α, MIP-2, IP-10, MCPs, GRO-α, and KC in mice are secreted by macrophages, bronchial epithelial cells, and PMNs and are transcriptionally or translationally upregulated during tuberculosis (van Crevel et al., 2002). In vivo experiments assessing the role of chemokines in tuberculosis, however, are still rare. Microarray analyses performed in our own laboratory revealed profound transcriptional upregulation of the chemokines MIG, RANTES, MCP-1, IP-10 and B-lymphocyte chemoattractant (BLC), and intermediate upregulation of MIP-3α, ITAC, and MIP-2 in vivo in the lungs of *M. tuberculosis*-infected mice (Seiler et al., 2003). Intranasal MIP-2 treatment of mice attracts neutrophils to the lung and decreases *Mycobacterium bovis* BCG titers to a small but measurable degree (Fulton et al., 2002). Yet mouse KO mutants deficient in the chemokines MIP-1α and MIP-2, which are secreted by alveolar macrophages and epithelial cells and attract monocytes, were not impaired in the control of *M. tuberculosis* infection. Definite proof of a critical role in tuberculosis has been obtained for chemokines signaling through CCR2 because CCR2$^{-/-}$ KO mice rapidly succumb to *M. tuberculosis* infection (Peters et al., 2001; Scott and Flynn, 2002). A role of MCP-1 in this context is likely (Lu et al., 1998; Rutledge et al., 1995).

In vivo depletion of PMNs by using the monoclonal antibody RB6-8C5 substantially impaired granuloma formation. Immunohistochemical as well as microarray analyses revealed that granuloma formation involved chemokines that signal through the chemokine receptor CXCR3, most prominently MIG. The findings are supported by impaired granuloma formation in CXCR3 gene-deficient KO mice and in mice treated with MIG-neutralizing antibodies (Seiler et al., 2003).

Apart from chemotaxis-mediated regulation, the contribution of PMNs to protective innate immunity against *M. tuberculosis* remains controversial. In mice, PMNs are rapidly attracted to the lung within 30 min postinfection. PMNs are found throughout the infection and form a prominent part of the granulomas, which are mostly composed of macrophages and monocytes and T lymphocytes. Although in vitro data are conflicting (Denis, 1991; Jones et al., 1990), our own studies argue against a direct microbicidal activity of PMNs. Neither isolated human PMNs, enriched human neutrophil granules, nor mouse PMNs killed mycobacteria in vitro. This lack of function could be due to the failure to induce an oxidative burst in human as well as murine PMNs in response to mycobacterial phagocytosis. Consistent with this, in vivo depletion of PMNs does not exacerbate murine tuberculosis (Pedrosa et al., 2000; Seiler et al., 2000).

Evidence is increasing that human neutrophil α-defensins contribute to the control of *M. tuberculosis* (Ashitani et al., 2002; Kisich et al., 2001, 2002; Miyakawa et al., 1996; Sharma and Khuller, 2001; Sharma et al., 2000, 2001). High concentrations of HNP-1 kill avirulent and virulent strains as well as clinical isolates of *M. tuberculosis* in vitro. Tuberculosis patients exhibit elevated levels of pleural neutrophil defensins. Human and mouse alveolar macrophages are devoid of defensins, in contrast to species more resistant to *M. tuberculosis* infection such as rabbit and cattle (Kisich et al., 2002); absence of the defensin response during the initial macrophage encounter could facilitate establishment of infection. This notion is supported by the identification of *Staphylococcus aureus mprF*-related genes in the *M. tuberculosis* genome (Lehrer and Ganz, 2002b; Peschel et al., 2001). In *S. aureus mprF* covalently modifies phosphatidylglycerols with L-lysine, thereby reducing the net negative charge and impairing binding of cationic, antibacterial peptides. The mprF homologs may account for similar activities in *M. tuberculosis*.

Human macrophages upregulate TNF-α and IL-1β, and murine spleen cells proliferate and secrete cytokines upon stimulation with human α-defensins in vitro. Administration of human α-defensins to mice in vivo enhances humoral and cellular immune responses (Tani et al., 2000). It is thus very likely that human α-defensins impact on the adaptive immune response against *M. tuberculosis* indirectly.

Contribution of PMN β-defensins to the control of *M. tuberculosis* is unclear. Recently, intimate intracellular colocalization of phagocytosed *M. tuberculosis* and HBD-1 within human PMNs has been described (Kisich et al., 2001, 2002). However, in vitro HBD-1 does not affect *M. tuberculosis* at concentrations present in PMNs. It remains to be determined whether this is due to an intrinsic failure of HBD-1 to kill mycobacteria or due to a lack of critical cofactors or posttranslational modification in the cell-free culture system employed. PMN myeloperoxidase (MPO) exerts limited but detectable activity to kill *M. tuberculosis* H37Rv and clinical isolates in vitro. However, in PMNs, as in macrophages, phagosomal maturation and subsequent intraphagosomal release of granular contents are hindered by *M. tuberculosis*, therefore allowing encounter of MPO with the pathogen only extracellularly or in endosomes. Under culture conditions representing in vivo extracellular conditions, human eosinophil peroxidase kills *M. tuberculosis* more efficiently than MPO due to the independence of this enzyme from the cosubstrate H_2O_2, representing the most potent effector molecule in the killing of *M. tuberculosis* in vitro described to date. Furthermore, eosinophil peroxidase may kill not only extracellularly after release from eosinophils, but also after subsequent phagocytosis by macrophages inside phagosomes. It remains to be clarified, however, to what extent eosinophils migrate to the site of *M. tuberculosis* infection in vivo (Borelli et al., 1999, 2003).

CONCLUDING REMARKS

In summary, the innate immune system appears to be organized into two major branches: (i) a local, immobile, tissue-specific system composed of innate effector molecules and cells for immediate recognition and restriction of the pathogen and (ii) a systemic, highly mobile immune system rapidly recruited to the site of infection, composed of highly mobile innate effector cells, notably PMNs and monocytes. The well-concerted interplay between the resident and the mobile innate immune system ensures host defense at a high cost and efficiency rate.

REFERENCES

Abel, B., N. Thieblemont, V. J. Quesniaux, N. Brown, J. Mpagi, K. Miyake, F. Bihl, and B. Ryffel. 2002. Toll-like receptor 4 expression is required to control chronic *Mycobacterium tuberculosis* infection in mice. *J. Immunol.* **169:**3155–3162.

Aichele, P., J. Zinke, L. Grode, R. A. Schwendener, S. H. Kaufmann, and P. Seiler. 2003. Macrophages of the splenic marginal zone are essential for trapping of blood-borne particulate antigen but dispensable for induction of specific T cell responses. *J. Immunol.* **171:**1148–1155.

Ansel, K. M., R. B. Harris, and J. G. Cyster. 2002. CXCL13 is required for B1 cell homing, natural antibody production, and body cavity immunity. *Immunity* **16:**67–76.

Arnold, R. R., J. E. Russell, W. J. Champion, M. Brewer, and J. J. Gauthier. 1982. Bactericidal activity of human lactoferrin: differentiation from the stasis of iron deprivation. *Infect. Immun.* **35:**792–799.

Ashitani, J., H. Mukae, T. Hiratsuka, M. Nakazato, K. Kumamoto, and S. Matsukura. 2002. Elevated levels of alpha-defensins in plasma and BAL fluid of patients with active pulmonary tuberculosis. *Chest* **121:**519–526.

Astarie-Dequeker, C., E. N. N'Diaye, V. Le Cabec, M. G. Rittig, J. Prandi, and I. Maridonneau-Parini. 1999. The mannose receptor mediates uptake of pathogenic and nonpathogenic mycobacteria and bypasses bactericidal responses in human macrophages. *Infect. Immun.* **67:**469–477.

Auerbuch, V., L. L. Lenz, and D. A. Portnoy. 2001. Development of a competitive index assay to evaluate the virulence of Listeria monocytogenes actA mutants during primary and secondary infection of mice. *Infect. Immun.* **69:**5953–5957.

Austyn, J. M. 1996. New insights into the mobilization and phagocytic activity of dendritic cells. *J. Exp. Med.* **183:**1287–1292.

Banchereau, J., and R. M. Steinman. 1998. Dendritic cells and the control of immunity. *Nature* **392:**245–252.

Barton, G. M., and R. Medzhitov. 2002. Toll-like receptors and their ligands. *Curr. Top. Microbiol. Immunol.* **270:**81–92.

Beharka, A. A., C. D. Gaynor, B. K. Kang, D. R. Voelker, F. X. McCormack, and L. S. Schlesinger. 2002. Pulmonary surfactant protein a up-regulates activity of the mannose receptor, a pattern recognition receptor expressed on human macrophages. *J. Immunol.* **169:**3565–3573.

Bevilacqua, M. P., J. S. Pober, M. E. Wheeler, R. S. Cotran, and M. A. Gimbrone, Jr. 1985. Interleukin 1 acts on cultured human vascular endothelium to increase the adhesion of polymorphonuclear leukocytes, monocytes, and related leukocyte cell lines. *J. Clin. Invest.* **76:**2003–2011.

Bleharski, J. R., V. Kiessler, C. Buonsanti, P. A. Sieling, S. Stenger, M. Colonna, and R. L. Modlin. 2003. A role for triggering receptor expressed on myeloid cells-1 in host defense during the early-induced and adaptive phases of the immune response. *J. Immunol.* **170:**3812–3818.

Borelli, V., F. Vita, S. Shankar, M. R. Soranzo, E. Banfi, G. Scialino, C. Brochetta, and G. Zabucchi. 2003. Human eosinophil peroxidase induces surface alteration, killing, and lysis of *Mycobacterium tuberculosis. Infect. Immun.* **71:**605–613.

Borelli, V., E. Banfi, M. G. Perrotta, and G. Zabucchi. 1999. Myeloperoxidase exerts microbicidal activity against Mycobacterium tuberculosis. *Infect. Immun.* **67:**4149–4152.

Brennan, P. J., and H. Nikaido. 1995. The envelope of mycobacteria. *Annu. Rev. Biochem.* **64:**29–63.

Brook, I. 1999. Bacterial interference. *Crit. Rev. Microbiol.* **25:**155–172.

Cameron, L. A., P. A. Giardini, F. S. Soo, and J. A. Theriot. 2000. Secrets of actin-based motility revealed by a bacterial pathogen. *Nat. Rev. Mol. Cell Biol.* **1:**110–119.

Chico-Calero, I., M. Suarez, B. Gonzalez-Zorn, M. Scortti, J. Slaghuis, W. Goebel, and J. A. Vazquez-Boland. 2002. Hpt, a bacterial homolog of the microsomal glucose-6-phosphate translocase, mediates rapid intracellular proliferation in Listeria. *Proc. Natl. Acad. Sci. USA* **99:**431–436.

Coconnier, M. H., E. Dlissi, M. Robard, C. L. Laboisse, J. L. Gaillard, and A. L. Servin. 1998. Listeria monocytogenes stimulates mucus exocytosis in cultured human polarized mucosecreting intestinal cells through action of listeriolysin O. *Infect. Immun.* **66:**3673–3681.

Cole, A. M., T. Ganz, A. M. Liese, M. D. Burdick, L. Liu, and R. M. Strieter. 2001. Cutting edge: IFN-inducible ELR-CXC chemokines display defensin-like antimicrobial activity. *J. Immunol.* **167:**623–627.

Conlan, J. W., and R. J. North. 1994. Neutrophils are essential for early anti-Listeria defense in the liver, but not in the spleen or peritoneal cavity, as revealed by a granulocyte-depleting monoclonal antibody. *J. Exp. Med.* **179:**259–268.

Cossart, P., M. F. Vicente, J. Mengaud, F. Baquero, J. C. Perez-Diaz, and P. Berche. 1989. Listeriolysin O is essential for virulence of Listeria monocytogenes: direct evidence obtained by gene complementation. *Infect. Immun.* **57:**3629–3636.

Cousens, L. P., and E. J. Wing. 2000. Innate defenses in the liver during Listeria infection. *Immunol. Rev.* **174:**150–159.

Cyster, J. G. 2000. B cells on the front line. *Nat. Immunol.* **1:**9–10.

Czuprynski, C. J., N. G. Faith, and H. Steinberg. 2003. A/J mice are susceptible and C57BL/6 mice are resistant to Listeria monocytogenes infection by intragastric inoculation. *Infect. Immun.* **71:**682–689.

Dalrymple, S. A., L. A. Lucian, R. Slattery, T. McNeil, D. M. Aud, S. Fuchino, F. Lee, and R. Murray. 1995. Interleukin-6-deficient mice are highly susceptible to Listeria monocytogenes infection: correlation with inefficient neutrophilia. *Infect. Immun.* **63:**2262–2268.

Decatur, A. L., and D. A. Portnoy. 2000. A PEST-like sequence in listeriolysin O essential for Listeria monocytogenes pathogenicity. *Science* **290:**992–995.

Denis, M. 1991. Human neutrophils, activated with cytokines or not, do not kill virulent Mycobacterium tuberculosis. *J. Infect. Dis.* **163:**919–920.

Dorner, B. G., A. Scheffold, M. S. Rolph, M. B. Huser, S. H. Kaufmann, A. Radbruch, I. E. Flesch, and R. A. Kroczek. 2002. MIP-1alpha, MIP-1beta, RANTES, and ATAC/lymphotactin function together with IFN-gamma as type 1 cytokines. *Proc. Natl. Acad. Sci. USA* **99:**6181–6186.

Edelson, B. T., and E. R. Unanue. 2002. MyD88-dependent but Toll-like receptor 2-independent innate immunity to Listeria: no role for either in macrophage listericidal activity. *J. Immunol.* **169:**3869–3875.

Ehlers, M. R., and M. Daffe. 1998. Interactions between Mycobacterium tuberculosis and host cells: are mycobacterial sugars the key? *Trends Microbiol.* **6:**328–335.

Ehlers, S., M. E. Mielke, T. Blankenstein, and H. Hahn. 1992. Kinetic analysis of cytokine gene expression in the livers of naive and immune mice infected with Listeria monocytogenes. The immediate early phase in innate resistance and acquired immunity. *J. Immunol.* **149:**3016–3022.

Engering, A., T. B. Geijtenbeek, and Y. van Kooyk. 2002. Immune escape through C-type lectins on dendritic cells. *Trends Immunol.* **23:**480–485.

Ernst, J. D. 1998. Macrophage receptors for Mycobacterium tuberculosis. *Infect. Immun.* **66:**1277–1281.

Falk, P. G., L. V. Hooper, T. Midtvedt, and J. I. Gordon. 1998. Creating and maintaining the gastrointestinal ecosystem: what we know and need to know from gnotobiology. *Microbiol. Mol. Biol. Rev.* **62:**1157–1170.

Fauroux, B., B. Delaisi, A. Clement, C. Saizou, D. Moissenet, C. Truffot-Pernot, G. Tournier, and T. H. Vu. 1997. Mycobacterial lung disease in cystic fibrosis: a prospective study. *Pediatr. Infect. Dis. J.* **16:**354–358.

Ferguson, J. S., and L. S. Schlesinger. 2000. Pulmonary surfactant in innate immunity and the pathogenesis of tuberculosis. *Tuber. Lung Dis.* **80:**173–184.

Fischer, K., D. Chatterjee, J. Torrelles, P. J. Brennan, S. H. Kaufmann, and U. E. Schaible. 2001. Mycobacterial lysocardiolipin is exported from phagosomes upon cleavage of cardiolipin by a macrophage-derived lysosomal phospholipase A2. *J. Immunol.* **167:**2187–2192.

Flynn, J. L., and J. Chan. 2001. Immunology of tuberculosis. *Annu. Rev. Immunol.* **19:**93–129.

Fox, E. S., P. Thomas, and S. A. Broitman. 1987. Comparative studies of endotoxin uptake by isolated rat Kupffer and peritoneal cells. *Infect. Immun.* **55:**2962–2966.

Fulton, S. A., S. M. Reba, T. D. Martin, and W. H. Boom. 2002. Neutrophil-mediated mycobacteriocidal immunity in the lung during Mycobacterium bovis BCG infection in C57BL/6 mice. *Infect. Immun.* **70:**5322–5327.

Furie, M. B., and D. D. McHugh. 1989. Migration of neutrophils across endothelial monolayers is stimulated by treatment of the monolayers with interleukin-1 or tumor necrosis factor-alpha. *J. Immunol.* **143:**3309–3317.

Fusunyan, R. D., N. N. Nanthakumar, M. E. Baldeon, and W. A. Walker. 2001. Evidence for an innate immune response in the immature human intestine: toll-like receptors on fetal enterocytes. *Pediatr. Res.* **49:**589–593.

Ganz, T. 2002a. Antimicrobial polypeptides in host defense of the respiratory tract. *J. Clin. Invest.* **109:**693–697.

Ganz, T. 2002b. Epithelia: not just physical barriers. *Proc. Natl. Acad. Sci. USA* **99**:3357–3358.

Ganz, T. 2003. Angiogenin: an antimicrobial ribonuclease. *Nat. Immunol.* **4**:213–214.

Gardam, M. A., E. C. Keystone, R. Menzies, S. Manners, E. Skamene, R. Long, and D. C. Vinh. 2003. Anti-tumour necrosis factor agents and tuberculosis risk: mechanisms of action and clinical management. *Lancet Infect. Dis.* **3**:148–155.

Gedde, M. M., D. E. Higgins, L. G. Tilney, and D. A. Portnoy. 2000. Role of listeriolysin O in cell-to-cell spread of *Listeria monocytogenes*. *Infect. Immun.* **68**:999–1003.

Geijtenbeek, T. B., S. J. Van Vliet, E. A. Koppel, M. Sanchez-Hernandez, C. M. Vandenbroucke-Grauls, B. Appelmelk, and Y. van Kooyk. 2003. Mycobacteria target DC-SIGN to suppress dendritic cell function. *J. Exp. Med.* **197**:7–17.

Geoffroy, C., J. L. Gaillard, J. E. Alouf, and P. Berche. 1987. Purification, characterization, and toxicity of the sulfhydryl-activated hemolysin listeriolysin O from *Listeria monocytogenes*. *Infect. Immun.* **55**:1641–1646.

Gewirtz, A. T., T. A. Navas, S. Lyons, P. J. Godowski, and J. L. Madara. 2001. Cutting edge: bacterial flagellin activates basolaterally expressed TLR5 to induce epithelial proinflammatory gene expression. *J. Immunol.* **167**:1882–1885.

Gough, P. J., and S. Gordon. 2000. The role of scavenger receptors in the innate immune system. *Microb. Infect.* **2**:305–311.

Gregory, S. H., and E. J. Wing. 2002. Neutrophil-Kupffer cell interaction: a critical component of host defenses to systemic bacterial infections. *J. Leukoc. Biol.* **72**:239–248.

Gregory, S. H., A. J. Sagnimeni, and E. J. Wing. 1996a. Bacteria in the bloodstream are trapped in the liver and killed by immigrating neutrophils. *J. Immunol.* **157**:2514–2520.

Gregory, S. H., X. Jiang, and E. J. Wing. 1996b. Lymphokine-activated killer cells lyse Listeria-infected hepatocytes and produce elevated quantities of interferon-gamma. *J. Infect. Dis.* **174**:1073–1079.

Gregory, S. H., E. J. Wing, K. L. Danowski, N. van Rooijen, K. F. Dyer, and D. J. Tweardy. 1998. IL-6 produced by Kupffer cells induces STAT protein activation in hepatocytes early during the course of systemic listerial infections. *J. Immunol.* **160**:6056–6061.

Guermonprez, P., J. Valladeau, L. Zitvogel, C. Thery, and S. Amigorena. 2002. Antigen presentation and T cell stimulation by dendritic cells. *Annu. Rev. Immunol.* **20**:621–667.

Guo, Y., D. W. Niesel, H. K. Ziegler, and G. R. Klimpel. 1992. *Listeria monocytogenes* activation of human peripheral blood lymphocytes: induction of non-major histocompatibility complex-restricted cytotoxic activity and cytokine production. *Infect. Immun.* **60**:1813–1819.

Guzman, C. A., M. Rohde, T. Chakraborty, E. Domann, M. Hudel, J. Wehland, and K. N. Timmis. 1995. Interaction of *Listeria monocytogenes* with mouse dendritic cells. *Infect. Immun.* **63**:3665–3673.

Havell, E. A., G. R. Beretich, Jr., and P. B. Carter. 1999. The mucosal phase of Listeria infection. *Immunobiology* **201**:164–177.

Hooper, L. V., T. S. Stappenbeck, C. V. Hong, and J. I. Gordon. 2003. Angiogenins: a new class of microbicidal proteins involved in innate immunity. *Nat. Immunol.* **4**:269–273.

Huang, Q., D. Liu, P. Majewski, L. C. Schulte, J. M. Korn, R. A. Young, E. S. Lander, and N. Hacohen. 2001. The plasticity of dendritic cell responses to pathogens and their components. *Science* **294**:870–875.

Janeway, C. A., Jr., and R. Medzhitov. 2002. Innate immune recognition. *Annu. Rev. Immunol.* **20**:197–216.

Jiao, X., R. Lo-Man, P. Guermonprez, L. Fiette, E. Deriaud, S. Burgaud, B. Gicquel, N. Winter, and C. Leclerc. 2002. Dendritic cells are host cells for mycobacteria in vivo that trigger innate and acquired immunity. *J. Immunol.* **168**:1294–1301.

Jones, G. S., H. J. Amirault, and B. R. Andersen. 1990. Killing of *Mycobacterium tuberculosis* by neutrophils: a nonoxidative process. *J. Infect. Dis.* **162**:700–704.

Juffermans, N. P., A. Verbon, S. J. van Deventer, W. A. Buurman, H. van Deutekom, P. Speelman, and T. van der Poll. 1998. Serum concentrations of lipopolysaccharide activity-modulating proteins during tuberculosis. *J. Infect. Dis.* **178**:1839–1842.

Kang, B. K., and L. S. Schlesinger. 1998. Characterization of mannose receptor-dependent phagocytosis mediated by *Mycobacterium tuberculosis* lipoarabinomannan. *Infect. Immun.* **66**:2769–2777.

Kaufmann, S. H. 2001. How can immunology contribute to the control of tuberculosis? *Nat. Rev. Immunol.* **1**:20–30.

Kaufmann, S. H., and U. E. Schaible. 2003. A dangerous liaison between two major killers: *Mycobacterium tuberculosis* and HIV target dendritic cells through DC-SIGN. *J. Exp. Med.* **197**:1–5.

Kisich, K. O., L. Heifets, M. Higgins, and G. Diamond. 2001. Antimycobacterial agent based on mRNA encoding human beta-defensin 2 enables primary macrophages to restrict growth of *Mycobacterium tuberculosis*. *Infect. Immun.* **69**:2692–2699.

Kisich, K. O., M. Higgins, G. Diamond, and L. Heifets. 2002. Tumor necrosis factor alpha stimulates killing of *Mycobacterium tuberculosis* by human neutrophils. *Infect. Immun.* **70**:4591–4599.

Knowles, M. R., and R. C. Boucher. 2002. Mucus clearance as a primary innate defense mechanism for mammalian airways. *J. Clin. Invest.* **109**:571–577.

Kolb-Maurer, A., I. Gentschev, H. W. Fries, F. Fiedler, E. B. Brocker, E. Kampgen, and W. Goebel. 2000. *Listeria monocytogenes*-infected human dendritic cells: uptake and host cell response. *Infect. Immun.* **68:**3680–3688.

Koski, G. K., L. A. Lyakh, P. A. Cohen, and N. R. Rice. 2001. CD14+ monocytes as dendritic cell precursors: diverse maturation-inducing pathways lead to common activation of NF-kappab/RelB. *Crit. Rev. Immunol.* **21:**179–189.

Kraal, G. 1992. Cells in the marginal zone of the spleen. *Int. Rev. Cytol.* **132:**31–74.

Ladel, C. H., C. Blum, A. Dreher, K. Reifenberg, M. Kopf, and S. H. Kaufmann. 1997. Lethal tuberculosis in interleukin-6-deficient mutant mice. *Infect. Immun.* **65:**4843–4849.

Lee, R. E., P. J. Brennan, and G. S. Besra. 1996. *Mycobacterium tuberculosis* cell envelope, p. 1–28. *In* T. M. Shinnick (ed.), *Tuberculosis.* Springer, Berlin, Germany.

Leemans, J. C., S. Florquin, M. Heikens, S. T. Pals, R. R. Neut, and P. T. van der Poll. 2003. CD44 is a macrophage binding site for *Mycobacterium tuberculosis* that mediates macrophage recruitment and protective immunity against tuberculosis. *J. Clin. Invest.* **111:**681–689.

Lehrer, R. I., and T. Ganz. 2002a. Cathelicidins: a family of endogenous antimicrobial peptides. *Curr. Opin. Hematol.* **9:**18–22.

Lehrer, R. I., and T. Ganz. 2002b. Defensins of vertebrate animals. *Curr. Opin. Immunol.* **14:**96–102.

Linde, C. M., S. E. Hoffner, E. Refai, and M. Andersson. 2001. In vitro activity of PR-39, a proline-arginine-rich peptide, against susceptible and multi-drug-resistant *Mycobacterium tuberculosis.* *J. Antimicrob. Chemother.* **47:**575–580.

Lorber, B. 1997. Listeriosis. *Clin. Infect. Dis.* **24:**1–9.

Lu, B., B. J. Rutledge, L. Gu, J. Fiorillo, N. W. Lukacs, S. L. Kunkel, R. North, C. Gerard, and B. J. Rollins. 1998. Abnormalities in monocyte recruitment and cytokine expression in monocyte chemoattractant protein 1-deficient mice. *J. Exp. Med.* **187:**601–608.

Matsuguchi, T., K. Takagi, T. Musikacharoen, and Y. Yoshikai. 2000. Gene expressions of lipopolysaccharide receptors, toll-like receptors 2 and 4, are differently regulated in mouse T lymphocytes. *Blood* **95:**1378–1385.

McCormack, F. X., and J. A. Whitsett. 2002. The pulmonary collectins, SP-A and SP-D, orchestrate innate immunity in the lung. *J. Clin. Invest.* **109:**707–712.

McGregor, D. D., H. H. Hahn, and G. B. Mackaness. 1973. The mediator of cellular immunity. V. Development of cellular resistance to infection in thymectomized irradiated rats. *Cell Immunol.* **6:**186–199.

Mengaud, J., H. Ohayon, P. Gounon, R.-M. Mege, and P. Cossart. 1996. E-cadherin is the receptor for internalin, a surface protein required for entry of *L. monocytogenes* into epithelial cells. *Cell* **84:**923–932.

Miyakawa, Y., P. Ratnakar, A. G. Rao, M. L. Costello, O. Mathieu-Costello, R. I. Lehrer, and A. Catanzaro. 1996. In vitro activity of the antimicrobial peptides human and rabbit defensins and porcine leukocyte protegrin against *Mycobacterium tuberculosis.* *Infect. Immun.* **64:**926–932.

Miyamoto, M., M. Emoto, Y. Emoto, V. Brinkmann, I. Yoshizawa, P. Seiler, P. Aichele, E. Kita, and S. H. Kaufmann. 2003. Neutrophilia in LFA-1-deficient mice confers resistance to listeriosis: possible contribution of granulocyte-colony-stimulating factor and IL-17. *J. Immunol.* **170:**5228–5234.

Nathan, C., and M. U. Shiloh. 2000. Reactive oxygen and nitrogen intermediates in the relationship between mammalian hosts and microbial pathogens. *Proc. Natl. Acad. Sci. USA* **97:**8841–8848.

Nigou, J., C. Zelle-Rieser, M. Gilleron, M. Thurnher, and G. Puzo. 2001. Mannosylated lipoarabinomannans inhibit IL-12 production by human dendritic cells: evidence for a negative signal delivered through the mannose receptor. *J. Immunol.* **166:**7477–7485.

Nozaki, Y., Y. Hasegawa, S. Ichiyama, I. Nakashima, and K. Shimokata. 1997. Mechanism of nitric oxide-dependent killing of *Mycobacterium bovis* BCG in human alveolar macrophages. *Infect. Immun.* **65:**3644–3647.

Ochsenbein, A. F., and R. M. Zinkernagel. 2000. Natural antibodies and complement link innate and acquired immunity. *Immunol. Today* **21:**624–630.

Ofek, I., and N. Sharon. 1988. Lectinophagocytosis: a molecular mechanism of recognition between cell surface sugars and lectins in the phagocytosis of bacteria. *Infect. Immun.* **56:**539–547.

Ohya, S., Y. Tanabe, M. Makino, T. Nomura, H. Xiong, M. Arakawa, and M. Mitsuyama. 1998. The contributions of reactive oxygen intermediates and reactive nitrogen intermediates to listericidal mechanisms differ in macrophages activated pre- and postinfection. *Infect. Immun.* **66:**4043–4049.

Oshiumi, H., M. Matsumoto, K. Funami, T. Akazawa, and T. Seya. 2003. TICAM-1, an adaptor molecule that participates in Toll-like receptor 3-mediated interferon-beta induction. *Nat. Immunol.* **4:**161–167.

Ouellette, A. J. 1997. Paneth cells and innate immunity in the crypt microenvironment. *Gastroenterology* **113:**1779–1784.

Ozinsky, A., D. M. Underhill, J. D. Fontenot, A. M. Hajjar, K. D. Smith, C. B. Wilson, L. Schroeder, and A. Aderem. 2000. The repertoire for pattern recognition of pathogens by the innate immune system is defined by cooperation between toll-like receptors. *Proc. Natl. Acad. Sci. USA* **97:**13766–13771.

Pedrosa, J., B. M. Saunders, R. Appelberg, I. M. Orme, M. T. Silva, and A. M. Cooper. 2000. Neutrophils play a protective nonphagocytic role in systemic *Mycobacterium tuberculosis* infection of mice. *Infect. Immun.* **68:**577–583.

Peschel, A., R. W. Jack, M. Otto, L. V. Collins, P. Staubitz, G. Nicholson, H. Kalbacher, W. F. Nieuwenhuizen, G. Jung, A. Tarkowski, K. P. van Kessel, and J. A. van Strijp. 2001. Staphylococcus aureus resistance to human defensins and evasion of neutrophil killing via the novel virulence factor MprF is based on modification of membrane lipids with l-lysine. *J. Exp. Med.* **193:**1067–1076.

Peters, W., H. M. Scott, H. F. Chambers, J. L. Flynn, I. F. Charo, and J. D. Ernst. 2001. Chemokine receptor 2 serves an early and essential role in resistance to *Mycobacterium tuberculosis. Proc. Natl. Acad. Sci. USA* **98:**7958–7963.

Pieters, J. 2001. Entry and survival of pathogenic mycobacteria in macrophages. *Microb. Infect.* **3:**249–255.

Pieters, J., and J. Gatfield. 2002. Hijacking the host: survival of pathogenic mycobacteria inside macrophages. *Trends Microbiol.* **10:**142–146.

Portnoy, D. A., V. Auerbuch, and I. J. Glomski. 2002. The cell biology of *Listeria monocytogenes* infection: the intersection of bacterial pathogenesis and cell-mediated immunity. *J. Cell Biol.* **158:**409–414.

Pron, B., C. Boumaila, F. Jaubert, S. Sarnacki, J. P. Monnet, P. Berche, and J. L. Gaillard. 1998. Comprehensive study of the intestinal stage of listeriosis in a rat ligated ileal loop system. *Infect. Immun.* **66:**747–755.

Pron, B., C. Boumaila, F. Jaubert, P. Berche, G. Milon, F. Geissmann, and J. L. Gaillard. 2001. Dendritic cells are early cellular targets of *Listeria monocytogenes* after intestinal delivery and are involved in bacterial spread in the host. *Cell. Microbiol.* **3:**331–340.

Reiling, N., C. Holscher, A. Fehrenbach, S. Kroger, C. J. Kirschning, S. Goyert, and S. Ehlers. 2002. Cutting edge: toll-like receptor (TLR)2- and TLR4-mediated pathogen recognition in resistance to airborne infection with *Mycobacterium tuberculosis. J. Immunol.* **169:**3480–3484.

Remoli, M. E., E. Giacomini, G. Lutfalla, E. Dondi, G. Orefici, A. Battistini, G. Uze, S. Pellegrini, and E. M. Coccia. 2002. Selective expression of type I IFN genes in human dendritic cells infected with *Mycobacterium tuberculosis. J. Immunol.* **169:**366–374.

Rich, E. A., M. Torres, E. Sada, C. K. Finegan, D. B. Hamilton, and Z. Toossi. 1997. *Mycobacterium tuberculosis* (MTB)-stimulated production of nitric oxide by human alveolar macrophages and relationship of nitric oxide production to growth inhibition of MTB. *Tuber. Lung Dis.* **78:**247–255.

Rogers, H. W., and E. R. Unanue. 1993. Neutrophils are involved in acute, nonspecific resistance to *Listeria monocytogenes* in mice. *Infect. Immun.* **61:**5090–5096.

Rosen, H., S. Gordon, and R. J. North. 1989. Exacerbation of murine listeriosis by a monoclonal antibody specific for the type 3 complement receptor of myelomonocytic cells. Absence of monocytes at infective foci allows Listeria to multiply in nonphagocytic cells. *J. Exp. Med.* **170:**27–37.

Roussel, P., G. Lamblin, M. Lhermitte, N. Houdret, J. J. Lafitte, J. M. Perini, A. Klein, and A. Scharfman. 1988. The complexity of mucins. *Biochimie* **70:**1471–1482.

Russell, D. G. 2001. TB comes to a sticky beginning. *Nat. Med.* **7:**894–895.

Rutledge, B. J., H. Rayburn, R. Rosenberg, R. J. North, R. P. Gladue, C. L. Corless, and B. J. Rollins. 1995. High level monocyte chemoattractant protein-1 expression in transgenic mice increases their susceptibility to intracellular pathogens. *J. Immunol.* **155:**4838–4843.

Salzman, N. H., D. Ghosh, K. M. Huttner, Y. Paterson, and C. L. Bevins. 2003. Protection against enteric salmonellosis in transgenic mice expressing a human intestinal defensin. *Nature* **422:**522–526.

Sato, K., H. Tomioka, T. Shimizu, T. Gonda, F. Ota, and C. Sano. 2002. Type II alveolar cells play roles in macrophage-mediated host innate resistance to pulmonary mycobacterial infections by producing proinflammatory cytokines. *J. Infect. Dis.* **185:**1139–1147.

Saunders, B. M., A. A. Frank, I. M. Orme, and A. M. Cooper. 2000. Interleukin-6 induces early gamma interferon production in the infected lung but is not required for generation of specific immunity to *Mycobacterium tuberculosis* infection. *Infect. Immun.* **68:**3322–3326.

Schaible, U. E., H. L. Collins, and S. H. Kaufmann. 1999. Confrontation between intracellular bacteria and the immune system. *Adv. Immunol.* **71:**267–377.

Schaible, U. E., H. L. Collins, F. Priem, and S. H. Kaufmann. 2002. Correction of the iron overload defect in beta-2-microglobulin knockout mice by lactoferrin abolishes their increased susceptibility to tuberculosis. *J. Exp. Med.* **196:**1507–1513.

Schlech, W. F., III. 2000. Foodborne listeriosis. *Clin. Infect. Dis.* **31:**770–775.

Schlesinger, L. S. 1998. *Mycobacterium tuberculosis* and the complement system. *Trends Microbiol.* **6:**47–49.

Schlesinger, L. S., T. M. Kaufman, S. Iyer, S. R. Hull, and L. K. Marchiando. 1996. Differences in mannose receptor-mediated uptake of lipoarabinomannan from virulent and attenuated strains of *Mycobacterium tuberculosis* by human macrophages. *J. Immunol.* **157:**4568–4575.

Schorey, J. S., M. C. Carroll, and E. J. Brown. 1997. A macrophage invasion mechanism of pathogenic mycobacteria. *Science* **277:**1091–1093.

Scott, H. M., and J. L. Flynn. 2002. *Mycobacterium tuberculosis* in chemokine receptor 2-deficient mice: influence of dose on disease progression. *Infect. Immun.* **70:**5946–5954.

Seiler, P., P. Aichele, B. Raupach, B. Odermatt, U. Steinhoff, and S. H. Kaufmann. 2000. Rapid neutrophil response controls fast-replicating intracellular bacteria but not slow-replicating *Mycobacterium tuberculosis. J. Infect. Dis.* **181:**671–680.

Seiler, P., P. Aichele, S. Bandermann, A. E. Hauser, B. Lu, N. P. Gerard, C. Gerard, S. Ehlers, H. J. Mollenkopf, and S. H. Kaufmann. 2003. Early granuloma formation after aerosol *Mycobacterium tuberculosis*-infection is regulated by neutrophils via CXCR3-signalling chemokines. *Eur. J. Immunol.* **33:**2676–2686.

Sharma, S., and G. Khuller. 2001. DNA as the intracellular secondary target for antibacterial action of human neutrophil peptide-I against *Mycobacterium tuberculosis* H37Ra. *Curr. Microbiol.* **43:**74–76.

Sharma, S., I. Verma, and G. K. Khuller. 2000. Antibacterial activity of human neutrophil peptide-1 against *Mycobacterium tuberculosis* H37Rv: in vitro and ex vivo study. *Eur. Respir. J.* **16:**112–117.

Sharma, S., I. Verma, and G. K. Khuller. 2001. Therapeutic potential of human neutrophil peptide 1 against experimental tuberculosis. *Antimicrob. Agents Chemother.* **45:**639–640.

Shiloh, M. U., J. D. MacMicking, S. Nicholson, J. E. Brause, S. Potter, M. Marino, F. Fang, M. Dinauer, and C. Nathan. 1999. Phenotype of mice and macrophages deficient in both phagocyte oxidase and inducible nitric oxide synthase. *Immunity* **10:**29–38.

Soilleux, E. J., L. S. Morris, G. Leslie, J. Chehimi, Q. Luo, E. Levroney, J. Trowsdale, L. J. Montaner, R. W. Doms, D. Weissman, N. Coleman, and B. Lee. 2002. Constitutive and induced expression of DC-SIGN on dendritic cell and macrophage subpopulations in situ and in vitro. *J. Leukoc. Biol.* **71:**445–457.

Tailleux, L., O. Schwartz, J. L. Herrmann, E. Pivert, M. Jackson, A. Amara, L. Legres, D.

Dreher, L. P. Nicod, J. C. Gluckman, P. H. Lagrange, B. Gicquel, and O. Neyrolles. 2003. DC-SIGN is the major *Mycobacterium tuberculosis* receptor on human dendritic cells. *J. Exp. Med.* **197:**121–127.

Tani, K., W. J. Murphy, O. Chertov, R. Salcedo, C. Y. Koh, I. Utsunomiya, S. Funakoshi, O. Asai, S. H. Herrmann, J. M. Wang, L. W. Kwak, and J. J. Oppenheim. 2000. Defensins act as potent adjuvants that promote cellular and humoral immune responses in mice to a lymphoma idiotype and carrier antigens. *Int. Immunol.* **12:**691–700.

Thiel, S., T. Vorup-Jensen, C. M. Stover, W. Schwaeble, S. B. Laursen, K. Poulsen, A. C. Willis, P. Eggleton, S. Hansen, U. Holmskov, K. B. Reid, and J. C. Jensenius. 1997. A second serine protease associated with mannan-binding lectin that activates complement. *Nature* **386:**506–510.

Unanue, E. R. 1996. Macrophages, NK cells and neutrophils in the cytokine loop of Listeria resistance. *Res. Immunol.* **147:**499–505.

van Crevel, R., T. H. Ottenhoff, and J. W. Der Meer. 2002. Innate immunity to *Mycobacterium tuberculosis. Clin. Microbiol. Rev.* **15:**294–309.

Weikert, L. F., J. P. Lopez, R. Abdolrasulnia, Z. C. Chroneos, and V. L. Shepherd. 2000. Surfactant protein A enhances mycobacterial killing by rat macrophages through a nitric oxide-dependent pathway. *Am. J. Physiol. Lung Cell Mol. Physiol.* **279:**L216–L223.

West, J. B. 1994. Ventilation, blood flow, and gas exchange, p. 51–89. *In* J. F. N. J. A. Murray (ed.), *Textbook of Respiratory Medicine.* W. B. Saunders, Philadelphia, Pa.

Zahrt, T. C., and V. Deretic. 2002. Reactive nitrogen and oxygen intermediates and bacterial defenses: unusual adaptations in *Mycobacterium tuberculosis. Antioxid. Redox. Signal.* **4:**141–159.

Zhang, L., W. Yu, T. He, J. Yu, R. E. Caffrey, E. A. Dalmasso, S. Fu, T. Pham, J. Mei, J. J. Ho, W. Zhang, P. Lopez, and D. D. Ho. 2002. Contribution of human alpha-defensin 1, 2, and 3 to the anti-HIV-1 activity of CD8 antiviral factor. *Science* **298:**995–1000.

Zimmerli, S., S. Edwards, and J. D. Ernst. 1996. Selective receptor blockade during phagocytosis does not alter the survival and growth of *Mycobacterium tuberculosis* in human macrophages. *Am. J. Respir. Cell Mol. Biol.* **15:**760–770.

INDEX